D1163068

WITHDRAWN

Signaling Networks and Cell Cycle Control

Cancer Drug Discovery and Development

Beverly A. Teicher, Series Editor

Signaling Networks and Cell Cycle Control

The Molecular Basis of Cancer and Other Diseases

Edited by

J. Silvio Gutkind

National Institute of Dental and Craniofacial Research,
National Institutes of Health,
Bethesda, MD

Humana Press ✳ Totowa, New Jersey

© 2000 Humana Press Inc.
999 Riverview Drive, Suite 208
Totowa, New Jersey 07512

For additional copies, pricing for bulk purchases, and/or information about other Humana titles,
contact Humana at the above address or at any of the following numbers: Tel.: 973-256-1699;
Fax: 973-256-8341; E-mail: humana@humanapr.com or visit our Website: http://humanapress.com

Cover illustration: From Fig. 1 in Chapter 14, "Discovery of TNP-470 and Other Angiogenesis Inhibitors," by Donald E.
Ingber, in *Cancer Therapeutics: Experimental and Clinical Agents*, Edited by Beverly A. Teicher, Humana Press, 1997.

Cover design by Patricia F. Cleary.

This publication is printed on acid-free paper. ∞
ANSI Z39.48-1984 (American National Standards Institute) Permanence of Paper for Printed Library Materials.

Printed in the United States of America. 10 9 8 7 6 5 4 3 2

Library of Congress Cataloging-in-Publication Data

Signaling networks and cell cycle control: the molecular basis of cancer and other diseases/edited by J. Silvio Gutkind.
    p. cm—(Cancer drug discovery and development)
  Includes bibliographical references and index.
  ISBN 0-89603-710-X (alk. paper)
    1. Cellular signal transduction. 2. Cell cycle. 3. Cellular control mechanisms.   4. Pathology, Molecular.
  I.   Gutkind, J. Silvio.   II. Series.
QP517.C45 S558 2000
571.6--dc   99-056127

Preface

In the last few years we have witnessed a real explosion in the knowledge of how cell surface receptors transmit signals to the nucleus, thereby controlling the expression of genetic programs involved in many cellular processes, including normal and aberrant cell growth. We learned that a unique repertoire of signaling molecules link each class of receptors to a variety of newly discovered kinase cascades, in many cases through the activation of small GTP-binding proteins of the Ras superfamily. In turn, these kinases phosphorylate key molecules, including transcription factors, which ultimately control gene expression. Furthermore, recent work is helping to unveil how these signals initiated at the level of the cell surface are integrated in space and time to control the orderly progression through the cell cycle or, alternatively, the exit from the cell cycle and the activation of cellular processes leading to phenotypic differentiation or to programmed cell death. Parallel efforts have revealed that subtle alterations in signal transduction pathways and cell cycle control are implicated in a number of pathological processes, including cancer. Thus, the recent identification of key signaling and cell-cycle-regulating molecules has provided a golden opportunity in the search for novel targets for therapeutic intervention and disease.

The present volume describes the up-to-date knowledge on signaling pathways and cell cycle control, as well as the efforts of several groups to design, synthesize, and evaluate the biochemical and biological activities of inhibiting molecules. Leading scientists in the field have summarized the most current information regarding biologically relevant cell surface receptors, their ligands, and their downstream pathways; inflammatory mediators; second messenger generating systems; small GTP-binding proteins and their effector molecules; components of novel protein kinase cascades and their newly identified substrates; nuclear receptors; biochemical routes controlling the activity of nuclear transcription factors; apoptotic pathways; cell cycle regulatory molecules and their dysfunction in neoplastic disease; and the most recent studies, including preclinical and clinical, addressing the potential use of inhibiting agents in a variety of disease states. In each case, the contributors have emphasized the areas that are still open for exploration, and have attempted to define the most likely molecular targets for pharmacological intervention. They have also provided graphic representations of this wealth of information, which will be invaluable for understanding the emerging principles in the field. These comprehensive reviews are also expected to provide a guiding tool for those involved in basic research in this fascinating area, as well as for those actively engaged in drug discovery efforts.

J. Silvio Gutkind

Contents

Contributors

STUART A. AARONSON, MD • *Derald H. Ruttenberg Cancer Center, Mount Sinai School of Medicine, New York, NY*

ROBERT T. ABRAHAM • *Division of Oncology Research, Mayo Clinic and Foundation, Rochester, MN*

PETER ACS, MD • *Laboratory of Cellular Carcinogenesis and Tumor Promotion, National Cancer Institute, Bethesda, MD*

GRANT D. BARISH, BS • *Varmus Laboratory, National Cancer Institute, National Institutes of Health, Bethesda, MD*

DIPAK K. BHATTACHARYYA, PHD • *Laboratory of Cellular Carcinogenesis and Tumor Promotion, National Cancer Institute, Bethesda, MD*

PETER M. BLUMBERG, PHD • *Laboratory of Cellular Carcinogenesis and Tumor Promotion, National Cancer Institute, Bethesda, MD*

LEWIS C. CANTLEY, PHD • *Division of Signal Transduction, Beth Israel Deaconess Medical Center, Harvard Institutes of Medicine, Boston, MA*

ESTHER H. CHANG, PHD • *Department of Otolaryngology, Lombardi Cancer Center, Georgetown University Medical Center, Washington, DC*

MARIO CHIARELLO, MD • *Oral and Pharangeal Cancer Branch, National Institute of Dental and Craniofacial Research, National Institutes of Health, Bethesda, MD*

YANFANG CHU • *Laboratory of Pathology, National Cancer Institute, National Institutes of Health, Bethesda, MD*

GEOFFREY J. CLARK, PHD • *Department of Pharmacology, Lineberger Comprehensive Cancer Center, University of North Carolina at Chapel Hill, NC*

ADRIENNE D. COX, PHD • *Departments of Radiation Oncology and Pharmacology, Lineberger Comprehensive Cancer Center, University of North Carolina at Chapel Hill, NC*

ERIK H. J. DANEN, PHD • *Craniofacial Developmental Biology and Regeneration Branch, National Institute of Dental and Craniofacial Research, National Institutes of Health, Bethesda, MD*

ROGER J. DAVIS, PHD • *Howard Hughes Medical Institute and Program in Molecular Medicine, Department of Biochemistry and Molecular Biology, University of Massachusetts Medical School, Worcester, MA*

MARK P. DE CAESTECKER, MD, PHD • *Laboratory of Cell Regulation and Carcinogenesis, National Cancer Institute, Bethesda, MD*

CHANNING J. DER, PHD • *Department of Pharmacology, Curriculum in Genetics and Molecular Biology, Lineberger Comprehensive Cancer Center, University of North Carolina at Chapel Hill, NC*

DAVID T. DUDLEY, PHD • *Department of Cell Biology, Parke-Davis Pharmaceutical Research, Ann Arbor, MI*

ERASTUS C. DUDLEY • *Laboratory of Immunology, National Institute of Allergy and Infectious Diseases, National Institutes of Health, Bethesda, MD*

GARY R. FANGER • *Program in Molecular Signal Transduction, Division of Basic Sciences, National Jewish Medical and Research Center, Denver, CO*

PAOLO FEDI, MD, PHD • *Derald H. Ruttenberg Cancer Center, Mount Sinai School of Medicine, New York, NY*

TOREN FINKEL, MD, PHD • *Cardiology Branch, National Heart, Lung and Blood Institute, National Institutes of Health, Bethesda, MD*

DAVID A. FRUMAN, PHD • *Division of Signal Transduction, Beth Israel Deaconess Medical Center, Harvard Institutes of Medicine, Boston, MA*

SHIGETOMO FUKUHARA, PHD • *Oral and Pharyngeal Cancer Branch, National Institute of Dental and Craniofacial Research, National Institutes of Health, Bethesda, MD*

J. SILVIO GUTKIND, PHD • *Oral and Pharyngeal Cancer Branch, National Institute of Dental and Craniofacial Research, National Institutes of Health, Bethesda, MD*

FELICITA HORNUNG • *Laboratory of Immunology, National Institute of Allergy and Infectious Diseases, National Institutes of Health, Bethesda, MD*

GARY L. JOHNSON • *Program in Molecular Signal Transduction, Division of Basic Sciences, National Jewish Medical and Research Center, Denver, CO*

ANDREW KEIGHTLEY, PHD • *Department of Immunology, Cleveland Clinic Research Foundation, Cleveland, OH*

KATHLEEN KELLY • *Laboratory of Pathology, National Cancer Institute, National Institutes of Health, Bethesda, MD*

DAVID H. KIRN, MD • *Vice President of Clinical Research, Onyx Pharmaceuticals, Richmond, CA, and Department of Medicine, University of California, San Francisco, CA*

ANDREW C. LARNER, MD, PHD • *Department of Immunology, Cleveland Clinic Research Foundation, Cleveland, OH*

ROBERT J. LECHLEIDER, MD • *Department of Pharmacology, Uniformed University of the Health Sciences, Bethesda, MD*

MICHAEL J. LENARDO • *Laboratory of Immunology, National Institute of Allergy and Infectious Diseases, National Institutes of Health, Bethesda, MD*

ALEXANDER LEVITZKI • *Department of Biological Chemistry, The Alexander Silberman Institute of Life Sciences, The Hebrew University of Jerusalem, Israel*

PATRICIA S. LORENZO, PHD • *Laboratory of Cellular Carcinogenesis and Tumor Promotion, National Cancer Institute, Bethesda, MD*

ANTHONY M. MANNING, PHD • *Signal Pharmaceuticals, Inc., San Diego, CA*

MARIA JULIA MARINISSEN, PHD • *Oral and Pharangeal Cancer Branch, National Institute of Dental and Craniofacial Research, National Institutes of Health, Bethesda, MD*

DAVID A. MARTIN • *Laboratory of Immunology, National Institute of Allergy and Infectious Diseases, National Institutes of Health, Bethesda, MD*

BRUCE J. MAYER, PHD • *Howard Hughes Medical Institute, Children's Hospital and Department of Microbiology and Molecular Genetics, Harvard Medical School, Boston, MA*

FRANK MERCURIO, PHD • *Signal Pharmaceuticals, Inc., San Diego, CA*

SHELDON MILSTIEN, PHD • *Laboratory of Cellular and Molecular Regulation, National Institute of Mental Health, National Institutes of Health, Bethesda, MD*

JOHN P. O'BRYAN, PHD • *Department of Pharmacology, Lineberger Comprehensive Cancer Center, University of North Carolina at Chapel Hill, NC*

MICHELE PAGANO, MD • *Department of Pathology and Kaplan Cancer Center, New York University Medical Center, New York, NY*

KATHLEEN F. PIROLLO, PHD • *Department of Otolaryngology, Lombardi Cancer Center, Georgetown University Medical Center, Washington, DC*

KATYA RAVID, PHD • *Department of Biochemistry and Witaker Cardiovascular Institute, Boston University School of Medicine, Boston, MA*

ANITA B. ROBERTS, PHD • *Laboratory of Cell Regulation and Carcinogenesis, National Cancer Institute, Bethesda, MD*

KEVIN M. RYAN, PHD • *ABL-Basic Research Program, Frederick Cancer Research and Development Center, National Cancer Institute, Frederick, MD*

ALAN R. SALTIEL, PHD • *Department of Cell Biology, Parke-Davis Pharmaceutical Research, Ann Arbor, MI*

LAWRENCE E. SAMELSON, MD • *Laboratory of Cellular and Molecular Biology, National Cancer Institute, Bethesda, MD*

EDWARD A. SAUSVILLE, MD, PHD • *Developmental Therapeutics Program, Division of Cancer Treatment and Diagnosis, National Cancer Institute, Bethesda, MD*

THOMAS K. SCHLESINGER • *Program in Molecular Signal Transduction, Division of Basic Sciences, National Jewish Medical and Research Center, Denver, CO*

PAMELA L. SCHWARTZBERG, MD, PHD • *Laboratory of Genetic Disease Research, National Human Genome Research Institute, National Institutes of Health, Bethesda, MD*

ADRIAN M. SENDEROWICZ, MD • *Developmental Therapeutics Program, Division of Cancer Treatment and Diagnosis, National Cancer Institute, Bethesda, MD*

RICHARD M. SIEGEL • *Laboratory of Immunology, National Institute of Allergy and Infectious Diseases, National Institutes of Health, Bethesda, MD*

REUBEN P. SIRAGANIAN, MD, PHD • *Receptors and Signal Transduction Section, OIIB, National Institute of Dental and Craniofacial Research, National Institutes of Health, Bethesda, MD*

JOANNE SLOAN-LANCASTER, PHD • *Research Technologies and Proteins, Eli Lilly and Company, Indianapolis, IN*

SARAH SPIEGEL, PHD • *Department of Biochemistry and Molecular Biology, Georgetown University Medical Center, Washington, DC*

DANIEL M. SULLIVAN, PHD • *Cardiology Branch, National Heart, Lung and Blood Institute, National Institutes of Health, Bethsda, MD*

MARC SYMONS, PHD • *The Picower Institute for Molecular Medicine, Manhasset, NY*

RANDAL S. TIBBETS • *Division of Oncology Research, Mayo Clinic and Foundation, Rochester, MN*

KAREN H. VOUSDEN, PHD • *ABL-Basic Research Program, Frederick Cancer and Development Center, National Cancer Institute, Frederick, MD*

JEAN Y. J. WANG, PHD • *Department of Biology, Center for Molecular Genetics and the Cancer Center, University of California San Diego, La Jolla, CA*

BART O. WILLIAMS, PHD • *Varmus Laboratory, National Cancer Institute, National Institutes of Health, Bethesda, MD*

LIANG XU, MD, PHD • *Department of Otolaryngology, Lombardi Cancer Center, Georgetown University Medical Center, Washington, DC*

KENNETH M. YAMADA, MD, PHD • *Craniofacial Developmental Biology and Regeneration Branch, National Institute of Dental and Craniofacial Research, National Institutes of Health, Bethesda, MD*

PETER R. YOUNG • *Department of Molecular Biology, SmithKline Beecham Pharmaceuticals, King of Prussia, PA*

LIXIN ZHENG • *Laboratory of Immunology, National Institute of Allergy and Infectious Diseases, National Institutes of Health, Bethesda, MD*

Integrin Signaling

Kenneth M. Yamada, MD, PhD and Erik H. J. Danen, PhD

1. INTRODUCTION

Integrins fulfill a multitude of functions in embryonic cell migration and tissue organization, inflammation, wound repair, tumor cell invasion, and a variety of other biological and pathological processes. Over the past decade, it has become clear that integrins play central roles not only in adhesion and cell migration, but also in the regulation of growth, gene expression, and differentiation. Concepts of integrins have evolved from considering these receptors as simple cell surface binding moieties for extracellular adhesion molecules to the realization that they also serve complex roles as activators or modulators of signal transduction. As summarized in Fig. 1, integrins can stimulate a surprising range of signal transduction pathways. Integrin–ligand interactions trigger or modulate a variety of kinases, lipid signaling pathways, ion fluxes, and gene transcription events, as well as helping to organize the cytoskeleton. This broad repertoire of responses is consistent with the current view that integrins are central mediators of information transfer between cells and the extracellular matrix, and sometimes other cells, both at the physical/structural level and at the level of signal transduction. Research on integrin signaling has been expanding rapidly (a few of the many recent reviews in the area include refs. *1–9*).

This chapter briefly reviews the structure and ligand-binding properties of integrins and then examines roles of conformational changes and integrin cytoplasmic domains, followed by an exploration of the organization and functions of integrin signaling and cytoskeletal complexes in a variety of signaling pathways. Mechanisms of synergy of integrins with growth factor receptors are described, as well as roles of integrins in cell cycle progression, survival, and gene regulation. We conclude with a consideration of the regulation of integrin signaling and then list many unanswered questions and future research opportunities in this new field.

2. INTEGRIN STRUCTURES AND FUNCTIONS

All integrins are composed of one α and one β subunit, which bind noncovalently to form a heterodimer (Fig. 1). Integrins have a characteristic globular head domain that binds to ligands, long legs that hold the head a substantial distance above the plasma membrane, transmembrane domains, and short cytoplasmic tails (roughly 1000

From: Signaling Networks and Cell Cycle Control: The Molecular Basis of Cancer and Other Diseases
Edited by: J. S. Gutkind © Humana Press Inc., Totowa, NJ

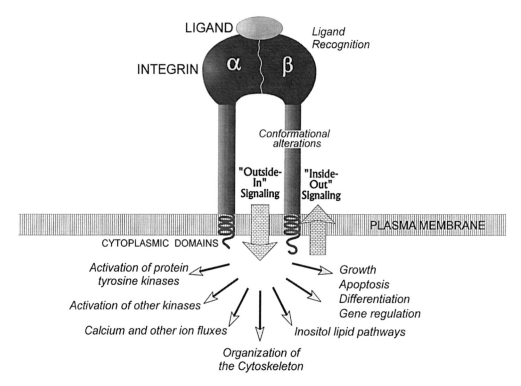

Fig. 1. Schematic overview of integrin signaling. Integrins consist of a heterodimer of one α and one β subunit that join to form an extracellular head domain that binds to specific ligands. Binding results in conformational changes in integrin structure and a process of information transfer or outside-in signaling across the plasma membrane to molecules that interact with the C-terminal cytoplasmic domains. Integrin affinity and ability to bind to specific target ligands can be modulated by cytoplasmic processes that result in inside-out signaling that affects binding by the head domain. As depicted, integrin signaling can result in a wide variety of effects on diverse signaling pathways or in organization of the actin-containing cytoskeleton.

residues for α subunits and 750 residues for β subunits, an exception being the very large $β_4$ cytoplasmic domain). The cytoplasmic domains, particularly the α tails, appear to be mediators of integrin intracellular signaling *(10,11)*. As depicted in Fig. 2, more than 20 integrin subunits are arranged in pairs—the α and β subunits each contribute to specificity of ligand binding. These ligands can be extracellular matrix molecules such as collagen, laminin or fibronectin, or they can be counter-receptors, such as intracellular cell adhesion molecules (ICAMs) or vascular cell adhesion molecules (VCAMs) on other cells. Consequently, integrins can mediate both cell-to-cell and cell-to-substrate adhesion, and either adhesive interaction can trigger specific forms of integrin signaling *(1–3,7)*.

2.1. Overlapping Ligand Specificities But Unique Roles for Individual Integrins

Figure 2 demonstrates that a specific integrin can have markedly overlapping ligand-binding activities as compared with those of other integrins. Nevertheless, mutations or loss of nearly any integrin α or β subunit leads to biological defects, as shown by

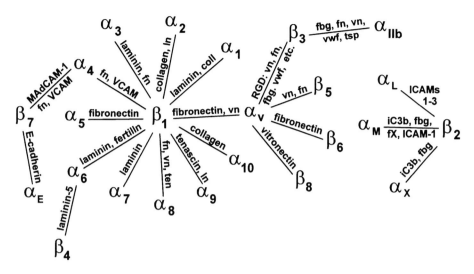

Fig. 2. Integrin heterodimers and ligands. Integrins form pairs between a specific α and β subunit as indicated; only certain combinations appear to occur. Each particular heterodimer binds to one or more ligands as indicated along the line connecting each partner of the pair. Abbreviations: coll, collagen; ln, laminin; fn, fibronectin; vn, vitronectin; ten, tenascin; RGD, ArgGlyAsp; fbg, fibrinogen; vwf, von Willebrand factor; tsp, thrombospondin; fX, factor X.

gene knockout studies in which the loss of most integrin subunits is lethal at embryonic stages or shortly after birth *(12,13)*. Subunits such as β_2 and β_3 are mutated in human genetic disorders, which affect leukocyte and platelet function, respectively. Thus, despite overlapping ligand-binding functions as determined by testing in vitro, it is clear that in the intact organism, most have unique and essential functions.

2.2. Integrin Recognition of Ligands by Binding to Specialized Peptide Sites

Integrins often bind to their ligands at key recognition sites composed of short peptide sequences *(14,15)*, although molecular recognition can sometimes require that key nonadjacent amino acid residues be displayed close together in a specific three-dimensional orientation *(16)*. For example, the $\alpha_5\beta_1$ fibronectin receptor binds to the Arg-Gly-Asp sequence in fibronectin, but also requires an Arg residue in the spatially very distant Pro-His-Ser-Arg-Asn synergy site for adequate affinity and specificity of binding *(15,17)*. Three-dimensional structural determinations of fibronectin and integrin antibody studies suggest a two-point recognition process for binding, with the α subunit potentially binding the Arg in the synergy sequence and the β subunit binding the Arg-Gly-Asp sequence *(18–20)*. It seems likely that this kind of multipoint, cooperative binding mechanism will be seen in other integrins—it provides a simple, effective mechanism for binding ligands directly with considerable specificity in order to trigger ligand-specific integrin signaling.

2.3. Crucial Functions of Integrin Cytoplasmic Tails

Although they lack enzymatic activity, the integrin cytoplasmic domains can trigger signaling. Molecular chimeras containing only the tails from several β, but not α, subunits are able to trigger focal adhesion kinase (FAK) phosphorylation after clustering, while an alternatively spliced version was inactive *(21,22)*. Although clustering of truncated β_1 integrins lacking cytoplasmic tails has been reported to trigger modest mitogen-activated protein (MAP) kinase activation *(23)*, clustering of chimeras with isolated β tails can produce striking activation (S. Miyamoto and K. M. Yamada, unpublished data).

Integrin β cytoplasmic tails also contain sufficient information to induce the physical localization of single-subunit chimeras to pre-existing focal contacts, presumably by binding to cytoskeletal components enriched at these sites *(24)*. This property may contribute to the organization of integrins into adhesion complexes. Although α cytoplasmic domains lack such direct activities, analyses using chimeras demonstrate that α tails can have strikingly distinct effects on cell adhesion, migration, growth, and differentiation *(25,26)*. Integrin cytoplasmic domains have also been implicated in the process of inside-out signaling (Fig. 1), in which cytoplasmic interactions alter the ability of the extracellular domain of an integrin to bind its ligand (*see* Section 12.).

More than two dozen spliced sequence variations of the originally described integrin cytoplasmic domain sequences are now known. For example, the β_{1C} and β_{1D} isoforms can inhibit DNA synthesis and cell proliferation, whereas the most common β_{1A} isoform supports normal substrate-dependent cell proliferation *(27)*. In primary myoblasts, the α_{6A} isoform inhibits cell proliferation, whereas the α_5 subunit stimulates growth (26). In general, splicing variants of integrin cytoplasmic domains affect intracellular interactions and functions, rather than the binding of ligands, although an example of a restriction of binding repertoire has been reported *(11,27)*.

2.4. Integrin Conformational Changes and Function

Conformational changes in integrins can be detected by antibodies that identify neoepitopes *(3,6,28)*. Such conformational alterations after the binding of ligands are currently thought to account for some aspects of integrin-mediated signaling. The clearest role for occupancy, however, is in the localization of integrins. If not occupied by a ligand, integrins tend to be distributed diffusely on the cell surface. After cells bind to a ligand immobilized on a surface, integrins accumulate at focal adhesions; in adherent cells with pre-existing focal adhesions, occupancy of integrins by even a soluble monomeric ligand triggers integrin accumulation at the focal adhesions (ref. *24* and citations therein). Current models of the mechanism of such integrin responses postulate that binding of ligand leads to conformational changes which either split apart α and β tails that normally bind to each other in nonoccupied integrins, or slide the α or β tail relative to each other to expose sites on the β tail (e.g., *see* ref. *29*). These models obviously need further rigorous testing *(30)*. A second major source of signaling, however, appears to be the clustering of integrins without ligand-induced conformational changes (*see* Section 3.1.).

3. INTEGRIN ADHESIVE AND SIGNALING COMPLEXES

Integrins bound to ligands, especially to fibrils of extracellular matrix proteins, form clusters in focal or fibrillar adhesions. A surprising recent finding has been that such clusters of integrins also contain more than 30 other molecules in large multimolecular complexes, which can even contain accumulations of mRNA involved in localized protein synthesis *(31,32)*.

3.1. Hierarchies of Signaling and Cytoskeletal Molecules

Integrin adhesion/signaling complexes contain a variety of cytoskeletal proteins, such as vinculin and paxillin, and an even larger variety of well-known signal transduction molecules. A functional relationship between cytoskeletal proteins and signaling by integrins is suggested by the marked effects of disruption of the actin cytoskeleton with cytochalasin D on integrin-mediated tyrosine phosphorylation events *(31,33,34)* without affecting growth factor-induced signaling.

The organization of signaling and cytoskeletal molecules appears to occur in a series of distinct steps or hierarchies of accumulation *(31,35–38)* (Fig. 3). Two separable inputs from integrins involve integrin occupancy by ligand and integrin aggregation or clustering. In addition, tyrosine phosphorylation of the type inhibited by herbimycin and genistein, as well as actin cytoskeletal integrity, are particularly important in determining the accumulation of signal transduction molecules *(31,39)*. Other factors including actions of Rho and actomyosin contractility, can also contribute to various steps *(40–42)*. The apparent net result is that integrins can respond to stimuli in a stepwise fashion.

As summarized in Fig. 3, occupancy of an integrin by even a monovalent ligand (e.g., a proteolytic fragment of fibronectin or a small synthetic peptide) causes physical redistribution of the occupied integrins in the plane of the membrane; they move from a diffuse distribution to local accumulations in pre-existing adhesion sites (focal adhesions). By contrast, active lateral aggregation or clustering of integrins (e.g., with a nonfunction-blocking antibody) results in a coclustering on the other side of the plasma membrane of tensin and FAK. In addition, FAK becomes phosphorylated on tyrosine residues. This process does not require integrin ligand occupancy, but only integrin clustering. The full accumulation of cytoskeletal molecules including F-actin and paxillin into adhesion/signaling complexes, appears to require both major stimuli, that is, a combination of integrin clustering and occupancy (e.g., by binding to intact fibronectin; *see* ref. 31 and citations therein).

Although the consequences of simple integrin occupancy without clustering generally appear quite limited in terms of signaling, an interesting exception occurs in certain embryonic cells. Interactions of isolated segmental plate or of neural crest cells with peptides containing the Arg-Gly-Asp integrin-binding motif results in a strong induction of cell-cell adhesion that is dependent on N-cadherin *(43,44)*. These findings indicate that, under special conditions, there is crosstalk between integrin and cadherin adhesion systems, in which a cell–substrate adhesion system can activate functions of a cell–cell adhesion system. Thus, even though simple integrin occupancy without integrin clustering generally does not activate many integrin functions, it can sometimes activate this unusual crosstalk signaling mechanism (Fig. 3).

3.2. Signaling Molecules in Integrin Complexes

Further studies have shown that integrin clustering can lead to co-clustering of a wide variety of signaling molecules. Molecules that accumulate at least transiently in such integrin adhesion/signaling complexes include MAP kinases, small GTPases, PI

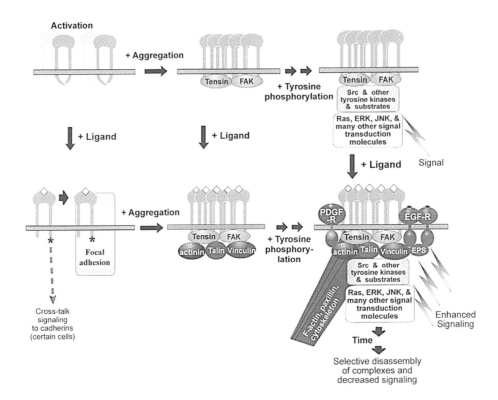

Fig. 3. Hierarchy and pathways of organization of integrin adhesion and signaling complexes. Integrins can undergo activation to bind ligands by inside-out signaling. Simple lateral aggregation in the plane of the plasma membrane (clustering) leads to accumulation of only certain cytoplasmic molecules. If tyrosine phosphorylation of the class inhibited by herbimycin or genistein occurs, a large number of signal transduction molecules accumulate and a signal is propagated. Conversely, occupancy of activated integrins by a soluble ligand results in a limited set of responses, particularly redistribution of laterally mobile integrins from a diffuse distribution in the plasma membrane to accumulation at previously existing adhesion sites termed *focal adhesions*. A key mechanism in this redistribution may involve enhanced accessibility or activation (*) of the β subunit cytoplasmic domain to bind to cytoskeletal proteins. In certain cases, simple ligand occupancy can induce crosstalk signaling that enhances cadherin-mediated cell–cell adhesion. A combination of aggregation and ligand occupancy leads to accumulation of at least four cytoskeletal proteins and focal adhesion kinase (FAK). A combination of all three parameters (ligand occupancy, integrin aggregation, and tyrosine phosphorylation) results in the full complex. These complexes transiently accumulate certain growth factor receptors, and binding of the appropriate growth factor results in an enhanced signal. Over time, the complexes lose certain components such as growth factor receptors and mitogen-activated protein (MAP) kinases, but not other components such as FAK, and signaling declines.

3-kinase, and a variety of other classical signal transduction proteins *(31,36)*. A substantial proportion of this accumulation can occur after simple integrin clustering, with a more limited contribution from concomitant occupancy of the integrin receptors by a ligand. With the exception of FAK, however, the clustering process requires kinase activity that is inhibited by the tyrosine kinase inhibitors herbimycin A and genistein. Nevertheless, the accumulation of a subset of cytoskeletal proteins including α-actinin and talin show immunity to these inhibitors if the integrins are both clustered and occupied *(31)*. As noted above, this stepwise hierarchy of organization would be expected to provide flexibility in the response of cells to external extracellular matrix and intracellular kinase signals in generating and organizing adhesion and signaling complexes (Fig. 3).

3.3. Integrin-Binding Proteins

A subset of the proteins associated with integrins or integrin-induced cytoskeletal and signaling complexes appear to be bound relatively directly to specific integrin molecules. Increasing numbers of such integrin-binding proteins have been identified, at least several of which appear to be involved in mediating or modulating signal transduction. The integrin-associated protein (IAP), or CD47, can associate with $\alpha_v\beta_3$ and has been implicated in phagocytosis, integrin-mediated changes in calcium fluxes, and T-cell tyrosine phosphorylation and co-mitogenic stimulation *(45,46)*. The urokinase-type plasminogen activator receptor (UPAR) associates with integrin $\alpha_v\beta_5$, and it can modulate cell migration *(47,48)*.

Another class of proteins associated with integrins involve the TM4 (transmembrane 4 or tetraspan) superfamily of proteins such as CD9 and CD81, which can bind to $\alpha_3\beta_1$, $\alpha_4\beta_1$, and $\alpha_6\beta_1$. The functions of these integrin-TM4 associations remain uncertain, but may include modulating signaling and cell migration *(49,50)*. The cytoplasmic protein cytohesin-1 serves as a mediator of PI 3-kinase activation of inside-out signaling affecting the functional activity of β_2 in lymphocytes *(51)*. Integrin-linked kinase (ILK) binds to β_1 integrins and has been implicated in cell adhesion, matrix assembly, and regulation of proliferation *(52,53)*. A variety of other intracellular molecules are known to bind to integrin β_1 cytoplasmic domains, including talin, α-actinin, FAK, and ICAP-1 *(54,55)*. In addition, filamin binds to β_2 integrins, β_3 endonexin interacts specifically with β_3 integrins, BP180 binds to β_4 integrins in hemidesmosomes, and (calcium- and integrin-binding [CIB] protein) binds to platelet α_{IIb} integrins *(56–59)*. In many cases, the biological functions of these specific binding proteins remain unknown, but many may modulate integrin signaling, affinity, or cytoskeletal effects.

An attractive biochemical mechanism by which the binding of certain cytoplasmic molecules to integrin cytoplasmic domains could be regulated would be through phosphorylation of the integrin tails themselves. Phosphorylation of integrin cytoplasmic domains can be detected; mutagenesis studies suggest potential roles for such posttranslational modifications; however, it is not entirely clear which biological results of mutating phosphorylation sites are caused by inducing conformational changes, as opposed to demonstrating a requirement for phosphorylation *per se* (e.g., *see* refs. *60,61* and citations therein). The β_4 integrin of hemidesmosomes is interesting, as it has sequences that resemble the "ITAM" motifs important for T-cell receptor signaling. Tyrosine phosphorylation of this particular integrin has been reported to be necessary for the formation of hemidesmosomes and for triggering the binding of Shc/Grb2 to initiate signaling *(8)* (*see also* ref. *58*).

4. FOCAL ADHESION KINASE

A striking early observation in the study of integrin signaling was the induction of specific tyrosine phosphorylation of FAK after cell adhesion to fibronectin or other integrin substrates. FAK phosphorylation has subsequently been used extensively to assay kinase-based integrin signaling (reviewed in *3,62–64*). As noted above, FAK has been reported to bind directly to β_1 integrin tails *(54)*. Even though FAK has been studied intensively, its actual functions and mechanism of action remain somewhat controversial. FAK kinase activity has been measured with a synthetic substrate or by autophosphorylation using the isolated protein, and integrin-mediated adhesion (with concomitant FAK phosphorylation) enhances its kinase activity *(34,65)*. In vitro substrates of FAK appear to include paxillin and tensin; the biological sequelae of this enhancement in vivo remain to be established.

The clearest biological effect of FAK is to enhance rates of cell migration, as shown by the opposing effects of gene ablation and overexpression *(66–68)*. The ability of FAK to accelerate integrin-dependent migration requires the autophosphorylation site Y397, to which c-Src can bind after phosphorylation. Conversely, FAK-null (knockout) mice die with defects in gastrulation at about the same time in development as fibronectin-deficient mice; cells from these mice show defective rates of migration *(66,69)*.

FAK has also been shown to bind to a number of interesting signaling and cytoskeletal proteins, including c-Src, CSK, PI 3-kinase, p130^Cas, Grb2, paxillin, talin, and α-actinin, (reviewed in *41,63,* and *64*). Although the binding of Src and Grb2 to FAK appears to be dependent on site-specific tyrosine phosphorylation *(70,71)*, many of the other proteins appear to bind even without induced phosphorylation of FAK. Thus, FAK is a major docking protein, which can potentially nucleate complexes of a number of the proteins found in integrin adhesive/signaling complexes. A dominant-negative form of FAK can, in fact, disrupt cell motility and proliferation *(68)*.

FAK also binds directly to integrin β cytoplasmic domains in vitro. It can be experimentally co-clustered along with integrins, suggesting a functional association in vivo as well *(35,54)*. Interestingly, FAK and Src respond to fibronectin stimulation by binding transiently to each other and by becoming incorporated into the Triton-insoluble cytoskeleton, which may prolong the kinase effects of these proteins *(34)*. Studies of FAK, like other signaling molecules, are potentially complicated by the need to use overexpression or null cells. Increased expression of any protein may induce novel effects; gene targeting can be accompanied by compensation: for example, FAK-null fibroblasts appear to induce FAK-B (Pyk2), a homolog of FAK. Nevertheless, FAK appears to be an interesting and important element of integrin-based signaling.

5. INTEGRIN MAP KINASE ACTIVATION

Integrins can stimulate both ERK and JNK MAP kinase activation *(31,72)*. The mechanisms of this activation has been controversial, with some published evidence favoring a pivotal role for FAK and Ras in ERK activation *(34,73,74)*, and yet other evidence showing that it is independent of FAK and Ras *(75,76)*.

5.1. Multiple Parallel and Intersecting Pathways

An explanation for these discrepancies appears to be the existence of more than a single linear pathway, in analogy to the increasing complexity and networking of signal transduction systems described elsewhere in this book. For integrin–mediated ERK activation, there are reportedly at least four mechanisms involving FAK, Src, Fyn, and

Shc *(34,76,77)*. As indicated in the schematic working model in Fig. 4A, integrin ligation or clustering can activate independent and mutually interacting pathways starting with FAK, c-Src, Fyn, and Shc. Evidence now exists for roles for each initiating mechanism, as well as for effects of c-Src on Shc as a downstream effector. Each potentially feeds into the classical Grb2, SOS, Ras, ERK pathway. In addition, c-Src and FAK can bind and potentially enhance each other's activity, and Shc can apparently be an upstream or more downstream effector, depending on the type of integrin and cell system studied.

An intriguing report has described the activation of Shc and ERK by a novel signaling pathway involving integrin α subunits, caveolin complexes, Fyn, and Shc phosphorylation *(76,77)*. This pathway may be cell-type specific and is reportedly specific to the α-subunit and the matrix molecule examined. A fourth pathway to activation of MAP kinases from integrins is via phosphatidylinositol (PI) 3-kinase *(78)*. This enzyme is necessary for Raf-1 stimulation of ERK activation, providing a fourth potential mechanism for integrin-based activation. Further complexity may still be discovered, and it is already clear that there are multiple paths from integrins to MAP kinase activation.

6. MORE INTERCONNECTIONS: OTHER DOCKING PROTEINS

At least several other proteins besides FAK with multiple protein-binding capabilities exist in adhesive/signaling complexes *(41)*. Paxillin can form complexes with FAK, vinculin, actin, Src family kinases, and CSK. The protein p130^{Cas} binds FAK. p130^{Cas} has been functionally linked to FAK as a potential downstream effector for enhancement of cell migration *(79)*. Vinculin can bind to other major cytoskeletal proteins *(41,80)*. Such remarkably pleiotropic binding capabilities of major components of these signaling and adhesive complexes provide a mechanism for massive networking, in which extremely complex and interconnected systems can assemble, and be modulated, by tyrosine phosphorylation. Other regulatory mechanisms are also possible, including serine phosphorylation (e.g., on FAK and paxillin), regulation by inositol phosphate lipids, such as PIP$_2$ (e.g., on vinculin and a variety of other structural and regulatory molecules) *(41,81)*, and phosphatases, such as PTEN (*see* Section 12.).

7. Rho AND LIPID SIGNALING PATHWAYS

The small GTPase Rho appears to function both upstream and downstream of integrins. Suppressing Rho functions can suppress integrin accumulation and the organization of focal adhesions *(82)*. By contrast, integrins can stimulate the activity of Rho and other small GTPases *(83,84)*. Integrin-activated Rho can stimulate a PIP 5-kinase, producing elevation of 4,5-PIP$_2$ *(83)*. This latter molecule is a substrate for PLC$_\gamma$, which can establish conditions for potential synergy with growth factor receptors. In addition, however, integrins can activate phosphatidylinositol (PI) 3-kinase *(63,78)*, or even PLC$_\alpha$ itself *(85,86)* to produce hydrolysis of 4,5-PIP$_2$, which leads into the well-known phosphoinositide signaling pathway involving diacylglycerol (DAG) and IP$_3$. Moreover, in at least one cell type, release of DAG is caused by the activation of phospholipase A$_2$ *(87,88)*. These steps can be required for cell spreading in some cells. Downstream

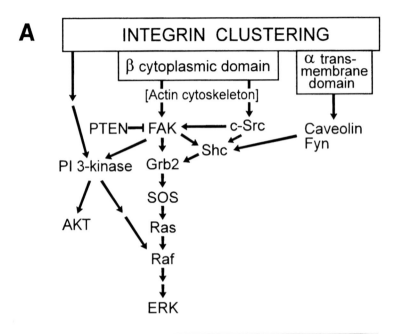

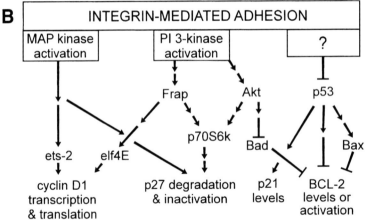

cell cycle progression and survival

Fig. 4. Schematic diagrams of integrin-mediated signaling. (**A**) For signal transduction, integrin clustering or aggregation is a particularly strong signal. Although most processes described to date appear to involve at least the β cytoplasmic domains, there is increasing evidence for important interactions involving the α transmembrane domain or tails. A role for the actin cytoskeleton in signaling is a recurring theme based on studies with cytochalasins, although the mechanisms remain obscure. Integrins induce complexes that include a variety of signaling molecules and activate or modulate the indicated pathways. In one, caveolin binds to some unknown additional component(s), and Fyn kinase is needed for proliferation-related functions. (**B**) A model for integrin- and adhesion-mediated effects on signaling that stimulate cell cycle progression or survival. In (A) and (B), arrows indicate positive effects and horizontal bars indicate negative effects on a process. Multiple arrows in a pathway indicate unknown or multiple intermediates; a dotted line indicates uncertainty about the source of triggering of the pathway. Note that in (**B**), integrin-mediated regulation of several of these steps is hypothetical and awaits experimental evidence (*see text*).

from DAG, PKC is translocated to the membrane *(87)* and is activated in a process also shown to be necessary for cell spreading and actin cytoskeletal organization *(89,90)*.

8. INTEGRINS USE OR MODULATE MANY SIGNALING PATHWAYS

In addition to the signal transduction pathways enumerated, integrins have been found to activate other classical signaling pathways, although the mechanisms are often not yet fully clarified. Induction of integrin clustering by antibodies or adhesion can trigger Ca^{2+} influxes that may depend on IP_3 mechanisms, or in one case on the integrin-associated protein IAP (for review, *see* ref. *3*). Even elevation of intracellular pH via activation of the Na-H antiporter can be triggered by integrin clustering *(91,92)*. It is important to stress that many descriptions of integrin signaling pathways are based on studies with only one to two cell types. It is consequently quite possible that a particular mechanism is not active in a specific cell type.

Nevertheless, some implications of this involvement of integrins in so many signal transduction systems are that (1) integrin modulation of signaling pathways appears to be widely pervasive and complex, and (2) cooperative and antagonistic interactions of integrins and various signaling systems may be a common event. A major gap in our current knowledge involves the precise mechanisms by which integrins modulate so many signaling systems. A working hypothesis is that at least some of these actions are the result of integrin functions in promoting the formation of macromolecular scaffolds and aggregates of a variety of signaling molecules. By bringing various kinases, substrates, docking molecules, and adapter proteins into close proximity, integrins may provide a physical mechanism for creating microdomains and microclusters of cytoplasmic signaling molecules, enhancing and modulating their functions.

9. MULTIPLE MECHANISMS OF INTEGRIN SYNERGY WITH GROWTH FACTOR RECEPTORS

Integrins are known to synergize biologically with a variety of growth factor and other regulatory systems *(2,3,93)*. Such synergism can occur by at least four distinct mechanisms:

Substrate availability: One system has been identified in which integrins increase levels of a substrate needed by an enzyme activated by growth factors. The PDGF receptor activates PLC_γ, and if its substrate 4,5-PIP_2 is limiting, integrin-mediated elevation of this substrate via Rho and 4-PIP 5-kinase activation produces a net synergistic enhancement of signaling *(83,94)*.

Modulation of the phosphorylation state of growth factor receptors: Integrin clustering and occupancy can produce a transient local accumulation of epidermal growth factor (EGF), platelet-derived growth factor (PDGF), and fibroblast growth factor (FGF) receptors *(36,37)*. Addition of the cognate growth factor results in a markedly enhanced level of receptor autophosphorylation *(37,95)*, which can then exert downstream effects on MAP kinase activation. The mechanism of this synergistic phosphorylation is unknown, but it may simply be the result of increasing the local concentrations of growth factor receptors, enhancing the likelihood of dimerization after addition of the growth factor ligand.

Binding of a cytoplasmic intermediary protein: IRS-1 appears to become bound to the $\alpha_v\beta_3$ integrin after cells adhere to vitronectin, which enhances the mitogenic effects of insulin

(96). The Eps8 downstream mediator of EGF receptor action becomes bound to integrin signaling complexes after integrins are clustered and occupied and EGF is bound to its receptor *(37)*. In these cases, the binding of a mediator of growth factor receptor action to integrin receptor complexes may produce cooperativity.

Targeting of a key intermediary step: Integrins and cell anchorage can be essential for MEK activity, and prolonged growth of cells in suspension can synergistically suppress growth factor signaling by inactivating this key signaling intermediate. As a consequence, growth factor-induced MAP kinase activation can depend on cell adhesion *(97)*. Because of the multiplicity of integrin interactions and the large number of signaling systems with which integrins can interact, other mechanisms for synergy are likely to be found.

10. CELL CYCLE PROGRESSION AND SURVIVAL

10.1. Anchorage-Dependent Cell Cycle Progression

It has long been known that cell attachment and spreading are required for cell proliferation and that loss of this requirement is related to tumorigenicity *(98,99)*. Control of growth by cell anchorage has been mapped to the G1 phase of the cell cycle *(100,101)*. Progression through G1 occurs via sequential activation of cyclin D-cdk4/6 and cyclin E-cdk2 kinase complexes, phosphorylation of the pocket proteins pRb, p107, and p130, release of the E2F transcription factor, and induction of cyclin A, the last cyclin to be induced before DNA synthesis *(102,103)*. The primary targets for regulation of G1 progression by cell anchorage are (1) transcription and translation of cyclin D, and (2) levels or distribution of the p21/p27 cdk inhibitors that determine cyclin E-cdk2 activity. By this mechanism, cell anchorage controls phosphorylation of the pocket proteins, availability of free E2F, and subsequent induction of cyclin A *(104–106)*. In parallel, cyclin A induction appears to be controlled by a mechanism that does not involve phosphorylation of the pocket proteins *(106–109)*. The small GTPase Ras is on the pathway of anchorage control of G1 cell cycle progression by targeting multiple downstream effector pathways *(110)*. Figure 4B shows a current model depicting integrin-mediated signals that connect with signal transduction cascades controlling cell proliferation and survival.

10.2. Anchorage-Dependent Cell Survival

Programmed cell death or apoptosis involves the action of a group of proteases termed ICE-like proteases or caspases *(111)*. This activity is regulated by the Bcl-2 family of proteins, which consists of pro-apoptotic proteins such as Bax and anti-apoptotic proteins such as Bcl-2 *(112)*. The tumor-suppressor protein p53 stimulates apoptosis when active, probably by promoting a low Bcl-2/Bax ratio and high levels of the p21 cdk inhibitor *(113)*. Integrin-mediated adhesion rescues many cell types from apoptosis *(114)*, and induction of apoptosis by loss of integrin-mediated adhesion has been termed anoikis *(115)*. Anoikis involves a positive feedback loop with activation of caspases that cleave (and activate) MEKK-1, which, in turn, activates more caspase activity *(116)*. The role of JNK-1 as the intermediate in this loop is still uncertain *(117, 118)*. Integrin-mediated adhesion appears to prevent anoikis by stimulating a high ratio of the levels of Bcl-2/Bax and by enhancing levels and activity of certain caspases *(119,120)*. For some cell types, maintaining low activity of the p53 tumor suppressor protein may be part of the survival pathway provided by integrin-mediated adhesion *(121)*.

Thus, integrin-mediated cell adhesion regulates cell cycle progression as well as cell survival. Moreover, there is evidence that control of both processes by anchorage may be connected at the level of Rb phosphorylation and Bcl-2 expression *(122)*. A major remaining question is how the various integrin-initiated signals actually connect to the signal transduction cascades that regulate cell survival and proliferation. There is evidence for a major role for cell spreading/stretching in this regulation, and mechanical links between integrins and the nucleus have been demonstrated. These findings have led to the suggestion that anchorage-dependent growth control is based indirectly on integrins by means of mechanotransduction *(123,124)*. By contrast, specificity for specific integrins has been demonstrated for anchorage control of cell cycle progression as well as survival *(26,76)* and intermediates of biochemical integrin signals such as FAK and Shc have been implicated in both processes *(68,76,125)*. Perhaps the best evidence for growth control by specific signals generated by integrin cytoplasmic tails is the fact that alternative splicing of the β1 subunit cytoplasmic domain can inhibit cell proliferation, without affecting cell spreading or the integrity of cell–substrate adhesions *(27,126)*.

10.3. MAP Kinases and Proliferation

Integrin signaling can activate MAP kinases and, perhaps more importantly, integrins can cooperate with growth factors at this level (*see* Sections 5. and 9.). The regulation of MAP kinase activity is one mechanism by which integrins may control proliferation, since ERK is an essential component of mitogenic signaling by various growth factors (reviewed in ref. *127*). In order for fibroblasts to pass the G1 restriction point, a persistent activation of the ERK type of MAP kinase is required. ERK activation can induce transcription of cyclin D1 mRNA through binding of the Ets-2 transcription factor *(128,129)*. Indeed, integrin stimulation results in a pattern of ERK activation that is more sustained than with growth factor activation alone, though the kinetics differ for different cell types (*see* Section 5. and references therein). In one case in vivo, the integrin $\alpha_v\beta_3$ induces sustained MAP kinase activity that lasts for more than 20 h and is required for angiogenesis *(130)*. However, another report demonstrates that even though $\alpha_v\beta_3$-induced endothelial cell survival involves Ras activation, it is independent of the ERK or the PI 3-kinase pathway *(131)*.

10.4. PI 3 Kinase and Growth Regulation

A second signaling event stimulated by integrins that may be highly relevant to growth control is the activation of PI 3-kinase and the downstream serine/threonine protein kinase PKB/Akt *(78,132)*. First, the stimulation of PKB/Akt activity can result in phosphorylation of Bad, which is then sequestered by 14-3-3 proteins, preventing Bad-induced Bcl-2 inhibition and subsequent stimulation of cell death *(112)*. Although Bcl-2 levels are indeed enhanced by integrin-mediated adhesion *(119,121)*, no direct evidence yet exists for regulation of the Bcl-2 pathway through this mechanism.

Another consequence of PI 3-kinase activation is the stimulation of FRAP, which phosphorylates p70 ribosomal S6 kinase and 4E-BP1 *(133)*. Phosphorylation of 4E-BP1 prevents its inhibitory binding to elf-4E. Because elf-4E regulates cyclin D1 translation, and integrin-mediated adhesion is required for cyclin D1 translation, this step may be involved in adhesion-mediated cell cycle control *(100,106,134)*. The phosphorylation of p70 ribosomal S6 kinase, which can be stimulated by integrin-mediated adhesion, has been postulated to be involved in the enhanced degradation of the p27 cdk inhibitor that occurs in suspended cells *(100,135)*. Indeed, a high level of p27 observed in smooth muscle cells plated on a collagen gel that did not support proliferation was paralleled by inhibited p70 S6 kinase activity *(136)*.

10.5. Connections of FAK to Proliferation and Apoptosis

FAK can mediate integrin-stimulated MAP kinase activation as well as PI 3-kinase activation. FAK has been implicated in regulating signals that control cell cycle progression as well as survival. Overexpression of a dominant-negative C-terminal FAK domain that inhibits FAK localization and decreases tyrosine phosphorylation inhibits DNA synthesis *(68)*. Moreover, constitutively activated (membrane-localized) FAK can transform MDCK cells *(125)*. The fact that FAK knockout fibroblasts do not show proliferative changes may be attributable to counteraction by the p53 mutation that is also present in those cells *(66)*. Although loss of matrix adhesion in untransformed fibroblasts typically leads to cell cycle arrest, one study has reported that inhibition of cell spreading by inhibition of FAK interaction with integrins can induce fibroblast apoptosis *(137)*. Interestingly, apoptosis-induced cell rounding has been associated with caspase cleavage of FAK *(138)*, suggesting a positive feedback loop: activation of caspases cleaving FAK, which results in loss of integrin-initiated signals inducing more caspase activity.

10.6. c-Abl and Cell Proliferation

A third mechanism that integrins may employ to control proliferation is to regulate the localization of proteins that can shuttle between the cytoplasm and the nucleus. The c-Abl protein is present in the nucleus, where its activity is regulated during the cell cycle by binding to Rb, as well as in the cytoplasm, where it appears to escape regulation *(139)*. Cell detachment followed by replating on extracellular matrix components induces a transient export into the cytoplasm and activation of this protein *(140)*. With time, the activated c-Abl returns to the nucleus. A tempting model would be that integrins somehow regulate the availability of active c-Abl in the nucleus and thus regulate genes involved in S-phase entry. However, the facts that oncogenic forms of Abl are cytoplasmic, and not nuclear, and that bcr-Abl (which induces anchorage independence) is found exclusively in the cytoplasm, where it binds actin filaments, suggests that integrins regulate functions of c-Abl in the cytoplasm *(141,142)*. A recent report that integrins regulate the phosphorylation of paxillin by c-Abl may be related to such functions *(143)*.

10.7. ILK and Growth Regulators

Finally, the serine/threonine kinase ILK has been implicated in anchorage-dependent growth, because its overexpression induces anchorage- but not serum-independent growth *(144)*. ILK overexpression was shown to enhance the level of cyclin D1 expression as well as cdk4 and cyclin E/cdk2 activity. However, the signal transduction pathway from ILK association with integrin cytoplasmic tails to these nuclear events is unknown. Whether ILK is involved in MAP kinase activation by integrins is unknown. By contrast, ILK has been suggested to play a role in regulation of expression of the

LEF-1 transcription factor by integrin-mediated adhesion *(145)*. Overexpression of ILK enhanced LEF-1 expression levels, as well as LEF-1/β-catenin complex formation and β-catenin nuclear translocation, resulting in enhanced LEF-1-dependent promoter activity. Because mutations that stabilize β-catenin (either directly or via inactivation of APC) can result in tumorigenicity *(146)*, this pathway may, in part, explain the oncogenic properties of ILK.

In conclusion, early signaling events initiated by integrin-mediated adhesion connect to signal transduction cascades that control cell cycle progression as well as cell survival. These connections are only just beginning to be understood. Future studies will fill in the many gaps that still exist. In fact, novel signaling pathways may be discovered in this search.

11. GENE EXPRESSION

Integrins can have striking downstream effects on specific gene expression (reviewed in refs. *2,3,* and *7*). For example, collagenase gene expression is triggered by altered integrin interactions with the fibronectin cell-binding domain on a substrate. The path of signaling from loss of binding to integrins to gene induction has been traced through Rac1 to a novel pathway involving reactive oxygen species, which induces nuclear translocation of the transcription factor NF-κB *(147)*. In rabbit synovial fibroblasts, this transcription factor is involved in induction of IL-1, which in turn serves as an autocrine stimulator of collagenase-1 synthesis. Although this particular pathway may be convoluted and specialized, it provides a model for beginning to trace the types of steps that lead from integrin ligation to regulation of specific gene expression.

A variety of other effects of integrin interactions with extracellular matrix proteins have been reported on differentiation, as in myoblast fusion *(26)*. The effects of integrin-dependent adherence to one type of substrate (e.g., fibronectin or collagen versus vitronectin) can be quite major in terms of the gene and protein expression patterns of cells. For example, >100 protein changes and >30 increases of gene expression within 6 h were found in an epithelial cells on different substrates *(148)*. In nearly all cases, the specific pathways and mechanisms of specific and global gene regulation by integrin interactions remain to be elucidated.

12. REGULATORS OF INTEGRIN SIGNALING AND FUNCTION

At least several mechanisms of regulating integrin signaling are likely to exist, including inside-out signaling governing integrin binding functions, modulation of the many specific pathways affected by integrins, and enzymes, such as phosphatases, that can selectively modulate subsets of integrin signaling molecules.

Inside-out signaling: Integrin function can be strongly regulated by a general process termed inside-out signaling. This process suppresses or activates the ability of the extracellular portion of integrins to bind to ligands via actions on their cytoplasmic domains. The most intensively studied system of this type of signaling is involved in platelet aggregation, in which some external signal (e.g., thrombin) activates integrins to bind fibrinogen and mediate platelet cell–cell adhesion *(28)*. Another system in which selective inside-out signaling appears to be important is in embryonic development. *Xenopus* gastrulation involves a switch in the ability of integrins to recognize adhesive sites in fibronectin: cells switch from only binding the Arg-Gly-Asp motif to induced recognition of a cell-binding synergy sequence, permitting cell migration *(149)*. In addition, integrins can regulate the functions of other integrins by incompletely understood receptor crosstalk mechanisms *(150–152)*. These effects may involve inside-out signaling without directly modifying integrin signaling (suppressing the binding of integrins to ligands), or they may also involve more complex effects on integrin signaling pathways.

General modulators of signaling pathways: In a sense, the many known modulators of classical signal transduction pathways will inevitably modify integrin signaling, because of the marked dependence of integrin signaling on other signaling systems. Although this form of regulation may appear trivial, it may permit major adjustments to the downstream effects of integrin signaling

Regulators of integrin signal transduction pathways: Increasing numbers of molecules that can more specifically regulate or modify integrin signaling will probably be identified in the near future. For example, the tumor suppressor PTEN has recently been shown to downmodulate integrin-dependent cell spreading and focal adhesion formation. One site of action appears to be directly on FAK, producing tyrosine dephosphorylation via its phosphatase domain *(153)*, although another target is the lipid mediator phosphatidylinositol 3,4,5-trisphosphate *(154)*. Interestingly, overexpression of FAK can restore FAK phosphorylation and rescue cell spreading as well as antagonizing the effects of PTEN on cell adhesion *(153)*. A second protein target of the tyrosine phosphatase activity of PTEN is Shc, and Shc dephosphorylation by PTEN can inhibit MAP kinase activation *(155)*. PTEN protein phosphatase activity also restrains cell migration by downregulating two parallel signaling pathways: a Shc/MAP kinase pathway that regulates random motility and a FAK/p130Cas pathway that promotes directionally persistent cell migration *(155,156)*. In contrast, the lipid phosphatase activity of PTEN appears particularly important for regulating apoptosis induced by a variety of agents, including the loss of integrin-mediated adhesion to extracellular matrix. PTEN transfection into tumor cell lines can restore this form of apoptosis, termed anoikis, which is characteristic of many normal cells. The mechanism involves PTEN dephosphorylation of PIP_3 and downstream effects on Akt/PKB *(157–159)*. In addition, PTEN dephosphorylation of FAK and a resulting decrease in PI 3′-kinase activity can also contribute to regulation of anoikis by PTEN *(159)*.

13. CONCLUSIONS AND FUTURE DIRECTIONS

The field of integrin signaling has grown explosively in just the past half-decade. Integrin-mediated regulatory effects are now known to modulate a remarkably wide array of well-known signal transduction pathways, including effects on kinases and tyrosine phosphorylation, lipid signaling, and ion fluxes. Although one general mechanism of integrin action in signaling appears to involve the ability of integrins to cluster cytoplasmic signaling and cytoskeletal proteins into large multimolecular complexes, other mechanisms exist. A major area of future research will involve determining the actual mechanisms of integrin activation or modulation of each known signaling pathway, and identifying and characterizing the individual cytoplasmic molecules and the intermediates involved.

Another major area of investigation should focus on the sources of signaling specificity as determined by each integrin α or β subunit. Besides the basic sequence differences between the different α and β cytoplasmic domains, there are now known to be more than two dozen spliced variants of these tails. Many of these splicing events are thought to affect cytoplasmic functions such as signaling, rather than extracellular ligand specificity. Understanding the molecular mechanisms that underlie the generation of different signals due to sequence variations of these short cytoplasmic α or β domains will be a fascinating approach to unraveling how different integrins selectively trigger specific signaling pathways.

It is also likely that cellular responses to ligation of the same type of integrin may differ depending on the cell type. These cell-specific differences may permit the identification of modifying signals (e.g. inside-out signals that modify the particular type of ligand that the same integrin can bind in one cell type versus another), as well as cell-type differences in the range of signaling pathways that can respond to an initial stimulus.

The biophysical mechanisms of signal transmission from the integrin-specific binding of a ligand to changes in the conformation of an integrin extracellular domain, and then to changes in the conformation or accessibility of an integrin cytoplasmic domain remain to be established. An attractive hypothesis that remains to be tested rigorously is that integrin specificity of signaling may be explained by differences in the specific cytoplasmic molecules that can bind to (1) a specific, noncovalently complexed α-β pair, and (2) a β tail after it is exposed after movement away of the α tail. More rigorous examinations of the specific molecules that bind to various chimeric constructs (e.g. α,β tail heterodimers and isolated α and β tails) before and after clustering may be particularly enlightening. Increasing numbers of cytoplasmic molecules are also being identified that appear to bind to only one type of integrin tail. Their roles in determining the specificity of signaling versus regulation of integrin location or affinity will also need to be resolved.

Regulation of integrin signaling pathways will remain another area of intensive investigation. One type of regulation that will require mechanistic explanation is the suppression or activation of one integrin by occupancy, or clustering of another type of integrin or both. In addition, many novel cytoplasmic regulators of integrin function will probably be found besides known modulators, such as Rho, R-Ras, and PTEN. Such molecules that modulate signaling from integrin tails or modify functions of adhesion/signaling complexes are likely to add daunting levels of sophistication and complexity to integrin signaling. Another important area of future research involves cell growth and survival. The links between initial integrin signaling and cell proliferation and prevention of apoptosis still need elucidation, especially to explain specificity in response to different integrins.

More generally, as for other signaling systems, it will eventually be necessary to combine quantitative characterizations of pathways in an integrated system. That is, the crosstalk between signaling systems and the quantitative activities of each system, when linked to others, will have to be determined. It seems likely that complex computer modeling will be necessary to represent such signaling networks. Such models will permit specific predictions and further testing to determine how integrin signaling is integrated with, and modulates, the many other signaling systems described in this book.

REFERENCES

1. Hynes RO. Integrins: Versatility, modulation, and signaling in cell adhesion. *Cell*, 1992; 69:11–25.
2. Clark EA, Brugge JS. Integrins and signal transduction pathways: The road taken. *Science* 1995; 268:233–239.

3. Schwartz MA, Schaller MD, Ginsberg MH. Integrins—emerging paradigms of signal-transduction. *Annu Rev Cell Dev Biol* 1995; 11:549–599.
4. Gumbiner BM. Cell adhesion: the molecular basis of tissue architecture and morphogenesis. *Cell* 1996; 84:345–357.
5. Ruoslahti E, and Obrink B. Common principles in cell adhesion. *Exp Cell Res* 1996; 227:1–11.
6. Humphries MJ. Integrin activation: The link between ligand binding and signal transduction. *Curr Opin Cell Biol* 1996; 8:632–640.
7. Lafrenie RM, Yamada KM. Integrin-dependent signal transduction. *J Cell Biochem* 1996; 61:543–553.
8. Giancotti FG. Integrin signaling: Specificity and control of cell survival and cell cycle progression. *Curr Opin Cell Biol* 1997; 9:691–700.
9. Yamada KM, ed. Mini-review series: integrin signaling. *Matrix Biol* 1997; 16:137–200.
10. Sastry SK, Horwitz AF. Integrin cytoplasmic domains: Mediators of cytoskeletal linkages and extra- and intracellular initiated transmembrane signaling. *Curr Opin Cell Biol* 1993; 5:819–831.
11. LaFlamme SE, Homan SM, Bodeau AL, Mastrangelo AM. Integrin cytoplasmic domains as connectors to the cell's signal transduction apparatus. *Matrix Biol* 1997; 16:153–163.
12. Hynes RO. Genetic analyses of cell–matrix interactions in development. *Curr Opin Genet Dev* 1994; 4:569–574.
13. Beauvais-Jouneau A, Thiery JP. Multiple roles for integrins during development. *Biol Cell* 1997; 89:5–11.
14. Yamada KM. Adhesive recognition sequences. *J Biol Chem* 1991; 266:12,809–12,812.
15. Ruoslahti E. RGD and other recognition sequences for integrins. *Ann Rev Cell Dev Biol* 1996; 12:697–715.
16. Eble JA, Golbik R, Mann K, Kuhn K. The alpha 1 beta 1 integrin recognition site of the basement membrane collagen molecule [alpha 1(IV)]2 alpha 2(IV). *EMBO J* 1993; 12:4795–4802.
17. Aota S, Nomizu M, Yamada KM. The short amino acid sequence Pro-His-Ser-Arg-Asn in human fibronectin enhances cell-adhesive function. *J Biol Chem* 1994; 269:24,756–24,761.
18. Leahy DJ, Aukhil I, Erickson HP. 2.0 Å crystal structure of a four-domain segment of human fibronectin encompassing the RGD loop and synergy region. *Cell* 1996; 84:155–164.
19. Copie V, Tomita Y, Akiyama SK, Aota S, Yamada KM, Venable RM, Pastor RW, Krueger S, Torchia DA. Solution structure and dynamics of linked cell attachment modules of mouse fibronectin containing the RGD and synergy regions: Comparison with the human fibronectin crystal structure. *J Mol Biol* 1998; 277:663–682.
20. Mould AP, Askari JA, Aota Si, Yamada KM, Irie A, Takada Y, Mardon HJ, Humphries MJ. Defining the topology of integrin alpha5 beta1–fibronectin interactions using inhibitory anti-alpha5 and anti-beta1 monoclonal antibodies. Evidence that the synergy sequence of fibronectin is recognized by the amino-terminal repeats of the alpha5 subunit. *J Biol Chem* 1997; 272:17,283–17,292.
21. Akiyama SK, Yamada SS, Yamada KM, LaFlamme SE. Transmembrane signal transduction by integrin cytoplasmic domains expressed in single-subunit chimeras. *J Biol Chem* 1994; 269:15,961–15,964.
22. Lukashev ME, Sheppard D, Pytela R. Disruption of integrin function and induction of tyrosine phosphorylation by the autonomously expressed beta 1 integrin cytoplasmic domain. *J Biol Chem* 1994; 269:18,311–18,314.
23. Lin TH, Aplin AE, Shen Y, Chen Q, Schaller M, Romer L, Aukhil I, Juliano RL. Integrin-mediated activation of MAP kinase is independent of FAK: Evidence for dual integrin signaling pathways in fibroblasts. *J Cell Biol* 1997; 136:1385–1395.

24. LaFlamme SE, Akiyama SK, Yamada KM. Regulation of fibronectin receptor distribution. *J Cell Biol* 1992; 117:437–447.

25. Hemler ME, Kassner PD, Chan BM. Functional roles for integrin alpha subunit cytoplasmic domains. *Cold Spring Harbor Symp Quant Biol* 1992; 57:213–220.

26. Sastry SK, Lakonishok M, Thomas DA, Muschler J, Horwitz AF. Integrin alpha subunit ratios, cytoplasmic domains, and growth factor synergy regulate muscle proliferation and differentiation. *J Cell Biol* 1996; 133:169–184.

27. Fornaro M, Languino LR. Alternatively spliced variants: A new view of the integrin cytoplasmic domain. *Matrix Biol* 1997; 16:185–193.

28. Shattil SJ, Kashiwagi H, Pampori N. Integrin signaling: The platelet paradigm. *Blood* 1998; 91:2645–2657.

29. Marcantonio EE, David FS. Integrin receptor signaling: The propagation of an alpha-helix model. *Matrix Biol* 1997; 16:179–184.

30. Bazzoni G, Hemler ME. Are changes in integrin affinity and conformation overemphasized? *Trends Biochem Sci* 1998; 23:30–34.

31. Miyamoto S, Teramoto H, Coso OA, Gutkind JS, Burbelo PD, Akiyama SK, Yamada KM. Integrin function: Molecular hierarchies of cytoskeletal and signaling molecules. *J Cell Biol* 1995; 131:791–805.

32. Chicurel ME, Singer RH, Meyer CJ, Ingber DE. Integrin binding and mechanical tension induce movement of mRNA and ribosomes to focal adhesions. *Nature* 1998; 392:730–733.

33. Shattil SJ, Haimovich B, Cunningham M, Lipfert L, Parsons JT, Ginsberg MH, Brugge JS. Tyrosine phosphorylation of pp125FAK in platelets requires coordinated signaling through integrin and agonist receptors. *J Biol Chem* 1994; 269:14,738–14,745.

34. Schlaepfer DD, Jones KC, Hunter T. Multiple Grb2-mediated integrin-stimulated signaling pathways to ERK2/mitogen-activated protein kinase: Summation of both c-Src-and focal adhesion kinase-initiated tyrosine phosphorylation events. *Mol Cell Biol* 1998; 18:2571–2585.

35. Miyamoto S, Akiyama SK, Yamada KM. Synergistic roles for receptor occupancy and aggregation in integrin transmembrane function. *Science* 1995; 267:883–885.

36. Plopper GE, McNamee HP, Dike LE, Bojanowski K, Ingber DE. Convergence of integrin and growth factor receptor signaling pathways within the focal adhesion complex. *Mol Biol Cell* 1995; 6:1349–1365.

37. Miyamoto S, Teramoto H, Gutkind JS, Yamada KM. Integrins can collaborate with growth factors for phosphorylation of receptor tyrosine kinases and MAP kinase activation: roles of integrin aggregation and occupancy of receptors. *J Cell Biol* 1996; 135:1633–1642.

38. Yamada KM, Miyamoto S. Integrin transmembrane signaling and cytoskeletal control. *Curr Opin Cell Biol* 1995; 7:681–689.

39. Burridge K, Turner CE, Romer LH. Tyrosine phosphorylation of paxillin and pp125FAK accompanies cell adhesion to extracellular matrix: A role in cytoskeletal assembly. *J Cell Biol* 1992; 119:893–903.

40. Defilippi P, Venturino M, Gulino D, Duperray A, Boquet P, Fiorentini C, Volpe G, Palmieri M, Silengo L, Tarone G. Dissection of pathways implicated in integrin-mediated actin cytoskeleton assembly. Involvement of protein kinase C, Rho GTPase, and tyrosine phosphorylation. *J Biol Chem* 1997; 272:21,726–21,734.

41. Yamada KM, Geiger B. Molecular interactions in cell adhesion complexes. *Curr Opin Cell Biol* 1997; 9:76–85.

42. Hato T, Pampori N, Shattil SJ. Complementary roles for receptor clustering and conformational change in the adhesive and signaling functions of integrin alphaIIb beta3. *J Cell Biol* 1998; 141:1685–1695.

43. Lash JW, Linask KK, Yamada KM. Synthetic peptides that mimic the adhesive recognition signal of fibronectin: Differential effects on cell–cell and cell–substratum adhesion in embryonic chick cells. *Dev Biol* 1987; 123:411–420.

44. Monier-Gavelle F, Duband JL. Cross talk between adhesion molecules: Control of N-cadherin activity by intracellular signals elicited by beta1 and beta3 integrins in migrating neural crest cells. *J Cell Biol* 1997; 137:1663–1681.
45. Schwartz MA, Brown EJ, Fazeli B. A 50-kDa integrin-associated protein is required for integrin-regulated calcium entry in endothelial cells. *J Biol Chem* 1993; 268:19,931–19,934.
46. Ticchioni M, Deckert M, Mary F, Bernard G, Brown EJ, Bernard A. Integrin-associated protein (CD47) is a comitogenic molecule on CD3-activated human T cells. *J Immunol* 1997; 158:677–684.
47. Yebra M, Parry GCN, Stromblad S, Mackman N, Rosenberg S, Mueller BM, Cheresh DA. Requirement of receptor-bound urokinase-type plasminogen activator for integrin alpha v beta5-directed cell migration. *J Biol Chem* 1996; 271:29,393–29,399.
48. Planus E, Barlovatz-Meimon G, Rogers RA, Bonavaud S, Ingber DE, Wang N. Binding of urokinase to plasminogen activator inhibitor type–1 mediates cell adhesion and spreading. *J Cell Sci* 1997; 110:1091–1098.
49. Berditchevski F, Zutter MM, Hemler ME. Characterization of novel complexes on the cell surface between integrins and proteins with 4 transmembrane domains (TM4 proteins). *Mol Biol Cell* 1996; 7:193–207.
50. Mannion BA, Berditchevski F, Kraeft SK, Chen LB, Hemler ME. Transmembrane-4 superfamily proteins CD81 (TAPA-1), CD82, CD63, and CD53 specifically associated with integrin alpha 4 beta 1 (CD49d/CD29). *J Immunol* 1996; 157:2039–2047.
51. Nagel W, Zeitlmann L, Schilcher P, Geiger C, Kolanus J, Kolanus W. Phosphoinositide 3-OH kinase activates the beta2 integrin adhesion pathway and induces membrane recruitment of cytohesin–1. *J Biol Chem* 1998; 273:14,853–14,861.
52. Hannigan GE, Leung-Hagesteijn C, Fitz-Gibbon L, Coppolino MG, Radeva G, Filmus J, Bell JC, Dedhar S. Regulation of cell adhesion and anchorage-dependent growth by a new beta 1-integrin-linked protein kinase. *Nature* 1996; 379:91–96.
53. Wu C, Keightley SY, Leung-Hagesteijn C, Radeva G, Coppolino M, Goicoechea S, McDonald JA, Dedhar S. Integrin-linked protein kinase regulates fibronectin matrix assembly, E-cadherin expression, and tumorigenicity. *J Biol Chem* 1998; 273:528–536.
54. Schaller MD, Otey CA, Hildebrand JD, Parsons JT. Focal adhesion kinase and paxillin bind to peptides mimicking beta integrin cytoplasmic domains. *J Cell Biol* 1995; 130:1181–1187.
55. Chang DD, Wong C, Smith H, Liu J. ICAP-1, a novel beta1 integrin cytoplasmic domain-associated protein, binds to a conserved and functionally important NPXY sequence motif of beta1 integrin. *J Cell Biol* 1997; 138:1149–1157.
56. Sharma CP, Ezzell RM, Arnaout MA. Direct interaction of filamin (ABP–280) with the beta 2-integrin subunit CD18. *J Immunol* 1995; 154:3461–3470.
57. Shattil SJ, O'Toole T, Eigenthaler M, Thon V, Williams M, Babior BM, Ginsberg MH. Beta 3-endonexin, a novel polypeptide that interacts specifically with the cytoplasmic tail of the integrin beta 3 subunit. *J Cell Biol* 1995; 131:807–816.
58. Schaapveld RQJ, Borradori L, Geerts D, van Leusden MR, Kuikman I, Nievers MG, Niessen CM, Steenbergen RDM, Snijders PJF, Sonnenberg A. Hemidesmosome formation is initiated by the beta4 integrin subunit, requires complex formation of beta4 and HD1/Plectin, and involves a direct interaction between beta4 and the bullous pemphigoid antigen 180. *J Cell Biol* 1998; 142:271–284.
59. Naik UP, Patel PM, Parise LV. Identification of a novel calcium-binding protein that interacts with the integrin alphaIIb cytoplasmic domain. *J Biol Chem* 1997; 272:4651–4654.
60. Schaffner-Reckinger E, Gouon V, Melchior C, Plancon S, Kieffer N. Distinct involvement of beta3 integrin cytoplasmic domain tyrosine residues 747 and 759 in integrin-mediated cytoskeletal assembly and phosphotyrosine signaling. *J Biol Chem* 1998; 273:12,623–12,632.

61. Jenkins AL, Nannizzi-Alaimo L, Silver D, Sellers JR, Ginsberg MH, Law DA, Phillips DR. Tyrosine phosphorylation of the beta3 cytoplasmic domain mediates integrin-cytoskeletal interactions. *J Biol Chem* 1998; 273:13,878–13,885.

62. Richardson A, Parsons JT. Signal transduction through integrins: A central role for focal adhesion kinase? *BioEssays* 1995; 17:229–236.

63. Guan JL. Focal adhesion kinase in integrin signaling. *Matrix Biol* 1997; 16:195–200.

64. Hanks SK, Polte TR. Signaling through focal adhesion kinase. *BioEssays* 1997; 19:137–145.

65. Guan JL, Shalloway D. Regulation of focal adhesion-associated protein tyrosine kinase by both cellular adhesion and oncogenic transformation. *Nature* 1992; 358:690–692.

66. Ilic D, Furuta Y, Kanazawa S, Takeda N, Sobue K, Nakatsuji N, Nomura S, Fujimoto J, Okada M, Yamamoto T. Reduced cell motility and enhanced focal adhesion contact formation in cells from FAK-deficient mice. *Nature* 1995; 377:539–544.

67. Cary LA, Chang JF, Guan JL. Stimulation of cell migration by overexpression of focal adhesion kinase and its association with Src and Fyn. *J Cell Sci* 1996; 109:1787–1794.

68. Gilmore AP, Romer LH. Inhibition of focal adhesion kinase (FAK) signaling in focal adhesions decreases cell motility and proliferation. *Mol Biol Cell* 1996; 7:1209–1224.

69. George EL, Georges-Labouesse EN, Patel-King RS, Rayburn H, Hynes RO. Defects in mesoderm, neural tube and vascular development in mouse embryos lacking fibronectin. *Development* 1993; 119:1079–1091.

70. Schlaepfer DD, Hunter T. Evidence for in vivo phosphorylation of the Grb2 SH2-domain binding site on focal adhesion kinase by Src-family protein-tyrosine kinases. *Mol Cell Biol* 1996; 16:5623–5633.

71. Schlaepfer DD, Broome MA, Hunter T. Fibronectin-stimulated signaling from a focal adhesion kinase-c-Src complex: Involvement of the Grb2, p130cas, and Nck adaptor proteins. *Mol Cell Biol* 1997; 17:1702–1713.

72. Schlaepfer DD, Hanks SK, Hunter T, van der Geer P. Integrin-mediated signal transduction linked to Ras pathway by GRB2 binding to focal adhesion kinase. *Nature* 1994; 372:786–791.

73. Schlaepfer DD, Hunter T. Focal adhesion kinase overexpression enhances ras-dependent integrin signaling to ERK2/mitogen-activated protein kinase through interactions with and activation of c-Src. *J Biol Chem* 1997; 272:13,189–13,195.

74. Clark EA, Hynes RO. Ras activation is necessary for integrin-mediated activation of extracellular signal-regulated kinase 2 and cytosolic phospholipase A2 but not for cytoskeletal organization. *J Biol Chem* 1996; 271:14,814–14,818.

75. Chen Q, Lin TH, Der CJ, Juliano RL. Integrin-mediated activation of mitogen-activated protein (MAP) or extracellular signal-related kinase kinase (MEK) and kinase is independent of Ras. *J Biol Chem* 1996; 271:18,122–18,127.

76. Wary KK, Mainiero F, Isakoff SJ, Marcantonio EE, Giancotti FG. The adaptor protein Shc couples a class of integrins to the control of cell cycle progression. *Cell* 1996; 87:733–743.

77. Wary KK, Mariotti A, Zurzolo C, Giancotti FG. A requirement for caveolin-1 and associated kinase Fyn in integrin signaling and anchorage-dependent cell growth. *Cell* 1998; 94:625–634.

78. King WG, Mattaliano MD, Chan TO, Tsichlis PN, Brugge JS. Phosphatidylinositol 3-kinase is required for integrin-stimulated AKT and Raf-1/mitogen-activated protein kinase pathway activation. *Mol Cell Biol* 1997; 17:4406–4418.

79. Cary LA, Han DC, Polte TR, Hanks SK, Guan JL. Identification of p130Cas as a mediator of focal adhesion kinase-promoted cell migration. *J Cell Biol* 1998; 140:211–221.

80. Jockusch BM, Bubeck P, Giehl K, Kroemker M, Moschner J, Rothkegel M, Rudiger M, Schluter K, Stanke G, Winkler J. The molecular architecture of focal adhesions. *Annu Rev Cell Dev Biol* 1995; 11:379–416.

81. Toker A. The synthesis and cellular roles of phosphatidylinositol 4,5-bisphosphate. *Curr Opin Cell Biol* 1998; 10:254–261.

82. Hotchin NA, Hall A. Regulation of the actin cytoskeleton, integrins and cell growth by the Rho family of small GTPases. *Cancer Surv* 1996; 27:311–322.

83. McNamee HP, Ingber DE, Schwartz MA. Adhesion to fibronectin stimulates inositol lipid synthesis and enhances PDGF-induced inositol lipid breakdown. *J Cell Biol* 1993; 121: 673–678.

84. Clark EA, King WG, Brugge JS, Symons M, Hynes RO. Integrin-mediated signals regulated by members of the rho family of GTPases. *J Cell Biol* 1998; 142:573–586.

85. Cybulsky AV, Carbonetto S, Cyr MD, McTavish AJ, Huang Q. Extracellular matrix-stimulated phospholipase activation is mediated by beta 1-integrin. *Am J Physiol* 1993; 264:C323–32.

86. Kanner SB, Grosmaire LS, Ledbetter JA, Damle NK. Beta 2-integrin LFA–1 signaling through phospholipase C-gamma 1 activation. *Proc Natl Acad Sci USA* 1993; 90:7099–7103.

87. Chun JS, Ha MJ, Jacobson BS. Differential translocation of protein kinase C epsilon during HeLa cell adhesion to a gelatin substratum. *J Biol Chem* 1996; 271:13,008–13,012.

88. Auer KL, Jacobson BS. Beta 1 integrins signal lipid second messengers required during cell adhesion. *Mol Biol Cell* 1995; 6:1305–1313.

89. Vuori K, Ruoslahti E. Activation of protein kinase C precedes alpha 5 beta 1 integrin-mediated cell spreading on fibronectin. *J Biol Chem* 1993; 268:21,459–21,462.

90. Lewis JM, Cheresh DA, Schwartz MA. Protein kinase C regulates alpha v beta 5-dependent cytoskeletal associations and focal adhesion kinase phosphorylation. *J Cell Biol* 1996; 134:1323–1332.

91. Schwartz MA, Lechene C, Ingber DE. Insoluble fibronectin activates the Na/H antiporter by clustering and immobilizing integrin alpha 5 beta 1, independent of cell shape. *Proc Natl Acad Sci USA* 1991; 88:7849–7853.

92. Schwartz MA, Ingber DE, Lawrence M, Springer TA, Lechene C. Multiple integrins share the ability to induce elevation of intracellular pH. *Exp Cell Res* 1991; 195:533–535.

93. Damsky CH, Werb Z. Signal transduction by integrin receptors for extracellular matrix: Cooperative processing of extracellular information. *Curr Opin Cell Biol* 1992; 4:772–781.

94. Chong LD, Traynor-Kaplan A, Bokoch GM, Schwartz MA. The small GTP-binding protein Rho regulates a phosphatidylinositol 4-phosphate 5-kinase in mammalian cells. *Cell* 1994; 79:507–513.

95. Cybulsky AV, McTavish AJ, Cyr MD. Extracellular matrix modulates epidermal growth factor receptor activation in rat glomerular epithelial cells. *J Clin Invest* 1994; 94:68–78.

96. Vuori K, Ruoslahti E. Association of insulin receptor substrate-1 with integrins. *Science* 1994; 266:1576–1578.

97. Renshaw MW, Ren XD, Schwartz MA. Growth factor activation of MAP kinase requires cell adhesion. *EMBO J* 1997; 16:5592–5599.

98. MacPherson IA, Montagnier L. Agar suspension culture for the selective assay of cells transformed by polyoma virus. *Virology* 1964; 23:291–294.

99. Freedman VH, Shin SI. Cellular tumorigenicity in nude mice: correlation with cell growth in semi-solid medium. 1974; *Cell* 3:355–359.

100. Bottazzi ME, Assoian RK. The extracellular matrix and mitogenic growth factors control G1 phase cyclins and cyclin-dependent kinase inhibitors. *Trends Cell Biol* 1997; 7:348–352.

101. Howe A, Aplin AE, Alahari SK, Juliano RL. Integrin signaling and cell growth control. *Curr Opin Cell Biol* 1998; 10:220–231.

102. Elledge SJ. Cell cycle checkpoints: Preventing an identity crisis. *Science* 1996; 274:1664–1672.

103. Morgan DO. Cyclin-dependent kinases: Engines, clocks, and microprocessors. *Annu Rev Cell Dev Biol* 1997; 13:261–291.

104. Fang F, Orend G, Watanabe N, Hunter T, Ruoslahti E. Dependence of cyclin E-CDK2 kinase activity on cell anchorage. *Science* 1996; 271:499–502.

105. Schulze A, Zerfass-Thome K, Berges J, Middendorp S, Jansen-Durr P, Henglein B. Anchorage-dependent transcription of the cyclin A gene. *Mol Cell Biol* 1996; 16:4632–4638.

106. Zhu XY, Ohtsubo M, Bohmer RM, Roberts JM, Assoian RK. Adhesion-dependent cell-cycle progression linked to the expression of cyclin D1, activation of cyclin E-CDK2, and phosphorylation of the retinoblastoma protein. *J Cell Biol* 1996; 133:391–403.

107. Guadagno TM, Ohtsubo M, Roberts JM, Assoian RK. A link between cyclin A expression and adhesion-dependent cell cycle progression. *Science* 1993; 262:1572–1575.

108. Chen Y, Knudsen ES, Wang JY. Cells arrested in G1 by the v-Abl tyrosine kinase do not express cyclin A despite the hyperphosphorylation of RB. *J Biol Chem* 1996; 271:19,637–19,640.

109. Kang JS, Krauss RS. Ras induces anchorage-independent growth by subverting multiple adhesion-regulated cell cycle events. *Mol Cell Biol* 1996; 16:3370–3380.

110. Vojtek AB, Der CJ. Increasing complexity of the ras signaling pathway. *J Biol Chem* 1998; 273:19,925–19,928.

111. Fraser A, Evan G. A license to kill. *Cell* 1996; 85:781–784.

112. Chao DT, Korsmeyer SJ. BCL–2 family: Regulators of cell death. *Annu Rev Immunol* 1198; 16:395–419.

113. Ko LJ, Prives C. p53: Puzzle and paradigm. *Genes Dev* 1996; 10:1054–1072.

114. Meredith JE, Schwartz MA. Integrins, adhesion and apoptosis. *Trends Cell Biol* 1997; 7:146–150.

115. Frisch SM, Ruoslahti E. Integrins and anoikis. *Curr Opin Cell Biol* 1997; 9:701–706.

116. Cardone MH, Salvesen GS, Widmann C, Johnson G, Frisch SM. The regulation of anoikis: MEKK–1 activation requires cleavage by caspases. *Cell* 1997; 90:315–323.

117. Frisch SM, Vuori K, Kelaita D, Sicks S. A role for Jun-N-terminal kinase in anoikis; suppression by bcl–2 and crmA. *J Cell Biol* 1996; 135:1377–1382.

118. Khwaja A, Downward J. Lack of correlation between activation of Jun-NH2-terminal kinase and induction of apoptosis after detachment of epithelial cells. *J Cell Biol* 1997; 139:1017–1023.

119. Zhang Z, Vuori K, Reed JC, Ruoslahti E. The alpha 5 beta 1 integrin supports survival of cells on fibronectin and up-regulates Bcl-2 expression. *Proc Natl Acad Sci USA* 1995; 92:6161–6165.

120. Boudreau N, Sympson CJ, Werb Z, Bissell MJ. Suppression of ICE and apoptosis in mammary epithelial cells by extracellular matrix. *Science* 1995; 267:891–893.

121. Stromblad S, Becker JC, Yebra M, Brooks PC, Cheresh DA. Suppression of p53 activity and p21WAF1/CIP1 expression by vascular cell integrin alphaVbeta3 during angiogenesis. *J Clin Invest* 1996; 98:426–433.

122. Day ML, Foster RG, Day KC, Zhao X, Humphrey P, Swanson P, Postigo AA, Zhang SH, Dean DC. Cell anchorage regulates apoptosis through the retinoblastoma tumor suppressor/E2F pathway. *J Biol Chem* 1997; 272:8125–8128.

123. Chen CS, Mrksich M, Huang S, Whitesides GM, Ingber DE. Geometric control of cell life and death. *Science* 1997; 276:1425–1428.

124. Maniotis AJ, Chen CS, Ingber DE. Demonstration of mechanical connections between integrins, cytoskeletal filaments, and nucleoplasm that stabilize nuclear structure. *Proc Natl Acad Sci USA* 1997; 94:849–854.

125. Frisch SM, Vuori K, Ruoslahti E, Chan-Hui PY. Control of adhesion-dependent cell survival by focal adhesion kinase. *J Cell Biol* 1996; 134:793–799.

126. Belkin AM, Retta SF. β1D integrin inhibits cell cycle progression in normal myoblasts and fibroblasts. *J Biol Chem* 1998; 273:15,234–15,240.

127. Robinson MJ, Cobb MH. Mitogen-activated protein kinase pathways. *Curr Opin Cell Biol* 1997; 9:180–186.

128. Pages G, Lenormand P, L'Allemain G, Chambard JC, Meloche S, Pouyssegur J. Mitogen-activated protein kinases p42mapk and p44mapk are required for fibroblast proliferation. *Proc Natl Acad Sci USA* 1993; 90:8319–8323.

129. Albanese C, Johnson J, Watanabe G, Eklund N, Vu D, Arnold A, Pestell RG. Transforming p21ras mutants and c-Ets–2 activate the cyclin D1 promoter through distinguishable regions. *J Biol Chem* 1995; 270:23,589–23,597.

130. Eliceiri BP, Klemke R, Stromblad S, Cheresh DA. Integrin alphavbeta3 requirement for sustained mitogen-activated protein kinase activity during angiogenesis. *J Cell Biol* 1998; 140:1255–1263.

131. Scatena M, Almeida M, Chaisson ML, Fausto N, Nicosia RF, Giachelli CM. NF-kappaB mediates alphavbeta3 integrin-induced endothelial cell survival. *J Cell Biol* 1998; 141:1083–1093.

132. Khwaja A, Rodriguez-Viciana P, Wennstrom S, Warne PH, Downward J. Matrix adhesion and Ras transformation both activate a phosphoinositide 3-OH kinase and protein kinase B/Akt cellular survival pathway. *EMBO J* 1997; 16:2783–2793.

133. Brown EJ, Schreiber SL. A signaling pathway to translational control. *Cell* 1996; 86: 517–520.

134. Rosenwald IB, Lazaris-Karatzas A, Sonenberg N, Schmidt EV. Elevated levels of cyclin D1 protein in response to increased expression of eukaryotic initiation factor 4E. *Mol Cell Biol* 1993; 13:7358–7363.

135. Malik RK, Parsons JT. Integrin-dependent activation of the p70 ribosomal S6 kinase signaling pathway. *J Biol Chem* 1996; 271:29,785–29,791.

136. Koyama H, Raines EW, Bornfeldt KE, Roberts JM, Ross R. Fibrillar collagen inhibits arterial smooth muscle proliferation through regulation of Cdk2 inhibitors. *Cell* 1996; 87:1069–1078.

137. Hungerford JE, Compton MT, Matter ML, Hoffstrom BG, Otey CA. Inhibition of pp125FAK in cultured fibroblasts results in apoptosis. *J Cell Biol* 1996; 135:1383–1390.

138. Wen LP, Fahrni JA, Troie S, Guan JL, Orth K, Rosen GD. Cleavage of focal adhesion kinase by caspases during apoptosis. *J Biol Chem* 1997; 272:26,056–26,061.

139. Wang JY. Abl tyrosine kinase in signal transduction and cell-cycle regulation. *Curr Opin Genet Dev* 1993; 3:35–43.

140. Lewis JM, Baskaran R, Taagepera S, Schwartz MA, Wang JY. Integrin regulation of c-Abl tyrosine kinase activity and cytoplasmic-nuclear transport. *Proc Natl Acad Sci USA* 1996; 93:15,174–15,179.

141. Jackson P, Baltimore D, Picard D. Hormone-conditional transformation by fusion proteins of c-Abl and its transforming variants. *EMBO J* 1993; 12:2809–2819.

142. McWhirter JR, Wang JY. Activation of tyrosinase kinase and microfilament-binding functions of c-abl by bcr sequences in bcr/abl fusion proteins. *Mol Cell Biol* 1991; 11:1553–1565.

143. Lewis JM, Schwartz MA. Integrins regulate the association and phosphorylation of paxillin by c-Abl. *J Biol Chem* 1998; 273:14,225–14,230.

144. Radeva G, Petrocelli T, Behrend E, Leung-Hagesteijn C, Filmus J, Slingerland J, Dedhar S. Overexpression of the integrin-linked kinase promotes anchorage-independent cell cycle progression. *J Biol Chem* 1997; 272:13,937–13,944.

145. Novak A, Hsu SC, Leung-Hagesteijn C, Radeva G, Papkoff J, Montesano R, Roskelley C, Grosschedl R, Dedhar S. Cell adhesion and the integrin-linked kinase regulate the LEF-1 and beta-catenin signaling pathways. *Proc Natl Acad Sci USA* 1998; 95:4374–4379.

146. Cadigan KM, Nusse R. Wnt signaling: A common theme in animal development. *Genes Dev.* 1997; 11:3286–3305.

147. Kheradmand F, Werner E, Tremble P, Symons M, Werb Z. Role of Rac1 and oxygen radicals in collagenase-1 expression induced by cell shape change. *Science* 1998; 280: 898–902.

148. Lafrenie RM, Bernier SM, Yamada KM. Adhesion to fibronectin or collagen I gel induces rapid, extensive, biosynthetic alterations in epithelial cells. *J Cell Physiol* 1998; 175: 163–173.

149. Ramos JW, Whittaker CA, DeSimone DW. Integrin-dependent adhesive activity is spatially controlled by inductive signals at gastrulation. *Development* 1996; 122:2873–2883.

150. Blystone SD, Graham IL, Lindberg FP, Brown EJ. Integrin alpha v beta 3 differentially regulates adhesive and phagocytic functions of the fibronectin receptor alpha 5 beta 1. *J Cell Biol* 1994; 127:1129–1137.

151. Huhtala P, Humphries MJ, McCarthy JB, Tremble PM, Werb Z, Damsky CH. Cooperative signaling by alpha 5 beta 1 and alpha 4 beta 1 integrins regulates metalloproteinase gene expression in fibroblasts adhering to fibronectin. *J Cell Biol* 1995; 129:867–879.

152. Diaz-Gonzalez F, Forsyth J, Steiner B, Ginsberg MH. Trans-dominant inhibition of integrin function. *Mol Biol Cell* 1996; 7:1939–1951.

153. Tamura M, Gu J, Matsumoto K, Aota S, Parsons R, Yamada KM. Inhibition of cell migration, spreading, and focal adhesions by tumor suppressor PTEN. *Science* 1998; 280:1614–1617.

154. Maehama T, Dixon JE. The tumor suppressor, PTEN/MMAC1, dephosphorylates the lipid second messenger, phosphatidylinositol 3,4,5-trisphosphate. *J Biol Chem* 1998; 273: 13,375–13,378.

155. Gu J, Tamura M, Yamada KM. Tumor suppressor PTEN inhibits integrin- and growth factor-mediated mitogen-activated protein (MAP) kinase signaling pathways. *J Cell Biol* 1998; 143:1375–1383.

156. Gu J, Tamura M, Pankov R, Danen EH, Takino T, Matsumoto K, Yamada KM. Shc and FAK differentially regulate cell motility and directionality modulated by PTEN. *J Cell Biol* 1999; 146:389–403.

157. Stambolic V, Suzuki A, de la Pompa JL, Brothers GM, Mirtsos C, Sasaki T, Ruland J, Penninger JM, Siderovski DP, Mak TW. Negative regulation of PKB/Akt-dependent cell survival by the tumor suppressor PTEN. *Cell* 1998; 95:29–39.

158. Davies MA, Lu Y, Sano T, Fang X, Tang P, LaPushin R, Koul D, Bookstein R, Stokoe D, Yung WK, Mills GB, Steck PA. Adenoviral transgene expression of MMAC/PTEN in human glioma cells inhibits Akt activation and induces anoikis. *Cancer Res* 1998; 58:5285–5290.

159. Tamura M, Gu J, Danen EH, Takino T, Miyamoto S, Yamada KM. PTEN interactions with focal adhesion kinase and suppression of the extracellular matrix-dependent phosphatidylinositol 3-kinase/Akt cell survival pathway. *J Biol Chem* 1999; 274:20,693–20,703.

2

Signal Transduction Through Tyrosine Kinase Growth Factor Receptors

Paolo Fedi, MD, PhD and Stuart A. Aaronson, MD

1. INTRODUCTION

The evolution of multicellular organisms has involved the development of intercellular communication required for development and differentiation, as well as systemic responses to wounds and infections. These complex signaling networks are in large part mediated by growth factors, cytokines, and hormones. Such factors can influence cell proliferation in positive or negative ways, as well as inducing a series of differentiated responses in appropriate target cells. The interaction of a growth factor with its receptor by specific binding, in turn, activates a cascade of intracellular biochemical events that is ultimately responsible for the biological responses observed. Cytoplasmic molecules that mediate these responses have been termed *second messengers.* The eventual transmission of biochemical signals to the nucleus leads to effects on the expression of cassettes of genes involved in mitogenic and differentiation responses. This chapter discusses the mechanisms of activation of receptor tyrosine kinases (RTKs) and their signaling pathways.

2. MECHANISMS OF ACTIVATION OF RECEPTOR TYROSINE KINASES

Growth factors mediate their diverse biological responses by binding to and activating cell surface receptors with intrinsic protein kinase activity (1). To date, more than 50 RTKs, which belong to at least 13 different receptor families, have been identified. All RTKs contain a large glycosylated extracellular ligand-binding domain, a single transmembrane region, and a cytoplasmic portion with a conserved protein tyrosine kinase domain. In addition to the catalytic domain, a juxtamembrane region and a C-terminal tail can be identified in the cytoplasmic portion. Because of their structure, RTKs can be visualized as membrane-associated allosteric enzymes with the ligand binding and protein tyrosine kinase domains separated by the plasma membrane (2). Their role is to catalyze the transfer of the γ-phosphate of ATP to tyrosine residues of protein substrates. Tyrosine phosphorylation represents the language used by these receptors to transduce the information carried by the growth factor.

From: Signaling Networks and Cell Cycle Control: The Molecular Basis of Cancer and Other Diseases
Edited by: J. S. Gutkind © Humana Press Inc., Totowa, NJ

On the basis of sequence similarity, it is possible to classify these receptors into related groups *(3)*. Characteristic structural features of the extracellular domains of these groups include, among others, cysteine-rich motifs, immunoglobulin-like repeats (Ig-like), fibronectin type III repeats (FNIII), and epidermal growth factor (EGF) motifs that can be present singly or in different combination. These different domains helps determine specificity for ligand binding.

There is substantial evidence that ligand-induced activation of the kinase domain and its signaling potential are mediated by receptor oligomerization (reviewed in refs. *2, 4,* and *5*). This event stabilizes interactions between adjacent cytoplasmic domains and control the activation of kinase activity. Receptor oligomerization appears to be a common phenomenon among growth factor receptors. Dimerization can take place between two identical receptors (homodimerization), between different members of the same receptor family, or in some cases between a receptor and an accessory protein (heterodimerization) *(5–8)*.

How ligands bind to the receptors and induce oligomerization appears to be specific for each class of RTKs (reviewed in refs. *6* and *9*). Platelet-derived growth factor (PDGF), for example, induce receptor dimerization by virtue of its dimeric nature *(10)*. By contrast, EGF possesses two binding sites for its receptor. In the proposed model, the ligand uses one site to bind monovalently to the receptor and the other to bridge two ligand–receptor complexes *(11)*. Fibroblast growth factor (FGF), which is also a monomeric ligand like EGF, needs instead an accessory molecule to induce receptor dimerization *(9)*. It is now well established that dimerization is sufficient for RTK activation (reviewed in ref. *5*).

The activation of intrinsic protein kinase activity results in autophosphorylation of specific tyrosine residues in the cytoplasmic portion of the RTK. Moreover, tyrosine phosphorylation in the kinase domain stimulates the intrinsic catalytic activity of the receptor. Recently, biochemical and structural studies have demonstrated some of the molecular mechanisms that mediate such activation. There is substantial evidence that autophosphorylation occurs in *trans* by a second receptor tyrosine kinase after dimerization induced by ligand binding. In the unphosphorylated state, the receptor possesses a low catalytic activity because of the particular conformation of a specific domain in the kinase region, which interferes with the phosphotransfer event. Phosphorylation of the kinase domain removes this inhibition, and the catalytic activity is enhanced and persists for some time independent of the presence of the ligand. In particular, it has been shown that phosphorylation of a tyrosine in the activation loop (A-loop) in the catalytic domain of the FGF receptor permits rotation of a proline residue in position 663 that normally interferes with the binding of substrates to the kinase domain and therefore maintains the kinase in an inactive state (reviewed in ref. *12*). Although kinase activity is at a low basal level in the monomeric state, this activity is sufficient to induce *trans*-autophosphorylation once the dimer forms.

Autophosphorylation also occurs outside the kinase domain and serves the important function of creating docking sites for downstream signal transduction molecules.

The main function of the transmembrane domain is to anchor the receptor in the plane of the plasma membrane, connecting the extracellular environment with internal compartments of the cell. It was initially thought that this domain represented a passive anchor of the receptor to the membrane *(2)*. However, point mutations in the transmembrane domain of one receptor, the *neu*/erbB-2, enhance its transforming properties *(13,14)*. The transmembrane mutation in *neu* may have a stabilizing effect on the conformation, which results in dimerization and constitutive activation of receptor signaling *(15)*. Genetic alterations in this domain have, in fact, demonstrated an active role of this region in RTK dimerization and demonstrated that dimerization is not sufficient, but proper alignment must also occur to permit activation and signaling *(16,17)*.

The juxtamembrane sequence that separates the transmembrane and cytoplasmic domains is not well conserved between different families of receptors. However, juxtamembrane sequences are highly similar among members of the same family. Studies indicate that this domain plays a role in modulating receptor functions by heterologous stimuli, a process termed *receptor transmodulation (2)*. For example, the addition of PDGF to many types of cells causes a rapid decrease in high affinity binding of EGF to its receptor. This has been shown to be a downstream effect of PDGF receptor activation in which protein kinase C, itself a serine protein kinase, is activated and, in turn, phosphorylates a site in the juxtamembrane domain of the EGF receptor *(14)*. This region may also play a role in signaling, as has been suggested by the capacity to bind specific substrates in a ligand-dependent manner. For example it has been shown that *eps8* directly binds to the juxtamembrane domain of EGFR in a phosphotyrosine- and SH2-independent manner *(18)*.

The tyrosine kinase domain is the most conserved among tyrosine kinase receptors, and an intact protein tyrosine kinase domain is absolutely required for receptor signaling. For example, mutation of a single lysine in the ATP binding site, which blocks the ability of the receptor to phosphorylate tyrosine residues, completely inactivates receptor biological function. The kinase domain of some receptor tyrosine kinases (e.g., PDGF and FGF receptors) is split by insertions of ≤ 100 mostly hydrophilic amino acid residues. Kinase insertion sequences are highly conserved between species suggesting an important role of this domain in receptor function. In fact, this region contains important autophosphorylation sites, which have the function of coupling with signal transducing molecules. Thus, it appears that the role of the kinase insert region is to mediate receptor interactions with second messengers *(2,5)*.

The C-terminal tail sequences are among the most divergent of the known RTKs *(14)*. The C-terminal domain of the receptor is thought to play an important role in regulating kinase activity. This region typically contains several tyrosine residues, which are phosphorylated by the activated kinase. In fact, the receptor itself is often the major tyrosine-phosphorylated species observed after ligand stimulation. The presence of specific amino acid sequences in this domain plays an important role in determining activation of specific signal-transducing molecules by RTKs. Tyrosine autophosphorylation of such sites represents an important biochemical event that allows receptors to couple with signal transducing molecules. Tyrosine phosphorylation determines high-affinity binding, whereas the amino acids surrounding the site provide specificity. Signaling molecules containing SH2 domains, and phosphotyrosine interaction domains or phosphotyrosine binding domains (PID/PBD or PTB) have the capacity to bind specific peptide sequences containing phosphotyrosine *(19,20)*. In particular, residues

C-terminal to the phosphotyrosine are important in determining specific recognition of SH2 domain residues, whereas sequences N-terminal to the phosphotyrosine are important for recognition of the PTB domain reviewed in *(21)*. Several modes of activation have been identified once a specific signaling molecule has bound the receptor:

2.1. Activation by Tyrosine Phosphorylation: PLCγ, STATs

Each molecule binds to the cytoplasmic tail of the receptor by phosphotyrosine interaction and becomes a substrate of the receptor kinase. It has been demonstrated that tyrosine phosphorylation of phospholipase C-γ (PLC–γ) increases its catalytic activity and is essential for its activation *(22–24)*. Activation of PLC-γ results in hydrolysis of membrane-associated phosphatidylinositol-4,5-phosphate (PIP2) to generate inositol triphosphate and diacylglycerol, two potent second messengers that activate several different signaling pathways.

Signal transducers and activators of transcription (STAT) molecules are latent transcription factors that can be activated as a result of tyrosine phosphorylation by RTKs. Although STATs were first identified as components of interferon signaling and are key signaling molecules used by the cytokine receptor superfamily, a number of RTKs have recently been shown to activate this pathway as well. EGF, PDGF, and colony-stimulating factor-1 (CSF-1) stimulate tyrosine phosphorylation and activation of STATs 1 and 3 *(25)*. EGF can also activate STAT5 *(26)*. It has been shown that the intrinsic tyrosine kinase functions of these receptors are absolutely required for STAT activation and that their catalytic activity is sufficient to phosphorylate STATs independent from activation of the Janus kinases (JAKs). The latter kinases are used by cytokine receptors that lack intrinsic kinase activity (reviewed in *27*) to phosphorylate STATs. Their SH2 domains first bind to receptor phosphotyrosines, followed by the STATs, themselves, becoming tyrosine phosphorylated. Once phosphorylated, these proteins form homo- or heterodimers through intermolecular SH2–phosphotyrosine interactions. They then translocate into the nucleus, where they bind to specific DNA elements, stimulating transcription of downstream genes *(27,28)*.

2.2. Activation by Conformational Change: p85 and SH-PTP2

Phosphatidylinositol (PI) 3-kinases constitute a family of enzymes that are capable of phosphorylating the D3 position of PI *(see* Chapter 14). RTKs can mediate activation of these enzymes, which are composed of a heterodimeric complex of a separate regulatory (p85) and catalytic (p110) subunits. Activation of enzymatic activity is initiated by binding of p85 to the receptor. In particular, the activity of p85/p110 has been shown to be increased when the p85 SH2 domains bind to phosphotyrosine within the context of a particular sequence motif within the RTKs *(29–31)*. As p85 remains bound to p110, presumably p85 binding to the receptor induces a conformational change, which is then transmitted to p110. Recently, evidence has been presented that p85 plays a role in stabilizing and inhibiting the function of the p110 catalytic subunit *(32)*. Thus, it is possible that the conformational change induced by p85 binding to receptor phosphopeptide may eliminate its inhibition of the catalytic subunit and, therefore, increase PI3-kinase activity. Binding of p85 to the RTK and activation of the catalytic subunit parallel translocation of the enzyme to the membrane, where its substrates are concentrated. As the p85 subunit is composed of more than its SH2 domains, it is possible that it may exert other functions in addition to coupling PI 3-kinase to RTKs.

Another example of activation by conformational change is represented by the cytoplasmic tyrosine phosphatase, SH-PTP2. This ubiquitously expressed protein, also known as Syp, PTP1D, or PTP2C, contains a C-terminal catalytic domain and two SH2 domains at its N-terminus *(33–36)*. SH-PTP2 is the human homolog of the *Drosophila corkscrew,* which has been shown to participate in transmission of signals from growth factor receptors (reviewed in *37* and *38*). SH-PTP2 associates with activated EGF, PDGF, insulin/IRS-1, and FGF receptors and becomes tyrosine phosphorylated upon ligand stimulation (*see* refs. *37* and *38,* and references within). In the case of the PDGFR, it has been shown that Tyr 1009 represents the binding site for SH-PTP2 to the receptor. Moreover, a synthetic phosphopeptide containing this site strongly increases its enzymatic activity *(39)*. SH-PTP2 may function also as an adapter protein for signaling from the growth factor receptor to the activation of Ras and mitogen-activated protein kinase (MAPK) and PI 3-kinase pathways. In fact, it has been demonstrated that tyrosine–phosphorylated SH-PTP2 associates with the SH2 domains of Grb2, p85 *(39)* and Grb7 *(40)* molecules. Although its precise role in signaling still needs to be defined, it has been shown that disruption of SH-PTP2 functions in living cells inhibited cell cycle progression in response to growth factor stimulation, implying a positive role in transducing mitogenic responses mediated by RTKs (reviewed in ref. *37*).

2.3. Translocation to the Plasma Membrane of a Signal Transducing Component by an Adapter Molecule: Grb2/Sos.

This modality of signal transduction by RTKs is well exemplified by the manner in which these receptors modulate activation of Ras. It has been shown that the small GTP-binding protein Ras is a crucial downstream effector of the signal transduction pathways used by growth factors to initiate cell growth and differentiation *(41,42)*. RTK stimulation by growth factors induce Ras to convert from an inactive GDP-bound to an active GTP-bound state. The adapter molecule, Grb2, is responsible for mediating a link between RTKs and Ras *(43,44)*. Grb2 belongs to a group of proteins which are composed virtually only of SH2 and SH3 domains *(45,46)*, and they are thought to function as adapters or regulatory components of specific catalytic subunits. The proteins c-crk, nck, and p85 also belong to this group (reviewed in refs. *45* and *46*). These molecules differ from other SH2-containing molecules because they do not exhibit a distinct enzymatic activity such as PLC-γ.

Grb2 is a 23-kDa protein that consists of one SH2 domain intercalated between two SH3 domains. Like other signaling proteins, Grb2 uses its SH2 domain to bind in a ligand-dependent manner to specific phosphorylated tyrosines in the cytoplasmic domain of the RTKs *(29)*. However, Grb2 does not itself become tyrosine phosphorylated. Moreover, Grb2 also associates through its SH3 domains to the proline-rich region in the C-terminal tail of the ubiquitously expressed protein, Sos *(47)*. Sos *(Son of Sevenless)* is a Ras guanine nucleotide exchange factor, which promotes the release of GDP from Ras and therefore facilitates the binding to GTP and generation of active Ras *(48)*. It appears that the accumulation of active Ras after growth factor stimulation is caused by the translocation of the Sos exchange factor to the plasma membrane by binding and recruitment of Grb2 to the cytoplasmic tail of RTKs, as no changes in the guanine nucleotide releasing activity of Sos can be detected after growth factor stimulation.

Activation of Ras is a necessary step for many RTKs to induce activation of the extracellular signal-regulated kinase (ERK) subfamily of mitogen-activated protein kinases (MAPK), a cascade of serine/threonine-specific protein kinases that are able to regulate gene transcription via phosphorylation of transcription factors (reviewed in refs. *49* and *50*). However, MAPK is not the only signaling pathway activated by Ras (reviewed in ref. *42*).

SHC proteins are another group of cytoplasmic adapter molecules that contain SH2 domains *(51)*. In growth factor-stimulated cells, SHC forms stable complexes with the activated receptors by means of their SH2 or PTB domains, or both, and becomes tyrosine phosphorylated. Such phosphorylation allows SHC to interact with other signaling molecules. It has been demonstrated that SHC can directly associate with Grb2 through direct binding of the Grb2 SH2 domain to the major SHC phosphorylation site *(52)*. Thus, SHC can function as an alternative docking site for recruiting the Grb2/Sos complex to the membrane *(53)*. Experiments in PC12 cells, have demonstrated that the EGFR can use both adapters to activate Ras signaling *(54)*. Why two different adapters might exist remains to be determined. It has been suggested that activation of Ras may imply different functions if mediated by SHC or by direct binding of the receptor to Grb2/Sos. Moreover, the adapter proteins, Grb2 and SHC, may be involved in the activation of other signaling pathways, while coupling RTKs to Ras activation (reviewed in refs. *55* and *56*).

FGF and nerve growth factor (NGF) receptors appear to use an alternative method to recruit Grb2/Sos. It has been demonstrated that after ligand stimulation, these receptors induce tyrosine phosphorylation of a novel lipid-anchored docking protein, FRS2 (FGF receptor substrate 2) *(57)*. This molecule corresponds to the previously identified FGF substrate SNT (Suc1-associated neurotrophic factor-induced tyrosine phosphorylation target), discovered by its capacity to bind to the protein p13*suc1* in differentiating neuronal cells *(58)*. FRS2/SNT is the major phosphorylated substrate visible in cells after stimulation with FGF and NGF and forms a complex with Grb2/Sos in a ligand dependent manner *(56,57,59–61)*. Therefore, this adaptor molecule links FGF-receptor activation to the Ras/MAPK signaling pathway and represents an alternative to SHC-mediated Grb2/Sos signaling *(57)*. Because tyrosine phosphorylation of FRS2 seems to be specifically associated with FGF and NGF receptor signaling, this new lipid-anchored adaptor may account for more specific responses mediated by these receptors *(57)*.

2.4. Recruitment of Multiadapter Proteins: Gab1

RKT activation and autophosphorylation can lead to the recruitment of multiadapter molecules, which in turn become phosphorylated and mediate recruitment of other signaling molecules. This is an important modality in signal transduction because it expands the repertoire of pathways that a single RTK can activate. Grb2-associated binder-1 (Gab1) is a member of a family of docking molecules that includes the insulin-receptor substrates 1 and 2 (IRS-1, -2), as well as the *Drosophila* protein DOS, associated with signaling of an expanding number of RTKs. This family is characterized by a pleckstrin-homology domain at the amino terminus of the protein and several binding sites for SH2 and SH3 domains. Gab1 was identified as a Grb2 binding protein as well as a protein involved in EGF and Insulin receptor signaling *(62)*. Tyrosine phosphorylation of Gab1 mediates interaction with several proteins that contain SH2 domains including PLC-γ, PI 3-kinase, and Syp2 *(62)*. Recent studies have demonstrated that Gab1 represents a major phosphorylated substrate of the activated HGF receptor and appears to mediate biological effects, including cell scattering and branching morphogenesis, in epithelial cells *(63)*. Moreover, in PC-12 cells, Gab1 has the role of associating the NGF receptor, TrkA, to PI 3-kinase pathways and, therefore, promoting cell survival by NGF stimulation *(64)*.

Tyrosine phosphorylation is the major biochemical event by which RTKs control signal transduction. Tyrosine phosphorylation favors association with SH2 and PTB-containing molecules and also provides signaling specificity, because these domains preferentially recognize residues within the context of a particular amino acid sequence (reviewed in *21*). However, it has been shown that RTKs may use other mechanisms for recruiting signaling molecules. A zinc finger-containing protein, ZPR1, was recently described. This molecule binds the EGFR in the catalytic domain using its zinc-finger domain. In this case, exposure of cells to EGF causes decreased binding of ZPR1 to the receptor and its accumulation in the nucleus, suggesting that ZPR1 may function as a transcription factor *(65)*. Another example is the protein *eps8*, which binds directly to the juxtamembrane domain of EGFR, but does not possess any phosphotyrosine binding domain *(18)*. Moreover, it has been shown that RTKs can also become phosphorylated in serine or threonine, or both, after ligand stimulation *(66,67,68*, and references within). Although the function of such phosphorylation is still unclear, it has been suggested that it may have a negative effect on RTK activity.

3. HETERODIMERS OF RELATED RTKS EXPAND SIGNALING DIVERSITY

RTKs can be activated as a result of heterodimer formation as well as after homodimerization. For example, different isoforms of PDGF, which is itself a dimer, induce different dimeric forms of the related PDGF receptors *(69)*. The PDGF A chain dimer binds only α receptors, while the B chain dimer binds both α and β receptors at high affinity. Thus, PDGF AA binds αα receptor homodimers, PDGF AB induces αα and αβ receptor heterodimers, and PDGF BB activates all three combinations of receptors. This results in an added complexity in ligand/receptor interactions, as there are differences in signals transduced by these three different receptor combinations. Thus, the response to PDGF depends both on the particular PDGF isoform and the number of α and β receptors expressed by the target cells.

The variety of responses is even more complex among members of other related families of RTKs. The EGFR is prototype for the erbB family of four related receptors that interact with an expanding family of ligands. The ligands induce different combinations of homo- or heterodimers between different erbB family members *(70)*. Moreover, two of the receptors have unusual properties. One, erbB2, appears to lack the ability to bind erbB ligands but forms heterodimers with other family members in response to ligands or can become constitutively activated as a result of overexpression. Another, erbB3, lacks certain highly conserved amino acid residues in its kinase domain and has little if any detectable intrinsic kinase activity. Thus, erbB3 may function in heterodimers as a substrate for an active erbB family member and to provide docking sites for downstream signaling molecules. Given that other structurally related receptor families exist and that there are multimember ligand families for such receptors, it is reasonable to assume that receptor heterodimers as well as homodimers occur among other RTK families.

4. NATURALLY OCCURRING RECEPTOR ANTAGONISTS

Signaling by RTKs can be antagonized by a number of mechanisms that impair ligand–receptor interactions. Receptor isoforms resulting from alternative transcripts or from post translational processing can create a secreted soluble receptor that could presumably act to bind and sequester the ligand *(71)*. Other studies have shown that inactivated receptor mutants, which retain ligand binding can act in a dominant negative manner to attenuate signals induced by ligands *(72,73)*. There are also naturally occurring ligand antagonists that are formed as products of alternative transcripts of the gene encoding the ligand as has been shown for HGF *(74)* or the product of a different gene *(75–77)*. These act as competitive antagonists of ligand binding.

5. CONCLUSIONS

The signaling cascades initiated by interactions of ligands with their receptors are complex, and many details remain to be elucidated. However, a general feature appears to be the formation of ligand-induced dimers. Moreover, the repertoire of responses is expanded by the ability of related ligands to activate different combinations of homodimers and heterodimers. Another important feature is that growth/differentiation signals by RTKs require activation of tyrosine kinase activity in the receptor complex. Finally, the resulting phosphorylation of tyrosine residues both on the receptor and on signal transducing molecules further amplifies and diversifies the signaling capacity through the formation of specific protein–protein interactions and signaling complexes. Thus, protein tyrosine phosphorylation by RTKs and its regulation by tyrosine phosphatases are crucial to the downstream events that transduce a ligand mediated signal cascades.

REFERENCES

1. Aaronson SA. Growth factors and cancer. *Science* 1991; 254:1146–1153.
2. Ullrich A, Schlessinger J. Signal transduction by receptor with tyrosine kinase activity. *Cell* 1990; 61:203–212.
3. Fantl WJ, Johnson DE, Williams LT. Signalling by receptor tyrosine kinases. *Annu Rev Biochem* 1993; 62:453–481.
4. Weiss A, Schlessinger J. Switching on or off by receptor dimerization. *Cell* 1998; 94: 277–280.
5. Heldin C-H. Dimerization of cell surface receptors in signal transduction. *Cell* 1995; 80: 213–223.
6. Heldin C-H, Ostman A. Ligand-induced dimerization of growth factor receptors: variation on the theme. *Cytokine Growth Factor Rev* 1996; 7:3–10.

7. Lemmon MA, Schlessinger J. Regulation of signal transduction and signal diversity by receptor oligomerization. *Trends Biochem Sci* 1994; 19:459–463.
8. Carraway KL III, Cantley LC. A neu acquaintance for erbB3 and erbB4: A role for receptor heterodimerization in growth signaling. *Cell* 1994; 78:5–8.
9. Schlessinger J. Direct binding and activation of receptor tyrosine kinases by collagen. *Cell* 1997; 91:869–872.
10. Heldin CH, Ostman A, Ronnstrand L. Signal transduction via platelet-derived growth factor receptors. *Biochim Biophys Acta* 1998; 1378:F79–F113.
11. Lemmon MA, Bu Z, Ladbury JE, Zhou M, Pinchasi D, Lax I, Engelman DM, Schlessinger J. Two EGF molecules contribute additively to stabilization of the EGFR dimer. *Embo J* 1997; 16:281–294.
12. Hubbard SR, Mohammadi M, Schlessinger J. Autoregulatory mechanisms in protein-tyrosine kinases. *J Biol Chem* 1998; 273:11,987–11,990.
13. Stern DF, Kamps MP, Cao H. Oncogenic activation of p185neu stimulates tyrosine phosphorylation in vivo. *Mol Cell Biol* 1988; 8:3969–3973.
14. Yarden Y, Ullrich A. Growth factor receptor tyrosine kinases. *Annu Rev Biochem* 1988; 57:443–478.
15. Weiner DB, Liu J, Cohen JA, Williams WV, Greene MI. A point mutation in the neu oncogene mimics ligand induction of receptor aggregation. *Nature* 1989; 339:230–231.
16. Burke CL, Lemmon MA, Coren BA, Engelman DM, Stern DF. Dimerization of the p185*neu* transmembrane domain is necessary but not sufficient for transformation. *Oncogene* 1997; 14:687–696.
17. Burke CL, Stern DF. Activation of Neu (ErbB-2) mediated by disulfide bond-induced dimerization reveals a receptor tyrosine kinase dimer interface. *Mol Cell Biol* 1998; 18:5371–5379.
18. Castagnino P, Biesova Z, Wong WT, Fazioli F, Gill GN, Di Fiore PP. Direct binding of *eps8* to the juxtamembrane domain of EGFR is phosphotyrosine- and SH2-independent. *Oncogene* 1995; 10:723–729.
19. Bork P, Margolis B. A phosphotyrosine interaction domain. Letter to the Editor. *Cell* 1995; 80:693–694.
20. Pawson T, Schlessinger J. SH2 and SH3 domains. *Curr Biol* 1993; 3:4345–4442.
21. Songyang Z, Cantley LC. Recognition and specificity in protein tyrosine kinase-mediated signalling. *Trends Biol Sci* 1995; 20:470–475.
22. Nishibe S, Wahl MI, Hernandez-Sotomayor SMT, Tonks NK, Rhee SG, Carpenter G. Increase of the catalytic activity of phospholipase C-γ1 by tyrosine phosphorylation. *Science* 1990; 250:1253–1256.
23. Goldschmidt-Clermont PJ, Kim JW, Machesky LM, Rhee SG, Pollard TD. Regulation of phospholipase C-γ1 by profilin and tyrosine phosphorylation. *Science* 1991; 251:1231–1233.
24. Kim HK, Kim JW, Zilberstein A, Margolis B, Kim JG, Schlessinger J, Rhee SG. PDGF stimulation of inositol phospholipid hydrolysis requires PLC-γ1 phosphorylation on tyrosine residues 783 and 1254. *Cell* 1991; 65:435–441.
25. Schindler C, Darnell JE Jr. Transcriptional responses to polipeptide ligands: The JAK-STAT pathway. *Annu Rev Biochem* 1995; 64:621–651.
26. Ruff-Jamison S, Chen K, Cohen S. Epidermal growth factor induces the tyrosine phosphorylation and nuclear translocation of STAT 5 in mouse liver. *Proc Natl Acad Sci USA* 1995; 92:4215–4218.
27. Leaman DW, Leung S, Li X, Stark GR. Regulation of STAT-dependent pathways by growth factors and cytokines. *FASEB J* 1996; 10:1578–1588.
28. Darnell JE Jr. STATs and gene regulation. *Science* 1997; 277:1630–1635.
29. Songyang Z, Shoelson SE, Chaudhuri M, Gish G, Pawson T, Haser WG, King F, Roberts T, Ratnofsky S, Lechleider RJ, et al. SH2 domains recognize specific phosphopeptide sequences. *Cell* 1993; 72:767–778.

30. Carpenter CL, Auger KR, Chanudhuri M, Yoakim M, Schaffhausen B, Shoelson S, Cantley LC. Phosphoinositide 3-kinase is activated by phosphopeptides that bind to the SH2 domains of the 85-kDa subunit. *J Biol Chem* 1993; 268:9478–9483.
31. Backer JM, Myers MG Jr, Shoelson SE, Chin DJ, Sun XJ, Miralpeix M, Hu P, Margolis B, Skolnik EY, Schlessinger J, et al. Phosphatidylinositol 3'-kinase is activated by association with IRS-1 during insulin stimulation. *EMBO J* 1992; 11:3469–3479.
32. Yu J, Zhang Y, McIlroy J, Rordorf-Nikolic T, Orr GA, Backer JM. Regulation of the p85/p110 phosphatidylinositol 3'-kinase: Stabilization and inhibition of the p110α catalytic subunit by the p85 regulatory subunit. *Mol Cell Biol* 1998; 18:1379–1387.
33. Feng GS, Hui CC, Pawson T. SH2-containing phosphotyrosine phosphatase as a target of protein-tyrosine kinases. *Science* 1993; 259:1607–1611.
34. Vogel W, Lammers R, Huang J, Ullrich A. Activation of a phosphotyrosine phosphatase by tyrosine phosphorylation. *Science* 1993; 259:1611–1614.
35. Ahmad S, Banville D, Zhao Z, Fischer EH, Shen SH. A widely expressed human protein-tyrosine phosphatase containing src homology 2 domains. *Proc Natl Acad Sci USA* 1993; 90:2197–2201.
36. Freeman RM Jr, Plutzky J, Neel BG. Identification of a human src homology 2-containing protein-tyrosine-phosphatase: A putative homolog of Drosophila corkscrew. *Proc Natl Acad Sci USA* 1992; 89:11,239–11,243.
37. Streuli M. Protein tyrosine phosphatases in signaling. *Curr Opin Cell Biol* 1996; 8:182–188.
38. Byon JCH, Kenner KA, Kusari AB, Kusari J. Regulation of growth factor-induced signaling by protein tyrosine phosphatases. *Proc Soc Exp Biol Med* 1997; 216:1–20.
39. Lechleider RJ, Sugimoto S, Bennett AM, Kashishian AS, Cooper JA, Shoelson SE, Walsh CT, Neel BG. Activation of the SH2-containing phosphotyrosine phosphatase SH-PTP2 by its binding site, phosphotyrosine 1009, on the human platelet-derived growth factor receptor. *J Biol Chem* 1993; 268:21,478–21,481.
40. Keegan K, Cooper JA. Use of the two hybrid system to detect the association of the protein-tyrosine-phosphatase, SHPTP2, with another SH2-containing protein, Grb7. *Oncogene* 1996; 12:1537–1544.
41. Egan SE, Giddings BW, Brooks MW, Buday L, Sizeland AM, Weinberg RA. Association of Sos Ras exchange protein with Grb2 is implicated in tyrosine kinase signal transduction and transformation. *Nature* 1993; 363:45–51.
42. Marshall CJ. Ras effectors. *Curr Biol* 1996; 8:197–204.
43. Schlessinger J. How receptor tyrosine kinases activate Ras. *Trends Biochem Sci* 1993; 18:273–275.
44. Margolis B, Skolnik EY. Activation of Ras by receptor tyrosine kinases. *J Am Soc Nephrol* 1994; 5:1288–1299.
45. Schlessinger J. SH2/SH3 signaling proteins. *Curr Opin Genet Dev* 1994; 4:25–30.
46. Schlessinger J, Ullrich A. Growth factor signaling by receptor tyrosine kinases. *Neuron* 1992; 9:383–391.
47. Bonfini L, Karlovich CA, Dasgupta C, Banerjee U. The Son of sevenless gene product: A putative activator of Ras. *Science* 1992; 255:603–606.
48. Boguski MS, McCormick F. Proteins regulating Ras and its relative. *Nature* 1993; 366:643–654.
49. Hill CS, Treisman R. Transcriptional regulation by extracellular signals: mechanisms and specificity. *Cell* 1995; 80:199–211.
50. Marshall CJ. MAP kinase kinase kinase, MAP kinase kinase and MAP kinase. *Curr Opin Genet Dev* 1994; 4:82–89.
51. Pelicci G, Lanfrancone L, Grignani F, McGlade J, Cavallo F, Forni G, Nicoletti I, Pawson T, Pelicci PG. A novel transforming protein (SHC) with an SH2 domain is implicated in mitogenic signal transduction. *Cell* 1992; 70:93–104.

52. Rozakis-Adcock M, McGlade J, Mbamalu G, Pelicci G, Daly R, Li W, Batzer A, Thomas S, Brugge J, Pelicci PG, et al. Association of the Shc and Grb2/Sem5 SH2-containing proteins is implicated in activation of the Ras pathway by tyrosine kinases. *Nature* 1992; 360:689–692.

53. Egan SE, Giddings BW, Brooks MW, Buday L, Sizeland AM, Weinberg RA. Association of Sos Ras exchange protein with Grb2 is implicated in tyrosine kinase signal transduction and transformation [see comments]. *Nature* 1993; 363:45–51.

54. Basu T, Warne PH, Downward J. Role of Shc in the activation of Ras in response to epidermal growth factor and nerve growth factor. *Oncogene* 1994; 9:3483–3491.

55. Bonfini L, Migliaccio E, Pelicci G, Lanfrancone L, Pelicci PG. Not all Shc's roads lead to Ras. *Trends Biochem Sci* 1996; 21:257–261.

56. Wang JK, Xu H, Li HC, Goldfarb M. Broadly expressed SNT-like proteins link FGF receptor stimulation to activators of Ras. *Oncogene* 1996; 13:721–729.

57. Kouhara H, Hadari YR, Spivak-Kroizman T, Schilling J, Bar-Sagi D, Lax I, Schlessinger J. A lipid-anchored Grb2-binding protein that links FGF-receptor activation to the Ras/MAPK signaling pathway. *Cell* 1997; 89:693–702.

58. Rabin SJ, Cleghon V, Kaplan DR. SNT, a differentiation-specific target of neurotrophic factor-induced tyrosine kinase activity in neurons and PC12 cells. *Mol Cell Biol* 1993; 13:2203–2213.

59. Mohammadi M, Dikic I, Sorokin A, Burgess WH, Jaye M, Schlessinger J. Identification of six novel autophosphorylation sites on fibroblast growth factor receptor 1 and elucidation of their importance in receptor activation and signal transduction. *Mol Cell Biol* 1996; 16:977–989.

60. Goh KC, Lim YP, Ong SH, Siak CB, Cao X, Tan YH, Guy GR. Identification of p90, a prominent tyrosine-phosphorylated protein in fibroblast growth factor-stimulated cells, as 80K-H. *J Biol Chem* 1996; 271:5832–5838.

61. Klint P, Kanda S, Claesson-Welsh L. Shc and a novel 89-kDa component couple to the Grb2–Sos complex in fibroblast growth factor-2-stimulated cells. *J Biol Chem* 1995; 270:23,337–23,344.

62. Holgado-Madruga M, Emlet DR, Moscatello DK, Godwin AK, Wong AJ. A Grb2-associated docking protein in EGF- and insulin-receptor signalling. *Nature* 1996; 379:560–564.

63. Weidner KM, Di Cesare S, Sachs M, Brinkmann V, Behrens J, Birchmeier W. Interaction between Gab1 and the c-Met receptor tyrosine kinase is responsible for epithelial morphogenesis. *Nature* 1996; 384:173–176.

64. Holgado-Madruga M, Moscatello DK, Emlet DR, Dieterich R, Wong AJ. Grb2-associated binder-1 mediates phosphatidylinositol 3-kinase activation and the promotion of cell survival by nerve growth factor. *Proc Natl Acad Sci USA* 1997; 94:12,419–12,424.

65. Galcheva-Gargova Z, Konstantinov KN, Wu IH, Klier FG, Barrett T, Davis RJ. Binding of zinc finger protein ZPR1 to the epidermal growth factor receptor. *Science* 1996; 272:1797–1802.

66. Theroux SJ, Stanley K, Campbell DA, Davis RJ. Mutational removal of the major site of serine phosphorylation of the epidermal growth factor receptor causes potentiation of signal transduction: Role of receptor down-regulation. *Mol Endocrinol* 1992; 6:1849–1857.

67. Countaway JL, Girones N, Davis RJ. Reconstitution of epidermal growth factor receptor transmodulation by platelet-derived growth factor in Chinese hamster ovary cells. *J Biol Chem* 1989; 264:13,642–13,647.

68. Countaway JL, Northwood IC, Davis RJ. Mechanism of phosphorylation of the epidermal growth factor receptor at threonine 669. *J Biol Chem* 1989; 264:10,828–10,835.

69. Heldin CH, Ostman A, Ronnstrand L. Signal transduction via platelet-derived growth factor receptors. *Biochim Biophys Acta* 1998; 1378:F79–113.

70. Riese DJ II, Stern DF. Specificity within the EGF family/ErbB receptor family signaling network. *BioEssays* 1998; 20:41–48.

71. Flickinger TW, Maihle NJ, Kung HJ. An alternatively processed mRNA from the avian c-erbB gene encodes a soluble, truncated form of the receptor that can block ligand-dependent transformation. *Mol Cell Biol* 1992; 12:883–893.

72. Dunn SE, Ehrlich M, Sharp NJ, Reiss K, Solomon G, Hawkins R, Baserga R, Barrett JC. A dominant negative mutant of the insulin-like growth factor-I receptor inhibits the adhesion, invasion, and metastasis of breast cancer. *Cancer Res* 1998; 58:3353–3361.

73. D'Ambrosio C, Ferber A, Resnicoff M, Baserga R. A soluble insulin-like growth factor I receptor that induces apoptosis of tumor cells in vivo and inhibits tumorigenesis. *Cancer Res* 1996; 56:4013–4020.

74. Chan AM, Rubin JS, Bottaro DP, Hirschfield DW, Chedid M, Aaronson SA. Identification of a competitive HGF antagonist encoded by an alternative transcript. *Science* 1991; 254:1382–1385.

75. Carter DB, Deibel MR Jr, Dunn CJ, Tomich CS, Laborde AL, Slightom JL, Berger AE, Bienkowski MJ, Sun FF, McEwan RN, et al. Purification, cloning, expression and biological characterization of an interleukin-1 receptor antagonist protein [see comments]. *Nature* 1990; 344:633–638.

76. Hannum CH, Wilcox CJ, Arend WP, Joslin FG, Dripps DJ, Heimdal PL, Armes LG, Sommer A, Eisenberg SP, Thompson RC. Interleukin-1 receptor antagonist activity of a human interleukin-1 inhibitor. *Nature* 1990; 343:336–340.

77. Eisenberg SP, Evans RJ, Arend WP, Verderber E, Brewer MT, Hannum CH, Thompson RC. Primary structure and functional expression from complementary DNA of a human interleukin-1 receptor antagonist. *Nature* 1990; 343:341–346.

3

Signaling from TGF-β Receptors

**Anita B. Roberts, PhD, Mark P. de Caestecker, MD, PhD
and Robert J. Lechleider, MD**

1. INTRODUCTION

Signaling from transforming growth factor-β (TGF-β) receptors involves biochemical mechanisms and molecular interactions unique to the transmembrane receptor serine-threonine kinases that bind and transduce signals from ligands belonging to the large family of peptides related to TGF-β *(1,2)*. Members of this family play key roles in regulation of a wide variety of biological end points ranging from early embryonic patterning events to the control of growth, differentiation, and gene expression in adult cells. Although approximately 40 ligands belong to this family, most of the information obtained thus far on signal transduction pathways has come either from genetic studies in *Drosophila* and *Caenorhabditis elegans (3,4)* or from study of the pathways activated by a restricted set of ligands expressed in vertebrates, including TGF-β, activin, and the bone morphogenetic proteins, BMPs 2 and 4. Although several pathways, including those involving ras and mitogen-activated protein kinases (MAP-kinases) have been implicated in signaling from TGF-β *(2,5)*, this brief review emphasizes the downstream signaling pathways of these ligands and their receptors attributable to one particular family of signaling intermediates, the recently identified SMAD proteins, which are phosphorylated by the receptor kinases and translocate to the nucleus, where they activate nuclear targets by participating in transcriptional complexes.

2. RECEPTOR SERINE-THREONINE KINASES OF THE TGF-β FAMILY

Receptor complexes mediating signaling from TGF-β family ligands are heterotetrameric and consist of two type II receptors (75–85 kDa), which bind ligand, and two signal transducing type I receptors (50–60 kDa), which, in most instances, cannot bind ligand directly and thus are considered to act downstream of the type II receptor *(2,5,6)*. Whereas the assembly of the heteromeric complex is initiated by ligand binding, the interaction of the two receptor types is also stabilized by interactions between their cytoplasmic domains *(7)*. This model for receptor activation involves potentiation of the kinase activity of the type I receptor by phosphorylation of several residues in a glycine-serine-rich juxtamembrane domain (GS domain) of the receptor by the type II receptor kinase. Mutation of a single threonine residue to glutamine (T204D) at the

From: Signaling Networks and Cell Cycle Control: The Molecular Basis of Cancer and Other Diseases
Edited by: J. S. Gutkind © Humana Press Inc., Totowa, NJ

interface between the GS domain and the kinase domain of the TGF-β type I receptor results in its constitutive activation, demonstrating that the type I kinase alone is sufficient to initiate signal transduction *(8)*. Mutationally activated type I receptors are now often used in studies of signal transduction by members of the TGF-β family, because they eliminate the need for ligand and the type II receptor.

Application of the yeast two-hybrid system resulted in identification of several proteins which interact specifically with type I and II serine/threonine kinase receptors. By far the most abundant interacting protein, and the only one for which a function has been demonstrated, is the immunophilin FKBP12, which binds all known type I receptors of the family through a Leu-Pro motif in the GS domain, and which may serve to protect against ligand-independent activation of receptors *(9,10)*. Other interacting proteins for which no functions have yet been ascribed include the α subunit of farnesyltransferase, which interacts specifically with the TGF-β type I receptor, and apolipoprotein J/clusterin *(11)* and TRIP-1, a WD-domain protein *(12)*, which interact specifically with the TGF-β type II receptor. Based on the inability to demonstrate roles for any of these proteins in signal transduction, it must be concluded that key signaling elements bind the receptors only transiently, or possibly bind only activated forms of the receptors.

3. DOWNSTREAM SIGNAL TRANSDUCTION PATHWAYS

The first clues to downstream signaling pathways from the TGF-β family serine/ threonine kinase receptors came from genetic studies in *Drosophila* demonstrating that effects of weak alleles of the TGF-β family ligand decapentaplegic (Dpp) could be enhanced by mutations in a maternally expressed gene called *mothers against dpp (Mad)*, *(13)* and that *Mad* could partially rescue the *dpp* null phenotype. Studies in *C. elegans* resulted in identification of 3 genes, *sma-2*, *sma-3*, and *sma-4*, homologous to *Mad*, which have a mutant phenotype similar to that of the mutant *daf-4* (a type II receptor serine-threonine kinase) *(4)*. Further studies clearly implicated these *Mad* and *sma* homologs in downstream signaling from the receptors *(3,14)*.

By consensus, the vertebrate homologues of the *Mad* and *sma* genes have been called *Smads*. All these genes encode proteins with highly conserved N- and C-terminal domains (called *Mad* homology 1 and 2, MH1 and MH2, respectively) connected by highly divergent proline-rich linker regions *(6)*. These proteins contain no recognizable protein–protein interaction motifs or enzymatic activities that would give a clue to their function. To date, 9 or 10 different *Smad* genes have been described that fall into three distinct functional sets: signal-transducing, receptor-activated SMADs, which includes *Smads 1, 2, 3, 5, 8,* and *9*; a single common mediator SMAD, *Smad 4/DPC4*, and inhibitory SMADS, *Smads 6* and *7* and the *Xenopus* protein, *Xsmad8* (Fig. 1).

The present model for downstream signaling emerging from these studies is that (1) receptor-activated SMADs bind to and are phosphorylated on two C-terminal serine residues in their MH2 domain by the type I receptor kinase *(15,16)*; (2) the phosphorylated, pathway-specific SMADS (SMAD-P) then form a heteromeric complex in the cytoplasm with the common mediator, Smad4 *(17)*; (3) the SMAD-P/ Smad4 complex is then translocated to the nucleus, where it participates in a transcriptional complex and mediates activation of the target gene *(18,19)* (Fig. 2). Inhibitory SMADS, induced

A Structural comparisons

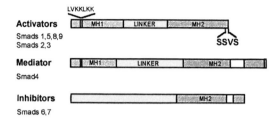

B Sequence features

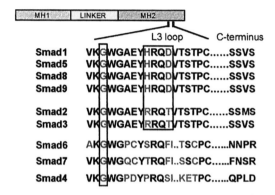

C Model for activation and oligomerization

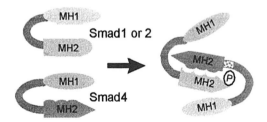

Fig. 1. General features of SMAD proteins important for their receptor binding and ligand-induced activation. (**A**) Structural features of the three subsets of SMAD proteins showing the common MAD-homology domains 1 and 2 (MH1 and MH2) and the proline-rich linker region. (**B**) Sequence characteristics of the SMAD proteins showing the C-terminal phosphorylation site, SSVS, common to receptor-activated SMAD proteins, and the L3 loop motif (HRQD) common to Smad1, 5, 8, and 9 downstream of BMP receptors or (RRQT) common to Smad2 and 3 downstream of either TGF-β or activin receptors. Note also the glycine residue in the L3 loop conserved in all SMADs, a target of naturally occurring inactivating mutations common to *Drosophila* and *Caenorhabditis elegans* and found in human cancers. (**C**) Model showing the internally repressive interactions of the MH1 and MH2 domains of both receptor-activated SMADs and the mediator, Smad4, which are relieved following ligand-dependent phosphorylationto to permit hetero-oligomerization. Note also the SAD, Smad-activating domain (stippled portion of the C-terminal region of the middle linker region) unique to Smad4 and critical to its functional activation.

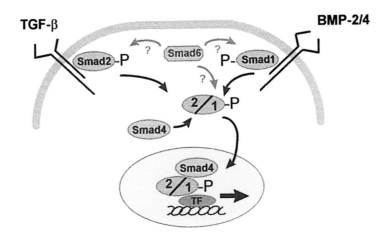

Fig. 2. Model for SMAD-mediated signal transduction from receptor serine-threonine kinases of the TGF-β family. Basic features include phosphorylation of the receptor activated SMAD proteins on their C-terminal SSXS motif by the type I receptor kinase, their hetero-oligomerization with the common mediator Smad4, and the translocation of the SMAD-P/Smad4 complex to the nucleus where it activates transcriptional targets either by direct DNA binding or via participation in transcriptional complexes. Ligand-inducible inhibitory SMADs (represented here by Smad6) block transcriptional activation either by interacting stably with the type I receptors to block phosphorylation of receptor-activated SMADs, or by competing with the common mediator Smad4 for binding to the activated SMADs.

by TGF-β family ligands, function in a negative feedback loop to terminate or reduce the strength of the signal *(20–23)*.

3.1. Assays Commonly Used for Signaling Responses

To date, the most commonly used endpoints to assess SMAD activity are luciferase reporter gene constructs known to be responsive to TGF-β, BMPs, or activin. Promoters used to assess transcriptional activity of TGF-β and other ligands include two highly inducible reporter constructs, p800luc, an 800 bp TGF-β–responsive region of the *plasminogen-activator inhibitor-1 (PAI-1)* gene promoter *(24)*, and the artificial 3TP-lux reporter, which contains three repeats of an AP-1 site from the collagenase promoter linked to a short region of the PAI-1 promoter *(25)*. TGF-β represses expression of pCAL2, which includes a 760-bp TGF-β–responsive region of the cyclin A promoter and is often used as a surrogate marker for growth inhibition *(26)*. Although these reporters are very useful, they are specific neither for the inducing ligand nor for the SMAD pathway, as demonstrated by induction of 3TP-lux by a MAP kinase signaling pathway *(27)*.

A more complex in vivo assay is based on the ability of various members of the TGF-β family to induce mesoderm in *Xenopus* embryos *(28)* and particularly on the differential effects of activin and BMPs to induce dorsal and ventral mesoderm, respectively. In this assay, mRNAs encoding SMAD proteins are injected into the animal pole of two cell embryos, and either whole embryos or excised and cultured animal caps are subsequently analyzed for expression of mesodermal markers. Interestingly, mammalian genes appear to function well in *Xenopus* embryos, even when the mammalian sequences are divergent from the nearest *Xenopus* ortholog *(29)*. The *Xenopus* system is however, only a crude indicator of signal specificity, as the ectodermal cells are poised to differentiate along one of two pathways. Only when particular transcriptional complexes in target genes are characterized can the specificity of each SMAD be determined precisely.

3.2. Receptor-Activated SMAD Proteins

Studies in both *Xenopus* embryos and mammalian cells have shown that the six receptor-activated SMADs identified thus far fall into two restricted pathways: Smad2 and 3 mediate signals from TGF-β and activin receptors *(30–33)* whereas Smad1 *(34–37)*, 5 *(38,39)*, 8 *(40)*, and 9 *(41)* mediate signals from BMP receptors, corresponding to induction of dorsal and ventral mesoderm, respectively, in *Xenopus* embryos. All six of these receptor-activated SMAD proteins share a common C-terminal motif, SSXS-COOH, in which the two-C-terminal serine residues are phosphorylated by the activated type I receptor kinase *(15,16,42)* (Fig. 1B). Mutations in this phosphorylation motif (3S>A) result in dominant negative function, because these mutants associate stably with the type I receptor and fail to translocate to the nucleus or transduce signals *(15,16,33)*.

The L3 loop, another motif in the MH2 domain predicted by analogy to the crystal structure of the C-terminal domain of Smad4 to protrude from the compact homotrimeric "pie-like" Smad complex *(43)*, has recently been shown to be an important determinant of the specificity of the receptor interaction of this subset of SMAD proteins *(44)*. The critical amino acids flank either side of an Arg-Gln which is conserved in all SMADs. For Smad1, 5, 8, and 9, activated by the BMP receptors, this sequence is HRQD, whereas for Smad2 and 3, activated by activin and TGF-β receptors, the corresponding sequence is RRQT (Fig. 1B). Interchanging the flanking amino acids from Smad1 and 2 permits activation of the mutated Smad1 by the TGF-β receptor and Smad2 by the BMP receptor, suggesting that these residues specify binding of the SMAD protein to its respective receptor *(44)*.

These receptor-activated SMAD proteins can act as transcriptional activators when fused to a heterologous GAL4 DNA-binding domain and assayed using a GAL4 reporter gene *(35)*. In this assay, full-length Smad1 or 2 require ligand activation, whereas C-terminal (MH2 domain) domains of these SMADs activate in a ligand-independent fashion. These and other results show that the MH1 domain interferes with the oligomer-izing and transcriptional activating activity of the MH2 domain and suggest that, in the absence of ligand, interactions of the MH1 and MH2 domains are mutually repressive *(45,46)* (Fig. 1C). Ligand-dependent relief of this autorepression can be blocked by mutation of the C-terminal serines (3S>A), mutation of a critical glycine residue in the L3 loop common to all SMADs (Fig. 1B), or mutation of a conserved arginine the MH1 domain which increases the strength of the intramolecular interaction *(46)*. Importantly, the use of Smad4 null cells has now conclusively demonstrated the additional requirement of Smad4 for this transcriptional activation *(19,47)*.

3.3. The Common Mediator—Smad4/DPC4

Smad4 is unique among all the SMADs. It was first identified as a tumor suppressor gene for pancreatic cancer, being either mutated or deleted in more than 80% of pancreatic cancers as well as a smaller percentage of colon cancers and breast cancers

(48). Based on our present understanding of the singular role of Smad4 in mediating signals from receptor serine-threonine kinases *(17,49),* it is clear that functional inactivation of this molecule affects most, if not all, transcriptional targets of the set of receptor-activated SMADs. Its essential role in signaling comes broadly from the demonstration that tumor cells null for Smad4 are insensitive to growth inhibition by TGF-β and that transfection with Smad4 restores responsiveness *(47,50).*

Smad4 is not phosphorylated upon receptor activation, nor does it have the critical C-terminal phosphorylation motif common to the receptor-activated SMADs *(17,31,50).* Biochemical evidence for its central role in the signaling pathways comes from the demonstration of its specific association with receptor-activated SMADs following their ligand-dependent phosphorylation *(17,39,45).* Recent data suggest that this funneling of multiple signals through a single node can serve to modulate crosstalk between different receptors of the TGF-β family in that the relative strength of each signal can be controlled by competition for a limited pool of Smad4 *(49).*

Determination of the tertiary structure of the C-terminal domain of Smad4 shows that it associates as a homotrimer. Key residues at the trimer protein–protein interfaces, which are targets for mutation in human cancers, interfere with homo- and hetero-oligomerization and nuclear translocation *(43,45,51).* Similar to the receptor-activated SMADs, the MH1 domain of Smad4 is inhibitory to the transcriptional activating activity of its MH2 domain, but, unique to Smad4, an activation domain (SAD) has been identified near the extreme C-terminal portion of the middle linker region *(47)* (Fig. 1C). Additional mutations of Smad4 found in human cancers localize to the MH1 domain, stabilizing autorepression *(46).*

Not surprisingly, deletion of the Smad4 gene has severe consequences for early embryonic patterning resulting in lethality at about d E7.5 from impaired differentiation of visceral mesoderm *(52).* A later role in anterior patterning was also demonstrated. However, the exact signaling pathways that have been interrupted cannot be determined, since so many TGF-β family ligands are known to be expressed early in embryogenesis and since all of them are presumed to require Smad4 for signaling.

3.4. Inhibitory SMADS

An important new development in our understanding of the mechanism of signal transduction by SMAD proteins has been the identification of inhibitory SMADs or anti-SMADs. Members of this SMAD protein subset, which presently includes Smad6, Smad7, and the *Xenopus* protein, XSmad8 *(20–23,53),* share the general features of having an N-terminal domain distinct from that of the MH1 domain shared by other SMADs and being more similar to Smad4 in the MH2 domain, in that neither the L3 loop receptor binding motif nor the C-terminal serine phosphorylation motif common to the receptor-activated SMADs are present (Fig. 1B). The conservation of the MH2 domain and the ability of Smads6 and 7 to interact with both the type I receptors and with other SMADs, suggest that this domain may represent a novel interaction domain specific for this pathway, analogous to the SH2/SH3 interaction domains which are hallmarks of tyrosine kinase signaling pathways *(54).* Identification in *Drosophila* of the product of a homologous gene called *Daughters against decapentaplegic (Dad),* which inhibits patterning by *dpp,* suggests that this inhibitory pathway evolved early and is basic to the mechanisms of signal transduction by this family of ligands and receptors *(55)*.

Smad7 mRNA is rapidly induced by treatment of cells with TGF-β, suggesting that anti-SMADs are direct effectors of a ligand-induced signal to suppress a response *(23)*. In this capacity, they may also be important in selective induction of target genes with requirements for different strengths or duration of signal input. Vascular endothelial cells subjected to laminar shear stress express an N-terminally truncated Smad6 *(20,21)*. Since this truncation changes the interaction pattern, resulting in non-specific interaction with Smad1, 2, and 4, the possibility exists that expression of the truncated version of this protein by endothelial cells may represent an adaptive response to mechanical stress, altering signaling from TGF-β family ligands.

There is a lack of consensus regarding the mechanism of action of these anti-SMADs. Anti-SMADs can associate with activated type I receptors and prevent the phosphorylation and nuclear translocation of receptor-activated SMADs. Thus, Smad7 overexpression blocked the phosphorylation of Smad1, 2, and 3 and Smad6 overexpression blocked the phosphorylation of Smad1 and 2, but not of Smad3 *(20,22,23)*. Other data suggest that the receptor interaction might not be functionally significant in that a G>S mutation in the L3 loop of Smad6, which eliminates its inhibitory effect on Smad1 signaling, does not interfere with its ability to bind the type I receptor *(56)*. There are also conflicting data on the ability of Smad6 and 7 to hetero-oligomerize selectively *(56)* or nonselectively with receptor-activated SMADs *(20)*. In *Xenopus*, Smad6 selectively blocks BMP-mediated responses, as supported by studies showing that it interacts selectively with Smad1 and prevents the binding and subsequent functional activation of Smad1 by Smad4 *(56)*. This mechanism would provide a basis for crossregulation of signals emanating from receptor serine-threonine kinases; that is, induction of Smad6 by TGF-β and its association with Smad1 would serve to block competing signals from BMP receptors and ensure favorable competition of Smad2 or Smad3 for a limited pool of Smad4 *(49)* (Fig. 2).

3.5. Transcriptional Activation of Nuclear Target Genes by SMADs

The nuclear translocation of receptor-activated SMADs in a phosphorylation-dependent manner suggests that they play a direct role in transcriptional activation of target genes *(33,35)*. However, unlike the specific *cis* elements that led to the identification of the Stat transducers of signals from receptor tyrosine kinases *(57)*, the diversity of response elements identified in target genes activated by activins and TGF-β has proved challenging in terms of understanding the mechanisms of transcriptional activation by SMADs *(58)*. Although certain of these response elements bind known transcription factors, such as AP1 or Sp1, others probably bind novel transcription factors. Studies are now beginning to provide insight into the mechanisms of transcriptional activation by SMAD proteins and suggest that although SMAD proteins can bind DNA directly, they likely require the cooperation of multiple, diverse, sequence-specific DNA-binding proteins to mediate their transcriptional effects.

The present model for the role of SMAD proteins in transcriptional activation is based on characterization of a complex (activin response factor, ARF) which binds to an activin-response element (ARE) in the promoter of the *Xenopus* Mix.2 homeobox gene and is rapidy induced by activin independently of new protein synthesis *(59)*. The essential component of the ARF, a forkhead/winged-helix transcription factor, FAST-1, binds the ARE directly *(60)*. Both Smad2 and Smad4 are also present in the complex although they do not directly bind the ARE: the MH2 domain of Smad2 interacts with the C-terminal domain (SMAD-interaction domain, SID) of FAST-1 directly, whereas the binding of Smad4 is assumed to be dependent on its association with activated Smad2, and not on direct binding to FAST-1 *(18,60)*. The identification of both Smad2 and 4 in the active transcriptional complex is consistent with the findings that receptor-activated SMADs require Smad4 for transcriptional activation, even though they can translocate to the nucleus in its absence *(19)*, and that nuclear translocation of Smad4 requires heteromeric association with a receptor-activated SMAD *(15)*. Reconstitution of the FAST-1/*Mix.2* system in mammalian cells shows that whereas the MH1 region of Smad2 is dispensable in formation of the ternary gel-shifted complex of Smad2, Smad4, and FAST-1, the MH1 region of Smad4 is required for activation of the promoter and appears to stabilize formation of the ternary complex *(19)*. Studies of two other distinct activin-response elements found in enhancers of genes regulating expression of mesoderm in *Xenopus, goosecoid,* and *XFKH1/pintallavis,* also show Smad2 involvement in the transcriptional complex, suggesting that SMADs act as transcriptional co-activators when complexed with sequence-specific transcription factors *(49,61)*.

Direct interactions of SMAD proteins with DNA may also be important in directing transcriptional activation. A concensus binding sequence, GCCCnCGc, which binds C-terminally truncated forms of *Drosophila* MAD, has been identified in Dpp response elements of the *vestigial, labial,* and *Ultrabithorax* genes *(62)*. Although this interaction is weak, it is specific and correlates with activation of these enhancer elements *in vivo*. In the absence of ligand activation, the DNA-binding activity of the MH1 domain of receptor activated SMADs is repressed by the MH2 domain, showing that these domains are mutually autorepressive *(62)*. In the 3TP-Lux promoter, Smad4 is involved both in direct binding to DNA through its MH1 domain, and with Smad3 in a TGF-β-induced gel-shifted complex that appears in a time course identical to that of SMAD phosphorylation, being maximal at about 15 min after ligand stimulation *(63)*.

Somewhat surprisingly, mutation or deletion of the Smad4 DNA binding elements changed neither the TGF-β nor the Smad3/4 inducibility of the reporter construct in this artificial setting, whereas mutation of the AP1 site in these constructs resulted in loss of inducibility by either *(63)*. Although it is possible that direct binding of Smad4 to DNA may be important in the context of the native promoter, these data also suggest that SMADs may be able to potentiate the activity of transcription factors, such as AP1, without directly binding it. This mechanistic complexity is consistent with the observations that the minimum DNA elements required for activation of the *Mix.2, goosecoid* and *XFKH1/pintallavis* enhancers, and the 3TP-Lux reporter are considerably longer than standard consensus transcription factor binding sites and appear to have bipartite elements *(60,63)*. Clearly, more investigations into the roles of SMAD proteins both as transcriptional coactivators in association with specific transcription factors and in direct binding to DNA are needed to resolve these questions.

4. RECEPTOR CROSSTALK MEDIATED BY SMAD PROTEINS

Depending on the context, TGF-β family ligands can either synergize or antagonize the actions of mitogenic growth factors such as epidermal growth factor (EGF) which signal through receptor tyrosine kinases *(64)*. Recent data now implicate SMADs in the cross-talk between signal transduction pathways downstream of certain receptor tyrosine kinase and TGF-β family signaling pathways. Specifically, it has been shown that Smad1 can be phosphorylated at several PXSP sites in its middle linker region, which are consensus sites for MAP kinases *(65)*. Treatment of cells with EGF or hepatocyte growth factor (HGF) results in phosphorylation of Smad1 on these sites by activation of the Erk subfamily of MAP kinases. This Erk-dependent phosphorylation is independent of phosphorylation of Smad1 on the C-terminal SSVS motif by the BMP type I receptor kinase and results in its retention in the cytoplasm, blocking the nuclear translocation and transcriptional activating activity of Smad1/Smad4 complexes *(65)*. In certain instances, SMADs may also mediate synergistic signals from these two receptor families *(66)*. These exciting findings suggest that receptor-activated SMADs may be sensors of the competing or synergistic inputs from receptor tyrosine and serine/threonine kinases and that activation of selected gene targets by SMADs may reflect an integrated signal input from these two distinct pathways.

5. CONCLUSIONS

An explosion of information during the past 2 yrs has resulted in the characterization of an entirely novel signal transduction pathway downstream of the type 1 receptor serine-threonine kinases of TGF-β family ligands. The SMAD protein transducers of signals from these receptors are inducibly phosphorylated to interact in both activated and inhibitory hetero-oligomeric complexes via C-terminal MH2 domains which, in the absence of an activated receptor kinase, are internally repressed by N-terminal MH1 domains. Nuclear translocation of activated heteromeric SMAD complexes results in transcriptional activation of target genes by mechanisms that probably involve both direct and indirect interactions with DNA, but that are still only poorly understood. Importantly, these proteins may also mediate certain aspects of crosstalk between receptors with either serine-threonine or tyrosine kinase activity. While the basic features of this signal transduction mechanism have now been elucidated, many aspects of the regulation of this pathway are still unclear. Present studies have focused on signaling of a limited set of the family of ligands and receptors related to TGF-β, and the manner in which specificity of signals from ligands to nuclear targets is determined is not yet known. Moreover, the genes identified thus far as regulated by SMAD-mediated pathways are all immediate-early gene targets, and the mechanisms of involvement of SMAD proteins in signals requiring longer duration or greater intensity, such as those resulting in inhibition of cell growth or apoptosis, are unknown. Clearly, there is still much to be learned.

REFERENCES

1. Kingsley DM. The TGF-beta superfamily: New members, new receptors, and new genetic tests of function in different organisms. *Genes Dev* 1994; 8:133–146.

 2. Derynck R, Feng XH. TGF-beta receptor signaling. *Biochim Biophys Acta* 1997; 1333: F105–150.
 3. Newfeld SJ, Chartoff EH, Graff JM, Melton DA, Gelbart WM. Mothers against dpp encodes a conserved cytoplasmic protein required in DPP/TGF-beta responsive cells. *Development* 1996; 122:2099–2108.
 4. Savage C, Das P, Finelli AL, Townsend SR, Sun CY, Baird SE, Padgett RW. *Caenorhabditis elegans* genes sma-2, sma-3, and sma-4 define a conserved family of transforming growth factor beta pathway components. *Proc Natl Acad Sci USA* 1996; 93:790–794.
 5. Attisano L, Wrana JL. Signal transduction by members of the transforming growth factor-beta superfamily. *Cytokine Growth Factor Rev* 1996; 7:327–339.
 6. Heldin CH, Miyazono K, ten Dijke P. TGF-beta signalling from cell membrane to nucleus through SMAD proteins. *Nature* 1997; 390:465–471.
 7. Feng XH, Derynck R. Ligand-independent activation of transforming growth factor (TGF) beta signaling pathways by heteromeric cytoplasmic domains of TGF-beta receptors. *J Biol Chem* 1996; 271:13,123–13,129.
 8. Wieser R, Wrana JL, Massague J. GS domain mutations that constitutively activate T beta R-I, the downstream signaling component in the TGF-beta receptor complex. *EMBO J* 1995; 4:2199–2208.
 9. Charng MJ, Kinnunen P, Hawker J, Brand T, Schneider MD. FKBP-12 recognition is dispensable for signal generation by type I transforming growth factor-beta receptors. 1996; *J Biol Chem* 271:22,941–22,944.
10. Chen YG, Liu F, Massague J. Mechanism of TGFbeta receptor inhibition by FKBP12. *EMBO J* 1997; 16:3866–3876.
11. Reddy KB, Jin G, Karode MC, Harmony JA, Howe PH. Transforming growth factor beta (TGF beta)-induced nuclear localization of apolipoprotein J/clusterin in epithelial cells. *Biochemistry* 1996; 35:6157–6163.
12. Chen RH, Miettinen PJ, Maruoka EM, Choy L, Derynck R. A WD-domain protein that is associated with and phosphorylated by the type II TGF-beta receptor. *Nature* 1995; 377:548–552.
13. Raftery LA, Wisotzkey RG. Characterization of Medea, a gene required for maximal function of the *Drosophila* BMP homolog Decapentaplegic. *Ann NY Acad Sci* 1996; 785:318–320.
14. Wiersdorff V, Lecuit T, Cohen SM, Mlodzik M. Mad acts downstream of Dpp receptors, revealing a differential requirement for dpp signaling in initiation and propagation of morphogenesis in the *Drosophila* eye. *Development* 1996; 122:2153–2162.
15. Souchelnytskyi S, Tamaki K, Engstrom U, Wernstedt C, ten Dijke P, Heldin CH. Phosphorylation of Ser465 and Ser467 in the C terminus of Smad2 mediates interaction with Smad4 and is required for transforming growth factor-beta signaling. *J Biol Chem* 1997; 272:28,107–28,115.
16. Abdollah S, Macias-Silva M, Tsukazaki T, Hayashi H, Attisano L, Wrana JL. TbetaRI phosphorylation of Smad2 on Ser465 and Ser467 is required for Smad2-Smad4 complex formation and signaling. *J Biol Chem* 1997; 272:27,678–27,685.
17. Lagna G, Hata A, Hemmati-Brivanlou A, Massague J. Partnership between DPC4 and SMAD proteins in TGF-beta signalling pathways. *Nature* 1996; 383:832–836.
18. Chen X, Weisberg E, Fridmacher V, Watanabe M, Naco G, Whitman M. Smad4 and FAST-1 in the assembly of activin-responsive factor. *Nature* 1997; 389:85–89.
19. Liu F, Pouponnot C, Massague J. Dual role of the Smad4/DPC4 tumor suppressor in TGFbeta-inducible transcriptional complexes. *Genes Dev* 1997; 11:3157–3167.
20. Hayashi H, Abdollah S, Qiu Y, Cai J, Xu YY, Grinnell BW, Richardson MA, Topper JN, Gimbrone MA Jr, Wrana JL, Falb D. The MAD-related protein Smad7 associates with the TGFbeta receptor and functions as an antagonist of TGFbeta signaling. *Cell* 1997; 89:1165–1173.

21. Topper JN, Cai J, Qiu Y, Anderson KR, Xu YY, Deeds JD, Feeley R, Gimeno CJ, Woolf EA, Tayber O, Mays GG, Sampson BA, Schoen FJ, Gimbrone MA Jr, Falb D. Vascular MADs: Two novel MAD-related genes selectively inducible by flow in human vascular endothelium. *Proc Natl Acad Sci USA* 1997; 94:9314–9319.

22. Imamura T, Takase M, Nishihara A, Oeda E, Hanai J, Kawabata M, Miyazono K. Smad6 inhibits signalling by the TGF-beta superfamily. *Nature* 1997; 389:622–626.

23. Nakao A, Afrakhte M, Moren A, Nakayama T, Christian JL, Heuchel R, Itoh S, Kawabata M, Heldin NE, Heldin CH, ten Dijke P. Identification of Smad7, a TGFbeta-inducible antagonist of TGF-beta signalling. *Nature* 1997; 389:631–635.

24. Keeton MR, Curriden SA, van Zonneveld AJ, Loskutoff DJ. Identification of regulatory sequences in the type 1 plasminogen activator inhibitor gene responsive to transforming growth factor beta. *J Biol Chem* 1991; 66:23,048–23,052.

25. Wrana JL, Attisano L, C:arcamo J, Zentella A, Doody J, Laiho M, Wang XF, Massague J. TGF beta signals through a heteromeric protein kinase receptor complex. *Cell* 1992; 71:1003–1014.

26. Feng XH, Filvaroff EH, Derynck R. Transforming growth factor-beta (TGF-beta)-induced down-regulation of cyclin A expression requires a functional TGF-beta receptor complex. Characterization of chimeric and truncated type I and type II receptors. *J Biol Chem* 1995; 270:24,237–24,245.

27. Shibuya H, Yamaguchi K, Shirakabe K, Tonegawa A, Gotoh Y, Ueno N, Irie K, Nishida E, Matsumoto K. TAB1: An activator of the TAK1 MAPKKK in TGF-beta signal transduction. *Science* 1996; 272:1179–1182.

28. Slack JM. Inducing factors in *Xenopus* early embryos. *Curr Biol* 1994; 4:116–126.

29. Baker JC, Harland RM. A novel mesoderm inducer, Madr2, functions in the activin signal transduction pathway. *Genes Dev* 1996; 10:1880–1889.

30. Nakao A, Roijer E, Imamura T, Souchelnytskyi S, Stenman G, Heldin CH, ten Dijke P. Identification of Smad2, a human Mad-related protein in the transforming growth factor beta signaling pathway. *J Biol Chem* 1997; 272:2896–2900.

31. Nakao A, Imamura T, Souchelnytskyi S, Kawabata M, Ishisaki A, Oeda E, Tamaki K, Hanai J, Heldin CH, Miyazono K, ten Dijke P. TGF-beta receptor-mediated signalling through Smad2, Smad3 and Smad4. *EMBO J* 1997; 16:5353–5362.

32. Eppert K, Scherer SW, Ozcelik H, Pirone R, Hoodless P, Kim H, Tsui LC, Bapat B, Gallinger S, Andrulis IL, Thomsen GH, Wrana JL, Attisano L. MADR2 maps to 18q21 and encodes a TGFbeta-regulated MAD-related protein that is functionally mutated in colorectal carcinoma. *Cell* 1996; 86:543–552.

33. Macias-Silva M, Abdollah S, Hoodless PA, Pirone R, Attisano L, Wrana JL. MADR2 is a substrate of the TGFbeta receptor and its phosphorylation is required for nuclear accumulation and signaling. *Cell* 1996; 87:1215–1224.

34. Hoodless PA, Haerry T, Abdollah S, Stapleton M, O'Connor MB, Attisano L, Wrana JL. MADR1, a MAD-related protein that functions in BMP2 signaling pathways. *Cell* 1996; 85:489–500.

35. Liu F, Hata A, Baker JC, Doody J, Carcamo J, Harland RM, Massague J. A human Mad protein acting as a BMP-regulated transcriptional activator. *Nature* 1996; 381:620–623.

36. Lechleider RJ, de Caestecker MP, Dehejia A, Polymeropoulos MH, Roberts AB. Serine phosphorylation, chromosomal localization, and transforming growth factor-beta signal transduction by human bsp-1. *J Biol Chem* 1996; 271:17,617–17,620.

37. Yingling JM, Das P, Savage C, Zhang M, Padgett RW, Wang XF. Mammalian dwarfins are phosphorylated in response to transforming growth factor beta and are implicated in control of cell growth. *Proc Natl Acad Sci USA* 1996; 93:8940–8944.

38. Suzuki A, Chang C, Yingling JM, Wang XF, Hemmati-Brivanlou A. Smad5 induces ventral fates in *Xenopus* embryo. *Dev Biol* 1997; 184:402–405.

39. Nishimura R, Kato Y, Chen D, Harris SE, Mundy GR, Yoneda T. Smad5 and DPC4 are

key molecules in mediating BMP-2-induced osteoblastic differentiation of the pluripotent mesenchymal precursor cell line C2C12. *J Biol Chem* 1998; 273:1872–1879.

40. Chen Y, Bhushan A, Vale W. Smad8 mediates the signaling of the receptor serine kinase. *Proc Natl Acad Sci USA* 1997; 4:12,938–12,943.

41. Watanabe TK, Suzuki M, Omori Y, Hishigaki H, Horie M, Kanemoto N, Fujiwara T, Nakamura Y, Takahashi E. Cloning and characterization of a novel member of the human Mad gene family (MADH6). *Genomics* 1997; 42:446–451.

42. Kretzschmar M, Liu F, Hata A, Doody J, Massagué J. The TGF-beta family mediator Smad1 is phosphorylated directly and activated functionally by the BMP receptor kinase. *Genes Dev* 1997; 11:984–995.

43. Shi Y, Hata A, Lo RS, Massague J, Pavletich NP. A structural basis for mutational inactivation of the tumour suppressor Smad4. *Nature* 1997; 388:87–93.

44. Lo RS, Chen Y-G, Shi Y, Pavletich NP, Massagué J. The L3 loop: A structural motif determining specific interactions between SMAD proteins and TGF-β receptors. *EMBO J*, 1998; 17:996–1005.

45. Wu RY, Zhang Y, Feng XH, Derynck R. Heteromeric and homomeric interactions correlate with signaling activity and functional cooperativity of Smad3 and Smad4/DPC4. *Mol Cell Biol* 1997; 17:2521–2528.

46. Hata A, Lo RS, Wotton D, Lagna G, Massagué J. Mutations increasing autoinhibition inactivate tumour suppressors Smad2 and Smad4. *Nature* 1997; 388:82–87.

47. de Caestecker MP, Hemmati P, Larisch-Bloch S, Ajmera R, Roberts AB, Lechleider RJ. Characterization of functional domains within Smad4/DPC4. *J Biol Chem* 1997; 272: 13,690–13,696.

48. Hahn SA, Schutte M, Hoque AT, Moskaluk CA, da Costa LT, Rozenblum E, Weinstein CL, Fischer A, Yeo CJ, Hruban RH, Kern SE. DPC4, a candidate tumor suppressor gene at human chromosome 18q21.1. *Science* 1996; 271:350–353.

49. Candia AF, Watabe T, Hawley SH, Onichtchouk D, Zhang Y, Derynck R, Niehrs C, Cho KW. Cellular interpretation of multiple TGF-beta signals: Intracellular antagonism between activin/BVg1 and BMP-2/4 signaling mediated by Smads. *Development* 1997; 124:4467–4480.

50. Zhang Y, Feng X, We R, Derynck R. Receptor-associated Mad homologues synergize as effectors of the TGF-beta response. *Nature* 1996; 383:168–172.

51. Zhang Y, Musci T, Derynck R. The tumor suppressor Smad4/DPC 4 as a central mediator of Smad function. *Curr Biol* 1997; 7:270–276.

52. Sirard C, de la Pompa JL, Elia A, Itie A, Mirtsos C, Cheung A, Hahn S, Wakeham A, Schwartz L, Kern SE, Rossant J, Mak TW. The tumor suppressor gene Smad4/Dpc4 is required for gastrulation and later for anterior development of the mouse embryo. *Genes Dev* 1998; 12:107–119.

53. Nakayama T., Snyder M., Grewal S., Tsuneizumi K., Tabata T., Christian J. *Xenopus* Smad8 acts downstream of BMP-4 to modulate its activity during vertebrate embryonic patterning. *Development* 1998; 125:857–867.

54. Pawson T, Scott JD. Signaling through scaffold, anchoring, and adaptor proteins. *Science* 1997; 278:2075–2080.

55. Tsuneizumi K, Nakayama T, Kamoshida Y, Kornberg TB, Christian JL, Tabata T. Daughters against dpp modulates dpp organizing activity in *Drosophila* wing development. *Nature* 1997; 389:627–631.

56. Hata A, Lagna G, Massague J, Hemmati-Brivanlou A. Smad6 inhibits BMP/Smad1 signaling by specifically competing with the smad4 tumor suppressor. *Genes Dev* 1998; 12:186–197.

57. Darnell JE Jr. STATs and gene regulation. *Science* 1997; 277:1630–1635.

58. Roberts AB. Molecular and cell biology of TGF-β. *Miner Electrolyte Metab* 1998; 24:111–119.

59. Huang HC, Murtaugh LC, Vize PD, Whitman M. Identification of a potential regulator of

early transcriptional responses to mesoderm inducers in the frog embryo. *EMBO J* 1995; 14:5965–5973.

60. Chen X, Rubock MJ, Whitman M. A transcriptional partner for MAD proteins in TGF-beta signalling [published erratum appears in *Nature* 1996; 19–26; 384(6610):648]. *Nature* 383:691–696.

61. Howell M, Hill CS. XSmad2 directly activates the activin-inducible, dorsal mesoderm gene XFKH1 in *Xenopus* embryos. *EMBO J* 1997; 16:7411–7421.

62. Kim J, Johnson K, Chen HJ, Carroll S, Laughon A. *Drosophila* Mad binds to DNA and directly mediates activation of vestigial by Decapentaplegic. *Nature* 1997; 388:304–308.

63. Yingling JM, Datto MB, Wong C, Frederick JP, Liberati NT, Wang XF. Tumor suppressor Smad4 is a transforming growth factor beta-inducible DNA binding protein. *Mol Cell Biol* 1997; 17:7019–7028.

64. Roberts AB, Anzano MA, Wakefield LM, Roche NS, Stern DF, Sporn MB. Type beta transforming growth factor: A bifunctional regulator of cellular growth. *Proc Natl Acad Sci USA* 1985; 82:119–123.

65. Kretzschmar M, Doody J, Massagué J. Opposing BMP and EGF signalling pathways converge on the TGF-beta family mediator Smad1. *Nature* 1997; 389:618–622.

66. de Caestecker MP, Parks WT, Frank CS, Castagnino P, Bottaro DP, Roberts AB, Lechleider RS. Smad2 transduces common signals from receptor serine–threonine and tyrosine kinases. *Genes Dev* 1998; 12:1587–1592.

4

The Wnt Signal Transduction Pathway

Grant D. Barish, BS and Bart O. Williams, PhD

1. GENERAL OVERVIEW

Wnt signaling plays a central role in the development of many phylogenetically diverse organisms including *Drosophila*, *Caenorhabditis elegans*, *Xenopus*, and higher vertebrates. In addition, genetic alterations of components in the pathway are associated with tumorigenesis in mice and humans, particularly melanomas and carcinomas of the breast and colon. This chapter reviews the characteristics of individual components of the pathway and discusses some of its unresolved issues.

In contrast to many of the signaling pathways described elsewhere in this volume, the mechanisms underlying Wnt signal transduction involve no known tyrosine kinases, SH2- or SH3-containing proteins, kinase cascades, or positively acting phosphorylation events. Instead, other types of regulation are involved. These include the inactivation of a constituitively active serine/threonine protein kinase, glycogen synthase kinase 3 (GSK-3), and the regulation of ubiquitin-dependent proteolysis. A schematic diagram of the Wnt signaling pathway is shown in Fig. 1 and a brief overview is presented in the following discussion.

The cysteine-rich glycoprotein Wnt is secreted and binds to the cell surface, initiating a signal. The reception of this signal is mediated, at least in part, by a member of the Frizzled family of seven transmembrane spanning receptors. The mechanisms underlying Wnt-induced activation of Frizzled are unclear but lead to the activation of Dishevelled, a cytosolic phosphoprotein of unknown function. Dishevelled then initiates poorly characterized cellular events that result in the downregulation of GSK-3 kinase activity. Normally, the constitutive kinase activity of GSK-3 results in the phosphorylation and subsequent ubiquitin-dependent degradation of β-catenin. Inhibition of GSK-3 leads to increased concentrations of β-catenin (and, in some cases, plakoglobin) in the cytosol and nucleus, allowing them to interact physically with the Tcf/Lef class of DNA binding proteins. These heterodimeric complexes modulate transcriptional activity of mostly unidentified target gene promoters. In addition to the components described above, other proteins regulate the activity of the pathway at several levels. Frizzled-related proteins (FRPs) or FRZBs, as well as other secreted inhibitors, such as Dickkopf, regulate signaling at the level of the Wnt/Frizzled interaction, whereas Axin, Conductin,

From: Signaling Networks and Cell Cycle Control: The Molecular Basis of Cancer and Other Diseases
Edited by: J. S. Gutkind © Humana Press Inc., Totowa, NJ

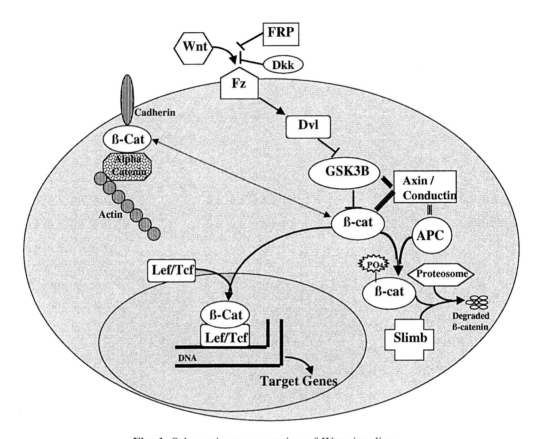

Fig. 1. Schematic representation of Wnt signaling.

Slimb/h-βTrCP, and APC, the product of the adenomatous polyposis coli tumor suppressor gene, control the pathway at the level of GSK-3 and β-catenin.

2. HISTORICAL BACKGROUND

The first Wnt gene was cloned in 1982 as a gene whose expression was upregulated in mouse mammary tumor virus (MMTV) induced breast tumors *(1)*. Since the gene was found next to newly integrated MMTV proviruses in the mouse genome, it was originally named *int-1*. Further analysis showed the locus encoded a secreted protein *(2–4)*. Work on *int-1* proceeded slowly, mainly because of the difficulty in obtaining purified, biologically active protein with which biochemical studies could be performed. An important advance came in 1987 with the report that the *Drosophila wingless (wg)* gene was a conserved homolog of the mouse *int-1* gene *(5)*. In fact, the phenotypes of *wg* mutants had been studied for over a decade *(6)*. The combination of the names *int-1* and *wg* led to the renaming of *int-1* as *Wnt-1*, the name used today to denote the first isolated member of the gene family *(7)*.

Because *wg* mutants had a well characterized developmental phenotype, *Drosophila* mutants with similar phenotypes, many of them isolated by Nusslein-Vohlhard and Wieschaus *(8)*, were linked to the Wg pathway. Epistasis experiments allowed the ordering of these components in the pathway. Many of these genes have subsequently

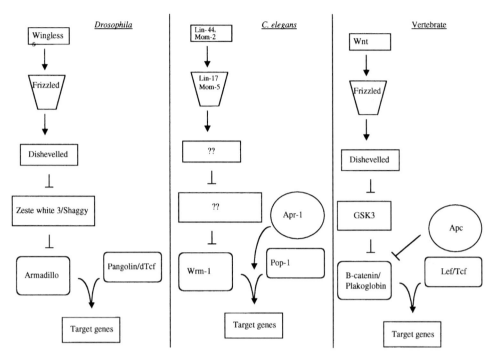

Fig. 2. Evolutionary conservation of the Wnt signaling pathway.

been linked to Wnt signaling in other systems and vertebrate homologs of each have been cloned (Fig. 2).

Several other genes not directly involved in Wg signaling cause similar phenotypes when mutated in *Drosophila*. Many of these genes are components of another signaling pathway, the hedgehog (*hh*) pathway *(9)*. The reason for the similarity in phenotypic manifestation is that, during segment development in *Drosophila*, *hh* and *wg* are necessary for the maintenance of each other's expression *(10)*. This coordinated relationship occurs in other systems as well, such as vertebrate limb development *(11,12)*.

3. ASSAYS OF WNT SIGNALING FUNCTION

Numerous assays are used to study the Wnt signaling pathway. These can be roughly grouped into three categories: genetic, phenotypic, and biochemical/cell biological.

3.1. Genetic Assays

As described above, the genetic analysis of *Drosophila* embryonic development has played a critical role in identifying and ordering components of the signaling pathway. Recently, genetic analysis of cell fate decisions in *C. elegans* has led to new insights on the roles of components in the pathway *(13–18)* (Fig. 2). Finally, as with almost all areas of biological study, the creation of mouse strains with targeted inactivations of specific genes has generated tremendous information on the physiological roles of these genes (Table 1).

Table 1
Phenotypes of Mouse Knockouts of Wnt Pathway Components

Gene	Phenotype	References
Wnt-1	Failure of midbrain structures to develop, perinatal death	*(214, 215)*
Wnt-1 (Swaying) Spontaneous frameshift mutation	Defects in cerebellar structure and function	*(216)*
Wnt-2	Defects in placental development, late gestational or perinatal death	*(217)*
Wnt-3A	Failure to form caudal somites and a tailbud, disrupted notochord; death at embryonic d 10	*(218)*
Wnt-3A (Vestigial tail)	Shortening of tail	*(219)*
Wnt-4	Failure to form kidney tubules; neonatal lethality	*(220)*
Wnt-7A	Improper limb formation; dorsoventral and anteroposterior transformations of limb fate; viable but sterile	*(221)*
Dvl-1	Viable and fertile; social interaction, and sensorimotor abnormalities	*(222)*
β-*Catenin*	Early embryonic death	*(159)*
Plakoglobin	Defects in heart and skin; death from midgestation until perinatally because of cardiac problems	*(161, 162)*
Axin (Spontaneous inactivating mutations)	Death at embryonic days 8–10; wide spectrum of developmental defects including cardiac malformations, neuroectodermal abnormalities, asymmetric vertebral fusions, and embryonic axis duplications	*(145)*
APC (Knockouts and chemically induced point mutation)	Early embryonic death; heterozygotes develop hundreds of intestinal polyps	*(223–226)*
LEF-1	Failure to form teeth, hair, or mammary glands; perinatal death	*(188)*
Tcf-1	Defects in T-cell maturation; otherwise viable and fertile	*(187)*

[a]All listed mouse models are targeted gene disruptions unless noted. In addition, all phenotypes listed are associated with homozygosity for the mutation unless noted.

3.2. Phenotypic Assays

Misexpression of components in the signaling pathway can induce profound phenotypic effects. For example, induction of a secondary axis in the developing *Xenopus* embryo is commonly used to examine Wnt signaling. McMahon and Moon *(19)* showed in 1988 that injection of Wnt-1 mRNA into the ventral side of a two- or four-cell *Xenopus* embryo leads to the formation of a complete secondary body axis. Injections of mRNA from other activating components in the pathway or dominant negative GSK-3 lead to similar body axis induction.

Another assay for testing Wnt function is based on the observation that the C57MG mammary gland cell line is morphologically transformed upon introduction of numerous Wnt genes *(20)*. This phenotypic effect has been used for structure/function analysis of Wnt genes as well as for comparisons of signaling among Wnt family members.

3.3. Biochemical/Cell Biological Assays

A common method for studying Wnt signaling is the measurement of armadillo or β-catenin protein levels, as the concentration of these proteins is increased by Wnt/Wg *(21–23)*. As described below, one immediate outcome of Wnt signaling is the inhibition of the serine/threonine kinase activity of GSK-3 *(24)*. Because this kinase activity is necessary for the phosphorylation and subsequent targeting of β-catenin for degradation, inhibition of GSK-3 causes β-catenin protein to accumulate in the cytosol *(24)*. Consequently, accumulation of armadillo or β-catenin is often used to measure the signaling activity of upstream components of the Wnt pathway.

Finally, the identification of LEF/TCF DNA binding proteins as mediators of Wnt signaling has permitted the use of reporter gene constructs with LEF/TCF binding sites to measure Wnt signaling activity.

4. SUMMARIES OF COMPONENTS

4.1. Wnt

Numerous Wnt genes have been identified since the discovery of the *int-1/Wnt-1* gene in 1982. For example, multiple Wnt genes have been found in mice (16 genes), humans *(13)*, *Xenopus (15)*, zebrafish *(9)*, *Drosophila* (four), and *C. elegans* (five) *(25)*. In fact, Wnt gene family members are found in all metazoans examined *(26)*. Most encode protein products with 350–400 amino acids *(25)*. All Wnt proteins contain several putative N-linked glycosylation sites with 22–24 cysteine residues arranged in a spatially conserved pattern. These cysteines are among a total of approximately 100 conserved amino acids distributed evenly throughout the proteins *(25)*. More detailed, continuously updated information on Wnt genes is accessible on the World Wide Web Wnt Window (WWWWW). This site is maintained by Roel Nusse and colleagues and can be accessed at the following URL: http://www.stanford.edu/~rnusse/wntwindow .html.

Analysis of Wnt proteins is technically challenging because of the difficulty in preparing purified, biologically active forms. As most tissue culture cells do not express large amounts of endogenous Wnt proteins *(27)*, biochemical characterization has used gene overexpression in cell culture. Within this context, large proportions of the protein are associated with the Golgi network *(2,4,28)*. Consistent with this, the endoplasmic reticulum (ER)-based chaperonin BiP physically interacts with Wnt-1 *(29)*. The small amount of secreted Wnt is tightly associated with components of the extracellular matrix. In fact, solubilization of the extracellular matrix, the addition of soluble heparin, or the presence of the polyanion suranim is usually necessary to recover detectable amounts of secreted protein *(3,4)*. However, there have been some reports of soluble, artially purified Wnts retaining biological activity *(30–32)*. This association of Wnts

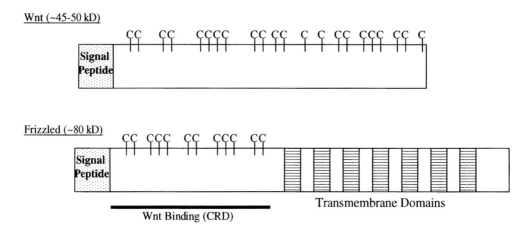

Fig. 3. Structural and functional domains of Wnt and Frizzled. The positions of cysteine residues are signified by the letter C. (Adapted from Dale, 1998, and Cadigan and Nusse, 1997.)

with the extracellular matrix is consistent with both genetic and biochemical studies showing that proteoglycans are necessary for efficient Wnt/Wg signaling *(33–37)*.

The presence of multiple Wnt genes suggests a great deal of specificity in expression and function (Fig. 3). Indeed, targeted disruptions (knockouts) of several Wnts reveal very specific phenotypic effects (Table 1). A related question is whether all Wnts signal in the same way. To test this, several laboratories introduced Wnt genes into C57MG cells and examined whether they had equivalent abilities to induce morphological transformation. Whereas the Wnt genes commonly referred to as the Wnt-1 class (including Wnt-1, Wnt-2, Wnt-3A, and Wnt-8) alter the morphology of C57MG cells, the expression of a second group, commonly referred to as the Wnt-5A class (including Wnt-5A, Wnt-4, and Wnt-11) does not *(20,28,38,39)*. Concordant with this, β-catenin protein levels are high in C57MG cells expressing Wnt-1 class members and low in those transfected with Wnt-5A family members *(40)*. Furthermore, Wnt-1 class members, but not those of the Wnt-5A group, induce an ectopic axis in *Xenopus (19,41–49)*. One interpretation is that the two groups of Wnt genes signal via different or perhaps antagonistic mechanisms. In support of this idea, some aspects of Wnt-1 signaling in *Xenopus* can be antagonized by coexpression with members of the Wnt-5A class *(50)*. Further studies in *Xenopus* have shown that Wnt-5A, but not Wnt-8, can induce changes in intracellular calcium levels *(51)*.

An alternative explanation for these differences is that the receptors necessary for Wnt-5A class signaling are not present in either the *Xenopus* or C57MG systems. Support for this model stems from other work in *Xenopus*. Injection of Wnt-5A, which alone has no effect, can induce a secondary axis when injected in combination with human Frizzled-5 mRNA *(52)*.

4.2. Frizzled

Identifying a cellular receptor for Wnt/Wg proteins proved technically challenging, mainly because of the difficulty in obtaining biologically active, purified Wnt proteins. In addition, no gene encoding a cell surface protein was identified during genetic screens for Wg pathway members in *Drosophila*. An important advance came in 1994, when methods to obtain conditioned media enriched for the *Drosophila* wingless (Wg) protein were reported *(32)*. This facilitated binding studies which, together with the use of the Armadillo stabilization assay in *Drosophila* cell lines, identified Frizzleds as putative Wnt receptors *(53)*.

The first Frizzled gene (*Dfz1* in *Drosophila*) was cloned in 1987 based on mutants in this gene which display defects in tissue polarity of the wing *(54)*. Normally, the hairs on the surface of the *Drosophila* wing point in the same direction, but in wing regions mutant for this gene, the pattern of wing hair is disorganized *(55)*. Additional work on *Dfz1* mutants demonstrated a defect in the chiral pattern of ommatidia in the eye *(56,57)*. Together, the wing hair and eye patterns in *Dfz1* mutants are referred to as planar or tissue polarity phenotypes *(58)*. Although *Dfz1* mutants were extensively characterized for planar polarity phenotypes, no evidence for their involvement in Wg signaling was observed.

A potential role for Frizzled genes in Wg signaling was further examined when several mammalian homologs and another family member in *Drosophila* (*Dfz2*) were identified *(53,59–63)*. However, since no *Dfz2* mutants are known, other assays to test its potential role in Wg signaling were used. Transfection of Frizzled genes into several cell lines permits Wg binding *(53)*. In addition, expression of Dfz2 in a *Drosophila* cell line normally unresponsive to added Wg confers a Wg-dependent stabilization of the armadillo protein *(53)*. Furthermore, expression of a rat Frizzled gene (*Rfz1*) in *Xenopus* induces the relocation of Xwnt-8 from the endoplasmic reticulum to the plasma membrane *(64)*. It is unclear whether Frizzled mediates these interactions by a direct or indirect association with Wg.

Genetic evidence for the involvement of Frizzled in Wnt signal transduction comes from studies in *C. elegans*. Mutations in a worm Frizzled homolog (*lin-17*) produce phenotypes related to those associated with mutations in a Wnt homolog (*lin-44*) *(13,14,65)*. In addition, mutations in another *C. elegans* Frizzled gene, *mom-5*, cause effects similar to those induced by mutations in *mom-2*, a Wnt family member *(17,18)*.

Whereas two Frizzled genes have been identified in *Drosophila* and *C. elegans*, at least eight are present in vertebrates *(53,59–63)*. All encode seven transmembrane spanning proteins and share extensive homology throughout their coding regions. The N-terminus, specifically the first extracellular domain, contains a cysteine-rich domain (CRD) with a spatially conserved pattern of cysteine residues. The CRD is sufficient for mediating the association of Wg protein with cells expressing Frizzled molecules *(53)*.

Seven-transmembrane spanning proteins typically signal via the activation of hetero-trimeric G-proteins *(66)*. Frizzleds are seven-transmembrane spanning proteins, it is therefore tempting to speculate that they signal through such a mechanism. Support for this model comes from studies in zebrafish *(67)*. In early zebrafish embryos, the injection of mRNA from rat Frizzled 2 *(Rfz2)* increases in intracellular calcium. This can be blocked by co-injection of either inositol monophosphatase inhibitors, pertussis toxin, α-transducin, or GDP-βS. This suggests that Rfz2 signals are transduced via heterotrimeric G-protein βγ subunits via the phosphatidylinositol pathway.

The final three residues of many Frizzled proteins are serine or threonine, followed by any amino acid and then by valine or isoleucine (Ser/Thr-Xxx-Val/Ile). This sequence is a strong consensus binding site for some PDZ domains *(68)*. The Dishevelled protein contains a PDZ domain; however, the Dishevelled PDZ domain belongs to a subclass of PDZ domains that may not bind to Ser/Thr-Xxx-Val/Ile *(69–71)*. Furthermore, deletion of the C-terminus of *lin-17* (a Frizzled homolog in *C. elegans*) to facilitate the fusion of a green fluorescence protein tag shows that it is not required for normal function *(65)*. Further studies will no doubt demonstrate whether PDZ-containing proteins (or other proteins) associate with the carboxyl terminus of Frizzleds.

The preferences of individual Wnts for binding to different Frizzleds are largely unknown. Wg protein has been shown to bind to cells transfected with some, but not all, Frizzled genes. Another example of Wnt/Frizzled specificity comes from work in *Xenopus,* where coinjection of mRNA from Wnt-5A and Frizzled 5 (neither of which induces a secondary axis on their own) is sufficient to induce a secondary axis *(52)*. Co-injection of several other Frizzled mRNAs with Wnt-5A does not have the same effect. Other work implies specificity between Wnt-5A and rat Frizzled-2 *(67)*. The increased intracellular calcium levels seen in zebrafish embryos injected with rat Frizzled 2 can be enhanced by co-injection with Wnt-5A. Obviously, the determination of binding specificities between Wnt and Frizzled components would be helpful in these considerations. Once again, however, the difficulty in obtaining pure, biologically active preparations of Wnt proteins precludes these experiments.

4.3. Frzbs/FRPs and Other Secreted Wnt Antagonists

Several laboratories recently identified genes encoding FRPs or FRZBs. These genes encode secreted proteins highly homologous to the first extracellular domain of Frizzleds. At least four FRPs are present in vertebrates and have been reported under various names *(72–80)*.

FRPs contain a CRD related to the CRD domain found in Frizzleds. In addition, FRPs share a domain homologous to one found in netrins *(25)*, a family of proteins involved in neural cell adhesion *(81)*. The CRD of FRP proteins is also present in at least two other otherwise unrelated proteins: carboxypeptidase Z *(82)* and several isoforms of collagen XVIII *(83)*. The function of the CRD is unclear, but it may bind and inhibit Wnts. Consistent with this, injection of FRP mRNAs can inhibit Wnt-induced axis duplication in *Xenopus (72–80)*. Whether this inhibition is mediated via direct Wnt/FRP interactions is the subject of disagreement.

Recently, another family of secreted Wnt antagonists, *Dickkopfs,* or *Dkks,* has been identified *(84)*. At least three *Dkk* genes are present in vertebrates. They are unrelated to any other known genes but do have two CRDs otherwise structurally unrelated to those found in Frizzleds and FRPSs. Dkks may play key roles during embryonic axis specification as injection of Dkk mRNA into the ventral side of *Xenopus* embryos is sufficient to induce a second head *(84)*.

4.4. Dishevelled

Like many components of the Wnt/Wg signaling pathway, Dishevelled was first studied in *Drosophila*. Mutants of *Drosophila Dishevelled* (*Dsh*) have segment polarity phenotypes similar to *wg* mutants *(85–88)*. Injection of Dishevelled mRNA into the ventral side of *Xenopus* embryos induces a complete secondary axis. In addition to its role in Wg signaling, Dishevelled is also involved in the establishment of planar polarity by genetically interacting with *Dfz1 (89)*. Furthermore, Dishevelled physically interacts

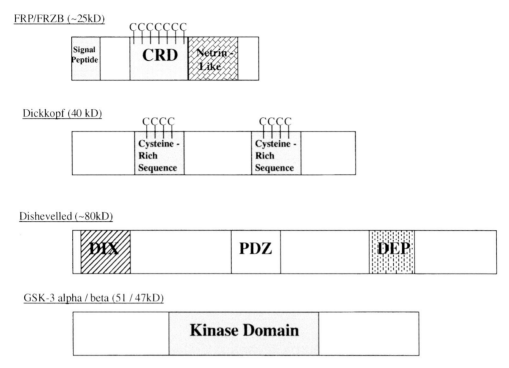

Fig. 4. Schematic representation of structural domains in FRP/FRZB, Dickkopf, Dishevelled, and GSK-3 proteins. Please refer to text for details. Positions of functionally important cysteine residues are noted by a C.

with the Notch protein *(90)*, which could explain the genetic interaction between the Wg and Notch pathways in *Drosophila (91–93)*.

The mechanisms underlying Dishevelled's activation and subsequent signaling are unknown. Phosphorylation of Dishevelled correlates with Wg activity *(94)*, but it is not sufficient to transduce Wnt signals *(95)*. One candidate for a Dishevelled kinase is casein kinase II *(95)*, but whether this is physiologically relevant is unknown.

One Dishevelled gene is present in *Drosophila*, and three highly related genes are present in vertebrates *(96–103)*. Sequence comparisons show three regions of high sequence homology among family members (Fig. 4). The PDZ domain in the central part of the protein is the best characterized and is required for Dishevelled function. Injection of Dishevelled mRNA lacking this domain not only fails to induce a secondary axis in *Xenopus* embryos, but it prevents axis duplication when coinjected with mRNAs derived from wild type Dishevelled or Wnt genes, which normally signal in this system *(104)*.

PDZ domains are 80–90 amino acid motifs found in many proteins *(68)*. Some of these domains bind to the Ser/Thr-Xxx-Val/Ile (where Xxx is any amino acid) sequences at or near the C-terminus of proteins *(68)*. In addition, PDZ domains can also mediate heterotypic interactions with PDZ domains in other proteins. It has been suggested that the PDZ domain in Dishevelled cannot bind to the canonical carboxyl terminal Ser/Thr-Xxx-Val/Ile motif found in many Frizzled proteins *(69–71)*; however, apart from casein kinase II and Notch, no Dishevelled-interacting proteins have been reported.

A second conserved domain in Dishevelled is also present in axin and conductin *(105,106)*, other proteins implicated in Wnt signaling. Thus, this domain is referred to as the DIX (Dishevelled and axin) domain *(25)*. Its function is unknown, but it may be responsible for specification of subcellular localization (J. Axelrod, personal communication).

The third shared region of homology is found near the carboxyl terminus of Dishevelleds and is known as the DEP domain *(107)*. It is found in a number of proteins, many of which are associated with G-protein signaling. This domain is dispensable for Wg signaling, but it is required to specify planar polarity (J. Axelrod, personal communication). This finding suggests that Dishevelled and, by extension, Frizzled, transduce separable signals for planar polarity and Wg signaling. In support of this, other studies show that specification of planar polarity in the *Drosophila* ommatidia is dependent on the normal function of *RhoA* and *basket* (the *Drosophila* homolog of Jun kinase) *(108)*. These genes have no known role in Wg signaling. Consistent with the idea of a separate planar polarity signaling pathway, mutations in the Wg signaling components *zeste-white 3* (the *Drosophila* version of GSK-3) and *armadillo* have no affect on planar polarity in the wing *(108)*.

4.5. GSK-3

GSK-3 is a serine/threonine protein kinase first identified on the basis of its ability to phosphorylate and inactivate glycogen synthase *(109)*. Subsequent analysis revealed that highly homologous isoforms of this kinase, GSK-3α (51 kDa) and GSK-3β (47 kDa), are encoded by two genes in vertebrates *(109)*. GSK-3 is very conserved phylogenetically with highly related genes present in *Drosophila (110,111)*, *Dictyostelium (112)*, *Saccharomyces cerevisiae (113,114)*, and *Arabidopsis (115)*.

Mutations in the *Drosophila* homolog of GSK-3 (*zeste white 3* or *shaggy*) cause phenotypes similar to those induced by ectopic expression of wingless *(110,111)*. This suggests that Wg acts by either directly inhibiting GSK-3 or somehow overcoming its activity. Consistent with this, co-injection of GSK-3α or GSK-3β mRNA blocks axis induction normally caused by injection of Dishevelled or Wnt-1 class mRNAs and ventral injection of mRNAs encoding putative dominant negative forms of GSK-3 causes axis duplication *(116–118)*.

Recent work with mouse 10T1/2 fibroblasts shows that addition of Wg-conditioned media can reduce GSK-3 kinase activity by one-half *(24,119)*. This suggests Wnt/Wg signaling directly inhibits GSK-3 kinase activity. Inhibitors of protein kinase C (PKC) can block the Wg-induced inhibition of GSK-3, suggesting that PKC mediates the Wnt/Wg-induced inhibition of GSK-3 activity *(119)*. Furthermore, some isoforms of PKC can phosphorylate GSK-3 and inhibit its activity in vitro *(120)*. Whether all Wnts will induce this reduction in GSK-3 activity remains unknown. In fact, recent work on GSK-3 regulation in *Dictyostelium* suggests that activation of different upstream seven transmembrane receptors may have opposing effects on GSK-3 activity *(121)*. This is an important consideration, in light of the possibility that the Wnt-1 and Wnt-5A classes may signal via different downstream mechanisms *(50)*.

GSK-3 kinase activity is also inhibited by signaling pathways that respond to insulin, insulin-like growth factor (IGF-1), and epidermal growth factor (EGF) *(24,119)*. Regulation of GSK-3 by these factors is pharmacologically distinct from that induced by Wg and mediated by protein kinase B/Akt or rsk-90 *(24,122)*. The monovalent cation lithium is also a potent inhibitor of GSK-3 kinase activity *(123,124)* and can induce a secondary axis in the *Xenopus* system *(125)*.

GSK-3 has many potential protein substrates including c-Jun, c-Myb, c-Myc, Tau, the eukaryotic initiation factor 2B, CREB, the regulatory subunit of cAMP-dependent kinase (RII), NFAT, and armadillo/β-catenin *(126)*. All these proteins contain at least one consensus site for GSK-3 phosphorylation in which the target serine or threonine residue is followed by any three amino acids followed by another serine or threonine that is usually prephosphorylated *(109)*. Both protein kinase A and casein kinase II are candidates to mediate this priming phosphorylation reaction *(109)*.

In the absence of Wnt ligands GSK-3 suppresses the Wnt pathway via its constituitive activity on β-catenin (and perhaps plakoglobin), targeting them for degradation by phosphorylation *(23,110)*. When Wnt is present, GSK-3 kinase activity is inhibited and β-catenin protein is stabilized in the cytoplasm *(23,110)*. Axin and Conductin are adapter proteins that bind to GSK-3, β-catenin, and APC *(106,127–129)*. This bridging of components may allow GSK-3 to come into close proximity with β-catenin, facilitating its phosphorylation.

4.6. APC

The *adenomatous polyposis coli (APC)* gene was originally identified as the tumor suppressor gene that is inactivated in humans with familial adenomatous polyposis (FAP) syndrome *(130,131)*. Such individuals develop hundreds to thousands of benign colorectal polyps, of which a small number progress to colorectal adenocarcinoma. FAP patients inherit one defective copy of the *APC* gene and subsequently lose their wild-type copy before polyp development (reviewed in ref. *132*).

Approximately 85% of all colorectal tumors have mutations in *APC (132)*. Approximately one-half of the remaining 15% contain mutations in β-catenin that result in the stabilization of β-catenin protein *(133)*. Such mutations are never observed in *APC*-deficient tumors. This is consistent with the idea that APC and β-catenin function in the same pathway involved in suppressing colorectal tumor growth. Functional support for this came from studies of *APC*-deficient colon tumor cell lines. These cell lines contain elevated levels of β-catenin protein and have high activity from LEF/TCF responsive reporter genes, both of which are dramatically reduced upon introduction of a wild-type *APC* gene *(134,135)*.

The APC gene encodes a large, 310-kDa protein containing numerous functionally defined domains (Fig. 5) (reviewed in *136*). Seven armadillo repeats, which are thought to function in mediating protein–protein interactions *(137)* are found near the N-terminus. Following this, several repeated homology regions shown to be necessary for binding to β-catenin or plakoglobin, or both, are present *(136)*. Interspersed within the putative β-catenin binding repeats are SAMP repeats (named for the central Ser-Ala-Met-Pro motif in each repeat). SAMP repeats mediate the interactions of APC with the RGS domain of conductin, and perhaps axin *(106)*. In addition, EB1 *(138)*, the human homolog of the *Drosophila* discs large protein (hDLG) *(139)*, and microtubules *(140,141)* bind to the C-terminus of APC.

The function of APC and its relationship to Wnt signaling has been genetically examined in several systems (Fig. 2). In *C. elegans* (Fig. 2), inactivation of an *APC*

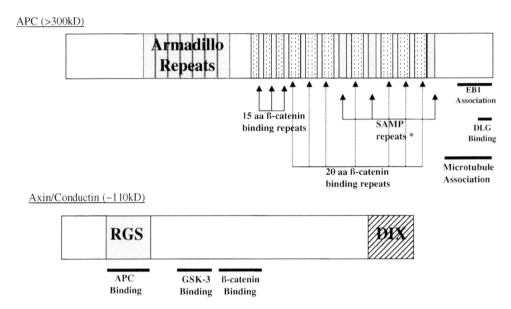

Fig. 5. Functionally important domains identified in APC and Axin/Conductin. Please consult text for details.

homolog *(Apr-1)* causes phenotypes similar to those associated with inactivation of a β-catenin homolog *(wrm-1) (17)*. Thus, *Apr-1* in the worm positively transduces either Wnt signals or those emanating from a parallel pathway. This is consistent with *Xenopus* studies in which injection of APC mRNA into the ventral side of the embryo causes axis duplication *(142)*. Thus, APC can positively or negatively regulate signaling of B-catenin-dependent signaling pathways depending on context. The reasons underlying these differences are not understood. Further complicating the picture, mutations in the *Drosophila APC (dAPC)* gene have no affect on embryonic patterning *(143)*. However, *dAPC* is still capable of downregulating β-catenin protein levels when introduced into a mammalian cell line *(143)*. Of note, the SAMP repeats found necessary for binding to conductin an axin are present in *C. elegans* and vertebrate *APC*, but absent in *Drosophila (106)*.

4.7. Axin/Conductin

Axin, an intracellular inhibitor of Wnt signaling, was discovered by analysis of the mouse *fused* locus *(105,144)*. Homozygous mouse *fused* mutants, first described during the 1940s, die *in utero* between embryonic days 8 and 10 *(see* ref. *145* and references therein). These mutant embryos exhibit a wide spectrum of developmental defects including cardiac malformations, neuroectodermal abnormalities, asymmetric vertebral fusions, and embryonic axis duplications (Table 1). This latter defect prompted investigation of the gene's role in axis formation. Dorsal injection of mRNA transcribed from the wild type *fused* gene was found to block normal axis formation in *Xenopus (105)*. Thus, the *fused* gene was renamed *axin* for its axis-inhibiting function *(105)*. A yeast two-hybrid screen for β-catenin interaction partners identified an Axin-related gene, known as Conductin (or Axil) *(106,128)*. Conductin is 45% identical to Axin and appears to be functionally analogous.

The involvement of Axin in Wnt signaling has been studied using the *Xenopus* axis induction assay *(105)*. Coinjection of Axin mRNA inhibits axis induction by *Xenopus* Wnt 8, *Xenopus* Dishevelled, and the dominant-negative form of GSK-3 mRNAs *(105)*. Axis induction by β-catenin and Siamois mRNAs, however, is not affected by coinjection with Axin. Conductin acts similarly to Axin in *Xenopus* assays *(146)*. Thus, Axin and Conductin regulate Wnt signaling downstream of *Dishevelled* and upstream of β-catenin.

Biochemical and comparative sequence analysis have identified several functional domains in Axin and Conductin (Fig. 5). A regulator of G-protein signaling (RGS) domain maps to the N-terminus and bears approximately 30% identity to RGS4 *(105)*, a GTPase activating protein for heterotrimeric G-proteins *(147)*. Although not demonstrated to work as a GTPase, the Axin and Conductin RGS domain has clear functional significance and binds to SAMP repeats in the APC protein *(106)*. In *Xenopus*, ventral injection of mRNA encoding Axin that lacks an RGS domain causes axis duplication, changing Axin from an axis inhibitor to an axis inducer, or so-called dominant negative Axin *(105)*. A region in the middle of the Axin and Conductin proteins binds to GSK-3β, and a contiguous region interacts physically with β-catenin *(106,127–129)*. The C-terminus of these proteins contains a DIX domain *(25)*, which has ~40% identity to the N-terminus of *Dishevelled* and unknown functional significance.

The mechanism underlying the inhibitory effect of Axin and Conductin on Wnt signaling is beginning to be understood. As previously described, Axin and Conductin bind several proteins, including APC, GSK-3, and β-catenin. Thus, Axin and Conductin may mediate the formation of multiprotein complexes that spatially approximate GSK-3 and β-catenin. This could promote GSK-3 directed phosphorylation of β-catenin, leading to its degradation. Axin and Conductin may also be phosphorylated by GSK-3, but the significance of this is uncertain, as binding affinities for GSK-3 and β-catenin are unaffected by such modification *(129)*. The significance of the interaction of APC with Axin and Conductin is also unclear, as the expression of Conductin fragments which cannot bind APC still downregulate β-catenin protein levels in wild-type and mutant APC-expressing cell lines *(106)*.

4.8. β-Catenin/Plakoglobin

β-Catenin and plakoglobin (also referred to as γ-catenin) were initially identified as components of the cadherin-based cell–cell adherence junctions *(148–150)*, where they play critical roles in cell-cell contact and cytoskeletal anchorage. Their homology to the *Drosophila* segment polarity gene Armadillo produce additional roles in Wnt signaling, as mutations in Armadillo cause a mutant Wingless-like phenotype *(151,152)*. Furthermore, injection of mRNA from β-catenin or plakoglobin into the ventral side of *Xenopus* embryos induces a secondary axis *(153,154)*.

Like other Wnt pathway components, β-catenin and plakoglobin have been highly conserved during evolution. The *Drosophila* segment polarity gene product Armadillo is functionally analogous and 70% identical to β-catenin, and β-catenin and plakoglobin have 68% sequence identity *(151,152)*. These related proteins share a common structure (Fig. 6). Their N-terminus contains a GSK-3 consensus phosphorylation site, in part

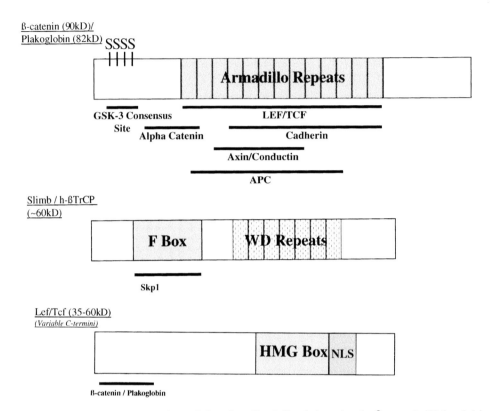

Fig. 6. Schematic representation of functionally defined domains in β-catenin/Plakoglobin, Slimb, and Lef/Tcfs.

composed of some of five serines and a threonine residue that map to this region. The central region of these proteins consists of 12–13 repeats ("armadillo repeats") of a 42-amino acid motif, which function as nonhomotypic protein interaction domains *(137)*. In the case of β-catenin, these mediate interactions with cadherin, Axin, Conductin, APC, LEF/TCFs and α-catenin *(155)*. The armadillo plakoglobin repeats can additionally bind to desmosomal plaque proteins known as desmogleins and desmocollins *(156)*. Although only examined in Armadillo protein, the C-terminus appears to be required for signaling activity, but it is dispensable for function at the adherens junction *(157)*.

In addition to their roles in Wnt/Wg signaling, Armadillo, β-catenin, and plakoglobin are also involved in cellular adhesion. There, they bind to the cytosolic tails of E- and N-cadherins and to α-catenin, indirectly linking cadherins to the actin cytoskeleton *(155)* (*see* Fig. 1). This tethering function is critical in the development and maintenance of tissue architecture. Deletion of the β-catenin binding domain of cadherin causes cell adhesion defects *(149,158)*, and *β-catenin* null mice manifest defects in ectoderm and mesoderm organization *(159)*. Similarly, *Armadillo* null *Drosophila* germ cells have collapsed cytoskeletons and are disconnected from follicle cells *(160)*, demonstrating the importance of Armadillo and related proteins in cytoskeletal anchorage and intercellular adhesion. Plakoglobin can also tether cadherins to the actin cytoskeleton, or it can help to anchor intermediate filaments to desmosomal plaques. *Plakoglobin*-deficient mice manifest critical structural deficits, dying from myocardial instability and ventricular rupture during embryogenesis *(161,162)*.

The nonmembranous fractions of β-catenin and plakoglobin are both involved in Wnt signaling, although research has focused more heavily on β-catenin. For simplicity, β-catenin is presented below, although plakoglobin is thought to signal analogously. In the absence of a Wnt stimulus, GSK-3 constitutively phosphorylates serine and threonine residues in the N-terminus of β-catenin *(22,23)*. Once phosphorylated, β-catenin is ubiquitinated and proteolytically degraded *(163,164)* through a process mediated by Slimb and possibly APC (see sections on Slimb and APC). With Wnt stimulation, GSK-3 activity is downmodulated *(119)*. Unphosphorylated β-catenin then accumulates, and it eventually translocates to the nucleus to signal as a heterodimer with LEF/TCF proteins *(165)*. The strength of the transduced signal correlates with the cytosolic levels of β-catenin.

Mutant forms of β-catenin were recently identified in human colorectal cancers and melanomas *(166–170)*. These mutants have altered or deleted GSK phosphorylation sites and consequently resist degradation. They are thought to drive oncogenesis by increasing β-catenin levels, thereby activating Wnt target genes. By contrast, no plakoglobin mutations have been identified in neoplasms.

β-Catenin signals through its actions in the nucleus. However, it lacks a classic nuclear localization signal. Two models have been proposed to explain its mechanism for nuclear translocation. One model contends that β-catenin binds to LEF/TCFs in the cytoplasm; then, guided by the nuclear localization signal of a LEF/TCF, it translocates to the nucleus. Indirect support for this derives from transfection studies in which the nuclear import of β-catenin is increased by co-expression of LEF/TCF *(146)*. Alternatively, other observations support a nuclear localization signal-independent import model in which β-catenin can bind directly to the nuclear envelope and mediate its own translocation *(171)*.

4.9. β-TrCP/Slimb

Genetic analysis of *Drosophila* adult patterning defects has implicated the *Drosophila slimb* gene in Wnt signaling *(172)*. Specifically, clones of *slimb*-deficient cells have phenotypes similar to those induced by the ectopic expression of Wg. In addition, these cells contain high levels of armadillo protein. This suggests slimb functions upstream of armadillo and is required for its degradation in the absence of Wg signaling. The slimb protein contains two recognizable motifs, an F-box and a series of seven WD (or β-transducin) repeats (Fig. 6). The F-box is found in several other proteins and mediates interactions with Skp1, a component of an E3 ubiquitin conjugating complex *(173,174)*. Thus, it is conceivable that slimb is required in targeting armadillo for ubiquitin-dependent degradation. WD (or β-transducin repeats) are found in many proteins with diverse functions *(175)*. Although the precise function of these repeats in the slimb protein is unknown, they mediate protein–protein interactions in other proteins *(175)*.

Studies of human immunodeficiency virus (HIV) proteins have unexpectedly shed light on the function of *slimb*. During a screen for proteins which could interact with the HIV-1 protein Vpu, a human homolog of *slimb* was isolated *(176)*. Slimb is also highly related to a *Xenopus* protein, β-transducin repeat containing protein (*X-βTrCP*) *(177,178)*, thus, the human gene was named *h-βTrCP*.

Previous work showed that Vpu was involved in the degradation of the human CD4 protein *(179)*. Recent work indicates it induces this degradation by serving as an adapter protein linking CD4 with h-BTrCP *(176)*. This ternary complex then targets CD4 for degradation. Of interest, the presence of two phosphoserine residues separated by three other amino acids is necessary for the binding of h-βTrCP to Vpu *(176)*. As a similar motif is necessary for β-catenin degradation, perhaps the serine phosphorylation of armadillo (and by extension β-catenin) mediated by GSK-3 allows it to associate with Slimb/h-βTrCP and be targeted for degradation. This model is consistent with the observation that point mutations in serine residues in β-catenin result in oncogenic proteins, which are presumably no longer able to undergo ubiquitin-dependent proteolysis.

4.10. LEF/TCF

Lymphoid enhancer factor (LEF) and T-cell factors (TCFs) belong to a group of proteins which bind to DNA via an HMG box domain, a region homologous to high-mobility group I proteins. LEF-1 and the TCFs were initially identified as lymphoid-specific transcription factors, based on the affinities of LEF-1 and TCF-1 for the enhancer regions of T-cell receptor α chain and CD3 ε, respectively *(180–183)*. It has subsequently become clear that these factors play far more global roles and are expressed in both lymphoid and nonhematopoietic tissues. To date, four vertebrate homologs have been identified: LEF-1, TCF-1, TCF-3, and TCF-4 *(165)*. *Xenopus TCF-3 (184)*, *C. elegans Pop-1 (16)*, and *Drosophila Pangolin (dTcf) (185,186)* are structural and functional analogs of the mammalian LEF/TCFs.

Structurally, LEF-1 and the TCFs can be divided into several regions (Fig. 6). For all LEF/TCFs, the N-terminus is both necessary and sufficient for binding to β-catenin or plakoglobin. An 85-amino acid HMG box is located towards the C-terminus and is highly conserved among all the LEF/TCFs. The HMG box binds to the consensus DNA nucleotide sequence 5'-CTTGAA and contains an overlapping nuclear localization signal. The C-terminus of LEF/TCFs is the most divergent region among family members, and it is often created by alternative splicing *(165)*.

The broad-ranging and distinct developmental roles of LEF-1 and the TCFs are evident by their different expression profiles and by the spectrum of abnormalities manifested by *LEF-1* and *Tcf-1* null mice (Table 1). Phenotypically, *TCF-1* gene disruption causes a severe T-cell developmental defect *(187)*. By contrast, *LEF-1* disruption has no immune system phenotype but results in perinatal death from abnormal development of skin appendages, teeth, and the trigeminal nucleus *(188)*. During mouse development, *TCF-3* is almost universally expressed at embryonic day 6.5, but it becomes almost undetectable after embryonic d 10.5 *(189)*. *TCF-4* is observed beginning on day 10.5 of mouse embryogenesis, with expression limited to the central nervous system and the intestinal epithelium *(189)*.

The connection between LEF/TCFs and Wnt signaling was discovered by a yeast two-hybrid screen for β-catenin interaction partners, which identified LEF-1 *(146)*. LEF-1 and the Tcfs are now known to bind and dimerize with β-catenin and plakoglobin *(106,184)*. In addition, injection of LEF-1 mRNA, but not mRNA from other Tcf family members *(184)*, induces a secondary axis in *Xenopus (146)*. These LEF/TCF–β-catenin/

plakoglobin heterodimeric complexes transduce the Wnt signal to the nucleus, where they are thought to alter transcription of Wnt-responsive genes.

An alternative hypothesis for the mechanism underlying LEF/TCF signaling is based on experiments which show that membrane-tethered forms of plakoglobin and β-catenin can induce a secondary axis in *Xenopus (190,191)*. Because these membrane-tethered proteins are excluded from the nucleus, it is proposed that they signal by binding to, and excluding, a transcriptional repressor from the nucleus *(190)*. This possibility that LEF/TCF family members may act in a repressive fashion suggests an additional level of complexity in signaling. However, other work suggests that these membrane-bound β-catenin/plakoglobin may signal by sequestering out the degradative machinery that regulates endogenous β-catenin *(191)*.

LEF-1 and the TCFs are believed to function by altering DNA bending and, accordingly, are described as architectural transcription factors. Circular permutation analysis shows that LEF-1 induces a 120 to 130° angle bend in the DNA double helix *(193)*. On the basis of mobility shift assays, it appears that heterodimerization with β-catenin decreases LEF-induced DNA bending by ~40° *(193)*. Presumably, the modification of DNA structure by β-catenin/plakoglobin–LEF/TCF heterodimers and recruitment of additional factors result in transcription of Wnt target genes.

4.11. Downstream Target Genes

Genetic analysis in *Drosophila* has identified numerous genes required to carry out Wg-induced functions (for examples, see *194* and *195*). In most cases, it is not clear whether Wg signaling has primary or secondary effects on the transcriptional activation of a target gene. With the identification of the LEF/TCFs as mediators of Wg/Wnt signaling, it is now possible to examine putative target gene promoters for LEF/TCF binding sites and test their responsiveness directly to Wnt/Wg signaling in cell culture or in the animal. One example is the *ultrabithorax* gene in *Drosophila*, where such binding sites have been mapped to the Wg-responsive element in the promoter *(196)*.

Xenopus studies also show several potential signaling targets including the homeobox genes *siamois* and *goosecoid (197–202)*, and a member of the transforming growth factor β (TGF-β) family *Xenopus nodal-related 3 (Xnr3) (203)*. The promoter for *siamois*, a gene sufficient to induce a secondary axis, has been extensively characterized *(204)*. Four LEF sites are present and some of these are necessary for the β-catenin-induced activation of reporter genes driven by this promoter. In addition, the *Xnr3* promoter contains a putative LEF/TCF binding site, which is required for response to Wnt signals *(203)*.

5. DISCUSSION

Our understanding of the mechanisms underlying Wnt signal transduction has increased dramatically during the past few years. However, several important questions remain, and many new questions have emerged.

5.1. A Potential Mechanistic Relationship for Wnt and Hh Signaling

As previously discussed, the Wnt/Wg and Hh pathways can coordinately regulate each other by maintaining the expression of each other in a variety of systems. There are also several indications that the two pathways, at least at some levels, may transduce signals in a similar manner. For example, the Smoothened seven-transmembrane protein, which is required for hedgehog signaling, is highly homologous to Frizzleds in several regions, including the putative intracellular loops *(205–207)*. This relationship may suggest a similar signaling mechanism. Consistent with this, genetic analysis in *Drosophila* shows that *slimb* negatively regulates both pathways *(172)*.

The homology between Frizzled and Smoothened is also important when considering potential interactions between Wnts and Frizzleds. In cells not exposed to hedgehog protein, the activity of smoothened is constitutively inhibited by its association with Patched, another multiple transmembrane spanning protein *(207)*. Upon secretion, the hedgehog protein is modified by the addition of a cholesterol moiety and is thought to bind directly to patched, and not to smoothened, *(207)*. This binding releases smoothened from the inhibitory effects of patched and activates the pathway *(207)*. It remains possible that Frizzled and Smoothened function similarly and that another protein functions analogously to Patched in Wnt signaling.

5.2. The Presence of a Large Multiprotein Regulatory Complex

Recent work shows that Wnt signaling is controlled by the interactions of a multiprotein complex containing GSK-3, APC, Axin or conductin, and β-catenin. In addition, APC associates both with numerous other proteins and with microtubules *(see above)*. An important area of future research will be how this multiprotein complex changes upon exposure to a Wnt signal and how Dishevelled and Frizzled deliver signals to this complex. Perhaps the DIX domain, a domain common to Dishevelled and Axin/Conductin will be a key to this mystery.

5.3. Coordinated Regulation of Cell Adhesion and Cell Growth by Wnt and Cadherin

The cell adhesion and signaling functions of β-catenin, although distinct, may be coordinately regulated. Overexpression of cadherin inhibits β-catenin signaling, presumably by binding up the cytosolic pool of β-catenin *(154,208–210)*. In addition, there may be β-catenin-mediated regulation of cadherin expression, as the mouse E-cadherin promoter region is reported to contain a LEF/TCF binding motif that can bind β-catenin-LEF/TCF dimers in vitro *(211)*. The distinct, yet potentially coordinated cellular roles of β-catenin are the focus of much research, and they highlight the complexity of β-catenin.

5.4. Downstream Targets of Signaling

Finally, an area where recent technological advances may allow the most immediate progress is in the identification of downstream target genes of Wnt signals. The availability of methods such as cDNA array analysis *(212,213)* for fast screening of potential targets will undoubtedly lead to new insights into the pathway.

ACKNOWLEDGMENTS

We thank Harold Varmus for critical reading of this manuscript and members of the Varmus laboratory for helpful discussions. We also thank Jeff Axelrod for communication of unpublished results and Roel Nusse for allowing us to cite his web site.

G.D.B. is a Howard Hughes Medical Institute–NIH Research Scholar. B.O.W. is a fellow of the Cancer Research Fund of the Damon Runyon–Walter Winchell Foundation.

REFERENCES

1. Nusse R, Varmus HE. Many tumors induced by the mouse mammary tumor virus contain a provirus integrated in the same region of the host genome. *Cell* 1982; 31:99–109.
2. Brown AM, Papkoff J, Fung YK, Shackleford GM, Varmus GV. Identification of protein products encoded by the proto-oncogene *int-1*. *Mol Cell Biol* 1987; 7:3971–3977.
3. Bradley RS, Brown AM. The proto-oncogene *int-1* encodes a secreted protein associated with the extracellular matrix. *EMBO J* 1990; 9:1569–1575.
4. Papkoff J, Brown AM, Varmus AV. The *int-1* proto-oncogene products are glycoproteins that appear to enter the secretory pathway. *Mol Cell Biol* 1987; 7:3978–3984.
5. Rijsewijk F, Schuermann M, Wagenaar E, Parren P, Weigel D, Nusse R. The *Drosophila* homolog of the mouse mammary oncogene *int-1* is identical to the segment polarity gene wingless. *Cell* 1987; 50:649–657.
6. Sharma RP, Chopra VL. Effect of the *Wingless* (*wg1*) mutation on wing and haltere development in *Drosophila* melanogaster. *Dev Biol* 1976; 48:461–465.
7. Nusse R, Brown A, Papkoff J, Scambler P, Shackleford G, McMahon A, Moon R, Varmus H. A new nomenclature for *int-1* and related genes: the Wnt gene family. *Cell* 1991; 64:231.
8. Nusslein-Volhard C, Wieschaus E. Mutations affecting segment number and polarity in *Drosophila*. *Nature* 1980; 287:795–801.
9. Hammerschmidt M, Brook A, McMahon AM. The world according to hedgehog. *Trends Genet* 1997; 13:14–21.
10. DiNardo S, Heemskerk J, Dougan S, O'Farrell SO. The making of a maggot: patterning the *Drosophila* embryonic epidermis. *Curr Opin Genet Dev* 1994; 4:529–534.
11. Munsterberg AE, Kitajewski J, Bumcrot DA, McMahon AP, Lassar AL. Combinatorial signaling by Sonic hedgehog and Wnt family members induces myogenic bHLH gene expression in the somite. *Genes Dev* 1995; 9:2911–2922.
12. Yang Y, Niswander L. Interaction between the signaling molecules WNT7a and SHH during vertebrate limb development: dorsal signals regulate anteroposterior patterning. *Cell* 1995; 80:939–947.
13. Harris J, Honigberg L, Robinson N, Kenyon C. Neuronal cell migration in *C. elegans*: regulation of Hox gene expression and cell position. *Development* 1996; 122:3117–3131.
14. Herman MA, Vassilieva LL, Horvitz HR, Shaw JE, Herman JH. The *C. elegans* gene lin-44, which controls the polarity of certain asymmetric cell divisions, encodes a Wnt protein and acts cell nonautonomously. *Cell* 1995; 83:101–110.
15. Lin R, Hill RJ, Priess RP. POP-1 and anterior-posterior fate decisions in *C. elegans* embryos. *Cell* 1998; 92:229–239.
16. Lin R, Thompson S, Priess SP. POP-1 encodes an HMG box protein required for the specification of a mesoderm precursor in early *C. elegans* embryos. *Cell* 1995; 83:599–609.
17. Rocheleau CE, Downs WD, Lin R, Wittmann C, Bei Y, Cha YH, Ali M, Priess JR, Mello JM. Wnt signaling and an APC-related gene specify endoderm in early *C. elegans* embryos [see comments]. *Cell* 1997; 90:707–716.
18. Thorpe CJ, Schlesinger A, Carter JC, Bowerman B. Wnt signaling polarizes an early *C. elegans* blastomere to distinguish endoderm from mesoderm. *Cell* 1997; 90:695–705.
19. McMahon AP, Moon RT. Ectopic expression of the proto-oncogene *int-1* in *Xenopus* embryos leads to duplication of the embryonic axis. *Cell* 1989; 58:1075–1084.
20. Brown AM, Wildin RS, Prendergast TJ, Varmus TV. A retrovirus vector expressing the putative mammary oncogene *int-1* causes partial transformation of a mammary epithelial cell line. *Cell* 1986; 46:1001–1009.

21. Miller JR, Moon RT. Signal transduction through beta-catenin and specification of cell fate during embryogenesis. *Genes Dev* 1996; 10:2527–2539.
22. Pai LM, Orsulic S, Bejsovec A, Peifer M. Negative regulation of Armadillo, a Wingless effector in *Drosophila*. *Development* 1997; 124:2255–2266.
23. Yost C, Torres M, Miller JR, Huang E, Kimelman D, Moon DM. The axis-inducing activity, stability, and subcellular distribution of beta-catenin is regulated in *Xenopus* embryos by glycogen synthase kinase 3. *Genes Dev* 1996; 10:1443–1454.
24. Dale TC. Signal transduction by the Wnt family of ligands. *Biochem J* 1998; 329:209–223.
25. Cadigan KM, Nusse R. Wnt signaling: a common theme in animal development. *Genes Dev* 1997; 11:3286–3305.
26. Sidow A. Diversification of the Wnt gene family on the ancestral lineage of vertebrates. *Proc Natl Acad Sci USA* 1992; 89:5098–5102.
27. Nusse R, Varmus HE. Wnt genes. *Cell* 1992; 69:1073–1087.
28. Blasband A, Schryver B, Papkoff J. The biochemical properties and transforming potential of human Wnt-2 are similar to Wnt-1. *Oncogene* 1992; 7:153–161.
29. Kitajewski J, Mason JO, Varmus JV. Interaction of Wnt-1 proteins with the binding protein BiP. *Mol Cell Biol* 1992; 12:784–790.
30. Austin TW, Solar GP, Ziegler FC, Liem L, Matthews W. A role for the Wnt gene family in hematopoiesis: expansion of multilineage progenitor cells. *Blood* 1997; 89:3624–3635.
31. Bradley RS, Brown AM. A soluble form of Wnt-1 protein with mitogenic activity on mammary epithelial cells. *Mol Cell Biol* 1995; 15:4616–4622.
32. van Leeuwen F, Samos CH, Nusse R. Biological activity of soluble wingless protein in cultured *Drosophila* imaginal disc cells. *Nature* 1994; 368:342–344.
33. Binari RC, Staveley BE, Johnson WA, Godavarti R, Sasisekharan R, Manoukian AS. Genetic evidence that heparin-like glycosaminoglycans are involved in wingless signaling. *Development* 1997; 124:2623–2632.
34. Hacker U, Lin X, Perrimon N. The *Drosophila* sugarless gene modulates Wingless signaling and encodes an enzyme involved in polysaccharide biosynthesis. *Development* 1997; 124:3565–3573.
35. Haerry TE, Heslip TR, Marsh JL, O'Connor JO. Defects in glucuronate biosynthesis disrupt Wingless signaling in *Drosophila*. *Development* 1997; 124:3055–3064.
36. Itoh K, Sokol SS. Heparan sulfate proteoglycans are required for mesoderm formation in *Xenopus* embryos. *Development* 1994; 120:2703–2711.
37. Reichsman F, Smith L, Cumberledge S. Glycosaminoglycans can modulate extracellular localization of the wingless protein and promote signal transduction. *J Cell Biol* 1996; 135:819–827.
38. Wong GT, Gavin BJ, McMahon BM. Differential transformation of mammary epithelial cells by Wnt genes. *Mol Cell Biol* 1994; 14:6278–6286.
39. Christiansen JH, Monkley SJ, Wainwright SW. Murine WNT11 is a secreted glycoprotein that morphologically transforms mammary epithelial cells. *Oncogene* 1996; 12:2705–2711.
40. Shimizu H, Julius MA, Giarre M, Zheng Z, Brown AM, Kitajewski J. Transformation by Wnt family proteins correlates with regulation of beta-catenin. *Cell Growth Differ* 1997; 8:1349–1358.
41. Sokol S, Christian JL, Moon RT, Melton RM. Injected Wnt RNA induces a complete body axis in *Xenopus* embryos. *Cell* 1991; 67:741–752.
42. Landesman Y, Sokol SY. Xwnt-2b is a novel axis-inducing *Xenopus* Wnt, which is expressed in embryonic brain. *Mech Dev* 1997; 63:199–209.
43. Wolda SL, Moody CJ, Moon CM. Overlapping expression of Xwnt-3A and Xwnt-1 in neural tissue of *Xenopus laevis* embryos. *Dev Biol* 1993; 155:46–57.
44. Ungar AR, Kelly GM, Moon GM. Wnt4 affects morphogenesis when misexpressed in the zebrafish embryo. *Mech Dev* 1995; 52:153–164.

45. Du SJ, Purcell SM, Christian JL, McGrew LL, Moon LM. Identification of distinct classes and functional domains of Wnts through expression of wild-type and chimeric proteins in *Xenopus* embryos. *Mol Cell Biol* 1995; 15:2625–2634.
46. Christian JL, McMahon JA, McMahon AP, Moon AM. Xwnt-8, a *Xenopus* Wnt-1/int-1-related gene responsive to mesoderm-inducing growth factors, may play a role in ventral mesodermal patterning during embryogenesis. *Development* 1991; 111:1045–1055.
47. Smith WC, Harland RM. Injected Xwnt-8 RNA acts early in *Xenopus* embryos to promote formation of a vegetal dorsalizing center. *Cell* 1991; 67:753–765.
48. Cui Y, Brown JD, Moon RT, Christian RC. Xwnt-8b: a maternally expressed *Xenopus* Wnt gene with a potential role in establishing the dorsoventral axis. *Development* 1995; 121:2177–2186.
49. Ku M, Melton MD. Xwnt-11: a maternally expressed *Xenopus* wnt gene. *Development* 1993; 119:1161–1173.
50. Torres MA, Yang-Snyder J, Purcell SM, DeMarais AA, McGrew LL, Moon LM. Activities of the Wnt-1 class of secreted signaling factors are antagonized by the Wnt-5A class and by a dominant negative cadherin in early *Xenopus* development. *J Cell Biol* 1996; 133:1123–1137.
51. Slusarski DC, Yang-Snyder J, Busa WB, Moon WM. Modulation of embryonic intracellular Ca2+ signaling by Wnt-5A. *Dev Biol* 1997; 182:114–120.
52. He X, Saint-Jeannet JP, Wang Y, Nathans J, Dawid I, Varmus H. A member of the Frizzled protein family mediating axis induction by Wnt-5A. *Science* 1997; 275:1652–1654.
53. Bhanot P, Brink M, Harryman Samos C, Hsieh J, Wang Y, Macke JP, Andrew D, Nathans J, Nusse R. A new member of the frizzled family from *Drosophila* functions as a Wingless receptor. *Nature* 1996; 382:225–230.
54. Vinson CR, Adler PN. Directional non-cell autonomy and the transmission of polarity information by the *frizzled* gene of *Drosophila*. *Nature* 1987; 329:549–551.
55. Adler PN. The genetic control of tissue polarity in *Drosophila*. *BioEssays* 1992; 14:735–741.
56. Tomlinson A, Strapps WR, Heemskerk J. Linking Frizzled and Wnt signaling in *Drosophila* development. *Development* 1997; 124:4515–4521.
57. Zheng L, Zhang J, Carthew JC. *frizzled* regulates mirror-symmetric pattern formation in the *Drosophila* eye. *Development* 1995; 121:3045–3055.
58. Eaton S. Planar polarization of *Drosophila* and vertebrate epithelia. *Curr Opin Cell Biol* 1997; 9:860–866.
59. Chan SD, Karpf DB, Fowlkes ME, Hooks M, Bradley MS, Vuong V, Bambino T, Liu MY, Arnaud CD, Strewler GJ, et al. Two homologs of the *Drosophila* polarity gene *frizzled (fz)* are widely expressed in mammalian tissues. *J Biol Chem* 1992; 267:25,202–25,207.
60. Zhao Z, Lee CC, Baldini A, Caskey AC. A human homologue of the *Drosophila* polarity gene *frizzled* has been identified and mapped to 17q21.1. *Genomics* 1995; 27:370–373.
61. Blankesteijn WM, Essers-Janssen YP, Ulrich MM, Smits MS. Increased expression of a homologue of *Drosophila* tissue polarity gene "*frizzled*" in left ventricular hypertrophy in the rat, as identified by subtractive hybridization. *J Mol Cell Cardiol* 1996; 28:1187–1191.
62. Wang Y, Macke JP, Abella BS, Andreasson K, Worley P, Gilbert DJ, Copeland NG, Jenkins NA, Nathans J. A large family of putative transmembrane receptors homologous to the product of the *Drosophila* tissue polarity gene frizzled. *J Biol Chem* 1996; 271:4468–4476.
63. Wang YK, Samos CH, Peoples R, Perez-Jurado LA, Nusse R, Francke U. A novel human homologue of the *Drosophila* frizzled wnt receptor gene binds wingless protein and is in the Williams syndrome deletion at 7q11.23. *Hum Mol Genet* 1997; 6:465–472.
64. Yang-Snyder J, Miller JR, Brown JD, Lai C, Moon JL. A *frizzled* homolog functions in a vertebrate Wnt signaling pathway. *Curr Biol* 1996; 6:1302–1306.

65. Sawa H, Lobel L, Horvitz LH. The *Caenorhabditis elegans* gene lin-17, which is required for certain asymmetric cell divisions, encodes a putative seven-transmembrane protein similar to the *Drosophila* frizzled protein. *Genes Dev* 1996; 10:2189–2197.
66. Bourne HR. How receptors talk to trimeric G proteins. *Curr Opin Cell Biol* 1997; 9:134–142.
67. Slusarski DC, Corces VG, Moon VM. Interaction of Wnt and a Frizzled homologue triggers G-protein-linked phosphatidylinositol signalling. *Nature* 1997; 390:410–413.
68. Saras J, Heldin CH. PDZ domains bind carboxy-terminal sequences of target proteins. *Trends Biochem Sci* 1996; 21:455–458.
69. Cabral JH, Petosa C, Sutcliffe MJ, Raza S, Byron O, Poy F, Marfatia SM, Chishti AH, Liddington AL. Crystal structure of a PDZ domain. *Nature* 1996; 382:649–652.
70. Doyle DA, Lee A, Lewis J, Kim E, Sheng M, MacKinnon R. Crystal structures of a complexed and peptide-free membrane protein-binding domain: molecular basis of peptide recognition by PDZ. *Cell* 1996; 85:1067–1076.
71. Songyang Z, Fanning AS, Fu C, Xu J, Marfatia SM, Chishti AH, Crompton A, Chan AC, Anderson JM, Cantley JC. Recognition of unique carboxyl-terminal motifs by distinct PDZ domains. *Science* 1997; 275:73–77.
72. Leyns L, Bouwmeester T, Kim SH, Piccolo S, De Robertis SD. Frzb-1 is a secreted antagonist of Wnt signaling expressed in the Spemann organizer. *Cell* 1997; 88:747–756.
73. Finch PW, He X, Kelley MJ, Uren A, Schaudies RP, Popescu NC, Rudikoff S, Aaronson SA, Varmus HE, Rubin HR. Purification and molecular cloning of a secreted, Frizzled-related antagonist of Wnt action. *Proc Natl Acad Sci USA* 1997; 94:6770–6775.
74. Mayr T, Deutsch U, Kuhl M, Drexler HC, Lottspeich F, Deutzmann R, Wedlich D, Risau W. Fritz: a secreted frizzled-related protein that inhibits Wnt activity. *Mech Dev* 1997; 63:109–125.
75. Pfeffer PL, De Robertis EM, Izpisua-Belmonte JC. Crescent, a novel chick gene encoding a Frizzled-like cysteine-rich domain, is expressed in anterior regions during early embryogenesis. *Int J Dev Biol* 1997; 41:449–458.
76. Rattner A, Hsieh JC, Smallwood PM, Gilbert DJ, Copeland NG, Jenkins NA, Nathans J. A family of secreted proteins contains homology to the cysteine-rich ligand-binding domain of frizzled receptors. *Proc Natl Acad Sci USA* 1997; 94:2859–2863.
77. Shirozu M, Tada H, Tashiro K, Nakamura T, Lopez ND, Nazarea M, Hamada T, Sato T, Nakano T, Honjo T. Characterization of novel secreted and membrane proteins isolated by the signal sequence trap method. *Genomics* 1996; 37:273–280.
78. Salic AN, Kroll KL, Evans LM, Kirschner LK. Sizzled: a secreted Xwnt8 antagonist expressed in the ventral marginal zone of *Xenopus* embryos. *Development* 1997; 124:4739–4748.
79. Wang S, Krinks M, Lin K, Luyten FP, Moos Jr, M. Frzb, a secreted protein expressed in the Spemann organizer, binds and inhibits Wnt-8. *Cell* 1997; 88:757–766.
80. Wolf V, Ke G, Dharmarajan AM, Bielke W, Artuso L, Saurer S, Friis R. *DDC-4,* an apoptosis-associated gene, is a secreted frizzled relative. *FEBS Lett* 1997; 417:385–389.
81. Guthrie S. Axon guidance: netrin receptors are revealed. *Curr Biol* 1997; 7:R6–9.
82. Song L, Fricker LD. Cloning and expression of human carboxypeptidase Z, a novel metallocarboxypeptidase. *J Biol Chem* 1997; 272:10,543–10,550.
83. Rehn M, Pihlajaniemi T. Identification of three N-terminal ends of type XVIII collagen chains and tissue-specific differences in the expression of the corresponding transcripts. The longest form contains a novel motif homologous to rat and *Drosophila* frizzled proteins. *J Biol Chem* 1995; 270:4705–4711.
84. Glinka A, Wu W, Delius H, Monaghan AP, Blumenstock C, Niehrs C. Dickkopf-1 is a member of a new family of secreted proteins and functions in head induction. *Nature* 1998; 391:357–362.

85. Theisen H, Purcell J, Bennett M, Kansagara D, Syed A, Marsh AM. *dishevelled* is required during *wingless* signaling to establish both cell polarity and cell identity. *Development* 1994; 120:347–360.

86. Klingensmith J, Nusse R, Perrimon N. The *Drosophila* segment polarity gene dishevelled encodes a novel protein required for response to the wingless signal. *Genes Dev* 1994; 8:118–130.

87. Rothbacher U, Laurent MN, Blitz IL, Watabe T, Marsh JL, Cho JC. Functional conservation of the Wnt signaling pathway revealed by ectopic expression of *Drosophila* dishevelled in *Xenopus*. *Dev Biol* 1995; 170:717–721.

88. Sokol SY, Klingensmith J, Perrimon N, Itoh K. Dorsalizing and neuralizing properties of Xdsh, a maternally expressed *Xenopus* homolog of *dishevelled*. *Development* 1995; 121:3487.

89. Krasnow RE, Wong LL, Adler LA. Dishevelled is a component of the frizzled signaling pathway in *Drosophila*. *Development* 1995; 121:4095–4102.

90. Axelrod JD, Matsuno K, Artavanis-Tsakonas S, Perrimon N. Interaction between Wingless and Notch signaling pathways mediated by dishevelled. *Science* 1996; 271:1826–1832.

91. Couso JP, Martinez Arias A. Notch is required for wingless signaling in the epidermis of *Drosophila*. *Cell* 1994; 79:259–272.

92. Micchelli CA, Rulifson EJ, Blair EB. The function and regulation of cut expression on the wing margin of *Drosophila*: Notch, Wingless and a dominant negative role for Delta and Serrate. *Development* 1997; 124:1485–1495.

93. Rulifson EJ, Blair SS. Notch regulates wingless expression and is not required for reception of the paracrine wingless signal during wing margin neurogenesis in *Drosophila*. *Development* 1995; 121:2813–2824.

94. Yanagawa S, van Leeuwen F, Wodarz A, Klingensmith J, Nusse R. The dishevelled protein is modified by wingless signaling in *Drosophila*. *Genes Dev* 1995; 9:1087–1097.

95. Willert K, Brink M, Wodarz A, Varmus H, Nusse R. Casein kinase 2 associates with and phosphorylates dishevelled. *EMBO J* 1997; 16:3089–3096.

96. Yang Y, Lijam N, Sussman DJ, Tsang M. Genomic organization of mouse Dishevelled genes. *Gene* 1996; 180:121–123.

97. Tsang M, Lijam N, Yang Y, Beier DR, Wynshaw-Boris A, Sussman DJ. Isolation and characterization of mouse dishevelled-3. *Dev Dyn* 1996; 207:253–262.

98. Sussman DJ, Klingensmith J, Salinas P, Adams PS, Nusse R, Perrimon N. Isolation and characterization of a mouse homolog of the *Drosophila* segment polarity gene dishevelled. *Dev Biol* 1994; 166:73–86.

99. Semenov MV, Snyder M. Human dishevelled genes constitute a DHR-containing multigene family. *Genomics* 1997; 42:302–210.

100. Lijam N, Sussman DJ. Organization and promoter analysis of the mouse dishevelled-1 gene. *Genome Res* 1995; 5:116–124.

101. Klingensmith J, Yang Y, Axelrod JD, Beier DR, Perrimon N, Sussman NS. Conservation of dishevelled structure and function between flies and mice: isolation and characterization of Dvl2. *Mech Dev* 1996; 58:15–26.

102. Greco TL, Sussman DJ, Camper DC. *Dishevelled-2* maps to human chromosome 17 and distal to Wnt3a and vestigial tail (vt) on mouse chromosome 11. *Mamm Genome* 1996; 7:475–476.

103. Bui TD, Beier DR, Jonssen M, Smith K, Dorrington SM, Kaklamanis L, Kearney L, Regan R, Sussman DJ, Harris DH. cDNA cloning of a human dishevelled *DVL-3* gene, mapping to 3q27, and expression in human breast and colon carcinomas. *Biochem Biophys Res Commun* 1997; 239:510–516.

104. Sokol SY. Analysis of Dishevelled signalling pathways during *Xenopus* development. *Curr Biol* 1996; 6:1456–1467.

105. Zeng L, Fagotto F, Zhang T, Hsu W, Vasicek TJ, Perry WLR, Lee JJ, Tilghman SM, Gumbiner BM, Costantini F. The mouse *Fused* locus encodes Axin, an inhibitor of the Wnt signaling pathway that regulates embryonic axis formation. *Cell* 1997; 90:181–192.

106. Behrens J, Jerchow BA, Wurtele M, Grimm J, Asbrand C, Wirtz R, Kuhl M, Wedlich D, Birchmeier W. Functional interaction of an axin homolog, conductin, with B-catenin, APC, and GSK3B. *Science* 1998; 280:596–599.

107. Ponting CP, Bork P. Pleckstrin's repeat performance: a novel domain in G-protein signaling? *Trends Biochem Sci* 1996; 21:245–246.

108. Strutt DI, Weber U, Mlodzik M. The role of RhoA in tissue polarity and Frizzled signalling. *Nature* 1997; 387:292–295.

109. Plyte SE, Hughes K, Nikolakaki E, Pulverer BJ, Woodgett BW. Glycogen synthase kinase-3: functions in oncogenesis and development. *Biochim Biophys Acta* 1992; 1114:147–162.

110. Peifer M, Pai LM, Casey M. Phosphorylation of the *Drosophila* adherens junction protein Armadillo: roles for wingless signal and zeste-white 3 kinase. *Dev Biol* 1994; 166:543–556.

111. Siegfried E, Wilder EL, Perrimon N. Components of wingless signalling in *Drosophila*. *Nature* 1994; 367:76–80.

112. Harwood AJ, Plyte SE, Woodgett J, Strutt H, Kay HK. Glycogen synthase kinase 3 regulates cell fate in *Dictyostelium*. *Cell* 1995; 80:139–148.

113. Plyte SE, Feoktistova A, Burke JD, Woodgett JR, Gould JG. *Schizosaccharomyces pombe* skp1+ encodes a protein kinase related to mammalian glycogen synthase kinase 3 and complements a cdc14 cytokinesis mutant. *Mol Cell Biol* 1996; 16:179–191.

114. Bianchi MW, Plyte SE, Kreis M, Woodgett MW. A Saccharomyces cerevisiae protein-serine kinase related to mammalian glycogen synthase kinase-3 and the *Drosophila* melanogaster gene shaggy product. *Gene* 1993; 134:51–56.

115. Bianchi MW, Guivarc'h D, Thomas M, Woodgett JR, Kreis M. Arabidopsis homologs of the shaggy and GSK-3 protein kinases: molecular cloning and functional expression in Escherichia coli. *Mol Gen Genet* 1994; 242:337–345.

116. Dominguez I, Itoh K, Sokol KS. Role of glycogen synthase kinase 3 beta as a negative regulator of dorsoventral axis formation in *Xenopus* embryos. *Proc Natl Acad Sci USA* 1995; 92:8498–8502.

117. He X, Saint-Jeannet JP, Woodgett JR, Varmus HE, Dawid HD. Glycogen synthase kinase-3 and dorsoventral patterning in *Xenopus* embryos. *Nature* 1995; 374:617–622.

118. Pierce SB, Kimelman, D. Regulation of Spemann organizer formation by the intracellular kinase Xgsk-3. *Development* 1995; 121:755–765.

119. Cook D, Fry MJ, Hughes K, Sumathipala R, Woodgett JR, Dale JD. Wingless inactivates glycogen synthase kinase-3 via an intracellular signalling pathway which involves a protein kinase C. *EMBO J* 1996; 15:4526–4536.

120. Goode N, Hughes K, Woodgett JR, Parker JP. Differential regulation of glycogen synthase kinase-3 beta by protein kinase C isotypes. *J Biol Chem* 1992; 267:16,878–16,882.

121. Ginsburg GT, Kimmel AR. Autonomous and nonautonomous regulation of axis formation by antagonistic signaling via 7-span cAMP receptors and GSK3 in *Dictyostelium*. *Genes Dev* 1997; 11:2112–2123.

122. Stambolic V, Woodgett JR. Mitogen inactivation of glycogen synthase kinase-3 beta in intact cells via serine 9 phosphorylation. *Biochem J* 1994; 303:701–704.

123. Klein PS, Melton DA. A molecular mechanism for the effect of lithium on development. *Proc Natl Acad Sci USA* 1996; 93:8455–8459.

124. Stambolic V, Ruel L, Woodgett LW. Lithium inhibits glycogen synthase kinase-3 activity and mimics wingless signalling in intact cells. *Curr Biol* 1996; 6:1664–1668.

125. Kao KR, Masui Y, Elinson YE. Lithium induced respecification of pattern in *Xenopus laevis* embryos. *Nature* 1986; 322:371–373.

126. Beals CR, Sheridan CM, Turck CW, Gardner P, Crabtree PC. Nuclear export of NF-ATc enhanced by glycogen synthase kinase-3. *Science* 1997; 275:1930–1934.

127. Sakanaka C, Weiss JB, Williams JW. Bridging of beta-catenin and glycogen synthase kinase-3beta by axin and inhibition of beta-catenin-mediated transcription. *Proc Natl Acad Sci USA* 1998; 95:3020–3023.

128. Yamamoto H, Kishida S, Uochi T, Ikeda S, Koyama S, Asashima M, Kikuchi A. Axil, a member of the axin family, interacts with glycogen synthase kinase 3B and B-catenin and inhibits axis formation of *Xenopus* embryos. *Mol Cell Biol* 1998; 18:2867–2875.

129. Ikeda S, Kishida S, Yamamoto H, Murai H, Koyama S, Kikuchi A. Axin, a negative regulator of the Wnt signaling pathway, forms a complex with GSK-3beta and beta-catenin and promotes GSK-3beta-dependent phosphorylation of beta-catenin. *EMBO J* 1998; 17:1371–1384.

130. Nishisho I, Nakamura Y, Miyoshi Y, Miki Y, Ando H, Horii A, Koyama K, Utsunomiya J, Baba S, Hedge P. Mutations of chromosome 5q21 genes in FAP and colorectal cancer patients. *Science* 1991; 253:665–669.

131. Groden J, Thliveris A, Samowitz W, Carlson M, Gelbert L, Albertsen H, Joslyn G, Stevens J, Spirio L, Robertson M, and et al. Identification and characterization of the familial adenomatous polyposis coli gene. *Cell* 1991; 66:589–600.

132. Kinzler KW, Vogelstein B. Lessons from hereditary colorectal cancer. *Cell* 1996; 87:159–170.

133. Sparks AB, Morin PJ, Vogelstein B, Kinzler BK. Mutational analysis of the APC/beta-catenin/Tcf pathway in colorectal cancer. *Cancer Res* 1998; 58:1130–1134.

134. Korinek V, Barker N, Morin PJ, van Wichen D, de Weger R, Kinzler KW, Vogelstein B, Clevers H. Constitutive transcriptional activation by a beta-catenin-Tcf complex in APC-/- colon carcinoma. *Science* 1997; 275:1784–1787.

135. Munemitsu S, Albert I, Souza B, Rubinfeld B, Polakis P. Regulation of intracellular beta-catenin levels by the adenomatous polyposis coli (APC) tumor-suppressor protein. *Proc Natl Acad Sci USA* 1995; 92:3046–3050.

136. Shoemaker AR, Gould KA, Luongo C, Moser AR, Dove AD. Studies of neoplasia in the *Min* mouse. *Biochim Biophys Acta* 1997; 1332:F25–48.

137. Peifer M, Berg S, Reynolds SR. A repeating amino acid motif shared by proteins with diverse cellular roles [letter]. *Cell* 1994; 76:789–791.

138. Su LK, Burrell M, Hill DE, Gyuris J, Brent R, Wiltshire R, Trent J, Vogelstein B, Kinzler BK. APC binds to the novel protein EB1. *Cancer Res* 1995; 55:2972–2977.

139. Matsumine A, Ogai A, Senda T, Okumura N, Satoh K, Baeg GH, Kawahara T, Kobayashi S, Okada M, Toyoshima K, Akiyama T. Binding of APC to the human homolog of the *Drosophila* discs large tumor suppressor protein. *Science* 1996; 272:1020–1023.

140. Munemitsu S, Souza B, Muller O, Albert I, Rubinfeld B, Polakis P. The APC gene product associates with microtubules *in vivo* and promotes their assembly *in vitro*. *Cancer Res* 1994; 54:3676–3681.

141. Smith KJ, Levy DB, Maupin P, Pollard TD, Vogelstein B, Kinzler BK. Wild-type but not mutant APC associates with the microtubule cytoskeleton. *Cancer Res* 1994; 54:3672–3675.

142. Vleminckx K, Wong E, Guger K, Rubinfeld B, Polakis P, Gumbiner PG. Adenomatous polyposis coli tumor suppressor protein has signaling activity in *Xenopus laevis* embryos resulting in the induction of an ectopic dorsoanterior axis. *J Cell Biol* 1997; 136:411–420.

143. Hayashi S, Rubinfeld B, Souza B, Polakis P, Wieschaus E, Levine EL. A *Drosophila* homolog of the tumor suppressor gene adenomatous polyposis coli down-regulates beta-catenin but its zygotic expression is not essential for the regulation of Armadillo. *Proc Natl Acad Sci USA* 1997; 94:242–247.

144. Vasicek TJ, Zeng L, Guan XJ, Zhang T, Costantini F, Tilghman FT. Two dominant mutations in the mouse *fused* gene are the result of transposon insertions. *Genetics* 1997; 147:777–786.

145. Perry WLI, Vasicek TJ, Lee JJ, Rossi JM, Zeng L, Zhang T, Tilghman SM, Costantini R. Phenotypic and molecular analysis of a transgenic insertional allele of the mouse *Fused* locus. *Genetics* 1995; 141:321–332.

146. Behrens J, von Kries JP, Kuhl M, Bruhn L, Wedlich D, Grosschedl R, Birchmeier W. Functional interaction of beta-catenin with the transcription factor LEF-1. *Nature* 1996; 382:638–642.

147. Koelle MR. A new family of G-protein regulators—the RGS proteins. *Curr Opin Cell Biol* 1997; 9:143–147.

148. Cowin P, Kapprell HP, Franke WW, Tamkun J, Hynes JH. Plakoglobin: a protein common to different kinds of intercellular adhering junctions. *Cell* 1986; 46:1063–1073.

149. Ozawa M, Baribault H, Kemler R. The cytoplasmic domain of the cell adhesion molecule uvomorulin associates with three independent proteins structurally related in different species. *EMBO J* 1989; 8:1711–1717.

150. Nagafuchi A, Takeichi, M. Transmembrane control of cadherin-mediated cell adhesion: a 94 kDa protein functionally associated with a specific region of the cytoplasmic domain of E-cadherin. *Cell Regul* 1989; 1:37–44.

151. McCrea PD, Turck CW, Gumbiner B. A homolog of the armadillo protein in *Drosophila* (plakoglobin) associated with E-cadherin. *Science* 1991; 254:1359–1361.

152. Peifer M, McCrea PD, Green KJ, Wieschaus E, Gumbiner EG. The vertebrate adhesive junction proteins beta-catenin and plakoglobin and the *Drosophila* segment polarity gene *armadillo* form a multigene family with similar properties. *J Cell Biol* 1992; 118:681–691.

153. Funayama N, Fagotto F, McCrea P, Gumbiner PG. Embryonic axis induction by the armadillo repeat domain of beta-catenin: evidence for intracellular signaling. *J Cell Biol* 1995; 128:959–968.

154. Karnovsky A, Klymkowsky MW. Anterior axis duplication in *Xenopus* induced by the over-expression of the cadherin-binding protein plakoglobin. *Proc Natl Acad Sci USA* 1995; 92:4522–4536.

155. Barth AI, Nathke IS, Nelson IN. Cadherins, catenins and APC protein: interplay between cytoskeletal complexes and signaling pathways. *Curr Opin Cell Biol* 1997; 9:683–690.

156. Cowin P, Burke B. Cytoskeleton-membrane interactions. *Curr Opin Cell Biol* 1996; 8:56–65.

157. Orsulic S, Peifer M. An *in vivo* structure-function study of armadillo, the beta-catenin homologue, reveals both separate and overlapping regions of the protein required for cell adhesion and for wingless signaling. *J Cell Biol* 1996; 134:1283–1300.

158. Nagafuchi A, Takeichi M. Cell binding function of E-cadherin is regulated by the cytoplasmic domain. *EMBO J* 1988; 7:3679–3684.

159. Haegel H, Larue L, Ohsugi M, Fedorov L, Herrenknecht K, Kemler R. Lack of *beta-catenin* affects mouse development at gastrulation. *Development* 1995; 121:3529–3537.

160. Peifer M. Cell adhesion and signal transduction: the Armadillo connection. *Trends in Cell Biology* 1995; 5:224–229.

161. Bierkamp C, McLaughlin KJ, Schwarz H, Huber O, Kemler R. Embryonic heart and skin defects in mice lacking *plakoglobin*. *Dev Biol* 1996; 180:780–785.

162. Ruiz P, Brinkmann V, Ledermann B, Behrend M, Grund C, Thalhammer C, Vogel F, Birchmeier C, Gunthert U, Franke WW, Birchmeier W. Targeted mutation of *plakoglobin* in mice reveals essential functions of desmosomes in the embryonic heart. *J Cell Biol* 1996; 135:215–225.

163. Aberle H, Bauer A, Stappert J, Kispert A, Kemler R. beta-catenin is a target for the ubiquitin-proteasome pathway. *EMBO J* 1997; 16:3797–3804.

164. Orford K, Crockett C, Jensen JP, Weissman AM, Byers AB. Serine phosphorylation-regulated ubiquitination and degradation of beta-catenin. *J Biol Chem* 1997; 272:24,735–24,738.

165. Clevers H, van de Wetering, M. TCF/LEF factor earn their wings. *Trends Genet* 1997; 13:485–489.
166. Ilyas M, Tomlinson IP, Rowan A, Pignatelli M, Bodmer MB. *Beta-catenin* mutations in cell lines established from human colorectal cancers. *Proc Natl Acad Sci USA* 1997; 94:10,330–10,334.
167. Peifer M. *Beta-catenin* as oncogene: the smoking gun. *Science* 1997; 275:1752–1753.
168. Rubinfeld B, Robbins P, El-Gamil M, Albert I, Porfiri E, Polakis P. Stabilization of beta-catenin by genetic defects in melanoma cell lines. *Science* 1997; 275:1790–1792.
169. Takahashi M, Fukuda K, Sugimura T, Wakabayashi K. *Beta-catenin* is frequently mutated and demonstrates altered cellular location in azoxymethane-induced rat colon tumors. *Cancer Res* 1998; 58:42–46.
170. Morin PJ, Sparks AB, Korinek V, Barker N, Clevers H, Vogelstein B, Kinzler BK. Activation of beta-catenin-Tcf signaling in colon cancer by mutations in *beta-catenin* or *APC. Science* 1997; 275:1787–1790.
171. Fagotto F, Gluck U, Gumbiner B. Nuclear localization signal-independent and importin/karyopherin-independent nuclear import of β-catenin. *Curr Biol* 1998; 8:181–190.
172. Jiang J, Struhl G. Regulation of the Hedgehog and Wingless signalling pathways by the F-box/WD40-repeat protein Slimb. *Nature* 1998; 391:493–496.
173. Bai C, Sen P, Hofmann K, Ma L, Goebl M, Harper JW, Elledge JE. SKP1 connects cell cycle regulators to the ubiquitin proteolysis machinery through a novel motif, the F-box. *Cell* 1996; 86:263–274.
174. Margottin F, Benichou S, Durand H, Richard V, Liu LX, Gomas E, Benarous R. Interaction between the cytoplasmic domains of HIV–1 Vpu and CD4: role of Vpu residues involved in CD4 interaction and *in vitro* CD4 degradation. *Virology* 1996; 223:381–386.
175. Neer EJ, Schmidt CJ, Nambudripad R, Smith RS. The ancient regulatory-protein family of WD-repeat proteins. *Nature* 1994; 371:297–300.
176. Margottin F, Bour SP, Durand H, Selig L, Benichou S, Richard V, Thomas D, Strebel K, Benarous R. A novel human WD protein, h-BTrCP, that interacts with HIV-1 Vpu connects CD4 to the ER degradation pathway through an F-box motif. *Mol Cell* 1998; 1:565–574.
177. Hudson JW, Alarcon VB, Elinson VE. Identification of new localized RNAs in the *Xenopus* oocyte by differential display PCR. *Dev Genet* 1996; 19:190–198.
178. Spevak W, Keiper BD, Stratowa C, Castanon CC. *Saccharomyces cerevisiae* cdc15 mutants arrested at a late stage in anaphase are rescued by *Xenopus* cDNAs encoding N-ras or a protein with beta-transducin repeats. *Mol Cell Biol* 1993; 13:4953–4966.
179. Chen MY, Maldarelli F, Karczewski MK, Willey RL, Strebel K. Human immunodeficiency virus type 1 Vpu protein induces degradation of CD4 *in vitro*: the cytoplasmic domain of CD4 contributes to Vpu sensitivity. *J Virol* 1993; 67:3877–3884.
180. Oosterwegel M, van de Wetering M, Dooijes D, Klomp L, Winoto A, Georgopoulos K, Meijlink F, Clevers H. Cloning of murine *TCF-1*, a T cell-specific transcription factor interacting with functional motifs in the CD3-epsilon and T cell receptor alpha enhancers. *J Exp Med* 1991; 173:1133–1142.
181. Travis A, Amsterdam A, Belanger C, Grosschedl R. LEF-1, a gene encoding a lymphoid-specific protein with an HMG domain, regulates T-cell receptor alpha enhancer function. *Genes Dev* 1991; 5:880–894.
182. van de Wetering M, Oosterwegel M, Dooijes D, Clevers H. Identification and cloning of *TCF-1*, a T lymphocyte-specific transcription factor containing a sequence-specific HMG box. *EMBO J* 1991; 10:123–132.
183. Waterman ML, Fischer WH, Jones WJ. A thymus-specific member of the HMG protein family regulates the human T cell receptor C alpha enhancer. *Genes Dev* 1991; 5:656–669.
184. Molenaar M, van de Wetering M, Oosterwegel M, Peterson-Maduro J, Godsave S, Korinek V, Roose J, Destree O, Clevers H. XTcf-3 transcription factor mediates beta-catenin-induced axis formation in *Xenopus* embryos. *Cell* 1996; 86:391–399.

185. Brunner E, Peter O, Schweizer L, Basler K. *pangolin* encodes a LEF-1 homologue that acts downstream of Armadillo to transduce the Wingless signal in *Drosophila*. *Nature* 1997; 385:829–833.

186. van de Wetering M, Cavallo R, Dooijes D, van Beest M, van Es J, Loureiro J, Ypma A, Hursh D, Jones T, Bejsovec A, Peifer M, Mortin M, Clevers H. Armadillo coactivates transcription driven by the product of the *Drosophila* segment polarity gene *dTCF*. *Cell* 1997; 88:789–799.

187. Verbeek S, Izon D, Hofhuis F, Robanus-Maandag E, te Riele H, van de Wetering M, Oosterwegel M, Wilson A, MacDonald HR, Clevers H. An HMG-box-containing T-cell factor required for thymocyte differentiation. *Nature* 1995; 374:70–74.

188. van Genderen C, Okamura RM, Farinas I, Quo RG, Parslow TG, Bruhn L, Grosschedl R. Development of several organs that require inductive epithelial-mesenchymal interactions is impaired in LEF-1-deficient mice. *Genes Dev* 1994; 8:2691–2703.

189. Korinek V, Barker N, Willert K, Molenaar M, Roose J, Wagenaar G, Markman M, Lamers W, Destree O, Clevers H. Two members of the Tcf family implicated in Wnt/beta-catenin signaling during embryogenesis in the mouse. *Mol Cell Biol* 1998; 18:1248–1256.

190. Merriam JM, Rubenstein AB, Klymkowsky MW. Cytoplasmically anchored plakoglobin induces a WNT-like phenotype in *Xenopus*. *Dev Biol* 1997; 185:67–81.

191. Miller JR, Moon RT. Analysis of the signaling activities of localization mutants of β-catenin during axis specification in *Xenopus*. *J Cell Biol* 1997; 139:229–243.

192. Salomon D, Sacco PA, Roy SG, Simcha I, Johnson KR, Wheelock MJ, Ben-Ze'ev A. Regulation of beta-catenin levels and localization by overexpression of plakoglobin and inhibition of the ubiquitin-proteasome system. *J Cell Biol* 1997; 139:1325–1335.

193. Giese K, Pagel J, Grosschedl R. Functional analysis of DNA bending and unwinding by the high mobility group domain of LEF-1. *Proc Natl Acad Sci USA* 1997; 94:12,845–12,850.

194. Klingensmith J, Nusse R. Signaling by *wingless* in *Drosophila*. *Dev Biol* 1996; 166:396–414.

195. Brook WJ, Diaz-Benjumea FJ, Cohen FC. Organizing spatial pattern in limb development. *Annu Rev Cell Dev Biol* 1996; 12:161–180.

196. Riese J, Yu X, Munnerlyn A, Eresh S, Hsu SC, Grosschedl R, Bienz M. LEF-1, a nuclear factor coordinating signaling inputs from wingless and decapentaplegic. *Cell* 1997; 88:777–787.

197. Lemaire P, Garrett N, Gurdon NG. Expression cloning of Siamois, a *Xenopus* homeobox gene expressed in dorsal-vegetal cells of blastulae and able to induce a complete secondary axis. *Cell* 1995; 81:85–94.

198. Brannon M, Kimelman D. Activation of Siamois by the Wnt pathway. *Dev Biol* 1996; 180:344–347.

199. Carnac G, Kodjabachian L, Gurdon JB, Lemaire P. The homeobox gene *Siamois* is a target of the Wnt dorsalisation pathway and triggers organiser activity in the absence of mesoderm. *Development* 1996; 122:3055–3065.

200. Cho KW, Blumberg B, Steinbeisser H, De Robertis RR. Molecular nature of Spemann's organizer: the role of the *Xenopus* homeobox gene goosecoid. *Cell* 1991; 67:1111–1120.

201. Steinbeisser H, De Robertis EM, Ku M, Kessler DS, Melton DM. *Xenopus* axis formation: induction of goosecoid by injected Xwnt-8 and activin mRNAs. *Development* 1993; 118:499–507.

202. Niehrs C, Keller R, Cho KW, De Robertis KD. The homeobox gene *goosecoid* controls cell migration in *Xenopus* embryos. *Cell* 1993; 72:491–503.

203. McKendry R, Hsu SC, Harland RM, Grosschedl R. LEF-1/TCF proteins mediate wnt-inducible transcription from the *Xenopus* nodal-related 3 promoter. *Dev Biol* 1997; 192:420–431.

Perhaps even more frequent than activating mutations, paracrine and autocrine stimulation of multiple GPCRs for neuropeptides and prostaglandins has been reported in a variety of human malignancies, including bombesin, gastrin-releasing peptide (GRP), neuromedin B, bradykinin, cholecystokinin (CCK), galanin, neurotensin, and vasopressin, in human small cell lung cancer (SCLC) *(24–28)*, as well as neuropeptide receptors and their agonists in colon adenomas and carcinomas *(29)* and gastric hyperplasia *(30)*. In this regard, the potential use of receptor antagonists or antibodies against these peptides has been successfully explored in certain in vitro and in vivo models for SCLC, providing the basis for the future development of new treatment modalities *(27,31,32)*.

Surprisingly, recent data suggest that functional GPCRs are also encoded by DNA viruses, including human cytomegalovirus (HCMV) *(33,34)*, herpes virus saimiri (HVS) *(35)*, and Kaposi's sarcoma-associated herpesvirus (KSHV) *(36)*. Most of these viral-encoded GPCRs are highly related to the chemokine receptor family *(37,38)*, and their function, although still unclear, might be to help elude natural host defenses through molecular mimicry of proteins normally involved in host defense mechanisms *(38)*. The most direct evidence linking these GPCRs to aberrant cell growth came from the observation that the expression of the KSHV-encoded GPCR, which is likely to represent a constitutively active chemokine receptor, is sufficient to transform murine fibroblasts in culture *(36)*. In addition, recent evidence has indicated that the KSHV-GPCR can actively participate in the angiogenic process *(39)*.

The ability of GPCRs to affect cell growth suggests that their immediate downstream targets, the heterotrimeric G proteins, would also harbor transforming potential if mutationally activated. Indeed, constitutively active mutants of $G\alpha_i$, $G\alpha_q$, $G\alpha_0$, $G\alpha_{12}$, and $G\alpha_{13}$ were shown to display oncogenic properties in a variety of cellular systems. Naturally occurring activated mutants were also identified in several disease states, including cancer (reviewed in *40*). These observations led to the designation of several activated Gα mutants as oncogenes, including $G\alpha_s$, $G\alpha_{i2}$, and $G\alpha_{12}$, referred to as the *gsp (41)*, *gip2 (42)*, and *gep* oncogene *(43,44)*, respectively.

3. MULTIPLE INTRACELLULAR PATHWAYS MEDIATE THE PROLIFERATIVE EFFECT OF G-PROTEIN-COUPLED RECEPTORS

Although certain mitogenic GPCRs, including those for LPA and thrombin, inhibit adenyl cyclases through G_i proteins, no direct correlation between decreased intracellular levels of cyclic adenosine monophosphate (cAMP) and cell proliferation was observed. By contrast, the activation of phospholipase C and enhanced phosphatidylinositol bisphosphate (PIP_2) hydrolysis has frequently been associated with mitogenesis *(16)*. However, the use of ectopically expressed mutants of certain tyrosine kinase receptors suggested that in some cellular settings PIP_2 hydrolysis may be neither necessary nor sufficient for cell proliferation *(45,46)*. Similarly, several agonists acting on GPCRs can effectively induce PIP_2-hydrolysis, but fail to stimulate growth when added alone to quiescent cells *(15)*. Although it is not possible to exclude that prolonged activation of the phospholipase C-PIP_2 hydrolysis pathway may stimulate cell-growth, and even cause cell transformation in certain cellular systems, currently available information suggests that additional biochemical routes participate in mitogenic signaling through GPCRs. As discussed in other chapters in this book, one such critical component of intracellular signaling pathway(s) controlling cell proliferation is represented by the family of extracellular signal-regulated kinases (ERKs) or mitogen-activated protein (MAP) kinases (*see* Chapter 9). Thus, during the past few years, considerable efforts have been made to elucidate how the G-protein-linked family of cell surface receptors activate MAPKs.

4. THE PATHWAY LINKING G-PROTEIN-COUPLED RECEPTORS TO MAPK

Many agonists acting on endogenously expressed GPCRs stimulate MAPK in a variety of cell types (*see* ref. *14* for a recent review). In this regard, both G_i-coupled, Ptx-sensitive, and G_q-coupled, Ptx-insensitive, receptors were found to activate MAPK by a poorly understood mechanism. In the case of G_q-coupled receptors, PKC-dependent and -independent pathways were both reported, but the expression in NIH 3T3 cells and other cells of mutationally activated $G\alpha_q$ did not result in enhanced MAPK activity (our unpublished results and *see below*). For G_i-coupled receptors, activation of MAPK was shown to be largely PKC independent *(47)*. As an approach to investigate the mechanism of MAPK activation by GPCRs, a number of laboratories have used the transient coexpression of an epitope-tagged form of MAPK together with GPCRs in readily transfectable cell lines, such as COS-7 and HEK-293 cells. An advantage of this system is that several proteins can be expressed simultaneously at very high levels, without the influence of biological changes that might be manifested during prolonged culturing of cells. In this system, 24–48 h after transfection of the corresponding expression plasmids the epitope tagged-MAPK can be immunoprecipitated with an anti-epitope monoclonal antibody, and its enzymatic activity assayed using standard in vitro kinase assays *(48,49)*. Using this approach, it was shown that both G_q- and G_i-coupled receptors could activate MAPK, respectively, in a Ptx-insensitive and -sensitive fashion *(49–51)*. By contrast, activated forms of $G\alpha_{i2}$, $G\alpha_q$, $G\alpha_s$, or $G\alpha_{12}$ did not induce any detectable increase in MAPK activity when assayed under identical experimental conditions *(49)*.

Activated GPCRs act as guanine-nucleotide exchange factors for heterotrimeric G proteins, inducing the release of GDP bound to $G\alpha$ and its replacement for GTP, leading to the subsequent dissociation of GTP-bound-$G\alpha$ from $\beta\gamma$ complexes *(52)*. Thus, the failure of mutationally activated $G\alpha$ subunits to activate MAPK, and the recent observation that free $\beta\gamma$ subunits can stimulate a variety of effector pathways *(52)* prompted the exploration of a role for $\beta\gamma$ heterodimers in signaling to the MAPK pathway. This led to the observation that membrane-bound forms of $\beta\gamma$ subunits can directly activate biochemical routes leading to MAPK activation *(49)*, and stimulated the search for molecules acting downstream of $G_{\beta\gamma}$ in this pathway. In this regard, it was shown that neither PLC-β nor PKC activation is necessary to stimulate MAPK activity by $\beta\gamma$ dimers, but Ras-interfering molecules prevented this response *(49,50)*, and $\beta\gamma$ subunits were later shown to be sufficient to induce the accumulation of Ras in the GTP-bound active form *(50)*. Taken together, these findings provided evidence that signaling from GPCRs to MAPK involves βγ heterodimers acting on a Ras-dependent pathway, thus suggesting that βγ subunits link heterotrimeric G proteins to small G proteins of the Ras superfamily.

The way in which GPCRs and $G_{\beta\gamma}$ subunits signal to Ras and MAPK is still being actively investigated. Pharmacological approaches using nonspecific tyrosine kinase blockers provided the first indication that tyrosine kinases might play a role in the activation of MAPKs by GPCRs *(53)* through the tyrosine phosphorylation of the adaptor protein Shc thereby causing the formation of Shc-GRB2 complexes *(54,55)*. Indeed, several non-receptor tyrosine kinases were later implicated in signaling from GPCR to MAPKs, including Src and several Src-like kinases, such as Fyn, Lyn, Yes, and Syk *(56,57)*, and a Ca^{2+} and PKC-dependent protein tyrosine kinase, Pyk2 *(58–60)*. Crosstalk with receptor tyrosine kinases, such PDGF and EGF receptors, was also found to participate in MAPK activation by GPCRs *(61,62)*. Thus, a number of receptor and nonreceptor tyrosine kinases might be able to link GPCRs to the Ras-MAPK pathway.

Several additional molecules were recently shown to participate in signaling from GPCRs to MAPK, including protein tyrosine phosphatases such as SH-PTP1 *(63)*, Ras-GRF *(64)*, and PI3Kγ *(65)*. Particularly for PI3Kγ, it was found to act downstream from $G_{\beta\gamma}$, and probably upstream of Src-like kinases and Shc, Grb2, Sos, and Ras, suggesting a potential mechanism whereby heterotrimeric G proteins can regulate nonreceptor tyrosine kinases and, in turn, control the MAPK pathway *(65)*. In addition, MAPK activation by GPCRs in a Ras-independent manner has also been reported *(66,67)*, suggesting that, in certain cellular settings, GPCRs may stimulate MAPKs by still to be identified biochemical routes that bypass the requirement for Ras.

One such example is the recent identification of a pathway linking $G\alpha_s$ and $G\alpha_i$ to the small GTP-binding protein Rap1A *(112,113)*. In these cases, MAP kinase can be stimulated by activating a Rap1A-dependent pathway that utilized B-Raf *(112)*, or by inhibiting a Rap1A-inhibitory pathway in other cellular systems *(113)*. Another example may involve PKCs, as direct activation of several PKC isoforms by phorbol esters has been shown to induce MAPK by a mechanism that remains unclear *(68)*. PKCs phosphorylate Raf *(69,70)*, but this does not result in increased Raf phosphorylating activity on its natural substrate, MEK *(71)*. In addition, PKC activation appears not to induce Ras-GTP accumulation in most cell types *(72)*; however, it activates MAPK in a Ras-dependent manner in many cellular settings *(47,73,74)*. Furthermore, recently available data suggest that PKCs stimulate Ras and MAPKs by a mechanism distinct from those known to mediate Ras activation by receptors of the tyrosine kinase class *(75)*. Nevertheless, because Ras alone is not sufficient to activate Raf fully in vitro *(71)* or when coexpressed in *Sf9* cells *(76)*, it is still possible that PKCs might facilitate the full activation of Raf upon binding to Ras *(74)*. Thus, PKC activation may play a critical role in MAPK stimulation under conditions of submaximal activation of Ras by cell surface receptors. Such a scenario might explain why G_q-coupled receptors can activate MAPK in a PKC-dependent *(47)*, fully PKC-independent *(77)*, or partially PKC-dependent *(78)* manner. These apparently conflicting results may depend on the cellular system and the level

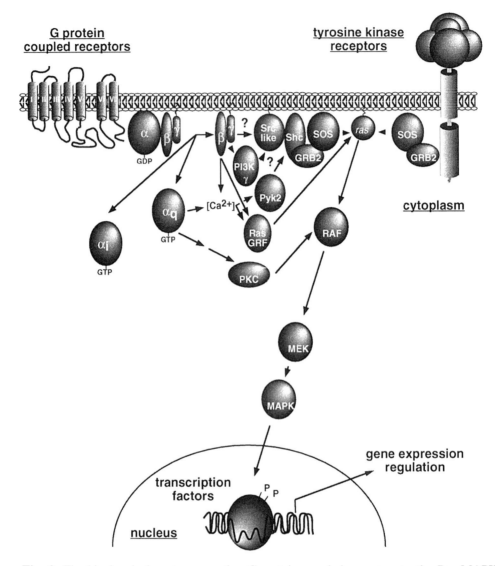

Fig. 2. The biochemical route connecting G-protein-coupled receptors to the Ras-MAPK signaling pathway (*see text* for details).

of receptor expression, which might determine the relative contribution of the $G\alpha_q$–phospholipase–C–PKC and the $Gq_{\beta\gamma}$–Ras pathways in signaling to MAPK from G_q-coupled GPCRs.

Additional signaling molecules may also participate in MAPK activation by GPCRs and $G_{\beta\gamma}$. However, many of the most likely candidates may have already been identified (Fig. 2). Of interest, many of the proteins suggested to participate in GPCR signaling exhibit a very restricted tissue distribution *(58,64,79)*. Thus, the nature of the molecules linking GPCRs and $G_{\beta\gamma}$ to MAPK stimulation would strictly depend on the repertoire of signaling molecules available in each particular tissue or cell type.

5. THE PATHWAY CONNECTING GPCRS TO THE C-JUN PROMOTER: NOVEL KINASE CASCADES

Once MAPKs are activated, they translocate to the nucleus, where they phosphorylate transcription factors, thereby enhancing their transactivating activity (*see* Chapter 9). Thus, as GPCRs and tyrosine kinases converge at the level of Ras to activate MAPKs, stimulation of both classes of cell surface receptors would be expected to lead to he same pattern of gene expression. However, that was found not to be the case *(80)*. In particular, c-*jun* expression was enhanced dramatically only in response to GPCR stimulation, and this response did not correlate with MAPK activation *(80)*. This observation suggested that GPCRs control a distinct biochemical route regulating gene expression. As described in Chapter 9, a novel family of enzymes structurally related to, but clearly distinct from, MAPKs, the jun kinases (JNKs) *(81)*, or stress activated-protein kinases (SAPKs) *(82)*, selectively phosphorylate the N-terminal transactivating domain of the c-*jun* protein, thereby increasing its transcriptional activity. Consistent with the idea that JNK regulates c-Jun activity and the earlier observation that c-Jun dimers enhance c-*jun* expression *(83)*, it was observed that GPCRs, but not tyrosine kinase receptors, potently activate JNK *(80)*.

An unexpected prediction from these studies was that distinct upstream signaling molecules might regulate JNK and MAPK. That, together with the observation that two small GTP-binding proteins of the Rho family, Rac and Cdc42, can control the activity of a serine-threonine kinase in a fashion analogous to that of Ras acting on Raf *(84)* (*see* Chapters 11 and 13), prompted investigators at several laboratories to examine whether the Rho family of GTPases participates in signaling to the JNK pathway. This led to the finding that Rac1 and Cdc42 can initiate an independent kinase cascade regulating JNK activity *(85)*. Many novel components of this pathway have been recently identified, and they include several members of the Ste20 family of serine-threonine kinases (*see* Chapter 11), members of the Ste11 family of kinases, including MEKK, and two members of the Ste7 class of kinases, including Sek/JNKK1/MKK4 and MKK7 *(86–88)*. Detailed examination of the pathway linking GPCRs to JNK provided evidence that free $\beta\gamma$ dimers *(89)* and, in some cellular systems, $G\alpha_{12}$ *(90)*, convey signals from this class of receptors to JNK.

The simplest model of how GPCRs induce c-*jun* expression involves the activation of Rac or Cdc42, or both, through $\beta\gamma$ dimers and $G\alpha_{12}$ and the consequent stimulation of a kinase cascade leading to JNK activation, which, in turn, phosphorylate c-Jun, and phospho-c-Jun would then enhance the transcription of c-*jun* by acting on an AP-1 site found in the c-*jun* promoter *(91)*. However, the idea that such a linear series of events regulate c-*jun* expression has been recently challenged *(92)*. Unexpectedly, it was observed that a critical regulatory element in the c-*jun* promoter binds members of the MEF2 family of transcription factors *(92)*, and one such MEF2 protein, MEF2C, was recently found to be regulated by the p38 MAPK *(93)*. Thus, expression of c-*jun* may be under the control of p38-related pathways. Further analysis of kinases acting on MEF2 led to the demonstration that a novel MAPK, ERK5, phosphorylate MEF2C thereby enhancing its transcriptional activity (*see* Chapter 9), and ongoing work in our laboratory strongly suggest that ERK5, p38 and ERK6 can stimulate the activity of

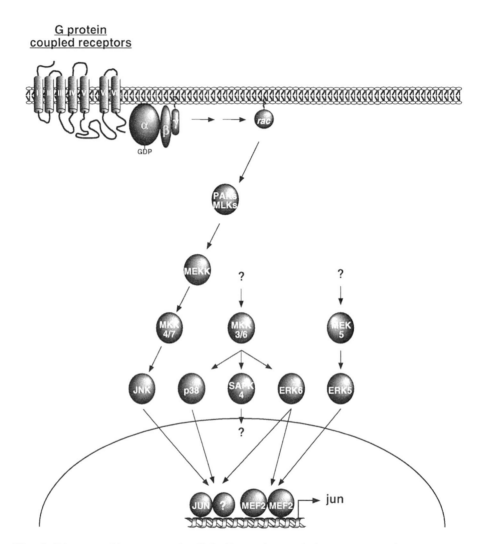

Fig. 3. Divergent kinase cascades link G-protein-coupled receptors to the c-*jun* promoter (*see text* for details).

the c-*jun* promoter by acting on its MEF2 site *(115)*. We can conclude that GPCRs control c-*jun* expression through several independent cytoplasmic MAPK cascades that converge in the nucleus to stimulate transcription factors acting on the c-*jun* promoter (*see* Fig. 3).

6. A NOVEL PATHWAY LINKING GPCRS TO Rho AND TO THE C-*Fos* SERUM RESPONSE ELEMENT

The complexity of regulatory molecules controlling the transcriptional activity of the c-*jun* promoter is not unique and can be also found in the promoter region of other early responsive genes. For example, several regulatory elements can be identified in the c-*fos* promoter *(94)*. Among them, the serum response element (SRE) is believed to play a central regulatory role *(95,96)*, as this sequence is necessary and sufficient for the rapid induction of *c-fos* by most growth-promoting stimuli *(97,98)*. A number of proteins that bind the c-*fos* SRE can mediate SRE-dependent transcription *(95,96)*, including serum response factor (SRF), which binds the SRE in vivo and in vitro as a dimer *(95,96)*. Another protein forms a ternary complex with SRE and the SRF dimer, and has been therefore termed ternary complex factor or p62[TCF] *(96)*. Interestengly, TCF can be phosphorylated by MAPK and JNK *(87,99,100)*, providing a mechanism whereby SRE activity can be regulated in response to the many external stimuli activating these MAPKs. SRE can also be regulated in a TCF-independent manner, and certain TCF-independent signaling pathways acting on SRE have been shown to be controlled by the small GTP-binding protein Rho *(101)* through a novel pathway independent of any MAPK described to date. The available data suggest that GPCRs can activate SRE through this TCF-independent pathway *(101)*. In addition, a recent report provided evidence to support that RhoA or other Rho-related proteins act as integral components of this biochemical route connecting GPCRs, acting either directly on Rho or through $G\alpha_{12}$, to both transcriptional activation of the SRE and neoplastic transformation *(102)*.

The mechanism whereby GPCRs and $G\alpha_{12}$ proteins activate the Rho family of small GTP-binding proteins was unknown, but recent findings have shed new light on this issue. It has been reported recently that $G\alpha_{13}$ interacts, in vitro, with a Rho exchange factor, p115 RhoGEF, through a region that shares similarity to RGS proteins (RGS domain) and stimulate its exchange activity toward Rho *(103)*. This RGS domain of p115 RhoGEF also displays GAP activity on both $G\alpha_{12}$ and $G\alpha_{13}$ *(104)*. Furthermore, we have recently identified a novel PDZ-domain containing exchange factor for Rho, which was termed PDZ-RhoGEF, that directly associates with $G\alpha_{12}$ and $G\alpha_{13}$ through its RGS domain in vivo, thereby mediating the Rho-dependent SRE activation *(116)*. Together, these findings suggest the existence of a novel mechanism whereby GPCRs can stimulate Rho-dependent pathways, involving the activation of $G\alpha_{12}$ and/or $G\alpha_{13}$ and their physical association with Rho-exchange factors containing RGS domains such as p115 RhoGEF and PDZ-RhoGEF. Of interest, recent work suggest that the effective coupling between receptors and $G\alpha_{12}/G\alpha_{13}$ and Rho-exchange factors may involve the activation of non-receptor tyrosine kinases, particularly from the Tec/Btk family *(105,106)*. How now the interplay between these signaling molecules result in Rho activation is likely to be fully elucidated in the foreseeable future.

Additional mechanisms linking GPCRs to Rho might also exist, as it has been reported that certain GPCRs carrying amino acid sequence Asn-Pro-X-X-Tyr in their seventh transmembrane domain can form molecular complexes with the small GTPases RhoA and ARF *(107)*. $G_{\beta\gamma}$ subunits might also affect Rho pathways, as they can interact with Rho proteins and ARF in vitro *(108,109)*, and a functional Rho binding domain (termed ROCK/Kinectin) has been described in G_β and in other signaling polypeptides *(110)*. Thus, through their interaction with Rho and Arf, $G_{\beta\gamma}$ complexes may play a role in intracellular vesicular trafficking and secretion, as recently reported *(111)*.

7. THE NEXT FRONTIER: FROM SIGNAL TRANSDUCTION TO SIGNAL INTEGRATION

The emerging picture is that GPCRs induce the activation of heterotrimeric G proteins, and then free βγ dimers or GTP-bound α subunits stimulate small GTP-binding proteins of the Ras superfamily which, in turn, control the activity of parallel kinase cascades resulting in the phosphorylation of critical nuclear transcription factors. However, stimulation of GPCRs also activate a variety of second messenger generating systems, including a phospholipase A_2, phospholipase C, phospholipase D, sphingomyelinases, sphingosine kinases, lipid kinases, calcium mobilizing systems, phosphodiesterases, adenylyl and guanylyl cylcases, certain ion channels and transporters, and oxidases, and even other cell surface receptors, such as PDGF and EGF receptors. These, in turn, stimulate a number of highly interconnected cytoplasmic signaling pathways that lead to a temporally distinct pattern of activation of members of the MAPK superfamily. Ultimately, these kinases will reach the nucleus and affect an intrincated balance of nuclear regulatory molecules controlling gene expression. The final biological outcome, including cell proliferation, will most likely result from the temporal integration of each of these signaling pathways, rather than resulting from a single series of sequential events. Recent advances in our understanding of the molecular mechanisms involved in signal transduction will now afford the possibility of unraveling the intricacies of how these signals are integrated to promote cell growth, and of how perturbation of this signaling network can result in malignant transformation. These efforts are expected to provide extraordinary opportunities to identify previously unsuspected molecular targets for pharmacological intervention in a number of disease states, including cancer.

REFERENCES

1. Dohlman HG, Caron MG, Lefkowitz RJ. A family of receptors coupled to guanine nucleotide regulatory proteins. *Biochemistry* 1987; 26:2657–2664.
2. Bourne HR. How receptors talk to trimeric G proteins. *Curr Opin Cell Biol* 1997; 9:134–142.
3. Wess J. G-protein-coupled receptors: Molecular mechanisms involved in receptor activation, selectivity of G-protein recognition. *FASEB J* 1997; 1:346–354.
4. Altenbach C, Yang K, Farrens K, Farahbakhsh KF, Khorana HG, Hubbell WL. Structural features, light-dependent changes in the cytoplasmic interhelical E-F loop region of rhodopsin: A site-directed spin-labeling study. *Biochemistry* 1996; 35:12,470–12,478.
5. Sondek J, Bohm A, Lambright A, Hamm AH, Sigler PB. Crystal structure of a G-protein beta gamma dimer at 2.1A resolution [see comments] [corrected] [published erratum appears in *Nature* 1996; 29;379(6568):847]. *Nature* 1996; 379:369–374.
6. Lambright DG, Sondek J, Bohm A, Skiba A, Hamm A, Sigler PB. The 2.0 Å crystal structure of a heterotrimeric G protein. *Nature* 1996; 379:311–319.
7. Sondek J, Lambright DG, Noel DN, Hamm HE, Sigler PB. GTPase mechanism of G proteins from the 1.7-A crystal structure of transducin alpha-GDP-AIF-4. *Nature* 1994; 372:276–279.
8. Lambright DG, Noel JP, Hamm JH, Sigler PB. Structural determinants for activation of the alpha-subunit of a heterotrimeric G protein. *Nature* 1994; 369:621–628.
9. Wilkie TM, Gilbert DJ, Olsen DO, Chen XN, Amatruda XA, Korenberg JR, Trask JT, de Jong P, Reed JP, Simon JS, et al. Evolution of the mammalian G protein alpha subunit multigene family. *Nature Genet* 1992; 1:85–91.
10. Ui M, Katada T. Bacterial toxins as probe for receptor-Gi coupling. *Adv Second Messenger Phosphoprotein Res* 1990; 24:63–69.
11. Chambard JC, Paris S, G LA, Pouyssegur J. Two growth factor signalling pathways in fibroblasts distinguished by pertussis toxin. *Nature* 1987; 326:800–803.

12. Pouyssegur J, Chambard JC, G LA, Magnaldo I, Seuwen K. Transmembrane signalling pathways initiating cell growth in fibroblasts. *Philos Trans R Soc Lond B Biol Sci* 1988; 320:427–436.

13. van Corven EJ, Groenink A, Jalink K, Eichholtz T, Moolenaar WH. Lysophosphatidate-induced cell proliferation: Identification, dissection of signaling pathways mediated by G proteins. *Cell* 1989; 59:45–54.

14. van Biesen T, Luttrell LM, Hawes LH, Lefkowitz RJ. Mitogenic signaling via G protein-coupled receptors. *Endocr Rev* 1996; 17:698–714.

15. Moolenaar WH. G-protein-coupled receptors, phosphoinositide hydrolysis, cell proliferation. *Cell Growth Differ* 1991; 2:359–364.

16. Rozengurt E. Early signals in the mitogenic response. *Science* 1986; 234:161–166.

17. Gutkind JS. The pathways connecting G protein-coupled receptors to the nucleus through divergent mitogen-activated protein kinase cascades. *J Biol Chem* 1998; 273:1839–1842.

18. Nagata A, Ito M, Iwata N, Kuno J, Takano H, Minowa O, Chihara K, Matsui T, Noda T. G protein-coupled cholecystokinin-B/gastrin receptors are responsible for physiological cell growth of the stomach mucosa in vivo. *Proc Natl Acad Sci USA* 1996; 93:11,825–11,830.

19. Young D, Waitches G, Birchmeier C, Fasano O, Wigler M. Isolation and characterization of a new cellular oncogene encoding a protein with multiple potential transmembrane domains. *Cell* 1986; 45:711–719.

20. Julius D, Livelli TJ, Jessell TJ, Axel R. Ectopic expression of the serotonin 1c receptor, the triggering of malignant transformation. *Science* 1989; 244:1057–1062.

21. Gutkind JS, Novotny EA, Brann EB, Robbins KC. Muscarinic acetylcholine receptor subtypes as agonist-dependent oncogenes. *Proc Natl Acad Sci USA* 1991; 88:4703–4707.

22. Allen LF, Lefkowitz RJ, Caron RC, Cotecchia S. G-protein-coupled receptor genes as protooncogenes: constitutively activating mutation of the alpha 1B-adrenergic receptor enhances mitogenesis, tumorigenicity. *Proc Natl Acad Sci USA* 1991; 88:11,354–11,358.

23. Parma J, Duprez L, Van Sande J, Cochaux P, Gervy C, Mockel J, Dumont J, Vassart G. Somatic mutations in the thyrotropin receptor gene cause hyperfunctioning thyroid adenomas. *Nature* 1993; 365:649–651.

24. Cuttitta F, Carney DN, Mulshine J, Moody TW, Fedorko J, Fischler A, Minna A. Bombesin-like peptides can function as autocrine growth factors in human small-cell lung cancer. *Nature* 1985; 316:823–826.

25. Schuller HM. Receptor-mediated mitogenic signals, lung cancer. *Cancer Cells* 1991; 3:496–503.

26. Schuller HM. Neuroendocrine lung cancer: A receptor-mediated disease? *Exp Lung Res* 1991; 17:837–852.

27. Sethi T, Langdon S, Smyth J, Rozengurt E. Growth of small cell lung cancer cells: Stimulation by multiple neuropeptides, inhibition by broad spectrum antagonists in vitro, in vivo. *Cancer Res* 1992; 52:2737s–2742s.

28. Moody TW, Cuttitta F. Growth factor, peptide receptors in small cell lung cancer. *Life Sci* 1993; 52:1161–1173.

29. Hoosein NM, Kiener PA, Curry PC, Rovati LC, McGilbra LM, Brattain MG. Antiproliferative effects of gastrin receptor antagonists, antibodies to gastrin on human colon carcinoma cell lines. *Cancer Res* 1988; 48:7179–7183.

30. Tahara E. Growth factors, oncogenes in human gastrointestinal carcinomas. *J Cancer Res Clin Oncol* 1990; 116:121–131.

31. Langdon S, Sethi T, Ritchie A, Muir M, Smyth J, Rozengurt E. Broad spectrum neuropeptide antagonists inhibit the growth of small cell lung cancer in vivo. *Cancer Res* 1992; 52:4554–4557.

32. Thomas F, Arvelo F, Antoine E, Jacrot M, Poupon M. Antitumoral activity of bombesin analogues on small cell lung cancer xenografts: relationship with bombesin receptor expression. *Cancer Res* 1992; 52:4872–4877.

33. Chee MS, Satchwell SC, Preddie E, Weston E, Barrell BG. Human cytomegalovirus encodes three G protein-coupled receptor homologues [see comments]. *Nature* 1990; 344:774–777.

34. Bankier AT, Beck S, Bohni R, Brown R, Cerny R, Chee MS, Hutchison CAD, Kouzarides T, Martignetti JA, Preddie E, et al. The DNA sequence of the human cytomegalovirus genome. *DNA Seq* 1991; 2:1–12.

35. Nicholas J, Cameron KR, Honess RW. Herpesvirus saimiri encodes homologues of G protein-coupled receptors, cyclins. *Nature* 1992; 355:362–365.

36. Arvanitakis L, Geras-Raaka E, Varma A, Gershengorn A, Cesarman E. Human herpesvirus KSHV encodes a constitutively active G-protein-coupled receptor linked to cell proliferation. *Nature* 1997; 385:347–350.

37. Neote K, DiGregorio D, Mak D, Horuk R, Schall R. Molecular cloning, functional expression, signaling characteristics of a C–C chemokine receptor. *Cell* 1993; 2:415–425.

38. Ahuja SK, Murphy PM. Molecular piracy of mammalian interleukin-8 receptor type B by herpesvirus saimiri. *J Biol Chem* 1993; 268:20,691–20,694.

39. Bais C, Santomasso B, Coso O, Arvanitakis L, Raaka L, Gutkind JS, Asch AS, Cesarman E, Gershengorn MC, Mesri MM. G-protein-coupled receptor of Kaposi's sarcoma-associated herpesvirus is a viral oncogene, angiogenesis activator. *Nature* 1998; 391:86–89.

40. Dhanasekaran N, Heasley LE, Johnson GL. G protein-coupled receptor systems involved in cell growth, oncogenesis. *Endocr Rev* 1995; 16:259–270.

41. Landis CA, Masters SB, Spada A, Pace AM, Bourne AB, Vallar L. GTPase inhibiting mutations activate the alpha chain of Gs, stimulate adenylyl cyclase in human pituitary tumours. *Nature* 1989; 340:692–696.

42. Lyons J, Landis CA, Harsh G, Vallar L, Grunewald K, Feichtinger H, Duh H, Clark HC, Kawasaki E, Bourne E, et al. Two G protein oncogenes in human endocrine tumors. *Science* 1990; 249:655–659.

43. Xu N, Voyno-Yasenetskaya T, Gutkind JS. Potent transforming activity of the G13 alpha subunit defines a novel family of oncogenes. *Biochem Biophys Res Commun* 1994; 201:603–609.

44. Xu N, Bradley L, Ambdukar I, Gutkind JS. A mutant alpha subunit of G12 potentiates the eicosanoid pathway, is highly oncogenic in NIH 3T3 cells. *Proc Natl Acad Sci USA* 1993; 90:6741–6745.

45. Mohammadi M, Dionne CA, Li W, Li N, Spivak T, Honegger T, Jaye M, Schlessinger J. Point mutation in FGF receptor eliminates phosphatidylinositol hydrolysis without affecting mitogenesis. *Nature* 1992; 358:681–684.

46. Coughlin SR, Escobedo JA, Williams LT. Role of phosphatidylinositol kinase in PDGF receptor signal transduction. *Science* 1989; 243:1191–1194.

47. Hawes BE, van Biesen T, Koch BT, Luttrell BL, Lefkowitz RJ. Distinct pathways of Gi-Gq-mediated mitogen-activated protein kinase activation. *J Biol Chem* 1995; 270:17,148–17,153.

48. Pages G, Lenormand P, L'Allemain G, Chambard G, Meloche S, Pouyssegur J. Mitogen-activated protein kinases p42mapk, p44mapk are required for fibroblast proliferation. *Proc Natl Acad Sci USA* 1993; 90:8319–8323.

49. Crespo P, Xu N, Simonds N, Gutkind JS. Ras-dependent activation of MAP kinase pathway mediated by G-protein beta gamma subunits. *Nature* 1994; 69:418–420.

50. Koch WJ, Hawes BE, Allen BA, Lefkowitz RJ. Direct evidence that Gi-coupled receptor stimulation of mitogen-activated protein kinase is mediated by G beta gamma activation of p21ras. *Proc Natl Acad Sci USA* 1994; 91:12,706–12,710.

51. Faure M, Voyno-Yasenetskaya TA, Bourne HR. cAMP, beta gamma subunits of heterotrimeric G proteins stimulate the mitogen-activated protein kinase pathway in COS-7 cells. *J Biol Chem* 1994; 269:7851–7854.

52. Clapham DE, Neer EJ. G protein beta gamma subunits. *Annu Rev Pharmacol Toxicol* 1997; 37:167–203.

53. Hordijk PL, Verlaan I, van Corven I, Moolenaar WH. Protein tyrosine phosphorylation induced by lysophosphatidic acid in Rat-1 fibroblasts. Evidence that phosphorylation of map kinase is mediated by the Gi-p21ras pathway. *J Biol Chem* 1994; 269:645–651.

54. van Biesen T, Hawes BE, Luttrell BL, Krueger KM, Touhara K, Porfiri E, Sakaue M, Luttrell M, Lefkowitz RJ. Receptor-tyrosine-kinase-, G beta gamma-mediated MAP kinase activation by a common signalling pathway. *Nature* 1995; 376:781–784.

55. Chen Y, Grall D, Salcini D, Pelicci DP, Pouyssegur J, Van Obberghen-Schilling E. Shc adaptor proteins are key transducers of mitogenic signaling mediated by the G protein-coupled thrombin receptor. *EMBO J* 1996; 15:1037–1044.

56. Ptasznik A, Traynor-Kaplan A, Bokoch GM. G protein-coupled chemoattractant receptors regulate Lyn tyrosine kinase.Shc adapter protein signaling. *J Biol Chem* 1995; 270:19,969–19,973.

57. Wan Y, Kurosaki T, Huang T. Tyrosine kinases in activation of the MAP kinase cascade by G-protein-coupled receptors. *Nature* 1996; 380:541–544.

58. Lev S, Moreno H, Martinez R, Canoll P, Peles E, Musacchio E, Plowman EP, Rudy B, Schlessinger J. Protein tyrosine kinase PYK2 involved in Ca^{2+}-induced regulation of ion channel, MAP kinase functions. *Nature* 1995; 376:737–345.

59. Dikic I, Tokiwa G, Lev S, Courtneidge S, Schlessinger J. A role for Pyk2, Src in linking G-protein-coupled receptors with MAP kinase activation. *Nature* 1996; 383:547–550.

60. Della Rocca GJ, van Biesen T, Daaka Y, Luttrell Y, Luttrell YL, Lefkowitz RJ. Ras-dependent mitogen-activated protein kinase activation by G protein-coupled receptors. Convergence of Gi-, Gq-mediated pathways on calcium/calmodulin, Pyk2, Src kinase. *J Biol Chem* 1997; 272:19,125–19,132.

61. Linseman DA, Benjamin CW, Jones DA. Convergence of angiotensin II, platelet-derived growth factor receptor signaling cascades in vascular smooth muscle cells. *J Biol Chem* 1995; 270:12,563–12,568.

62. Daub H, Weiss FU, Wallasch C, Ullrich A. Role of transactivation of the EGF receptor in signalling by G-protein-coupled receptors. *Nature* 1996; 379:557–560.

63. Gaits F, Li RY, Bigay J, Ragab A, Ragab-Thomas A, Chap H. G-protein beta gamma subunits mediate specific phosphorylation of the protein-tyrosine phosphatase SH-PTP1 induced by lysophosphatidic acid. *J Biol Chem* 1996; 271:20,151–20,155.

64. Mattingly RR, Macara IG. Phosphorylation-dependent activation of the Ras-GRF/CDC25Mm exchange factor by muscarinic receptors, G-protein beta gamma subunits. *Nature* 1996; 382:268–272.

65. Lopez-Ilasaca M, Crespo P, Pellici P, Gutkind JS, Wetzker R. Linkage of G protein-coupled receptors to the MAPK signaling pathway through PI 3-kinase gamma. *Science* 1997; 275:394–397.

66. Pace AM, Faure M, Bourne M. Gi2-mediated activation of the MAP kinase cascade. *Mol Biol Cell* 1995; 6:1685–1695.

67. Takahashi T, Kawahara Y, Okuda M, Ueno H, Takeshita A, Yokoyama M. Angiotensin II stimulates mitogen-activated protein kinases, protein synthesis by a Ras-independent pathway in vascular smooth muscle cells. *J Biol Chem* 1997; 272:16,018–16,022.

68. Schonwasser DC, Marais RM, Marshall RM, Parker PJ. Activation of the mitogen-activated protein kinase/extracellular signal- regulated kinase pathway by conventional, novel, atypical protein kinase C isotypes. *Mol Cell Biol* 1998; 18:790–798.

69. Kolch W, Heidecker G, Kochs G, Hummel R, Vahidi H, Mischak H, Finkenzeller G, Marme D, Rapp D. Protein kinase C alpha activates RAF-1 by direct phosphorylation. *Nature* 1993; 364:249–252.

70. Heidecker G, Kolch W, Morrison W, Rapp UR. The role of Raf-1 phosphorylation in signal transduction. *Adv Cancer Res* 1992; 58:53–73.

71. Macdonald SG, Crews CM, Wu L, Driller J, Clark R, Erikson R, McCormick F. Reconstitution of the Raf-1-MEK-ERK signal transduction pathway in vitro [published erratum appears in *Mol Cell Biol* 1994; 14:2223–2224]. *Mol Cell Biol* 1993; 13:6615–6620.

72. Bos JL. p21ras: An oncoprotein functioning in growth factor-induced signal transduction. *Eur J Cancer* 31A, 1051–1054.

73. Thomas SM, DeMarco M, D'Arcangelo G, Halegoua S, Brugge S. Ras is essential for nerve growth factor-, phorbol ester-induced tyrosine phosphorylation of MAP kinases. *Cell* 1992; 68:1031–1040.

74. Burgering BM, Bos JL. Regulation of Ras-mediated signalling: More than one way to skin a cat. *Trends Biochem Sci* 1995; 20:18–22.

75. Marais R, Light Y, Mason C, Paterson H, Olson H, Marshall CJ. Requirement of Ras-GTP-Raf complexes for activation of Raf-1 by protein kinase C. *Science* 1998; 280:109–112.

76. Williams NG, Roberts TM. Signal transduction pathways involving the Raf proto-oncogene. *Cancer Metastasis Rev* 1994; 13:105–116.

77. Charlesworth A, Rozengurt E. Bombesin, neuromedin B stimulate the activation of p42(mapk), p74(raf-1) via a protein kinase C-independent pathway in Rat-1 cells. *Oncogene* 1997; 14:2323–2329.

78. Crespo P, Xu N, Daniotti N, Troppmair J, Rapp J, Gutkind JS. Signaling through transforming G protein-coupled receptors in NIH 3T3 cells involves c-Raf activation. Evidence for a protein kinase C-independent pathway. *J Biol Chem* 1994; 269:21,103–21,109.

79. Stoyanov B, Volinia S, Hanck T, Rubio I, Loubtchenkov M, Malek D, Stoyanova S, Vanhaesebroeck B, Dhand R, Nurnberg B, et al. Cloning, characterization of a G protein-activated human phosphoinositide-3 kinase. *Science* 1995; 269:690–693.

80. Coso OA, Chiariello M, Kalinec G, Kyriakis G, Woodgett J, Gutkind JS. Transforming G protein-coupled receptors potently activate JNK (SAPK). Evidence for a divergence from the tyrosine kinase signaling pathway. *J Biol Chem* 1995; 270:5620–5624.

81. Derijard B, Hibi M, Wu M, Barrett T, Su B, Deng T, Karin M, Davis M. JNK1: A protein kinase stimulated by UV light, Ha-Ras that binds, phosphorylates the c-Jun activation domain. *Cell* 1994; 76:1025–1037.

82. Kyriakis JM, Banerjee P, Nikolakaki E, Dai T, Rubie T, Ahmad TA, Avruch J, Woodgett J. The stress-activated protein kinase subfamily of c-Jun kinases. *Nature* 1994; 369:156–160.

83. Karin M. Signal transduction from the cell surface to the nucleus through the phosphorylation of transcription factors. *Curr Opin Cell Biol* 1994; 6:415–424.

84. Manser E, Leung T, Salihuddin H, Zhao H, Lim L. A brain serine/threonine protein kinase activated by Cdc42, Rac1. *Nature* 1994; 367:40–46.

85. Coso OA, Chiariello M, Yu M, Teramoto H, Crespo P, Xu N, Miki T, Gutkind JS. The small GTP-binding proteins Rac1, Cdc42 regulate the activity of the JNK/SAPK signaling pathway. *Cell* 1995; 81:1137–1146.

86. Tournier C, Whitmarsh AJ, Cavanagh J, Barrett T, Davis T. Mitogen-activated protein kinase kinase 7 is an activator of the c-Jun NH2-terminal kinase. *Proc Natl Acad Sci USA* 1997; 94:7337–7342.

87. Whitmarsh AJ, Yang SH, Su SS, Sharrocks AD, Davis RJ. Role of p38, JNK mitogen-activated protein kinases in the activation of ternary complex factors. *Mol Cell Biol* 1997; 17:2360–2371.

88. Fanger GR, Gerwins P, Widmann C, Jarpe C, Johnson GL. MEKKs, GCKs, MLKs, PAKs, TAKs, tpls: Upstream regulators of the c-Jun amino-terminal kinases? *Curr Opin Genet Dev* 1997; 7:67–74.

89. Coso OA, Teramoto H, Simonds H, Gutkind JS. Signaling from G protein-coupled receptors to c-Jun kinase involves beta gamma subunits of heterotrimeric G proteins acting on a Ras, Rac1-dependent pathway. *J Biol Chem* 1996; 271:3963–3966.

90. Prasad MV, Dermott JM, Heasley JH, Johnson GL, Dhanasekaran N. Activation of Jun kinase/stress-activated protein kinase by GTPase-deficient mutants of G alpha 12, G alpha 13. *J Biol Chem* 1995; 270:18,655–18,659.

91. Karin M. The regulation of AP-1 activity by mitogen-activated protein kinases. *J Biol Chem* 1995; 270:16,483–16,486.

92. Coso OA, Montaner S, Fromm C, Lacal C, Prywes R, Teramoto H, Gutkind JS. Signaling from G protein-coupled receptors to the c-jun promoter involves the MEF2 transcription factor. Evidence for a novel c-jun amino-terminal kinase-independent pathway. *J Biol Chem* 1997; 272:20,691–20,697.

93. Han J, Jiang Y, Li Z, Kravchenko Z, Ulevitch RJ. Activation of the transcription factor MEF2C by the MAP kinase p38 in inflammation. *Nature* 1997; 386:296–299.

94. Hipskind RA, Nordheim A. Functional dissection in vitro of the human c-fos promoter. *J Biol Chem* 1991; 266:19,583–19,592.

95. Treisman R. Ternary complex factors: Growth factor regulated transcriptional activators. *Curr Opin Genet Dev* 1994; 4:96–101.

96. Treisman R. Journey to the surface of the cell: Fos regulation, the SRE. *EMBO J* 1995; 14:4905–4913.

97. Johansen FE, Prywes R. Two pathways for serum regulation of the c-fos serum response element require specific sequence elements, a minimal domain of serum response factor. *Mol Cell Biol* 1994; 14:5920–5928.

98. Greenberg ME, Siegfried Z, Ziff Z. Mutation of the c-fos gene dyad symmetry element inhibits serum inducibility of transcription in vivo, the nuclear regulatory factor binding in vitro. *Mol Cell Biol* 1987; 7:1217–1225.

99. Cavigelli M, Dolfi F, Claret F, Karin M. Induction of c-fos expression through JNK-mediated TCF/Elk-1 phosphorylation. *EMBO J* 1995; 14:5957–5964.

100. Gille H, Strahl T, Shaw T. Activation of ternary complex factor Elk-1 by stress-activated protein kinases. *Curr Biol* 1995; 5:1191–1200.

101. Hill CS, Wynne J, Treisman R. The Rho family GTPases RhoA, Rac1, CDC42Hs regulate transcriptional activation by SRF. *Cell* 1995; 81:1159–1170.

102. Fromm C, Coso OA, Montaner S, Xu N, Gutkind JS. The small GTP-binding protein Rho links G protein-coupled receptors, Galpha12 to the serum response element, to cellular transformation. *Proc Natl Acad Sci USA* 1997; 94:10,098–10,103.

103. Hart MJ, Jiang X, Kozasa T, Roscoe W, Singer W, Gilman WG, Sternweis PC, Bollag G. Direct Stimulation of the Guanine Nucleotide Exchange Activity of p115 RhoGEF by Galpha13. *Science* 1998; 280:2112–2114.

104. Kozasa T, Jiang X, Hart X, Sternweis XS, Singer WD, Gilman WG, Bollag G, Sternweis G. p115 RhoGEF, a GTPase Activating Protein for Galpha12, Galpha13. *Science* 1998; 280:2109–2111.

105. Mao J, Xie W, Yuan H, Simon W, Mano H, Wu D. Tec/Bmx non-receptor tyrosine kinases are involved in regulation of rho, serum response factor by Galpha12/13. *EMBO J* 1998; 17:5638–5646.

106. Jiang Y, Ma W, Wan Y, Kozasa T, Hattori S, Huang S. The G protein G alpha12 stimulates Bruton's tyrosine kinase, a rasGAP through a conserved PH/BM domain. *Nature* 1998; 395:808–813.

107. Mitchell R, McCulloch D, Lutz E, Johnson M, MacKenzie C, Fennell M, Fink G, Zhou W, Sealfon W. Rhodopsin-family receptors associate with small G proteins to activate phospholipase D. *Nature* 1998; 392:411–414.

108. Harhammer R, Gohla A, Schultz G. Interaction of G protein Gbetagamma dimers with small GTP-binding proteins of the Rho family. *FEBS Lett* 1996; 399:211–214.

109. Colombo MI, Inglese J, D'Souza-Schorey C, Beron W, Stahl W. Heterotrimeric G proteins interact with the small GTPase ARF. Possibilities for the regulation of vesicular traffic. *J Biol Chem* 1995; 270:24,564–24,571.
110. Alberts AS, Bouquin N, Johnston N, Treisman R. Analysis of RhoA-binding proteins reveals an interaction domain conserved in heterotrimeric G protein beta subunits, the yeast response regulator protein Skn7. *J Biol Chem* 1998; 273:8616–8622.
111. Jamora C, Takizawa PA, Zaarour PZ, Denesvre C, Faulkner C, Malhotra V. Regulation of Golgi structure through heterotrimeric G proteins. *Cell* 1997; 91:617–626.
112. de Rooij J, Zwartkruis FJ, Verheijen MH, Cool RH, Nijman SM, Wittinghofer A, Bos JL. Epac is a Rap1 guanine-nucleotide-exchange factor directly activated by cyclic AMP. *Nature* 1998; 396:474–477.
113. Mochizuki N, Ohba Y, Kiyokawa E, Kurata T, Murakami T, Ozaki T, Kitabatake A, Nagashima K, Matsuda M. Activation of the ERK/MAPK pathway by an isoform of rap1GAP associated with G α(i). *Nature* 1999; 400:891–894.
114. York RD, Yao H, Dillon T, Ellig CL, Eckert SP, McCleskey EW, Stork PJ. Rap1 mediates sustained MAP kinase activation induced by nerve growth factor. *Nature* 1998; 392:622–626.
115. Marinissen MJ, Chiariello M, Pallante M, Gutkind JS. A network of mitogen-activated protein kinases links G protein-coupled receptors to the c-jun promoter: a role for c-Jun NH2-terminal kinase, p38s, and extracellular signal-regulated kinase 5. *Mol Cell Biol* 1999; 19:4289–4301.
116. Fukuhara S, Murga C, Zohar M, Igishi T, Gutkind JS. A novel PDZ domain containing guanine nucleotide exchange factor links heterotrimeric G proteins to Rho. *J Biol Chem* 1999; 274:5868–5879.

6

Proximal Events in T-Cell Activation

Joanne Sloan-Lancaster, PhD and Lawrence E. Samelson, MD

1. INTRODUCTION

Engagement of the T cell antigen receptor (TCR) triggers complex intracellular signaling cascades, leading to new gene expression, initiation of protein synthesis, induction of effector functions, and clonal expansion. Characterization of the details of TCR-mediated activation has been an intense and fruitful area of investigation in recent years. Such studies have demonstrated the central involvement of protein tyrosine kinases (PTKs) and phosphatases (PTPs) in T cell signaling. Rapid tyrosine phosphorylation mediated by the PTKs leads to multiple events, including molecular translocation to the TCR and PTKs, initiation of protein–protein interactions, enzyme activation, cytoskeletal changes, and translocation of signals to the nucleus. The focus of this review is on the early events of TCR engagement and activation, with particular emphasis on some of the most recent discoveries, adding further light to the sequential steps of T-cell signaling.

2. T-CELL ANTIGEN RECEPTOR

The TCR has a multisubunit structure, composed of the polymorphic αβ heterodimer and the invariant CD3 γ, δ, ε and TCRζ subunits (1–3). Physiological T cell activation occurs upon engagement by the αβ pair of a short linear peptide bound in the pocket of a cell surface MHC molecule (4–7). The CD3 and TCRζ chains contain sequences required for TCR-mediated signal transduction (8–10). Since none of these molecules contains any intrinsic enzymatic activity, they recruit and bind signaling molecules by means of their conserved immunoreceptor tyrosine-based activation motifs (ITAMs), represented once in each of the CD3 chains and in triplicate in TCRζ (8,9,11). Such ITAMs, characterized by the sequence $YXXL(X)_{6-8}YXXL$, become phosphorylated on the tyrosine residues upon TCR engagement (12) and serve as docking sites for multiple SH2 domain-containing proteins, including both kinases and adaptor molecules (2,13,14). Thus, a multicomponent complex forms at the plasma membrane of the ligand-bound TCR; this structure either includes or recruits all the additional necessary components to initiate the biochemical pathways required to successfully activate the cell.

From: Signaling Networks and Cell Cycle Control: The Molecular Basis of Cancer and Other Diseases
Edited by: J. S. Gutkind © Humana Press Inc., Totowa, NJ

3. INTERPRETATION OF TCR ENGAGEMENT
ACROSS THE PLASMA MEMBRANE

During thymic development, thymocytes undergo a stringent differentiation process, which selects against cells that express TCRs capable of interacting with high affinity against self major histocompatibility complex (MHC) molecules combined with a peptide derived from a self antigen (15). T cells with TCRs of low affinity for self MHC molecules and peptide are positively selected and are allowed to exit the thymus (16). In light of this, it is perhaps not surprising that the estimated affinities of TCRs for their native ligands, the foreign antigenic peptide displayed in the groove of an MHC molecule, are of much lower affinity than are other receptor-ligand pairs (17,18). Moreover, the kinetics of such binding events reveal very rapid off-rates between the receptor and its ligand (17,18). Such properties present an apparent paradox, as it is difficult to comprehend how such weak and transient interactions can lead to productive translocation of a signal across the plasma membrane. Furthermore, several reports have presented certain criteria that must be met for a T cell to become activated after seeing its specific antigen. Several lines of evidence shed light on the mechanisms used by the immune system, which result in successful activation.

It appears that a T cell requires only about 100, and possibly fewer, TCRs to be engaged by specific ligand at any one time to initiate cellular activation (19–21). With an estimated 30,000 surface TCRs displayed by a T cell, as few as 0.3% need a coincident productive interaction. However, the engagement of this critical threshold number of TCRs has to persist long enough for signal transduction to be initiated (22). Recalling the fast off-rates calculated for these interactions, a problem is posed to the T cell. The combination of two sets of observations shows how a T cell meets these criteria. First, engaged TCRs tend to form a contact cap in a small area of the membrane, effectively concentrating the stimulated receptors in close proximity to each other, as is best demonstrated upon anti-CD3 stimulation. Second, the interaction of a TCR with ligand is apparently a dynamic one, with each TCR engaging multiple peptide/MHC pairs in a short period of time (23). Thus, by continually sampling the peptides displayed by the MHC molecules on the cognate APC, a T cell increases the likelihood that the critical number of productive interactions will be maintained in the contact cap for activation to be initiated. This cap of crosslinked TCRs results in aggregation of molecules associated via the TCR cytosolic tails, thus forming the multiprotein complex responsible for starting the biochemical signaling cascade.

4. INTRACELLULAR SIGNALING

4.1. Cooperation Between Protein Tyrosine Kinases and Phosphatases

One of the earliest events to occur after productive TCR engagement is the phosphory-lation of the CD3 and TCRζ molecules on the tyrosine residues of their ITAMs (12,24). This is achieved by the activated Src family PTKs Lck and Fyn (25–27). Their activity on their substrates is necessarily tightly regulated to prevent any aberrant T cell activation in the absence of antigenic stimulation. Two levels of control can be defined: localization and activation of the enzymes. Although Fyn is constitutively associated with the TCR by direct interactions with CD3ε and TCRζ (28,29), Lck plays the more important role in ITAM phosphorylation (30), and can be recruited to the bound TCR via CD8 or CD4 when these coreceptors bind sites on the antigen-bound MHC class I or II molecules, respectively *(31,32)*.

Src PTK kinase activity is kept in check by phosphorylation of a C-terminal tyrosine residue *(33)*. In the phosphorylated state, this site likely interacts intramolecularly with the upstream SH_2 domain, folding the catalytic domain back on itself, inhibiting the enzyme. By contrast, when this regulatory site is dephosphorylated, the protein can unfold, allowing activation. In T cells, the Src kinases Lck and Fyn are regulated by two other enzymes with specificity for this C-terminal tyrosine residue. These enzymes include the PTK Csk, responsible for negative regulation, and the PTP CD45, which activates these Src kinases *(9)*. Csk directly phosphorylates the C-terminal tyrosine in Lck and Fyn, maintaining them in an inactive state as described above. By contrast, CD45 dephosphorylates this site, permitting activation of the kinases. Thus, the competing activities of Csk and CD45 determine the status of Lck and Fyn activity and of TCR/CD3 phosphorylation. What "tips the balance" toward Lck/Fyn activation is unclear, but it appears to be required for subsequent steps.

4.2. ZAP-70 Activation

A primary role of the activated Src kinases is to phosphorylate the ITAMs of the CD3/TCR chains, allowing multiple downstream components to bind *(8)*. The first, most critical of these is ZAP-70, a member of the Syk family of PTKs, expressed exclusively in T cells, thymocytes, and some natural killer (NK) cells *(34)*. ZAP-70 recruitment and activation leads to the subsequent events that characterize successful T cell activation. This was clearly demonstrated by the phenotypes of ZAP-70-negative mice and patients with ZAP-70 mutations who present with severe combined immunodeficiency syndrome (SCID) *(35–38)*. The primary structure of this kinase predicts a cytosolic protein; biochemical data have shown that it rapidly and transiently translocates to the TCR upon ligand engagement *(34,39,40)*. A more recent study, using ZAP-70 fused to the green fluorescent protein (GFP), visually confirmed the biochemical observations. The fusion protein clears from the cytosolic compartment and moves to the cell surface quickly upon pharmacologic stimulation *(41)*. Surprisingly, a large pool of the ZAP-70 GFP chimera was located in the nucleus, a phenotype confirmed for the native ZAP-70 by antibody staining. The function of nuclear ZAP-70 is unclear, but a role in cell cycle regulation is conceivable, as the ultimate effect of T cell activation is clonal expansion.

ZAP-70 binding to the ITAMs is a high affinity interaction *(42,43)* and requires both the tandem SH2 domains of ZAP-70 and a doubly phosphorylated ITAM *(25,40,44)*. The crystal structure of the SH_2 domains of ZAP-70 bound to a phospho-ITAM highlights the molecular nature of this interaction. It is shown that, whereas the C-terminal SH_2 domain of ZAP-70 binds the N-terminal phosphotyrosine, both SH_2 domains are required to bind the C-terminal phosphotyrosine *(45)*. Furthermore, the spacing between the phosphotyrosines is important in allowing the tandem SH_2 domains of ZAP-70 to bind to a single ITAM. Because of this high-affinity interaction, one would assume that ZAP-70 converts from a freely diffusing to a more immobile state as it attaches at the cell surface. Such a phenotype has recently been directly confirmed using the ZAP-70 GFP fusion protein and a TCRζ chimera *(45a)*. Taking advantage of the GFP experimental system, we compared the mobility of the different pools of ZAP-70 in living cells and were able to generate diffusion coefficients for the protein at these intracellular locations. The results showed that, when ZAP-70 locates to the cell surface, it quickly becomes less mobile and stable, suggesting that it may become part of a higher-order structure involving many proteins. However, the diffusion of ZAP-70 in the membrane was around 20-fold faster than that of the ζ chimera. Although several studies have reported a pool of TCRζ associated with the cytoskeleton *(46)*, the membrane-bound ZAP-70 did not require intact actin filaments. This observation suggests that the interaction between ZAP-70 and the TCR/CD3 components is a dynamic one, with the ZAP-70 continually coming off and on, in a manner analogous to the TCR with its ligand. If correct, this model provides a potential mechanism for the transient nature of the interaction, and ultimately for returning the cell to a quiescent phenotype, as tyrosine phosphatases would have access to the phospho-ITAMs and would be able to compete with ZAP-70 for binding. As more ITAMs become dephosphorylated, fewer ZAP-70 molecules would be able to re-engage the TCR/CD3 molecules, and the positive signaling in the cell would eventually cease.

Soon after its recruitment and binding to the phospho-ITAMs, ZAP-70 itself both becomes phosphorylated and acquires kinase activity *(47–51)*. There are several tyrosines within the primary sequence of the protein, and the phosphorylation of each has different consequences for ZAP-70 activity. The initial phosphorylation is at site Y493 in the kinase domain, and is dependent on active Lck or Fyn. The results of this phosphorylation event are twofold: it correlates and reflects ZAP-70 activation, and it is followed by phosphorylation on additional sites, most prominently at the adjacent Y492, and Y292, in the second interdomain *(48,51)*. The enzyme responsible for phosphorylating these sites is unknown, but an accepted model is that active ZAP-70 molecules crossphosphorylate one another *(52)*. Y292 and Y492, in their phosphorylated states, have negative regulatory influences on the kinase, likely direct in the case of Y492, and perhaps via binding of an inhibitory protein for Y292 *(49,50)*. Several other tyrosines were shown to be phosphorylated in vitro, including Y69, Y126, and Y178, although their role in activating ZAP-70 is not well understood *(47)*. However, they could potentially provide the binding sites for the many proteins that associate only after phosphorylation of ZAP-70 *(52–59)*. Other sites in the hinge region between the SH$_2$ and kinase domains are candidates for phosphorylation and, if so, might bind Vav or other signaling molecules. The significance of tyrosine phosphorylation in the regulation of ZAP-70 activity is highlighted by the observation that, in murine thymocytes and freshly isolated lymph node T cells, ZAP-70 is constitutively associated with basally phosphorylated TCRζ *(60,61)*. This ZAP-70 is not phosphorylated, nor does it acquire kinase activity until the thymocytes or T cells are stimulated. Perhaps, under physiological conditions, some ZAP-70 is already situated at the cell surface, creating an anticipatory state for the T cell, which can very rapidly initiate signaling upon ligand engagement by the TCR.

4.3. Link Between PTKs and Downstream Pathways

Soon after the initial events have occurred, multiple biochemical events ensue. The membrane-proximal early activity is linked to downstream pathways through *adaptor proteins,* molecules that contain multiple domains that mediate protein–protein association, but that themselves have no enzymatic activity. These proteins serve to recruit and bind additional critical linkers and enzymes required for successful T-cell activation. Thus, they are the basis of a large multiprotein lattice forming at the plasma membrane site of TCR engagement *(62)*. The best characterized adaptor protein is Grb2, which has a structure of two SH3 domains, for binding proteins containing polyproline sequences, separated by an SH_2 domain, for binding phosphotyrosine residues in proteins *(63)*. In several receptor PTK systems, as well as in T-cell signaling, Grb2 couples these membrane-associated kinases to the guanine-nucleotide exchange factor SOS, and thus to pathways mediated by activated Ras *(63,64)*. Consistent with its central function in connecting the cell surface activity to cytosolic and nuclear pathways, Grb2 also interacts with multiple other substrates of the TCR-associated PTKs. These include the 120-kDa proto-oncogene Cbl via the Grb2 N-terminal SH3, the adaptor protein SLP-76 via the Grb2 C-terminal SH3 domain, the adaptor Shc, and a prominent tyrosine phosphorylated 36 kDa membrane-associated protein, pp36, via the Grb2 SH2 domain *(10,65–67)*.

Although it is clear that Grb2 serves to recruit molecules necessary to activate Ras and its downstream effectors *(68)*, multiple other signaling pathways are initiated independent of Grb2, including the hydrolysis of membrane phospholipids resulting in elevation of intracellular calcium ions (Ca^{2+}) and the activation of protein kinase C *(69,70)*. Moreover, Grb2 itself is not a membrane-associated protein. Thus, a central piece of information lacking until recently was the identification of molecules that serve to bridge the activated TCR and its associated PTKs to the kinase substrates. However, the cloning and identification of pp36 demonstrate that it satisfies all criteria for such a molecule *(71)*.

Pp36 is a prominent PTK substrate that is phosphorylated quickly after TCR engagement. It is named for its apparent molecular weight on sodium dodecyl sulfate–polyacrylamide gel electrophoresis (SDS-PAGE) and its abundance of phosphotyrosine as visualized by Western blotting *(72)*. It was assumed to play a critical role in T-cell signaling, as it not only binds the SH2 domain of Grb2, but also directly associates with phospholipase Cγ1 (PLCγ1) and phosphatidylinositol 3-kinase (PI_3K), in addition to having a tight membrane localization *(67,73,74)*. All these properties pointed to pp36 as the missing link in T-cell signaling, serving as the bridge between the kinases at the cell surface and their substrates. This was recently demonstrated, as the purification and cloning of pp36 exhibited a molecule of 233 amino acids, predicting a molecular weight of 24,985 Daltons *(71)*. The primary amino acid sequence allows it to be classified as a type III transmembrane protein. It has a long intracellular region containing 10 tyrosines in SH2-binding motifs as its only functional domains. A substrate of active ZAP-70, it associates with Grb2, PI_3K, and PLCγ1, upon tyrosine phosphorylation. The critical function of this protein in connecting the early cell surface events to the intracellular signaling cascades was confirmed when overexpression of a mutant, in which two tyrosines predicted to bind Grb2 upon phosphorylation were changed to phenylalanine. The mutant molecule did bind Grb2, PI_3K, or PLCγ1, and its expression inhibited AP-1 and NF-AT activation in Jurkat T cells. Because pp36 likely functions as the major docking protein coupling the TCR to critical downstream signaling events, it was named linker for activation of T (LAT) cells. Its central role in recruiting signaling molecules is depicted in Fig. 1, in which LAT, already situated at the plasma membrane, is quickly tyrosine phosphorylated by activated ZAP-70 and subsequently

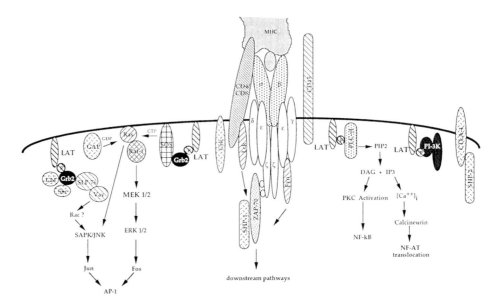

Fig. 1. Molecular interactions proximal to the plasma membrane occurring after TCR ligation. Engagement of the TCR by specific ligand results in phosphorylation of the tyrosines in the ITAMs of TCRζ and the CD3 molecules. This is achieved by Lck and Fyn, whose activities are regulated by the opposing influences of Csk and CD45. Once phosphorylated, the ITAMs bind ZAP-70, which quickly becomes phosphorylated on Y493, allowing it to acquire kinase activity. Subsequent phosphorylation on other tyrosines in ZAP-70 ensues, along with transloca-tion and binding of multiple adaptor and signaling molecules proximal to the membrane. One critical substrate of ZAP-70 is LAT, which, when phosphorylated on its tyrosine residues, binds Grb2, PLCγ1, and PI₃K, initiating the formation of a large multiprotein lattice under the plasma membrane at the region of the engaged TCR. Grb2 binds several proteins involved in different signaling pathways in the cell. These include SOS, which initiates the Ras/MAPK pathways, SLP-76 which, when associated with Vav, may play a role in Rac activation, and Cbl and Shc whose precise roles in T-cell signaling remain unclear. The LAT association with PLCγ1 allows initiation of phosphoinositol hydrolysis, resulting in NF-κB and NFAT translocation to the nucleus. The tyrosine phosphatases SHP-1 and SHP-2 most likely have negative regulatory roles in T-cell signaling, which is important for returning the cell to its quiescent state at the termination of an immune response.

recruits and binds the enzymes and adaptors known to be required for initiation of intracellular pathways.

5. DOWNSTREAM SIGNALING PATHWAYS

Several intracellular pathways used in other receptor signaling systems are common to TCR activation *(10)*. These include the activation of Ras and related small GTP-binding proteins, which, in turn, stimulate the mitogen-activated protein kinase (MAPK) and c-jun N-terminal kinase/stress-activated protein kinase (JNK/SAPK) pathways, the hydrolysis of inositol-containing phospholipids, and Ca²⁺ mobilization *(69,75,76)*. Each of these pathways is directly regulated by upstream PTKs, as illustrated in Fig. 1. Each of these cascades is briefly summarized in the following discussion (for further details, see other chapters of this book).

Ras activity commences when a Grb2–SOS complex is brought in close proximity to the plasma membrane *(63,64)*. We now understand that this probably occurs by a direct association of Grb2 with LAT, which in turn has been phosphorylated by active ZAP-70 at the engaged TCR *(71)*. Ras is regulated by the opposing influences of the guanine-nucleotide exchange factor, SOS, allowing formation of active Ras-GTP, and GTPase activating factors (GAPs), which convert Ras back to its inactive, GDP-bound state *(75)*. The most well-characterized small G protein-activated pathway is that leading to activation of the MAPKs/ERKs, which consist of a three-kinase sequence that includes a MAPK, which is activated by a MAPK/ERK kinase (MEK), which in turn is activated by a MEK kinase (MEKK) *(76)*. The first and best characterized MAPK cascade consists of Raf (the MEKK), MEK 1/2, and extracellular signal-regulated protein kinase (ERK 1/2), stimulated by agonists such as growth factors and tumor-promoting phorbol esters. Another group of MAPKs also play a role in T-cell signaling. These are activated by stressful stimuli or proinflammatory cytokines, and hence are called the stress-activated protein kinases (SAPKs). Whereas all the components in the SAPK pathway have not yet been identified, Rac most likely plays a major initiating role, although Ras also has some influence, and Raf is not the activating MEKK for the SAPKs *(76)*. The SAPKs serve to phosphorylate and activate c-Jun and are therefore also called Jun kinases (JNK). Although c-Jun is not a substrate for the ERKs, both SAPKs and ERKs are able to phosphorylate Fos. Together, these kinase cascades lead to the formation of the AP-1 complex *(77)*, which plays a critical role in the transcriptional activation of several cytokines in the T cell.

The hydrolysis of inositol-containing phospholipids is regulated by PLCγ1, which is activated by PTKs and is probably also maintained at the plasma membrane by directly binding LAT *(10)*. PLCγ1 cleaves phosphatidylinositol to diacylglycerol (DAG) and inositol triphosphate (IP$_3$). IP$_3$ subsequently increases intracellular Ca^{2+} concentration. Elevation of intracellular Ca^{2+} stimulates the phosphatase calcineurin, which in turn dephosphorylates the cytosolic nuclear factor of activated T cells (NFAT) and allows it to enter the nucleus, where it serves as a transcription factor. DAG activates protein kinase C (PKC), a serine/threonine kinase, which in turn activates the transcription factor NF-κB. The combination of the transcription factors AP-1, NFAT, and NF-κB act upon promoters of several cytokines in the T cell nucleus, resulting in differentiation, proliferation, and effector function induction.

Several other molecules most likely play a role in T cell signaling, although their precise functions remain unclear. Two of these include the proto-oncogene Vav and the adaptor protein SLP-76. With the formation of a LAT-Grb2-SLP-76 complex in activated Jurkat T cells, SLP-76 and Vav are probably brought in close proximity to the engaged TCR indirectly by LAT *(71)*. Whereas Vav$^{-/-}$ mice display an arrest in T-cell development and defective TCR signaling, overexpressing this protein in T cells results in basal activation of NFAT and interleukin-2 (IL-2) transcription, which are both enhanced even further upon TCR crosslinking *(78–81)*. SLP-76 overexpression also results in enhanced TCR-mediated NFAT induction and IL-2 transcription. Overexpression of both Vav and SLP-76 has a synergistic effect on NFAT activity *(82,83)*. Both proteins are tyrosine phosphorylated upon TCR engagement, at which point they associate with each other through the SH2 domain of Vav and tyrosine residues in SLP-76 *(83)*. Thus, the evidence suggests that Vav and SLP-76 participate jointly in T-cell signaling, although their precise role remains to be defined.

Finally, several other PTPs and PTKs are involved to some extent in the initiation or regulation of T-cell signaling. The two recently identified and characterized PTPs— SHP-1 and SHP-2—probably have negative regulatory functions. Both phosphatases have two N-terminal SH2 domains and a C-terminal phosphatase domain; they are also involved in B-cell and NK cell signaling pathways *(84–86)*. One investigative group has shown that SHP-1 associates with ZAP-70 and that this interaction results in an increase in SHP-1 activity and a decrease in ZAP-70 activity *(56)*. Thus, perhaps SHP-1 serves to dephosphorylate ZAP-70 and bring it back to its quiescent state in order to terminate a T-cell response. By contrast, SHP-2 binds to CTLA-4, a cell surface co-receptor expressed late on T cells after TCR stimulation, and whose ligands are members of the B7 family *(84)*. CTLA-4 is known to have negative regulatory roles in T cell activation, probably likely mediated by the associated SHP-2 *(87)*. A third phosphatase, SHIP, is also worth mentioning. This protein was shown to associate with Syk in B cells and is also present in T cells, acquiring phosphotyrosine upon TCR engagement *(88)*. It is a phosphoinositide phosphatase and dephosphorylates various inositol phosphates and phospholipids. One member of the Tec family of PTKs, Itk, is preferentially expressed in T cells. Mice that have developed in the absence of this enzyme have fewer thymocytes and CD4$^+$ T cells than are found in normal mice; and TCR signaling is also defective in these mice *(89)*. The mechanism by which Itk regulates T-cell activation remains to be discovered.

6. CONCLUSIONS

Several recent advances have contributed to a better understanding of the proximal events involved in TCR signaling. The most revealing of these is the identification and characterization of LAT, which serves to bridge the gap between the membrane-associated PTKs and the intracellular signaling molecules. Moreover, the results from the diffusion mobility studies of ZAP-70 shed further light on the way in which such tightly controlled downmodulation of a T-cell response might occur. Several key issues to be addressed in the near future: (1) what is the extent of the role of LAT, and are any signaling pathways initiated in its absence?; (2) what are the targets of SHP-1, SHP-2, and SHIP?; and (3) in which signaling cascades are Vav and SLP-76 involved? Ongoing studies will no doubt provide answers to these questions.

REFERENCES

1. Jorgensen JL, Reay PA, Ehrich EW, Davis MM. Molecular components of T-cell recognition. *Annu Rev Immunol* 1992; 10:835–873.
2. Weiss A. T cell antigen receptor signal transduction: A tale of tails and cytoplasmic protein-tyrosine kinases. *Cell* 1993; 73:209–212.
3. Weissman AM. The T-cell antigen receptor: A multisubunit signaling complex. *Chem Immunol* 1994; 59:1–18.
4. Garcia KC, Degano M, Stanfield RL, Brunmark A, Jackson MR, Peterson PA, Teyton L, Wilson IA. An αβ T cell receptor structure at 2.5 Å and its orientation in the TCR–MHC complex. *Science* 1996; 274:209–219.

5. Townsend ARM, Rothbard J, Gotch FM, Bahadur G, Wraith D, McMichael AJ. The epitopes of influenza nucleoprotein recognized by cytotoxic T lymphocytes can be defined with short synthetic peptides. *Cell* 1986; 44:959–968.

6. Babbitt BP, Allen PM, Matsueda G, Haber E, Unanue ER. Binding of immunogenic peptides to Ia histocompatibility molecules. *Nature* 1985; 317:359–361.

7. Bentley GA, Mariuzza RA. The structure of the T cell antigen receptor. *Annu Rev Immunol* 1996; 14:563–590.

8. Wange RL, Samelson LE. Complex complexes: Signaling at the TCR. *Immunity* 1996; 5:197–205.

9. Weiss A, Littman DR. Signal transduction by lymphocyte antigen receptors. *Cell* 1994; 76:263–274.

10. Cantrell D. T cell antigen receptor signal transduction pathways. *Annu Rev Immunol* 1996; 14:259–274.

11. Reth M. Antigen receptor tail clue. *Nature* 1989; 338:383–384.

12. Baniyash M, Garcia-Morales P, Luong E, Samelson LE, Klausner RD. The T cell antigen receptor ζ chain is tyrosine phosphorylated upon activation. *J Biol Chem* 1988; 263:18,225–18,230.

13. Samelson LE, Klausner RD. Tyrosine kinases and tyrosine-based activation motifs. *J Biol Chem* 1992; 267:24,913–24,916.

14. Chan AC, Desai DM, Weiss A. The role of protein tyrosine kinases and protein tyrosine phosphatases in T cell antigen receptor signal transduction. *Annu Rev Immunol* 1994; 12:555–592.

15. von Boehmer H. Positive selection of lymphocytes. *Cell* 1994; 76:219–228.

16. Nossal GJV. Negative selection of lymphocytes. *Cell* 1994; 76:229–239.

17. Matsui K, Boniface JJ, Steffner P, Reay PA, Davis MM. Kinetics of T-cell receptor binding to peptide/I-E^k complexes: Correlation of the dissociation rate with T-cell responsiveness. *Proc Natl Acad Sci USA* 1994; 91:12,862–12,866.

18. Corr M, Salnetz AE, Boyd LF, Jelonek MT, Khilko S, Al-Ramadi BK, Kim YS, Maher SE, Bothwell ALM, Margulies DH. T cell receptor-MHC class I peptide interactions: Affinity, kinetics, and specificity. *Science* 1994; 265:946–949.

19. Heemels MT, Ploegh H. Generation, translocation, and presentation of MHC class I-restricted peptides. *Annu Rev Biochem* 1995; 64:463–491.

20. Harding CV, Unanue ER. Quantitation of antigen-presenting cell MHC class II/peptide complexes necessary for T-cell stimulation. *Nature* 1990; 346:574–576.

21. Sykulev Y, Joo M, Vturina I, Tsomides TJ, Eisen HN. Evidence that a single peptide–MHC complex on a target cell can elicit a cytolytic T cell response. *Immunity* 1996; 4:565–571.

22. Valitutti S, Dessing M, Aktories K, Gallati H, Lanzavecchia A. Sustained signaling leading to T cell activation results from prolonged T cell receptor occupancy. Role of T cell actin cytoskeleton. *J Exp Med* 1995; 181:577–584.

23. Valitutti S, Müller S, Cella M, Padovan E, Lanzavecchia A. Serial triggering of many T-cell receptors by a few peptide–MHC complexes. *Nature* 1995; 375:148–151.

24. Samelson LE, Patel MD, Weissman AM, Harford JB, Klausner RD. Antigen activation of murine T cells induces tyrosine phosphorylation of a polypeptide associated with the T cell antigen receptor. *Cell* 1986; 46:1083–1090.

25. Iwashima M, Irving BA, van Oers NSC, Chan AC, Weiss A. Sequential interactions of the TCR with two distinct cytoplasmic tyrosine kinases. *Science* 1994; 263:1136–1139.

26. van Oers NS, Killeen N, Weiss A. Lck regulates the tyrosine phosphorylation of the T cell receptor subunits and ZAP-70 in murine thymocytes. *J Exp Med* 1996; 183:1053–1062.

27. Howe LR, Weiss A. Multiple kinases mediate T-cell-receptor signaling. *Trends Biochem Sci* 1995; 20:59–64.

28. Samelson LE, Phillips AF, Luong ET, Klausner RD. Association of the fyn protein-tyrosine kinase with the T-cell antigen receptor. *Proc Natl Acad Sci USA* 1990; 87:4358–4362.

29. Gauen LKT, Tony Kong A-N, Samelson LE, Shaw AS. p59[fyn] tyrosine kinase associates with multiple T-cell receptor subunits through its unique amino-terminal domain. *Mol Cell Biol* 1992; 12:5438–5446.

30. van Oers NSC, Killeen N, Weiss A. Lck regulates the tyrosine phosphorylation of the T cell receptor subunits and ZAP-70 in murine thymocytes. *J Exp Med* 1996; 183:1053–1062.

31. Turner JM, Brodsky MH, Irving BA, Levin SD, Perlmutter RM, Littman DR. Interaction of the unique N-terminal region of tyrosine kinase p56[lck] with cytoplasmic domains of CD4 and CD8 is mediated by cysteine motifs. *Cell* 1990; 60:755–765.

32. Glaichenhaus N, Shastri N, Littman DR, Turner JM. Requirement for association of p56[lck] with CD4 in antigen-specific signal transduction in T cells. *Cell* 1991; 64:511–520.

33. Cooper JA, Howell B. The when and how of Src regulation. *Cell* 1993; 73:1051–1054.

34. Chan AC, Iwashima M, Turck CW, Weiss A. ZAP-70: A 70 kd protein-tyrosine kinase that associates with the TCR zeta chain. *Cell* 1992; 71:649–662.

35. Arpaia E, Shahar M, Dadi H, Cohen A, Roifman CM. Defective T cell receptor signaling and CD8[+] thymocyte selection in humans lacking ZAP-70 kinase. *Cell* 1994; 76:947–958.

36. Chan AC, Kadlecek TA, Elder ME, Filipovich AH, Kuo W-L, Iwashima M, Parslow TG, Weiss A. ZAP-70 deficiency in an autosomal recessive form of severe combined immunodeficiency. *Science* 1994; 264:1599–1601.

37. Elder ME, Lin D, Clever J, Chan AC, Hope TJ, Weiss A, Parslow TG. Human severe combined immunodeficiency due to a defect in ZAP-70, a T cell tyrosine kinase. *Science* 1994; 264:1596–1599.

38. Negishi I, Motoyama N, Nakayama K-i, Nakayama K, Senju S, Hatakeyama S, Zheng Q, Chan AC, Loh DY. Essential role for ZAP-70 in both positive and negative selection of thymocytes. *Nature* 1995; 376:435–438.

39. Wange RL, Kong A-N, Samelson LE. A tyrosine-phosphorylated 70-KDa proten binds a photoaffinity analogue of ATP and associates with both the ζ chain and CD3 components of the activated T cell antigen receptor. *J Biol Chem* 1992; 267:11,685–11,688.

40. Wange RL, Malek SN, Desiderio S, Samelson LE. Tandem SH2 domains of ZAP-70 bind to T cell antigen receptor ζ and CD3ε from activated jurkat T cells. *J Biol Chem* 1993; 268:19,797–19,801.

41. Sloan-Lancaster J, Zhang W, Presley J, Williams BL, Abraham RT, Lippincott-Schwartz J, Samelson LE. Regulation of ZAP-70 intracellular localization: visualization with the green fluorescent protein. *J Exp Med* 1997; 186:1713–1724.

42. Isakov N, Wange RL, Burgess WH, Watts JD, Aebersold R, Samelson LE. ZAP 70 binding specificity to T cell receptor tyrosine-based activation motifs: The tandem SH2 domains of ZAP-70 bind distinct tyrosine-based activation motifs with varying affinity. *J Exp Med* 1995; 181:375–380.

43. Bu J-Y, Shaw AS, Chan AC. Analysis of the interaction of ZAP-70 and syk protein-tyrosine kinases with the T-cell antigen receptor by plasmon resonance. *Proc Natl Acad Sci USA* 1995; 92:5106–5110.

44. Koyasu S, Tse AGD, Moingeon P, Hussey RE, Mildonian A, Hannisian J, Clayton LK, Reinherz EL. Delineation of a T-cell activation motif required for binding of protein tyrosine kinases containing tandem SH2 domains. *Proc Natl Acad Sci USA* 1994; 91:6693–6697.

45. Hatada MH, Lu X, Laird ER, Green J, Morgenstern JP, Lou M, Marr CS, Phillips TB, Ram MK, Theriault K, Zoller MJ, Karas JL. Molecular basis for interaction of the protein tyrosine kinase ZAP-70 with the T-cell receptor. *Nature* 1995; 377:32–38.

45a. Sloan-Lancaster J, Presley J, Ellenberg J, Yamazaki T, Lippincott-Schwartz J, Samelson LE. ZAP-70 association with the TRCζ: Fluorescence imaging of dynamic changes upon cellular stimulation. *J Cell Biol* 1998; 143:613–624.

46. Caplan S, Zeliger S, Wang L, Baniyash M. Cell-surface-expressed T-cell antigen-receptor ζ chain is associated with the cytoskeleton. *Proc Natl Acad Sci USA* 1995; 92:4768–4772.

47. Watts JD, Affolter M, Krebs DL, Samelson LE, Aebersold R. Identification by electrospray ionization mass spectrometry of the sites of tyrosine phosphorylation induced in activated Jurkat T cells on the protein tyrosine kinase ZAP-70. *J Biol Chem* 1994; 269:29,520–29,529.

48. Wange RL, Guitian R, Isakov N, Watts JD, Aebersold R, Samelson LE. Activating and inhibitory mutations in adjacent tyrosines in the kinase domain of ZAP-70. *J Biol Chem* 1995; 270:18,730–18,733.

49. Kong G, Dalton M, Wardenburg JB, Straus D, Kurosaki T, Chan AC. Distinct tyrosine phosphorylation sites within ZAP-70 mediate activation and negative regulation of antigen receptor function. *Mol Cell Biol* 1996; 16:5026–5035.

50. Zhao Q, Weiss A. Enhancement of lymphocyte responsiveness by a gain-of-function mutation of ZAP-70. *Mol Cell Biol* 1996; 16:6765–6774.

51. Chan AC, Dalton M, Johnson R, Kong GH, Wang T, Thoma R, Kurosaki T. Activation of ZAP-70 kinase activity by phosphorylation of tyrosine 493 is required for lymphocyte antigen receptor function. *EMBO J* 1995; 14:2499–2508.

52. Neumeister EN, Zhu Y, Richars S, Terhorst C, Chan AC, Shaw AS. Binding of ZAP-70 to phosphorylated T-cell receptor ζ and ν enhances its autophosphorylation and generates specific binding sites for SH2 domain-containing proteins. *Mol Cell Biol* 1995; 15:3171–3178.

53. Huby RDJ, Carlile GW, Ley SC. Interactions between the protein-tyrosine kinase ZAP-70, the proto-oncoprotein Vav, and tubulin in Jurkat T cells. *J Biol Chem* 1995; 270:30,241–30,244.

54. Thome M, Duplay P, Guttinger M, Acuto O. Syk and ZAP-70 mediate recruitment of p56[lck]/CD4 to the activated T cell receptor/CD3/ζ complex. *J Exp Med* 1995; 181:1997–2006.

55. Katzav S, Sutherland M, Packham G, Yi T, Weiss A. The protein tyrosine kinase ZAP-70 can associate with the SH2 domain of proto-vav. *J Biol Chem* 1994; 269:32,579–32,585.

56. Plas DR, Johnson R, Pingel JT, Matthews RJ, Dalton M, Roy G, Chan AC, Thomas ML. Direct regulation of ZAP-70 by SHP-1 in T cell antigen receptor signaling. *Science* 1996; 272:1173–1176.

57. Fournel M, Davidson D, Weil R, Veillette A. Association of tyrosine protein kinase ZAP-70 with the protooncogene product p120c-cbl in T lymphocytes. *J Exp Med* 1996; 183:301–306.

58. Lupher MLJ, Reedquist KA, Miyake S, Langdon WY, Band H. A novel phosphotyrosine-binding domain in the N-terminal transforming region of Cbl interacts directly and selectively with ZAP-70 in T cells. *J Biol Chem* 1996; 271:24,063–24,068.

59. Weil R, Cloutier JF, Fournel M, Veillette A. Regulation of ZAP-70 by Src family tyrosine protein kinases in an antigen-specific T-cell line. *J Biol Chem* 1995; 270:2791–2799.

60. Lander ES, Schork NJ. Genetic dissection of complex traits. *Science* 1994; 265:2037–2048.

61. Wiest A, Ashe JM, Abe R, Bolen JB, Singer A. TCR activation of ZAP-70 is impaired in CD4⁺CD8⁺ thymocytes as a consequence of intrathymic interactions that diminish available p56lck. *Immunity* 1996; 4:495–504.

62. Pawson T. Protein modules and signalling networks. *Nature* 1995; 373:573–580.

63. Downward J. The GRB-2/Sem-5 adaptor protein. *FEBS Lett* 1994; 338:113–117.

64. Holsinger LJ, Spencer DM, Austin DJ, Schreiber SL, Crabtree GR. Signal transduction in T lymphocytes using a conditional allele of Sos. *Proc Natl Acad Sci USA* 1995; 92:9810–9814.

65. Donovan JA, Wange RL, Langdon WY, Samelson LE. The protein product of the c-cbl protooncogene is the 120-kDa tyrosine-phosphorylated protein in Jurkat cells activated via the T cell antigen receptor. *J Biol Chem* 1994; 269:22,921–22,924.

66. Jackman JK, Motto DG, Sun Q, Tanemoto M, Turck CW, Peltz GA, Koretsky GA, Findell PR. Molecular cloning of SLP-76, a 76-kDa tyrosine phosphoprotein associated with Grb-2 in T cells. *J Biol Chem* 1995; 270:7029–7032.

67. Buday L, Egan SE, Rodriguez-Viciana P, Cantrell DA, Downward J. A complex of Grb2 adaptor protein, Sos exchange factor, and a 36-kDa membrane-bound tyrosine phosphoprotein is implicated in ras activation in T cells. *J Biol Chem* 1994; 269:9019–9023.

68. Lowenstein EJ, Daly RJ, Batzer AG, Li W, Margolis B, Lammers R, Ullrich A, Skolnick D, Bar-Sagi D, Schlessinger J. The SH2 and SH3 domain-containing protein Grb2 links receptor tyrosine kinases to Ras signaling. *Cell* 1992; 70:431–442.

69. Rhee SG, Bae YS. Regulation of phosphoinositide-specific phospholipase C isoenzymes. *J Biol Chem* 1997; 272:15,045–15,048.

70. Newton AC. Regulation of protein kinase C. *Curr Opin Cell Biol* 1997; 9:161–167.

71. Zhang W, Sloan-Lancaster J, Kitchen J, Trible RP, Samelson LE. LAT: The ZAP-70 tyrosine kinase substrate that links T cell receptor to cellular activation. *Cell* 1998; 92:83–92.

72. June CH, Fletcher MC, Ledbetter JA, Samelson LE. Increases in tyrosine phosphorylation are detectable before phospholipase C activation after T cell receptor stimulation. *J Immunol* 1990; 144:1591–1599.

73. Fukazawa T, Reedquist KA, Panchamoorthy G, Soltoff S, Trub T, Druker B, Cantley L, Shoelson SE, Band H. T cell activation-dependent association between the p85 subunit of the phosphatidyl 3-kinase and Grb2/phospholipase C-γ1-binding phosphotyrosyl protein pp36/38. *J Biol Chem* 1995; 270:20,177–20,182.

74. Sieh M, Batzer A, Schlessinger J, Weiss A. Grb2 and phospholipase C-γ1 associate with a 36-38-kilodalton phosphotyrosine protein after T-cell receptor stimulation. *Mol Cell Biol* 1994; 14:4435–4442.

75. Marshall CJ. Ras effectors. *Curr Opin Cell Biol* 1996; 8:197–204.

76. Robinson MJ, Cobb MH. Mitogen-activated protein kinase pathways. *Curr Opin Cell Biol* 1997; 9:180–186.

77. Karin M, Lui Z, Zandi E. AP-1 function and regulation. *Curr Opin Cell Biol* 1997; 9:240–246.

78. Fischer K-D, Zmuidzinas A, Gardner S, Barbacid M, Bernstein A, Guidos C. Defective T-cell receptor signalling and positive selection of Vav-deficient CD4+CD8+ thymocytes. *Nature* 1995; 374:474–476.

79. Tarakhovsky A, Turner M, Schaal S, Mee PJ, Duddy LP, Rajewsky K, Tybulewicz VLJ. Defective antigen receptor-mediated proliferation of B and T cells in the absence of Vav. *Nature* 1995; 374:467–470.

80. Zhang R, Alt FW, Davidson L, Orkin SH, Swat W. Defective signalling through the T- and B-cell antigen receptors in lymphoid cells lacking the *vav* proto-oncogene. *Nature* 1995; 374:470–473.

81. Wu J, Katzav S, Weiss A. A functional T cell receptor signaling pathway is required for p95vav activity. *Mol Cell Biol* 1995; 15:4337–4346.

82. Motto DG, Ross SE, Wu J, Hendricks-Taylor LR, Korwtsky GA. Implication of the Grb2-associated phosphoprotein SLP-76 in T cell receptor-mediated interleukin 2 production. *J Exp Med* 1996; 183:1937–1943.

83. Wu J, Motto DG, Koretsky GA, Weiss A. Vav and SLP-76 interact and functionally cooperate in IL-2 gene activation. *Immunity* 1996; 4:593–602.

84. Marengere LE, Waterhouse P, Duncan GS, Mittrucker HW, Feng GS, Mak TW. Regulation of T cell receptor signaling by tyrosine phosphatase SYP association with CTLA-4. *Science* 1996; 272:1170–1173.

85. Burshtyn DN, Scharenberg AM, Wagtmann N, Rajagopalan S, Berrada K, Yi T, Kinet J-P, Long EO. Recruitment of tyrosine phosphatase HCP by the killer cell inhibitory receptor. *Immunity* 1996; 4:77–85.

86. Fry AM, Lanier LL, Weiss A. Phosphotyrosine in the killer cell inhibitory receptor motif of NKB1 are required for negative signaling and for association with protein tyrosine phosphatase 1C. *J Exp Med* 1996; 184:295–300.

87. Walunas TL, Lenschow DJ, Bakker CY, Linsley PS, Freeman GJ, Green JM, Thompson CB, Bluestone JA. CTLA-4 can function as a negative regulator of T cell activation. *Immunity* 1994; 1:405–413.

88. Chacko GW, Tridandapani S, Damen JE, Liu L, Krystal G, Coggeshall KM. Negative

signaling in B lymphocytes induces tyrosine phosphorylation of the 145-kDa inositol poly-phosphate 5-phosphatase, SHIP. *J Immunol* 1996; 157:2234–2238.
89. Liao XC, Littman DR. Altered T cell receptor signaling and disrupted T cell development in mice lacking Itk. *Immunity* 1995; 3:757–769.

7

Signal Transduction
from the High Affinity IgE Receptor

Reuben P. Siraganian, MD, PhD

1. INTRODUCTION

Mast cells and basophils synthesize and store histamine, proteoglycans, and proteases in their granules and have surface receptors (FcεRI) that bind IgE with high affinity. The interaction of multivalent antigen with this cell-bound IgE results in aggregation of FcεRI and activation of the cells to release an array of inflammatory mediators. These mediators include the granular contents, arachidonic acid from phospholipids produced by the action of phospholipase enzymes, and cytokines such as tumor necrosis factor (TNF-α). Unlike the rapid release within minutes of preformed mediators, release of most cytokines is a slow process that requires several hours. This chapter reviews the current understanding of these intracellular pathways; most of this information is based on studies with the rat basophilic leukemia RBL-2H3 cultured mast cell line.

The FcεRI consists of four noncovalently linked polypeptide chains: an IgE binding α chain of 45–60 kDa, a 33-kDa β subunit and a homodimer formed of disulfide linked γ chains (1). As these subunits lack any known enzymatic activity, the receptor depends on associated molecules for transducing intracellular signals. The extracellular domain of the α chain of FcεRI binds IgE, whereas its relatively short cytoplasmic domain probably does not play a role in cell signaling. The C-terminal cytoplasmic domains of both the β and the γ subunits contain a motif with the amino acid sequence (D/E)$x_2Yx_2Lx_{6-8}Yx_2$(L/I) that is critical for cell activation (2). This immunoreceptor tyrosine-based activation motif (ITAM) is also present in the immune receptor complex on B and T-cells (3). The aggregation of these receptors results in phosphorylation of the tyrosine residues within the ITAM that is critical for cell signaling. The γ component of FcεRI appears to be the essential receptor subunit for signaling cells for secretion, whereas the β subunit functions as a regulator or an amplifier (4).

Besides FcεRI, basophils and mast cells have a number of other receptors for immunoglobulins that include FcγRII and FcγRIII. The FcγRII and FcγRIII bind IgG with much lower affinity than the binding of IgE to the FcεRI. These receptors for IgG may activate or regulate the FcεRI-induced mast cell secretion (3,5,6). Mast cells/basophils are also activated to release by complement component C5a or formyl-methionine

From: Signaling Networks and Cell Cycle Control: The Molecular Basis of Cancer and Other Diseases
Edited by: J. S. Gutkind © Humana Press Inc., Totowa, NJ

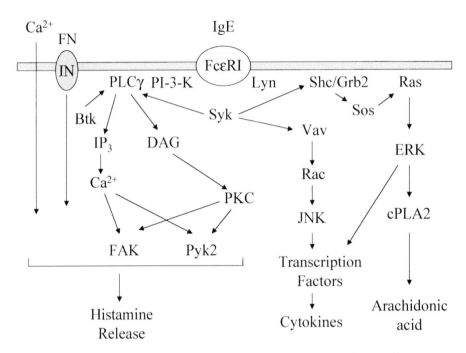

Fig. 1. Signaling pathways and molecules in basophils/mast cells.

containing small peptides that bind and activate receptors of the seven-transmembrane family.

2. PRESENT MODEL FOR FcεRI SIGNALING (FIG. 1)

In the present model for mast cell signaling, aggregation of FcεRI results in the tyrosine phosphorylation of the ITAMs of the β and γ subunits of the receptor, probably by Lyn or another Src family kinase. The tyrosine phosphorylated ITAM then functions as a scaffold for binding of additional signaling molecules. One of these molecules is the cytoplasmic protein tyrosine kinase Syk, which binds predominantly to the γ subunit of FcεRI. The binding of Syk to the tyrosine phosphorylated ITAM results in a conformational change in Syk, with an increase in its enzymatic activity and the downstream propagation of signals, such as the tyrosine phosphorylation of phospholipase C-γ1 (PLC), phospholipase C-γ2, and the influx of Ca^{2+}.

There is activation of phosphatidylinositol 3-kinase (PI-3-K) which results in the formation of phosphatidylinositol (3,4,5)-phosphate (PIP_3). This recruits the tyrosine phosphorylated PLC-γ1 and PLC-γ2 to the membrane. This activated PLC-γ catalyzes the hydrolysis of phosphatidylinositol 4,5-bisphosphate (PIP_2) with the generation of inositol 1,4,5-trisphosphate (IP_3) and 1,2,diacylglycerol (DAG). These second messengers release Ca^{2+} from internal stores and activate protein kinase C (PKC) respectively, both events are essential for FcεRI-mediated secretion. The IP_3 binds to specific intracellular receptors, which results in the mobilization of Ca^{2+} from intracellular stores and an increase in the cytoplasmic Ca^{2+} concentration $[Ca^{2+}]_i$. This initial rise in $[Ca^{2+}]_i$ is followed by the sustained influx of Ca^{2+} from the extracellular medium. The increase in $[Ca^{2+}]_i$ regulates Ca^{2+}/calmodulin dependent events, including calcineurin, a Ca^{2+}/calmodulin dependent serine phosphatase.

Aggregation of FcεRI also activates other cytoplasmic protein tyrosine kinases. One of these is Bruton's tyrosine kinase (Btk), which probably plays a role in the sustained influx of Ca^{2+}. Other protein tyrosine kinases are focal adhesion kinase (FAK), pp125[FAK], and the related kinase Pyk2, which are present in many cells and are activated by adhesion. Both tyrosine kinases are tyrosine phosphorylated after FcεRI stimulation and may play a role in the late steps of degranulation. The aggregation of FcεRI also induces the tyrosine phosphorylation of many other proteins that are important for the further propagation of intracellular signals.

The early tyrosine phosphorylation of such proteins as Shc and Vav then stimulate the Ras protein kinase cascades including the ERK, JNK, and p38 pathways which then phosphorylate and activate proteins including transcription factors and cytoplasmic phospholipase A2. This results in the synthesis or release, or both, of more inflammatory mediators such as arachidonic acid and cytokines.

The PKC family of molecules is an essential transducer of signals for secretion. The RBL-2H3 mast cells contain the α, β, δ, ϵ, and ζ isoforms of PKC. Activated PKC translocates to the membrane and phosphorylates several proteins, including the myosin light chain and the γ subunit of FcεRI. In studies with permeabilized cells, the β or δ isozymes of PKC were found to be essential for optimal FcεRI-mediated secretion.

Cytoskeletal reorganization is important for the degranulation process. These changes are secondary to the rise in $[Ca^{2+}]_i$, phosphorylation of cellular proteins and/or activation of GTP-binding proteins. Two *ras*-related small GTPases, Rho and Rac, appear to play a role in these cytoskeleton and morphological changes. The degranulation of mast cells results in swelling of the individual granules, a change in the electron-dense granular contents and the formation of interconnected granules with the granule closest to the cell surface fusing with the plasma membrane and thus open to the extracellular medium. An ion exchange mechanism then results in the release of the biogenic amines *(7)*.

The following sections describe in more detail the molecules involved in these pathways.

3. THE MOLECULES INVOLVED IN THE FcεRI SIGNALING PATHWAYS

Mast cells are stimulated to secrete mediators by antigen aggregating the IgE molecules bound to FcεRI on the cell surface. Optimal conditions for the reaction depend on the concentration of IgE on the basophil/mast cell surface, the concentration of the antigen and the affinity of the IgE for the antigen. Stimulation of the cell is by the bridging of two IgE molecules on the cell surface, which requires the aggregation of a very small proportion of the total surface IgE (probably bridging less than 100 IgE molecules representing 1% of the total receptors on the cell surface).

3.1. Lyn

Protein tyrosine phosphorylation is an early and critical signal for FcεRI-induced degranulation *(8–10)*. Lyn, a member of the Src family of kinases, is associated with

the inner surface of the plasma membrane and with the β subunit of FcεRI in nonstimulated cells *(11–14)*. The enzymatic activity of Lyn is downregulated by Csk, which
phosphorylates the tyrosine in the regulatory site *(15)*. Aggregation of the receptor
results in rapid phosphorylation of the tyrosine residues in the ITAMs of both the β
and γ subunits of the FcεRI *(16,17)* probably by Lyn or another Src family kinase
that associates with the receptor *(11,18,19)*. Some activation of Lyn occurs, possibly
attributable to the dephosphorylation of Lyn at its regulatory site by a protein tyrosine
phosphatase, such as CD45 (*see* Section 3.3). There is also an increase in the association
of Lyn with the receptor after receptor aggregation probably as a result of binding of
Lyn with the phosphorylated ITAMs. Tyrosine phosphorylation of the receptor subunits
is by a transphosphorylation reaction whereby Lyn associated with one FcεRI phosphorylates the ITAM of another FcεRI, both of which have been brought together by
aggregation *(13,18,19)*. The evidence is equivocal whether other tyrosine kinases can
replace the function of Lyn. For example, when Lyn is inactivated by homologous
recombination, one group reported that in vivo FcεRI-mediated degranulation is absent,
whereas another group observed that in vitro bone marrow derived mast cells secrete
normally *(20,21)*.

3.2. Syk

Phosphorylation of the two tyrosines in the ITAMs of FcεRI allows both the β and
γ subunits to function as scaffolds for binding of additional SH2-containing molecules
(22). Among these molecules is Syk which associates predominantly after receptor
phosphorylation and is critical for propagating the downstream signals. The association
of Syk with FcεRI is caused by the interaction of the two SH2 domains of Syk with
the two phosphorylated tyrosines in the ITAM, mainly of the γ subunit and less to that
of the β subunit *(12,22–25)*. Analysis of the crystal structure of the tandem SH2 domains
of ZAP-70 bound to a diphosphorylated ITAM peptide has led to a model showing
the interaction of Syk with ITAM *(26)*. The C-terminal SH2 domain binds to the N-
terminal YxxL sequence of the ITAM, whereas the N-terminal SH2 domain binds the
C-terminal YxxL of the ITAM.

The binding of Syk to the tyrosine phosphorylated ITAM results in a conformational
change in Syk, with an increase in its enzymatic activity *(27–29)*. This results in
autophosphorylation of Syk, which may be due to inter- and/or intramolecular reactions.
Syk located in the membrane together with the change in its conformation may also
allow it to be further phosphorylated by Lyn or other kinases, resulting in further
activation of Syk *(30)*. Therefore, Syk activation may involve several mechanisms that
include conformational changes caused by ITAM binding, autophosphorylation and
phosphorylation by other kinases. Whatever the mechanism, phosphorylation of the
two tyrosines in the activation loop of Syk is important for the capacity of Syk to
phosphorylate other molecules and to induce signal transduction in cells *(31)*.

Syk bound to FcεRI and activated may then phosphorylate other proteins in the
vicinity of the receptor such as proteins that have been recruited to the tyrosine-
phosphorylated subunits of the receptor. For example, the tyrosine-phosphorylated
ITAM of FcεRIβ binds not only Syk, but also other proteins that have SH2 domains,
including Shc, PLC-γ1, the SH2-domain containing inositol 5-phosphatase (SHIP),

and the SH2 containing protein tyrosine phosphatases SHP-2 *(12,22,25)*. Tyrosine-phosphorylated Syk could also recruit proteins such as Lyn or other kinases that bind to it through their own SH2 domains and may phosphorylate Syk and regulate its activity *(12,32,33)*. Other molecules such as p120$^{c\text{-}cbl}$ (Cbl) and protein tyrosine phosphatases associate with Syk and may control its tyrosine phosphorylation and kinase activity *(34,35)*.

The Syk protein tyrosine kinase is essential for degranulation in mast cells. In a Syk-negative variant of the RBL-2H3 cell line, FcεRI aggregation induced minimal increase in protein tyrosine phosphorylations of total cellular proteins *(36)*. Although some proteins are tyrosine phosphorylated independent of Syk, most of the FcεRI-induced cellular protein tyrosine phosphorylations require Syk. The phosphorylation of the following proteins is downstream of Syk: PLC-γ1 and PLC-γ2, Vav, SLP-76, Shc, MAP kinase, JNK kinase, the FAK, the protein tyrosine kinase Pyk2, paxillin, the adhesion molecule PECAM-1 (CD31), Cbl, rasGAP, and HS-1. However, these results do not imply that Syk is directly responsible for phosphorylating these proteins.

There are two alternatively spliced forms of Syk cDNA that result in two distinct isoforms that differ by the presence of a 23-amino acid insert located between the second SH2 and the catalytic domain *(37,38)*. Both mRNAs encode functional protein tyrosine kinases and the proteins are present in RBL-2H3 cells. When expressed by transfection in the Syk-negative mast cells, the isoform lacking the 23-amino acid insert is much less efficient in coupling FcεRI aggregation to cellular activation, although both forms have similar in vitro enzymatic activity *(39,40)*. This functional defect in the shorter Syk isoform correlates with its reduced capacity to bind phosphorylated ITAMs.

The FcεRI-induced tyrosine phosphorylation of a number of other proteins is independent of Syk. These include the β and γ subunits of FcεRI, the SH2-domain containing inositol 5-phosphatase (SHIP), and the SH2 containing protein tyrosine phosphatases SHP-1 and SHP-2 *(36,41,42)*. Some of these molecules are negative regulators of signaling in B cells and mast cells. Signal transduction may be regulated by SHIP, by controlling the level of inositol phosphates, and by SHP-1/SHP-2 regulating the extent of tyrosine phosphorylation of the receptor. Therefore, the pathways that generate signals that induce secretion and the pathway for regulating those signals diverge at an early step after receptor aggregation.

3.3. Protein Tyrosine Phosphatases

Several protein tyrosine phosphatases have been detected in basophils or mast cells *(43)*. CD45 is present on some basophils and mast cells, but there is contradictory evidence as to whether it plays any role in signal transduction from FcεRI *(44)*. Evidence for a role for CD45 comes from the observation that the addition of monoclonal antibodies to CD45 to human basophils blocked IgE-mediated histamine release *(45)* and that mast cells derived from mice in which the CD45 was genetically inactivated failed to secrete after FcεRI stimulation *(44)*. Evidence that CD45 may not be essential for signal transduction in mast cells is provided by the observation that certain variants of RBL-2H3 cell line lack CD45 but release histamine normally *(43)*.

There are several other protein tyrosine phosphatases in basophils and mast cells *(43)*. The two cytoplasmic SH2 domain containing protein tyrosine phosphatases SHP-1 and SHP-2 are present in RBL-2H3 cells, become tyrosine phosphorylated after FcεRI aggregation and associate with FcεRI. Whereas SHP-1 is constitutively associated with the receptor by a non-tyrosine-dependent mechanism, SHP-2 associates with FcεRI only after receptor aggregation because of the interaction of its SH2 domain with tyrosine-phosphorylated β subunit *(42)*. Phosphatases that associate with FcεRI can dephosphorylate both the tyrosine phosphorylated β and γ subunits *(46)*. Altogether these data suggest that protein tyrosine phosphatases play critical roles in the FcεRI-mediated signaling in basophils and mast cells.

3.4. PI Hydrolysis

As with many other receptors, the activation of FcεRI stimulates the hydrolysis of PIP_2 by activation of PLC-γ isoforms. The two products of this reaction, the intracellular second messengers IP_3 and DAG, mediate the release of Ca^{2+} from intracellular stores and activation of PKC, respectively *(47,48)*. There is evidence for the activation of PI-3-K in mast cells. The inhibitor, wortmannin, blocks the function of this kinase and, in parallel, the translocation of PLC-γ1 to the membrane, its activation, and therefore the formation of IP_3 *(49–51)*.

The PLC-γ1 and PLC-γ2 isoforms are activated by stimulation of both receptor and nonreceptor protein tyrosine kinases *(52)*. PLC-γ activity is regulated by tyrosine phosphorylation and by the lipid products of PI-3-K. Stimulation of PI-3-K results in the formation of PIP_3, which by binding the SH2 and the PH domains of PLC-γ both recruit it to the membrane and increase its enzymatic activity *(53,54)*. The translocation of PLC-γ1 to the plasma membrane increases its local concentration in the vicinity of its substrate, PIP_2. This membrane or receptor-associated PLC-γ, or both, could then be tyrosine phosphorylated by the FcεRI-associated and -activated Syk. PLC-γ1 may also directly associate with phosphorylated tyrosine residues in the linker region of Syk *(32,55,56)*.

3.5. Calcium

After FcεRI aggregation, the level of cytoplasmic Ca^{2+} increases rapidly. Part of the initial rise in intracellular Ca^{2+} is caused by the release of Ca^{2+} from the endoplasmic reticulum resulting from IP_3 binding to specific receptors *(57–61)*. The release of Ca^{2+} from the endoplasmic reticulum is followed by an increase in the influx of Ca^{2+} into the cell. Electrophysiological measurements have characterized a Ca^{2+}-selective current (I_{CRAC}) that is activated by depletion of the intracellular Ca^{2+} stores *(62–64)*. This current is very selective for Ca^{2+}; cyclic adenosine monophosphate (cAMP), cyclic guanosine monophosphate (cGMP), guanosine triphosphate (GTP), InsP4, or several other molecules do not activate it. However, the biochemical nature of this channel is unknown. There is a marked difference in the activation of I_{CRAC} compared with the Ca^{2+} release from intracellular stores: low concentrations of InsP3 induce substantial Ca^{2+} release without any activation of I_{CRAC}, whereas higher concentrations of InsP3-activated Ca^{2+} influx *(58)*. This suggests that there are functionally distinct stores controlling Ca^{2+} release and influx: one set of stores involved in Ca^{2+} release, and the other lower affinity store for Ca^{2+} entry. However, despite maximal activation of I_{CRAC}, Ca^{2+} influx can be graded due to changes in membrane potential or as a result of inhibitory signals such as PKC that are activated after receptor stimulation *(65)*. Although an increase in $[Ca^{2+}]_i$ is a prominent signal in mast cells or basophils, it alone is not sufficient to trigger degranulation. Similarly, activation of PKC together with the increase of $[Ca^{2+}]_i$ is not enough of a secretory signal. Therefore, multiple signals are essential for optimal degranulation.

3.6. Tec Family Protein Tyrosine Kinases (Btk and Itk/Emt)

Both Btk and Emt are present in some mast cells and are rapidly tyrosine phosphory-lated and activated after FcεRI aggregation *(66,67)*. Btk is tyrosine phosphorylated by Src family kinases, which then activate it and permit autophosphorylation *(68)*. There-fore, after FcεRI aggregation, Lyn probably tyrosine phosphorylates Btk, which leads to its activation and translocation from the cytosol to the membrane. Both Btk and Emt are also phosphorylated on Ser and Thr residues and associate with and are substrates of PKC, independent of FcεRI aggregation *(69)*. The PKC-mediated phos-phorylation results in the down regulation of the enzymatic activity of Btk.

Mast cells from Btk-negative mice degranulate, although they are less sensitive to FcεRI-mediated activation *(70)*. These cells exhibit a more dramatic decrease in the release of cytokines and defective FcεRI-mediated activation of the JNK pathway, although the ERK activation is normal *(71)*. These changes result in defective activation of transcription. The mechanism for these effects of Btk is probably its role in the influx of Ca^{2+} from the medium. In an avian B-cell line with targeted deletion of Btk, there is decreased tyrosine phosphorylation of PLC-γ2 and no BCR-mediated increase in intracellular Ca^{2+} *(72)*. In Btk-deficient mammalian B cells, there is still a defect in Ca^{2+} influx, although the effect of the lack of Btk is less dramatic *(73,74)*. In these cells, the initial rise in intracellular Ca^{2+} is normal, but the sustained release, attributable to the influx from extracellular sources, is defective. These effects of Btk/Tec are downstream of PI-3-K. Therefore, in normal cells the activation of PI-3-K results in the formation of PIP_3. Btk binds by its PH domain to the PIP_3 and is activated, which induces an increase in the tyrosine phosphorylation of PLC-γ. The formation of IP_3 by PLC-γ then controls the intracellular Ca^{2+} stores and the I_{CRAC}-mediated Ca^{2+} entry.

3.7. Vav

Vav is tyrosine phosphorylated after activation of receptors such as the BCR, TCR, FcγR, and FcεRI *(75,76)*. Vav serves as a GDP-GTP exchange factor for the Rac/Rho family of small GTP-binding proteins *(77)*. Tyrosine-phosphorylated Vav, but not the nonphosphorylated protein, catalyses GDP/GTP exchange on Rac-1 that links FcεRI to the JNK pathway *(77–79)*. Rho regulates the assembly of focal adhesion and actin stress fibers, whereas Rac regulates membrane ruffling *(80)*; both Rac and Rho regulate mast cell secretion *(see below)*. The tyrosine phosphorylation of Vav is downstream of Syk *(81–83)*. By regulating the function of Rac-1, tyrosine-phosphorylated Vav may affect downstream events, such as the changes in cell morphology, membrane ruffles, and secretion.

Vav interacts with molecules such as Grb2, Lck, ZAP-70, Syk, SLP-76, and tubulin. Vav associates with both ZAP-70 and Syk *(84,85)*. The SH2 domain of Vav binds to two tyrosines in the linker region of Syk when they are phosphorylated. Vav is also coprecipitated with FcεRI, which may be mediated indirectly by the binding of Syk to the γ subunit of FcϵRI *(76)*. However, the major tyrosine phosphorylated protein that associates with Vav is SLP-76, a protein that also associates with Grb2 *(86)*. SLP-76 is tyrosine-phosphorylated after FcϵRI aggregation downstream of Syk *(87)*.

3.8. Protein Kinase C

The RBL-2H3 cells contain the Ca^{2+}-dependent α and β and the Ca^{2+}-independent δ, ϵ, and ζ isoforms of PKC *(88,89)*. In nonstimulated cells, most of the PKC is in the cytoplasm but, after FcϵRI activation, the PKC isoforms, except for ζ, translocate to various extents to the membrane *(89,90)*. PKC isozymes are probably necessary for optimal FcϵRI-mediated secretion as shown by the following experiments. There is no secretion in washed permeabilized RBL-2H3 cells, which lose all the PKC isozymes *(89)*. The secretory response is reconstituted by the addition of either the β or δ isozymes of PKC, but the response still requires the presence of Ca^{2+}. In these permeabilized cells, the addition of α and ϵ isozymes of PKC inhibits hydrolysis of FcϵRI-induced PtdIns probably by reducing the tyrosine phosphorylation of PLC-γ1 *(91)*. These results suggest that there are distinct roles for both Ca^{2+} and PKC in the secretory pathway.

The activation of PKC results in phosphorylation on Ser or Thr, or both, of several proteins including the myosin light and heavy chains *(92,93)*. These phosphorylations closely parallel degranulation. The γ chain of FcϵRI is also phosphorylated by PKC on Thr residues after receptor aggregation, probably due to the Ca^{2+} independent PKC δ that associates with the β subunit of the receptor *(94)*. PKC could also play a role in the modulation of secretion. Treatment of RBL-2H3 cells with phorbol esters results in inhibition of both PtdIns hydrolysis and Ca^{2+} influx but in enhanced exocytosis *(95)*. This effect is seen with RBL-2H3 cells in suspension, but not when they are adherent to fibronectin *(96)*.

3.9. Ras and the MAP Kinase Pathways

Recruitment of the Grb2-Sos complex to the FcϵRI receptor may be mediated by binding of the adaptor protein Shc to the tyrosine phosphorylated FcϵRIβ or by another adapter protein (p33) *(22,97,98)*. The adapter protein Shc is constitutively tyrosine phosphorylated in RBL-2H3 cells cultured with fetal serum, probably as a result of c-Kit activation. However, when the cells are cultured in low serum concentrations the tyrosine phosphorylation of Shc is dependent on Syk *(78,97)*.

The ERK, JNK, and p38 MAP kinase pathways are activated after FcϵRI aggregation *(42,79,81,99–105)*. The activation of ERK and of p38 is rapid, reaching a peak within 1–5 minutes, whereas that of JNK is slower. As in many other cells, Ca^{2+} mobilizing agents, PKC activators and stress factors can also activate these pathways.

FcϵRI-induced activation of the ERK pathway is downstream of Syk *(81–83,106)*, although only JNK activation, but not ERK, includes Vav and Rac1 *(78)*. This would suggest a pathway that is FcϵRI→Syk→Vav→Rac1→JNK. The defect in JNK activation in Btk deficient mast cells suggests that the PH domain mediated recruitment of Btk to PIP_3 may also play a role in this activation pathway *(105)*. The activation of JNK in mast cells also probably involves MEKK1 *(79)*. Much less is known about the pathways that lead to the activation of p38; however, there is some overlap with the JNK pathway.

The activation of the ERK1 pathway results in the phosphorylation and stimulation of cytoplasmic phospholipase A2 (cPLA2). The activation of this phospholipase leads to the release of arachidonic acid that is then metabolized into inflammatory mediators. The use of inhibitors suggests that the MAP kinase pathways are critical for arachidonic acid release, but not for degranulation *(102,103,107)*. The activation of the Ras pathway therefore leads to the activation of ERK1 and cPLA2, but degranulation is independent of these two events.

The substrates of ERK, JNK, and the p38 pathways include transcription factors, such as c-Jun, Elk-1, and ATF-2. The phosphorylation of transcription factors and their nuclear migration regulates cytokine genes and proliferation that is induced by activation of FcεRI. Thus the activation of the Ras pathway leads to both the release of arachidonic acid and the nuclear events such as the induction of cytokine genes *(103)*. There are several different pathways to Ras-induced transcriptional regulation in mast cells. Activation of the transcription factor NFAT (nuclear factor of activated T cells) in the context of the IL-4 gene is controlled by Rac-1 in parallel with or by Ras, whereas the Ras/Raf-1/MAPK cascade alone is sufficient for activation of the Elk-1 transcription factor *(108)*.

3.10. Phospholipase D

FcεRI aggregation, calcium ionophore, phorbol 12-myristate 13-acetate (PMA) and compound 48/80 activate the PLD pathway in mast cells, suggesting that PLD stimulation is downstream of the Syk-mediated rise in intracellular Ca^{2+} and the activation of PKC *(109,110)*. The major substrate of phospholipase D in mast cells is phosphatidylcholine, the hydrolysis of which results in the formation of phosphatidic acid that is rapidly dephosphorylated by phosphatidate phosphohydrolyase to form DAG *(111)*. This PLD pathway is the major source of the DAG formed in mast cells after receptor aggregation, and as discussed in previous sections, the DAG activates PKC. The DAG can also be a substrate for DAG lipase for the release of arachidonic acid.

PLD activity is regulated by at least four factors: the phospholipids PIP_2 and PIP_3, PKC and the Ras related proteins Arf and Rho *(112)*. In mast cells, brefeldin A, an inhibitor of Arf, blocks the FcεRI- and calcium ionophore A23187-induced activation of PLD *(113,114)*. However, FcεRI-induced secretion is more easily inhibited than the activation of PLD. The activation of PLD and secretion are also blocked by *Clostridium difficile* toxin B that inhibits the Rho family proteins RhoA, Rac1, and Cdc42 *(115,116)*. However, activation of PLD without a concomitant rise in intracellular Ca^{2+} does not result in degranulation *(113,117,118)*. Altogether, these results suggest that PLD plays a role in FcεRI-mediated secretion.

3.11. Arachidonic Acid Release

Arachidonic acid is released either by the direct action of phospholipase A2 on cellular phospholipids or by the DAG lipase pathway. As discussed above, the activity of cytosolic phospholipase A2 is regulated by phosphorylation by MAP kinase and protein kinase C. Either the cyclo-oxygenase or the lipoxygenase pathway then metabolizes the arachidonic acid. The products of the lipoxygenase pathway are the monhydroxyl fatty acids and the leukotrienes (e.g., the cysteinal leukotrienes LTC4 and the two peptidolytic products LTD4 and LTE4), whereas the cyclo-oxygenase pathway results in the formation of prostaglandin D2. Formation of some thromboxane A2 and prostacyclin occurs as well.

3.12. Small GTP Binding Proteins and Cytoskeletal Changes

Aggregation of FcεRI induces cytoskeletal reorganization and transforms the micro-villous surface of basophils to a plicated ruffled appearance; the cells also spread and become more adherent. These changes are downstream of Syk and precede degranulation. The cytoskeleton is also involved in the large-scale clustering and capping of aggregated FcεRI. These morphological changes are secondary to the rise in intracellular Ca^{2+}, phosphorylation of cellular proteins, and/or activation of GTP-binding proteins. Among the Ras family of small GTP-binding proteins, members of the Ras, Rab, Rho, and Arf families are thought to play a role in secretion in mast cells. Activation of the Ras pathway that leads to the MAP kinase pathways as well as the role of Arf in regulating PLD have been discussed. This section discusses some of the other small GTP proteins.

3.12.1. Rab3

Rab3 isoforms are associated with secretory organelles, including synaptic and mast cell secretory granules *(119)*. They interact with vesicle specific proteins and may play a role in the docking and regulation of exocytosis in cells. RBL-2H3 cells express Rab3a and Rab3d isoforms. The majority of Rab3a is in the cytosol, whereas Rab3d is in the membrane fraction *(120)*. The intracellular perfusion of mast cells with Rab3a or with a 16 amino acid peptide based on the amino-terminal sequence of Rab3 induces secretion *(121)*. Furthermore, the over-expression of wild type or a dominant-negative form of Rab3a or Rab3d in RBL-2H3 cells inhibits secretion *(120,122)*. These results suggest that Rab3 plays a role in granule fusion and exocytosis.

3.12.2. Rho

The Rho family of GTPase mediate signals from cell surface receptors to the cytoskel-eton. As discussed in previous sections, Vav has guanine nucleotide exchange factor activity toward Rac1, whereas Rho/Cdc42 and Arf stimulate PLD activity. One of the downstream targets of the Rho family of GTPases is Rho kinase, which by phosphorylat-ing both myosin light chain phosphatase and myosin light chain regulates actin organiza-tion in the cells. The phosphorylation of both myosin heavy and light chains by PKC and by myosin light chain kinase correlates with antigen or calcium ionophore/PMA-induced secretion in RBL-2H3 cells *(92,93,123)*. Inhibition of either of the two kinases blocks phosphorylation as well as secretion *(93)*. Therefore, Rho-kinase probably partici-pates in the control of myosin in these cells, although the relationship of this to secretion remains unclear.

Both Rac and Rho appear to play a role in signaling from FcεRI aggregation. Inhibitors of endogenous Rac and Rho reduce secretory responses of permeabilized rat peritoneal mast cells, whereas constitutively active Rac or Rho mutant proteins enhance secretion and increase the level of F-actin *(124,125)*. The F-actin becomes rearranged into membrane ruffles and also associates with myosin in a cytoplasmic meshwork

(126). Although degranulation is independent of actin polymerization, cytoskeletal reorganization and secretion are still strongly correlated *(125)*. There is further evidence to suggest a role for these molecules in signal transduction. First, in permeabilized mast cells secretion is reconstituted by the addition of a complex of Rac and RhoGDI *(127)*. Second, RhoGDI, which inhibits Rho activity, when introduced into rat mast cells, inhibits the GTP-γ-S induced release *(128)*. Third, *Clostridium botulinum* C3 toxin, an inhibitor of Rho, blocks FcεRI secretion from permeabilized RBL-2H3 cells *(129)*. By contrast, *C. difficile* toxin B, which inactivates Rho, Rac1, and Cdc42, inhibits FcεRI-, GTP-γ-S-, or PMA-induced activation of phospholipase D both in intact and in permeabilized RBL-2H3 cells *(115)*. Studies with these toxins in intact cells suggest that Cdc42 is the GTPase that participates in degranulation *(116)*. Similarly, overexpression of the dominant-negative mutant form of Cdc42 in RBL-2H3 cells inhibits FcεRI-induced degranulation *(130)*. Altogether, these results suggest that the different small GTP binding proteins control distinct pathways that affect cytoskeletal change and are involved in degranulation.

4. INHIBITORY SIGNALS

Both intracellular and membrane molecules in basophils/mast cells can regulate or inhibit FcεRI-mediated signaling. Some of the membrane molecules are in close proximity to FcεRI. Inhibitory signals by the membrane molecules require that they be aggregated. In the case of one group, which includes a unique ganglioside, CD63, mast cell function-associated antigen (MAFA), and CD81, this inhibition is when the molecules are crosslinked, whereas in the case of gp49 and FcγRIIB the molecules have to be coligated with FcεRI. Recent studies have suggested the biochemical mechanism for this group that requires coligation with FcεRI.

The cytoplasmic domain of FcγRIIB and gp49 contains an immunoreceptor tyrosine-based inhibition motif (ITIM), which consists of 13-amino acids, I/V-X-pY-X2-L/V, also found in the cytoplasmic domain of other inhibitory receptors *(131,132)*. The cytoplasmic domain of MAFA includes the YSTL sequence that is part of the canonical ITIM sequence *(133)*. Studies with FcγRIIB have shown that the inhibitory activity requires the tyrosine residue, which probably becomes tyrosine phosphorylated after cell activation *(134)*. This phosphorylation is caused by Lyn and results in the recruitment of inhibitory molecules. Although in vitro, the phosphorylated ITIM of FcγRIIB binds SHIP and the two protein tyrosine phosphatases, SHP-1 and SHP-2, experimental evidence suggests that the inhibitory effect of coaggregation of FcγRIIB with FcεRI is attributable to SHIP.

4.1. SHIP

SHIP is a 145-kDa protein expressed in hematopoietic cells *(135)*. It is tyrosine phosphorylated after stimulation of FcεRI independent of Syk *(41)*. SHIP dephosphorylates the D-5 position of PIP_3 or inositol 1,3,4,5-tetraphosphate. This reduces the concentration of PIP_3, the product of PI-3-K. Both Btk and PLC-γ are recruited to the membrane by binding through their PH domains to PIP_3, which also results in the activation of PLC-γ *(136)*. SHIP would therefore decrease the recruitment and activation of Btk and PLC-γ, which would then result in a reduction in the formation of IP$_3$ *(137)*. This then would effect the IP$_3$ induced release of intracellular Ca^{2+} and ultimately Ca^{2+} influx.

4.2. Cbl (p120$^{c\text{-}cbl}$)

Cbl (p120$^{c\text{-}cbl}$), a protein expressed in many hematopoetic cells, may also regulate mast cell secretion *(34,35)*. Cbl associates with a variety of signaling molecules including PI-3-K, Lyn, Fyn, Crk, Grb2, and Syk. Cbl is tyrosine phosphorylated predominantly downstream of Syk. The transient overexpression of Cbl in RBL-2H3 cells inhibits the receptor-induced tyrosine phosphorylation and activation of Syk, decreasing the downstream phosphorylation of other proteins and secretion. Thus, Cbl may control the kinase activity of Syk by regulating the level of its tyrosine phosphorylation.

Interestingly, a synthetic tyrosine phosphorylated peptide based on the ITAM sequence of the β subunit, but not the γ subunit of FcϵRI, precipitates SHIP and SHP-2, in addition to some other signaling molecules *(22,41,42)*. These molecules are tyrosine-phosphorylated independent of Syk and may regulate or modulate FcϵRI-mediated signal transduction. This suggests that the different subunits of FcϵRI recruit both activating and regulatory molecules; the γ subunit recruits Syk, which is crucial for downstream activating signals, whereas the β subunit recruits molecules such as SHIP and SHP-2, which may either regulate or reverse the signals generated by receptor aggregation.

5. MODULATION OF THE MAST CELL RESPONSE BY CELL ADHESION

Basophils and mast cells have surface adhesion receptors (e.g., integrins) that are involved in the binding of these cells to other cells or to the extracellular matrix *(138)*. Adherence results in intracellular signals that induce changes in the cytoskeleton, cell spreading, and the redistribution of secretory granules to the periphery of the cell and the tyrosine phosphorylation of several proteins. These proteins include the FAK, the related kinase Pyk2, the adhesion molecule platelet/endothelial cell adhesion molecule 1 (PECAM-1, or CD31), and the cytoskeletal protein paxillin *(138–141)*. Adhesion may also change the activity of PKC *(96)*. These changes induced by cell adherence may play an important role in modulating the intracellular signaling that leads to degranulation. For example, there is enhanced secretion from RBL-2H3 cells that are adherent to surfaces coated with fibronectin *(139)*.

The aggregation of FcϵRI results in tyrosine phosphorylation of the protein tyrosine kinases FAK and Pyk2 which are downstream of the activaiton of PKC and the rise in intracellular Ca^{2+} and therefore downstream of Syk *(142,143)*. This receptor-induced phosphorylation of FAK and Pyk2 is dramatically enhanced by adherence of the cells to fibronectin and as noted above, this adherence also results in enhanced secretion *(139,142)*. Therefore, adherence may regulate the extent of mast cell degranulation by modulating intracellular protein tyrosine phosphorylations.

FAK and Pyk2 interact with signaling molecules such as paxillin, Cas, the p85 subunit of PI-3-K, Grb2, Crk, and Csk, suggesting that the FcϵRI induced phosphorylation of these molecules may further propagate signaling in the late steps of degranulation.

FAK, Pyk2, and paxillin become coordinately tyrosine phosphorylated after FcεRI aggregation and this phosphorylation is downstream of Syk and is enhanced by adherence of the cells *(144)*. Paxillin forms complexes with many proteins including Lyn, Csk, Crk, FAK, vinculin, α-actinin, and talin which may help direct actin filament interactions with the membrane *(145)*. Tyrosine phosphorylation of paxillin, FAK, and Pyk2 may be important in the development of actin stress fibers and the reorganization of F-actin and thus may play a role in signal transduction from receptors to the cytoskeleton *(146)*.

Experimental evidence suggests that FAK plays an important role during the late stages of signaling leading to degranulation. A monoclonal antibody to an FcεRI-associated ganglioside induces tyrosine phosphorylation of Lyn, PLC-γ1, Syk and the β and γ subunits of FcεRI, but not of FAK *(147,148)*. This antibody, however, does not induce significant degranulation, suggesting a role for FAK tyrosine phosphorylation in secretion from mast cells. Further evidence for an important function of FAK in degranulation are recent studies with a FAK deficient variant of the RBL-2H3 cells *(149)*. FcεRI, but not ionophore mediated secretion, is defective in these variant cells that have decreased levels of FAK. The stable transfection of FAK markedly enhances the FcεRI mediated secretion. This enhancement does not require the catalytic activity or the autophosphorylation site of FAK, suggesting that FAK is functioning as an adapter or linker molecule. However, the catalytically inactive FAK is still tyrosine phosphorylated after FcεRI aggregation. Tyrosine phosphorylation of the kinase-inactive FAK may still permit binding to it of other proteins mediated by SH2 domains; therefore, the mutated FAK can still function to transduce FcεRI-initiated signals.

The signals generated by FcεRI aggregation also result in enhanced cell adherence, indicating that it regulates adhesion molecules that could be secondary to tyrosine phosphorylations. For example, FcεRI aggregation results in tyrosine phosphorylation of the cell surface adhesion molecule PECAM-1 (CD31), which then binds the protein tyrosine phosphatase SHP-2 *(141,150)*. PECAM-1 is a cell adhesion molecule that functions in the transmigration of cells across the endothelium into sites of inflammation *(151)*. Therefore, the level of the tyrosine phosphorylation of PECAM-1 may modulate its interaction with other molecules, thereby regulating the migration of basophils into inflammatory sites.

6. CONCLUDING REMARKS

The signal transduction pathways initiated by FcεRI in basophils or mast cells are similar to that induced by aggregation of other immune receptors on T cells, B cells, or monocytes. In mast cells, Syk is critical for initiating signal transduction for secretion, although several molecules are tyrosine phosphorylated independent of Syk. Some of these molecules may regulate the extent of signal transduction. Secretion is also regulated by adhesion receptors that can activate other kinases, such as FAK.

REFERENCES

1. Metzger H. Receptor for IgE and initiation of allergic reactions, in *Allergy*, 2nd Ed (Kaplan AP, ed), WB Saunders, Philadelphia, 1997, pp. 92–98.
2. Reth M. Antigen receptor tail clue. *Nature* 1989; 338:383, 384.

3. Daeron M. Fc receptor biology. *Annu Rev Immunol* 1997; 15:203–234.
4. Lin SQ, Cicala C, Scharenberg AM, JP Kinet. The FcεRIβ subunit functions as an amplifier of FcεRIγ-mediated cell activation signals. *Cell* 1996; 85:985–995.
5. Daeron M, Malbec O, Latour S, Arock M, Fridman WH. Regulation of high-affinity IgE receptor-mediated mast cell activation by murine low-affinity IgG receptors. *J Clin Invest* 1995; 95:577–585.
6. Vivier E, Daeron M. Immunoreceptor tyrosine-based inhibition motifs. *Immunol Today* 1997; 18:286–291.
7. Marszalek PE, Farrell B, Verdugo P, Fernandez JM. Kinetics of release of serotonin from isolated secretory granules. 2. Ion exchange determines the diffusivity of serotonin. *Biophys J* 1997; 73:1169–1183.
8. Benhamou M, Gutkind JS, Robbins KC, Siraganian RP. Tyrosine phosphorylation coupled to IgE receptor-mediated signal transduction and histamine release. *Proc Natl Acad Sci USA* 1990; 87:5327–5330.
9. Benhamou M, Siraganian RP. Protein-tyrosine phosphorylation: An essential component of FcεRI signaling. *Immunol Today* 1992; 13:195–197.
10. Siraganian RP, Zhang J, Kimura T. Regulation and function of protein tyrosine Syk in FcεRI-mediated signaling, in *Signal Transduction in Mast Cells and Basophils*. Razin E, Rivera J, eds. Springer, New York, 1999; pp. 115–133.
11. Eiseman E, Bolen JB. Engagement of the high-affinity IgE receptor activates src protein-related tyrosine kinases. *Nature* 1992; 355:78–80.
12. Kihara H, Siraganian RP. Src homology 2 domains of Syk and Lyn bind to tyrosine-phosphorylated subunits of the high affinity IgE receptor. *J Biol Chem* 1994; 269:22,427–22,432.
13. Jouvin MH, Adamczewski M, Numerof R, Letourneur O, Valle A, Kinet JP. Differential control of the tyrosine kinases Lyn and Syk by the two signaling chains of the high affinity immunoglobulin E receptor. *J Biol Chem* 1994; 269:5918–5925.
14. Vonakis BM, Chen HX, Haleem-Smith H, Metzger H. The unique domain as the site on Lyn kinase for its constitutive association with the high affinity receptor for IgE. *J Biol Chem* 1997; 272:24,072–24,080.
15. Honda Z, Suzuki T, Hirose N, Aihara M, Shimizu T, Nada S, Okada M, Ra CS, Morita Y, Ito K. Roles of C-terminal Src kinase in the initiation and the termination of the high affinity IgE receptor-mediated signaling. *J Biol Chem* 1997; 272:25,753–25,760.
16. Paolini R, Jouvin MH, Kinet JP. Phosphorylation and dephosphorylation of the high-affinity receptor for immunoglobulin E immediately after receptor engagement and disengagement. *Nature* 1991; 353:855–858.
17. Pribluda VS, Pribluda C, Metzger H. Biochemical evidence that the phosphorylated tyrosines, serines, and threonines on the aggregated high affinity receptor for IgE are in the immunoreceptor tyrosine-based activation motifs. *J Biol Chem* 1997; 272:11,185–11,192.
18. Pribluda VS, Pribluda C, Metzger H. Transphosphorylation as the mechanism by which the high-affinity receptor for IgE is phosphorylated upon aggregation. *Proc Natl Acad Sci USA* 1994; 91:11,246–11,250.
19. Yamashita T, S-Y Mao, Metzger H. Aggregation of the high-affinity IgE receptor and enhanced activity of p53/56^{lyn} protein-tyrosine kinase. *Proc Natl Acad Sci USA* 1994; 91:11,251–11,255.
20. Hibbs ML, Tarlinton DM, Armes J, Grail D, Hodgson G, Maglitto R, Stacker RA, Dunn AR. Multiple defects in the immune system of Lyn-deficient mice, culminating in autoimmune disease. *Cell* 1995; 83:301–311.
21. Nishizumi H, Yamamoto T. Impaired tyrosine phosphorylation and Ca^{2+} mobilization, but not degranulation, in Lyn-deficient bone marrow-derived mast cells. *J Immunol* 1997; 158:2350–2355.

22. Kimura T, Kihara H, Bhattacharyya S, Sakamoto H, Appella E, Siraganian RP. Downstream signaling molecules bind to different phosphorylated immunoreceptor tyrosine-based activation motif (ITAM) peptides of the high affinity IgE receptor. *J Biol Chem* 1996; 271:27,962–27,968.

23. Hutchcroft JE, Geahlen RL, Deanin GG, Oliver JM. FcεRI-mediated tyrosine phosphorylation and activation of the 72-kDa protein-tyrosine kinase, PTK72, in RBL-2H3 rat tumor mast cells. *Proc Natl Acad Sci USA* 1992; 89:9107–9111.

24. Benhamou M, Ryba NJP, Kihara H, Nishikata H, Siraganian RP. Protein-tyrosine kinase p72syk in high affinity IgE receptor signaling. Identification as a component of pp72 and association with the receptor γ chain. *J Biol Chem* 1993; 268:23,318–23,324.

25. Shiue L, Green J, Green OM, Karas JL, Morgenstern JP, Ram MK, Taylor MK, Zoller MJ, Zydowsky LD, Bolen JB, Brugge JS. Interaction of p72syk with the γ and β subunits of the high-affinity receptor for immunoglobulin E, FcεRI. *Mol Cell Biol* 1995; 15: 272–281.

26. Hatada MH, Lu X, Laird ER, Green J, Morgenstern JP, Lou M, Marr CS, Phillips TB, Ram MK, Theriault K. Molecular basis for interaction of the protein tyrosine kinase ZAP-70 with the T-cell receptor. *Nature* 1995; 377:32–38.

27. Kimura T, Sakamoto H, Appella E, Siraganian RP. Conformational changes induced in the protein tyrosine kinase p72syk by tyrosine phosphorylation or by binding of phosphorylated immunoreceptor tyrosine-based activation motif peptides. *Mol Cell Biol* 1996; 16:1471–1478.

28. Rowley RB, Burkhardt AL, Chao HG, Matsueda GR, Bolen JB. Syk protein-tyrosine kinase is regulated by tyrosine- phosphorylated Ig alpha/Ig beta immunoreceptor tyrosine activation motif binding and autophosphorylation. *J Biol Chem* 1995; 270:11,590–11,594.

29. Shiue L, Zoller MJ, Brugge JS. Syk is activated by phosphotyrosine-containing peptides representing the tyrosine-based activation motifs of the high affinity receptor for IgE. *J Biol Chem* 1995; 270:10,498–10,502.

30. El-Hillal O, Kurosaki T, Yamamura H, Kinet JP, Scharenberg AM. Syk kinase activation by a Src kinase-initiated activation loop phosphorylation chain reaction. *Proc Natl Acad Sci USA* 1997; 94:1919–1924.

31. Zhang J, Kimura T, Siraganian RP. Mutations in the activation loop tyrosines of protein tyrosine kinase Syk abrogate intracellular signaling but not kinase activity. *J Immunol* 1998; 161: 4366–4374.

32. Sidorenko SP, Law CL, Chandran KA, Clarke EA. Human spleen tyrosine kinase p72syk associates with the Src-family kinase p53/56lyn and a 120-kDa phosphoprotein. *Proc Natl Acad Sci USA* 1995; 92:359–363.

33. Aoki Y, Kim YT, Stillwell R, Kim TJ, Pillai S. The SH2 domains of Src family kinases associate with Syk. *J Biol Chem* 1995; 270:15,658–15,663.

34. Ota Y, Beitz LO, Scharenberg AM, Donovan JA, Kinet JP, Samelson LE. Characterization of Cbl tyrosine phosphorylation and a Cbl-Syk complex in RBL-2H3 cells. *J Exp Med* 1996; 184:1713–1723.

35. Ota Y, Samelson LE. The product of the proto-oncogene c-cbl: A negative regulator of the Syk tyrosine kinase. *Science* 1997; 276:418–420.

36. Zhang J, Berenstein EH, Evans RL, Siraganian RP. Transfection of Syk protein tyrosine kinase reconstitutes high affinity IgE receptor mediated degranulation in a Syk negative variant of rat basophilic leukemia RBL-2H3 cells. *J Exp Med* 1996; 184:71–79.

37. Yagi S, Suzuki K, Hasegawa A, Okumura K, Ra C. Cloning of the cDNA for the deleted Syk kinase homologous to ZAP-70 from human basophilic leukemia cell line (KU812) *Biochem Biophys Res Commun* 1994; 200:28–34.

38. Rowley RB, Bolen JB, and Fargnoli J. Molecular cloning of rodent p72syk. Evidence of alternative mRNA splicing. *J Biol Chem* 1995; 270:12,659–12,664.

39. Latour S, Chow LML, Veillette A. Differential intrinsic enzymatic activity of Syk and Zap-70 protein-tyrosine kinases. *J Biol Chem* 1996; 271:22,782–22,790.

40. Latour S, Zhang J, Siraganian RP, Veillette A. A unique insert in the linker domain of Syk is necessary for its function in immunoreceptor signalling. *EMBO J* 1998; 17:2584–2595.

41. Kimura T, Sakamoto H, Appella E, Siraganian RP. The negative signaling molecule inositol polyphosphate 5-phosphatase, SHIP, binds to tyrosine phosphorylated beta subunit of the high affinity IgE receptor. *J Biol Chem* 1997; 272:13,991–13,996.

42. Kimura T, Zhang J, Sagawa K, Sakaguchi K, Appella E, Siraganian RP. Syk independent tyrosine phosphorylation and association of the protein tyrosine phosphatase SHP-1 and SHP-2 with the high affinity IgE receptor. *J Immunol* 1997; 159:4426–4434.

43. Swieter M, Berenstein EH, Swaim WD, Siraganian RP. Aggregation of IgE receptors in rat basophilic leukemia 2H3 cells induces tyrosine phosphorylation of the cytosolic protein-tyrosine phosphatase HePTP. *J Biol Chem* 1995; 270:21,902–21,906.

44. Berger SA, Mak TW, Paige CJ. Leukocyte common antigen (CD45) is required for immunoglobulin E- mediated degranulation of mast cells. *J Exp Med* 1994; 180:471–476.

45. Hook WA, Berenstein EH, Zinsser FU, Fischler C, Siraganian RP. Monoclonal antibodies to the leukocyte common antigen (CD45) inhibit IgE-mediated histamine release from human basophils. *J Immunol* 1991; 147:2670–2676.

46. Swieter M, Berenstein EH, Siraganian RP. Protein tyrosine phosphatase activity associates with the high affinity IgE receptor and dephosphorylates the receptor subunits, but not Lyn or Syk. *J Immunol* 1995; 155:5330–5336.

47. Berridge MJ. Inositol trisphosphate and calcium signalling. *Nature* 1993; 361:315–325.

48. Nishizuka Y. Protein kinase C and lipid signaling for sustained cellular responses. *FASEB J* 1995; 9:484–496.

49. Yano H, Nakanishi S, Kimura K, Hanai N, Saitoh Y, Fukui Y, Nonomura Y, Matsuda Y. Inhibition of histamine secretion by wortmannin through the blockade of phosphatidyl-inositol 3-kinase in RBL-2H3 cells. *J Biol Chem* 1993; 268:25,846–25,856.

50. Barker SA, Caldwell KK, Hall A, Martinez AM, Pfeiffer JR, Oliver JM, Wilson BS. Wortmannin blocks lipid and protein kinase activities associated with PI 3-kinase and inhibits a subset of responses induced by FcεRI cross-linking. *Mol Biol Cell* 1995; 6:1145–1158.

51. Barker SA, Caldwell KK, Pfeiffer JR, Wilson BS. Wortmannin-sensitive phosphorylation, translocation, and activation of PLC γ1, but not PLC γ2, in antigen-stimulated RBL-2H3 mast cells. *Mol Biol Cell* 1998; 9:483–496.

52. Rhee SG, Bae YS. Regulation of phosphoinositide-specific phospholipase C isozymes. *J Biol Chem* 1997; 272:15,045–15,048.

53. Bae YS, Cantley LG, Chen CS, Kim SR, Kwon KS, Rhee SG. Activation of phospholipase C-γ by phosphatidylinositol 3,4,5-trisphosphate. *J Biol Chem* 1998; 273:4465–4469.

54. Falasca M, Logan SK, Lehto VP, Baccante G, Lemmon MA, Schlessinger J. Activation of phospholipase Cγ by PI 3-kinase-induced PH domain-mediated membrane targeting. *EMBO J* 1998; 17:414–422.

55. Sillman AL, Monroe JG. Association of p72^{syk} with the src homology-2 (SH2) domains of PLC γ1 in B lymphocytes. *J Biol Chem* 1995; 270:11,806–11,811.

56. Law CL, Chandran KA, Sidorenko SP, Clark EA. Phospholipase C-γ1 interacts with conserved phosphotyrosyl residues in the linker region of Syk and is a substrate for Syk. *Mol Cell Biol* 1996; 16:1305–1315.

57. Matthews G, Neher E, Penner R. Second messenger-activated calcium influx in rat perito-neal mast cells. *J Physiol* 1989; 418:105–130.

58. Parekh AB, Fleig A, Penner R. The store-operated calcium current I$_{(CRAC)}$: Nonlinear activation by InsP3 and dissociation from calcium release. *Cell* 1997; 89:973–980.

59. Kim TD, Eddlestone GT, Mahmoud SF, Kuchtey J, Fewstrell C. Correlating Ca²⁺ responses and secretion in individual RBL-2H3 mucosal mast cells. *J Biol Chem* 1997; 272:31,225–31,229.

60. Watras J, Moraru I, Costa DJ, Kindman LA. Two inositol 1,4,5-trisphosphate binding sites in rat basophilic leukemia cells: Relationship between receptor occupancy and calcium release. *Biochemistry* 1994; 33:14,359–14,367.

61. Hirata M, Takeuchi H, Riley AM, Mills SJ, Watanabe Y, Potter BL. Inositol 1,4,5-trisphosphate receptor subtypes differentially recognize regioisomers of D-myo-inositol 1,4,5-trisphosphate. *Biochem J* 1997; 328:93–98.

62. Zweifach A, Lewis RS. Mitogen-regulated Ca²⁺ current of T lymphocytes is activated by depletion of intracellular Ca²⁺ stores. *Proc Natl Acad Sci USA* 1993; 90:6295–6299.

63. Hoth M, Penner R. Depletion of intracellular calcium stores activates a calcium current in mast cells. *Nature* 1992; 355:353–356.

64. Parekh AB, Penner R. Regulation of store-operated calcium currents in mast cells. *Soc Gen Physiol Ser* 1996; 51:231–239.

65. Parekh AB, Penner R. Depletion-activated calcium current is inhibited by protein kinase in RBL-2H3 cells. *Proc Natl Acad Sci USA* 1995; 92:7907–7911.

66. Kawakami Y, Yao L, Miura T, Tsukada S, Witte ON, Kawakami T. Tyrosine phosphorylation and activation of Bruton tyrosine kinase upon FcεRI cross-linking. *Mol Cell Biol* 1994; 14:5108–5113.

67. Kawakami Y, Yao L, Tashiro M, Gibson S, Mills GB, Kawakami T. Activation and interaction with protein kinase C of a cytoplasmic tyrosine kinase, Itk/Tsk/Emt, on FcεRI cross-linking on mast cells. *J Immunol* 1995; 155:3556–3562.

68. Mahajan S, Fargnoli J, Burkhardt AL, Kut SA, Saouaf SJ, Bolen JB. Src family protein tyrosine kinases induce autoactivation of Bruton's tyrosine kinase. 1995; *Mol Cell Biol* 15:5304–5311.

69. Yao L, Kawakami Y, Kawakami T. The pleckstrin homology domain of Bruton tyrosine kinase interacts with protein kinase C. *Proc Natl Acad Sci USA* 1994; 91:9175–9179.

70. Hata D, Kawakami Y, Inagaki N, Lantz CS, Kitamura T, Khan WN, Maeda-Yamamoto M, Miura T, Han W, Hartman SE, Yao L, Nagai H, Goldfeld AE, Alt FW, Galli SJ, Witte ON, Kawalami. T Involvement of Bruton's tyrosine kinase in FcεRI-dependent mast cell degranulation and cytokine production. *J Exp Med* 1998; 187:1235–1247.

71. Kawakami Y, Miura T, Bissonnette R, Hata D, Khan WN, Kitamura T, Maeda-Yamamoto M, Hartman SE, Yao LB, Alt FW, Kawakami T. Bruton's tyrosine kinase regulates apoptosis and JNK/SAPK kinase activity. *Proc Natl Acad Sci USA* 1997; 94:3938–3942.

72. Takata M, Kurosaki T. A role for Bruton's tyrosine kinase in B cell antigen receptor-mediated activation of phospholipase C-γ2. *J Exp Med* 1996; 184:31–40.

73. Fluckiger AC, Li ZM, Kato RM, Wahl MI, Ochs HD, Longnecker R, Kinet JP, Witte ON, Scharenberg AM, Rawlings DJ. Btk/Tec kinases regulate sustained increases in intracellular Ca²⁺ following B-cell receptor activation. *EMBO J* 1998; 17:1973–1985.

74. Scharenberg AM, El-Hillal O, Fruman DA, Beitz LO, Li ZM, Lin SQ, Gout I, Cantley LC, Rawlings DJ, Kinet JP. Phosphatidylinositol-3,4,5-trisphosphate (PtdIns-3,4,5-P-3) Tec kinase-dependent calcium signaling pathway: A target for SHIP-mediated inhibitory signals. *EMBO J* 1998; 17:1961–1972.

75. Margolis B, Hu P, Katzav S, Li W, Oliver JM, Ullrich A, Weiss A, Schlessinger J. Tyrosine phosphorylation of *vav* proto-oncogene product containing SH2 domain and transcription factor motifs. *Nature* 1992; 356:71–74.

76. Song JS, Gomez J, Stancato LF, Rivera J. Association of a p95 Vav-containing signaling complex with the FcεRIγ chain in the RBL-2H3 mast cell line. Evidence for a constitutive in vivo association of Vav with Grb2, Raf-1, and ERK2 in an active complex. *J Biol Chem* 1996; 271:26,962–26,970.

77. Crespo P, Schuebel KE, Ostrom AA, Gutkind JS, Bustelo XR. Phosphotyrosine-dependent activation of Rac-1 GDP/GTP exchange by the *vav* proto-oncogene product. *Nature* 1997; 385:169–172.

78. Teramoto H, Salem P, Robbins KC, Bustelo XR, Gutkind JS. Tyrosine phosphorylation of the *vav* proto-oncogene product links FcεRI to the Rac1-JNK pathway. *J Biol Chem* 1997; 272:10,751–10,755.

79. Ishizuka T, Terada N, Gerwins P, Hamelmann E, Oshiba A, Fanger GR, Johnson GL, Gelfand EW. Mast cell tumor necrosis factor α production is regulated by MEK kinases. *Proc Natl Acad Sci USA* 1997; 94:6358–6363.

80. Hall A. Small GTP-binding proteins and the regulation of the actin cytoskeleton. *Annu Rev Cell Biol* 1994; 10:31–54.

81. Hirasawa N, Scharenberg A, Yamamura H, Beaven MA, Kinet JP. A requirement for Syk in the activation of the microtubule-associated protein kinase/phospholipase A2 pathway by FcεRI is not shared by a G protein-coupled receptor. *J Biol Chem* 1995; 270:10,960–10,967.

82. Costello PS, Turner M, Walters AE, Cunningham CN, Bauer PH, Downward J, Tybulewicz VLJ. Critical role for the tyrosine kinase Syk in signalling through the high affinity IgE receptor of mast cells. *Oncogene* 1996; 13:2595–2605.

83. Zhang J, Swaim WD, Berenstein EH, Siraganian RP. Syk protein tyrosine kinase is essential for high affinity IgE receptor-induced cytoskeletal changes in mast cells. *J Allergy and Clin Immunol* 1997; 99:S93.

84. Katzav S, Sutherland M, Packham G, Yi T, Weiss A. The protein tyrosine kinase ZAP-70 can associate with the SH2 domain of proto-Vav. *J Biol Chem* 1994; 269:32,579–32,585.

85. Deckert M, Tartare-Deckert S, Couture C, Mustelin T, Altman A. Functional and physical interactions of Syk family kinases with the Vav proto-oncogene product. *Immunity* 1996; 5:591–604.

86. Wu J, Motto DG, Koretzky GA, Weiss A. Vav and SLP-76 interact and functionally cooperate in IL-2 gene activation. *Immunity* 1996; 4:593–602.

87. Hendricks-Taylor LR, Motto DG, Zhang J, Siraganian RP, Koretzky GA. SLP-76 is a substrate of the high affinity IgE receptor stimulated protein tyrosine kinases in RBL-2H3 cells. *J Biol Chem* 1997; 271:1363–1367.

88. Huang FL, Yoshida Y, Cunha-Melo JR, Beaven MA, Huang KP. Differential down-regulation of protein kinase C isozymes. *J Biol Chem* 1989; 264:4238–4243.

89. Ozawa K, Szallasi Z, Kazanietz MG, Blumberg PM, Mischak H, Mushinski JF, Beaven MA. Ca^{2+}-dependent and Ca^{2+}-independent isozymes of protein kinase C mediate exocytosis in antigen-stimulated rat basophilic RBL-2H3 cells. Reconstitution of secretory responses with Ca^{2+} and purified isozymes in washed permeabilized cells. *J Biol Chem* 1993; 268:1749–1756.

90. Buccione R, Di Tullio G, Caretta M, Marinetti MR, Bizzarri C, Francavilla S, Luini A, De Matteis MA. Analysis of protein kinase C requirement for exocytosis in permeabilized rat basophilic leukaemia RBL-2H3 cells: A GTP-binding protein(s) as a potential target for protein kinase C. *Biochem J* 1994; 298:149–156.

91. Ozawa K, Yamada K, Kazanietz MG, Blumberg PM, Beaven MA. Different isozymes of protein kinase C mediate feedback inhibition of phospholipase C and stimulatory signals for exocytosis in rat RBL-2H3 cells. *J Biol Chem* 1993; 268:2280–2283.

92. Ludowyke RI, Peleg I, Beaven MA, Adelstein RS. Antigen-induced secretion of histamine and the phosphorylation of myosin by protein kinase C in rat basophilic leukemia cells. *J Biol Chem* 1989; 264:12,492–12,501.

93. Choi OH, Adelstein RS, Beaven MA. Secretion from rat basophilic RBL-2H3 cells is associated with diphosphorylation of myosin light chains by myosin light chain kinase as well as phosphorylation by protein kinase C. *J Biol Chem* 1994; 269:536–541.

94. Germano P, Gomez J, Kazanietz MG, Blumberg PM, Rivera J. Phosphorylation of the γ chain of the high affinity receptor for immunoglobulin E by receptor-associated protein kinase C-Delta. *J Biol Chem* 1994; 269:23,102–23,107.

95. Gat-Yablonski G, Sagi-Eisenberg R. Differential down-regulation of protein kinase C selectively affects IgE-dependent exocytosis and inositol trisphosphate formation. *Biochem J* 1990; 270:679–684.

96. Wolfe PC, Chang EY, Rivera J, Fewtrell C. Differential effects of the protein kinase C activator phorbol 12-myristate 13-acetate on calcium responses and secretion in adherent and suspended RBL-2H3 mucosal mast cells. *J Biol Chem* 1996; 271:6658–6665.

97. Jabril-Cuenod B, Zhang C, Scharenberg AM, Paolini R, Numerof R, Beaven MA, Kinet JP. Syk-dependent phosphorylation of Shc—A potential link between FcεRI and the Ras/mitogen-activated protein kinase signaling pathway through Sos and Grb2. *J Biol Chem* 1996; 271:16,268–16,272.

98. Turner H, Reif K, Rivera J, Cantrell DA. Regulation of the adapter molecule Grb2 by the FcεRI in the mast cell line RBL2H3. *J Biol Chem* 1995; 270:9500–9506.

99. Offermanns S, Jones SVP, Bombien E, Schultz G. Stimulation of mitogen-activated protein kinase activity by different secretory stimuli in rat basophilic leukemia cells. *J Immunol* 1994; 152:250–261.

100. Santini F, Beaven MA. Tyrosine phosphorylation of a mitogen-activated protein kinase-like protein occurs at a late step in exocytosis. Studies with tyrosine phosphatase inhibitors and various secretagogues in rat RBL-2H3 cells. *J Biol Chem* 1993; 268:22,716–22,722.

101. Fukamachi H, Takei M, Kawakami T. Activation of multiple protein kinases including a MAP kinase upon FcεRI cross-linking. *Int Arch Allergy Immunol* 1993; 102:15–25.

102. Hirasawa N, Santini F, Beaven MA. Activation of the mitogen-activated protein kinase/cytosolic phospholipase A2 pathway in a rat mast cell line. Indications of different pathways for release of arachidonic acid and secretory granules. *J Immunol* 1995; 154:5391–5402.

103. Zhang C, Baumgartner RA, Yamada K, Beaven MA. Mitogen-activated protein (MAP) kinase regulates production of tumor necrosis factor-α and release of arachidonic acid in mast cells—Indications of communication between p38 and p42 MAP kinases. *J Biol Chem* 1997; 272:13,397–13,402.

104. Zhang C, Hirasawa N, Beaven MA. Antigen activation of mitogen-activated protein kinase in mast cells through protein kinase C-dependent and independent pathways. *J Immunol* 1997; 158:4968–4975.

105. Ishizuka T, Oshiba A, Sakata N, Terada N, Johnson GL, Gelfand EW. Aggregation of the FcεRI on mast cells stimulates c-Jun amino-terminal kinase activity—A response inhibited by Wortmannin. *J Biol Chem* 1996; 271:12,762–12,766.

106. Rivera VM, Brugge JS. Clustering of Syk is sufficient to induce tyrosine phosphorylation and release of allergic mediators from rat basophilic leukemia cells. *Mol Cell Biol* 1995; 15:1582–1590.

107. Rider LG, Hirasawa N, Santini F, Beaven MA. Activation of the mitogen-activated protein kinase cascade is suppressed by low concentrations of dexamethasone in mast cells. *J Immunol* 1996; 157:2374–2380.

108. Turner H, Cantrell DA. Distinct Ras effector pathways are involved in FcεRI regulation of the transcriptional activity of Elk-1 and NFAT in mast cells. *J Exp Med* 1997; 185:43–53.

109. Kennerly DA. Diacylglycerol metabolism in mast cells. Analysis of lipid metabolic pathways using molecular species analysis of intermediates. *J Biol Chem* 1987; 262:16,305–16,313.

110. Lin P, Fung WJC, Li S, Chen R, Repetto B, Huang KS, Gilfillan AM. Temporal regulation of the IgE-dependent 1,2-diacylglycerol production by tyrosine kinase activation in a rat (RBL 2H3) mast-cell line. *Biochem J* 1994; 299:109–114.

111. Exton JH. New developments in phospholipase D. *J Biol Chem* 1997; 272:15,579–15,582.
112. Singer WD, Brown HA, Sternweis PC. Regulation of eukaryotic phosphatidylinositol-specific phospholipase C and phospholipase D. *Annu Rev Biochem* 1997; 66:475–509.
113. Nakamura Y, Nakashima S, Kumada T, Ojio K, Miyata H, Nozawa Y. Brefeldin A inhibits antigen- or calcium ionophore-mediated but not PMA-induced phospholipase D activation in rat basophilic leukemia (RBL-2H3) cells. *Immunobiology* 1996; 195:231–242.
114. Ishimoto T, Akiba S, Sato T. Importance of the phospholipase D-initiated sequential pathway for arachidonic acid release and prostaglandin D2 generation by rat peritoneal mast cells. *J Biochem* 1996; 120:616–623.
115. Ojio K, Banno Y, Nakashima S, Kato N, Watanabe K, Lyerly DM, Miyata H, Nozawa Y. Effect of *Clostridium difficile* Toxin B on IgE receptor-mediated signal transduction in rat basophilic leukemia cells: Inhibition of phospholipase D activation. *Biochem Biophys Res Commun* 1996; 224:591–596.
116. Prepens U, Just I, Von Eichel-Streiber C, Aktories K. Inhibition of FcεRI-mediated activation of rat basophilic leukemia cells by *Clostridium difficile* toxin B (monoglucosyltransferase) *J Biol Chem* 1996; 271:7324–7329.
117. Lin P, Gilfillan AM. The role of calcium and protein kinase C in the IgE-dependent activation of phosphatidylcholine-specific phospholipase D in a rat mast (RBL 2H3) cell line. *Eur J Biochem* 1992; 207:163–168.
118. Cissel DS, Fraundorfer PF, Beaven MA. Thapsigargin-induced secretion is dependent on activation of a cholera toxin-sensitive and phosphatidylinositol-3-kinase-regulated phospholipase D in a mast cell line. *J Pharmacol Exp Ther* 1998; 285:110–118.
119. Oberhauser AF, Balan V, Fernandez-Badilla CL, Fernandez JM. RT-PCR cloning of Rab3 isoforms expressed in peritoneal mast cells. *FEBS Lett* 1994; 339:171–174.
120. Roa M, Paumet F, Le Mao J, David B, Blank U. Involvement of the ras-like GTPase rab3d in RBL-2H3 mast cell exocytosis following stimulation via high affinity IgE receptors (FcεRI) *J Immunol* 1997; 159:2815–2823.
121. Oberhauser AF, Monck JR, Balch WE, Fernandez JM. Exocytotic fusion is activated by Rab3a peptides. *Nature* 1992; 360:270–273.
122. Smith J, Thompson J, Armstrong J, Hayes B, Crofts A, Squire J, Teahan C, Upton L, Solari R. Rat basophilic leukaemia (RBL) cells overexpressing Rab3a have a reversible block in antigen-stimulated exocytosis. *Biochem J* 1997; 323:321–328.
123. Ludowyke RI, Scurr LL, McNally CM. Calcium ionophore-induced secretion from mast cells correlates with myosin light chain phosphorylation by protein kinase C. *J Immunol* 1996; 157:5130–5138.
124. Price LS, Norman JC, Ridley AJ, Koffer A. The small GTPases Rac and Rho as regulators of secretion in mast cells. *Curr Biol* 1995; 5:68–73.
125. Norman JC, Price LS, Ridley AJ, Koffer A. The small GTP-binding proteins, Rac and Rho, regulate cytoskeletal organization and exocytosis in mast cells by parallel pathways. *Mol Biol Cell* 1996; 7:1429–1442.
126. Ludowyke RI, Kawasugi K, French PW. ATP-γ-S induces actin and myosin rearrangement during histamine secretion in a rat basophilic leukemia cell line (RBL-2H3). *Eur J Cell Biol* 1994; 64:357–367.
127. O'Sullivan AJ, Brown AM, Freeman HNM, Gomperts BD. Purification and identification of FOAD-II, a cytosolic protein that regulates secretion in streptolysin-O permeabilized mast cells, as a Rac/RhoGDI complex. *Mol Biol Cell* 1996; 7:397–408.
128. Mariot P, O'Sullivan AJ, Brown AM, Tatham PER. Rho guanine nucleotide dissociation inhibitor protein (RhoGDI) inhibits exocytosis in mast cells. *EMBO J* 1996; 15:6476–6482.
129. Yonei SG, Oishi K, Uchida MK. Regulation of exocytosis by the small GTP-binding protein rho in rat basophilic leukemia (RBL-2H3) cells. *Gen Pharmacol* 1995; 26:1583–1589.

Table 1
Death Receptors and Their Ligands

Receptor	Other names	Chromosomal location (human)	Ligand	Interacting signaling molecules	Comments	References
Fas	DR1, APO-1, CD95	10q23	FasL	FADD–and others see table 2	Most consistently pro-apoptotic	(11–13)
TNFR1	DR2, CD120a	12p13	TNF	TRADD, RIP FADD (INDIRECT)	Cytotoxicity can be modulated by NFkB	(Loetscher et al., 1990; Schall et al., 1990)
DR3	TRAMP/WSL/ APO2/LARD	12p13	TWEAK (APO-3)	TRADD, FADD (INDIRECT), TNFR1	Expression restricted to lymphocytes	(Chinnaiyan et al., 1996; Kitson et al., 1996; Screaton et al., 1997)
DR4	TRAIL-R1	8p21	TRAIL	?	May bind FADD but no requirement for FADD in DR4-induced death found in FADD knockout mice.	(Schneider et al., 1997; Schneider et al., 1997; Yeh et al., 1998)
DR5	TRAIL-R2	8p21	TRAIL	?	Can heterodimerize with DR4	(Pan et al., 1997; Walczak et al., 1997)
TRID	TRAIL-R3, DcR1	8p21	TRAIL	No intracellular domain	GPI-linked extracellular receptor; Blocks TRAIL-induced apoptosis	(Degli-Esposti et al., 1997; Pan et al., 1997; Sheridan et al., 1997)
TRAIL-R4	DcR2	8p21	TRAIL	?	Incomplete Death Domain; Blocks TRAIL-induced apoptosis	(Degli-Esposti et al., 1997; Marsters et al., 1997)

Table 2
Fas-Interacting Proteins

Name	Fas Binding Site	Description	Methods	Effects of Overexpression	References
FADD	Death Domain	C-terminal Death Domain; N-terminal Death Effector domain	Yeast 2-Hybrid 293T cell overexpression/ Found in endogenous Fas signalling complex	Death domain protects from Fas-mediated apoptosis Death Effector Domain induces apoptosis without Fas crosslinking	(Boldin et al., 1995; Chinnaiyan et al., 1995)
RIP	Death Domain	74 kD serine-threonine Kinase with C-terminal Death Domain	Yeast 2-Hybrid	Induces cell death via death domain	(Stanger et al., 1995; Ting et al., 1996)
FAF1	Dimerized Death Domain	74 kD protein. Contains regions with homology to ubiquitin	Yeast 2-Hybrid Cos Cell overexpression	Potentiates Fas-induced apoptosis	(Chu et al., 1995)
UBC9/ UBC-FAP	Fas intracellular domain proximal to death domain	20 kD protein identical to human UBC9 Yeast 2-Hybrid HeLa cell overexpression	No effect on Fas signaling when overexpressed	(Becker et al., 1997; Wright et al., 1996)
DAXX	Fas or TNF-R1 death domains	81 kD protein	Yeast 2-Hybrid GST pull-down 293T cell overexpression	Activates JNK, synergizes with Fas for induction of apoptosis	(Yang et al., 1997)
Sentrin	Fas or TNF-R1 death domains 10 kD protein with homology to ubiquitin -	Yeast 2-Hybrid GST pull-down		inhibits Fas-induced apoptosis (Okura et al., 1996)	
FAP-1	COOH-terminal 15 AA of Fas	250 kD Tyrosine Phosphatase with 3 PDZ domains	Yeast 2-Hybrid GST pull-down	Protects Jurkat cells from Fas-mediated apoptosis	(Sato et al., 1995)

microsequenced as a Fas-associated protein and was genetically isolated in yeast two-hybrid screens (9,27,28). It is a 220-amino acid protein with a death domain at the C-terminal end and a region named the death-effector domain (DED) at the N-terminus. The DED was originally defined by its ability to induce apoptosis after overexpression in a number of cell types. This 80-amino acid motif forms a structure similar to that of the death domain (29). In a large number of cell lines tested, including primary T cells, Fas only associates with the death domain of FADD after Fas crosslinking with agonistic antibodies (9). In addition, a number of lines of evidence, including results from FADD-deficient mice have shown that the FADD pathway is required for Fas-induced apoptosis (30–33). The physiological roles of the other Fas-binding proteins have yet to be defined.

The next critical discovery was the identification of a caspase in the Fas signaling complex itself. FLICE/MACH/Caspase-8 was identified by yeast two-hybrid screening for proteins interacting with FADD as well as by direct biochemical purification (34,35). This protein consists of tandem DED domains in its N-terminus and a caspase enzyme domain in its C-terminal end. Upon ligation of the CD95 receptor, pro-caspase-8 is recruited to the cytoplasmic tail of CD95 through the FADD adapter molecule, as shown in Fig. 1. After recruitment, the caspase-8 enzyme is cleaved from the prodomain and processed to release the active caspase into the cytoplasm (36). The main function of the Fas signaling complex seems to be activation of caspase-8, as transfection of active caspase-8 can induce all of the hallmarks of apoptosis (27,34). Moreover, oligomerization of the caspase-8 enzymatic domain at the cell membrane can itself induce apoptosis, replacing the function of Fas and FADD (37,38). Thymocytes and embryonic fibroblasts from FADD-deficient mice are resistant to Fas-induced apoptosis, showing that this pathway is essential for apoptosis (30,32).

Unexpectedly, mature lymphocytes from FADD-deficient mice failed to proliferate in response to T-cell receptor (TCR) crosslinking. This block was downstream of interleukin-2 (IL-2) secretion, and could not be reversed with exogenous IL-2. Similar results were obtained with transgenic mice that overexpressed a dominant-negative form of human FADD (31). Earlier experiments had also suggested a paradoxical role for Fas signaling in T-cell activation, as Fas crosslinking of resting T cells could promote proliferation with suboptimal TCR stimulation (39). These results suggest a role for FADD in cell growth, perhaps because of crosstalk between the Fas apoptotic pathway and elements of the cell cycle control mechanism or IL-2 signaling.

The role of Fas binding proteins other than FADD is less clear. Although the protein kinase RIP was originally identified as a Fas-interacting protein in yeast two-hybrid experiments, recent experiments have shown that its primary physiological role may be to couple TNF signaling to NF-κB activation. Thymocytes from RIP knockout mice are hypersensitive to TNF-induced apoptosis, there is no defect in Fas-induced death (40). The Daxx protein binds noncompetitively with FADD to the Fas death domain, and in transfection experiments appeared to enhance Fas-induced apoptosis (41), perhaps through the activation of JNK kinases. However, Daxx has yet to be demonstrated in the native Fas signaling complex. FAP, a tyrosine phosphatase, binds a motif in the 15 AA C-terminal tail of Fas, previously shown to function as an inhibitory domain in Fas signaling (42). Although FAP-1 overexpression blocked Fas-induced apoptosis in susceptible cell lines, it is not known whether this effect is attributable to direct

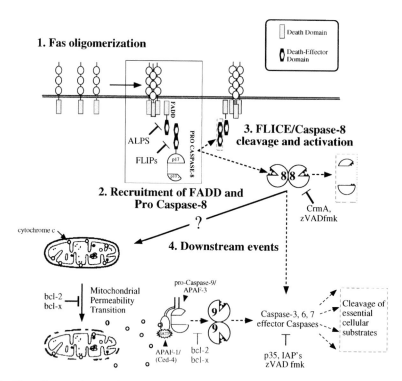

Fig. 1. Signaling pathways in Fas-mediated apoptosis: The diagram outlines the essential known steps that lead to apoptosis after Fas cross-linking. In step 1, Fas receptors are oligomerized by the trimeric ligand. Oligomerization leads to recruitment of the adaptor molecule FADD and the pro-caspase FLICE *(2)*. Recruited FLICE undergoes cleavage, probably by autoproteolysis, and active caspase-8 is produced *(3)*. Downstream events *(4)*, proceed by two routes: direct activation of effector caspases and/or amplification of the death signal via mitochondrial release of cytochrome c. The solid box indicates the components of the DISC (death-inducing signal complex), and the dashed boxes indicate proteolytic fragments which can be detected as indicators of activation of the Fas pathway. Dashed arrows indicate proteolytic steps in the pathway. I symbols indicate inhibitory interactions. Abbreviations: ALPS, autoimmune lymphoproliferative syndrome; FLIPs, Flice Inhibitory Proteins, APAF, apoptosis activating factor; IAP, inhibitor of apoptosis.

binding of Fas in vivo or to indirect effects on phosphorylation of other regulatory proteins. The proteins FAF-1, UBC/FAP, and Sentrin were also isolated in yeast two-hybrid screens with the Fas intracellular domain, and are all in the ubiquitin–proteasome pathway. Their physiological roles have yet to be defined. Sentrin has been localized to the nucleus, making it difficult to understand how it could affect proximal Fas signaling *(43)*. These studies illustrate the general point that a candidate signaling molecule isolated by the yeast-two hybrid technique must be rigorously evaluated before any conclusions can be drawn regarding its physiological role. Typically, a demonstration of in vivo binding to the receptor of interest, preferably in nontransfected cells, should be performed. In the Fas pathway, effects caused by overexpression experiments are not sufficient to implicate molecules in the direct Fas signaling cascade, as other regulatory pathways may independently modify cell viability.

4. CONNECTIONS WITH DOWNSTREAM MEDIATORS OF APOPTOSIS

After activation of caspase-8, there are potentially two pathways by which the death signal is amplified in the cytoplasm. The first is direct cleavage of caspase-3 (CPP32), 6 (Mch2) and 7 (Mch3, ICE-LAP3), members of the *effector* caspase subfamily. Caspases 3, 6, 9, and 10 have been shown to be substrates for caspase-8 in vitro *(44)*, but it is unclear to what extent this occurs in living cells. Effector caspases are known to proteolyze substrates involved in essential cellular processes such as DNA repair and cell cycle control. Examples include nuclear lamins *(45,46)*, DNA-dependent protein kinase, U1-70-K protein *(47)*, and the RB protein *(48)*. The characteristic DNA degradation seen in apoptosis may be mediated by the enzyme caspase-activated deoxyribonuclease (CAD), which is activated by cleavage of the inhibitor iCAD/DFF-45 *(49,50)*.

In some cell types, one possibility is that efficient Fas-induced apoptosis requires a mitochondrial amplification step. This occurs at least in part through caspase-dependent release of cytochrome c from mitochondria. Cytochrome c is known to be an essential cofactor along with the ced-4 homolog APAF-1 in the activation of caspase-9. Once activated, caspase-9 can cleave caspase-3/CPP32 and other effector caspases, which may trigger an irreversible positive feedback loop, as caspase-9 is itself a substrate for active caspase-3 *(51)*. Antiapoptotic Bcl-2 family proteins can block this step by blocking release of cytochrome c *(52,53)*. There may be additional effects of bcl-2 downstream of cytochrome c release as well, perhaps through interaction with the APAF-1/Ced-4 homolog *(54–56)*.

It is unclear what distinguishes cells with and without a requirement for mitochondrial amplification of apoptotic signals. One factor may be the amount of caspase-8 processed in the Fas signaling complex. Cells that rapidly produce large amounts of active caspase-8 may be able to bypass mitochondrial amplification and would thus be insensitive to the blocking effects of bcl-2 family members, whereas those that produce only small amounts of active caspase-8 may be dependent on this step *(57,58)*. However, it should be stressed that bcl-2 family proteins protect cells from a wider spectrum of apoptotic events than does blockade of the Fas pathway. Apoptosis resulting from cytokine withdrawal, γ-irradiation, and chemotherapeutic agents can be more readily protected against by bcl-2 than by blockade of the Fas pathway. In mouse lymphocytes, the bcl-2 and Fas pathways have been shown to be functionally distinct, perhaps because these cells use the direct caspase activation pathway, bypassing mitochondria and bcl-2 *(59–61)*.

Although a role for the interleukin-1β converting enzyme (ICE) subfamily of caspases (caspases 1, 2, 4, and 11) in Fas-mediated apoptosis was initially suggested *(62)*, experiments with ICE-deficient mice have shown that these caspases have little or no effect on Fas signaling *(63,63a)*. Rather than mediating apoptosis, the major role of the ICE subfamily of caspases is in the regulation of inflammation through processing of the cytokines IL-1β and interferon-γ (IFN-γ) *(64–66)*. Other biochemical changes, such as ceramide generation, have also been observed after Fas crosslinking *(67,68)*, but more recent experiments have shown that the presence of ceramide is probably a result, and not a cause, of apoptosis *(69,70)*.

5. VIRAL AND CELLULAR INHIBITORS OF Fas SIGNALING

Tight regulation of an irreversible pathway, such as Fas signaling, is clearly of great importance to maintaining appropriate homeostasis of Fas-expressing tissues. Uncontrolled Fas-induced apoptosis could be detrimental as a result of the elimination of protective lymphocytes or irreplaceable neurons. Indeed, increased Fas-mediated apoptosis may be a factor in the loss of CD4+ lymphocytes in HIV infection *(71–73)*, although direct lymphocyte killing by the virus does not require Fas *(74)*. It is not surprising that a number of viral and cellular proteins that inhibit Fas-induced apoptosis have been described. These molecules fall into two families: those that inhibit assembly and activation of the signaling complex, and those that inhibit downstream caspase activity. While the first class of molecules is specific for the Fas and related death receptors, downstream inhibitors have been shown to block apoptosis induced by many stimuli.

The most specific inhibitors of Fas-induced death prevent the assembly of signaling molecules on the intracellular tail of the Fas receptor. Several viral proteins contain DED-homologous domains. The E8 molecule from equine herpesvirus-2 and the MC159L protein from the human molluscum contagiosum virus have been found to bind strongly to the FADD DED and inhibit Fas-induced apoptosis *(75,76)*. These molecules are called FLICE inhibitory proteins (FLIPs). Analysis of the Fas signaling complex in E8-transfected cells showed that the viral DED-containing protein had largely replaced FLICE/pro-caspase 8 and prevented its activation *(75,76)*. A cellular homolog of the viral FLIP molecules was identified by a number of groups and given a variety of names (c-FLIP, Casper, MRIT, FLAME, Usurpin, or I-FLICE) *(77–82)*. This protein (refered to here as c-FLIP) consists of two tandem DED domains, followed by a caspase domain with several inactivating amino acid substitutions. The gene for c-FLIP maps to human chromosome 2, in linkage with caspase-8 and the related caspase-10. Overexpression of this protein protects cells against Fas-induced apoptosis, although very high levels of expression may actually induce apoptosis. The physiological role of this protein is uncertain, although there is a correlation between the level of c-FLIP and resistance to Fas-induced apoptosis in T cells at different stages of activation *(80)*.

Inhibitors of conserved downstream elements of the caspase pathway may also inhibit Fas-induced apoptosis in a less specific manner. Several viral and cellular proteins inhibit active caspases directly. The prototype of this family is the poxvirus crmA protein, a member of the serpin family of protease inhibitors that blocks caspase activity by a pseudosubstrate mechanism. The baculovirus p35 protein blocks *Drosophila* caspases by a similar mechanism. CrmA most efficiently blocks caspase-8 and caspase-1 activity, whereas p35 has a much broader spectrum of inhibition *(83)*. CrmA overexpression in transgenic mice impairs Fas-mediated apoptosis but interestingly does not lead to features of Fas-deficient mice, such as lymphadenopathy or autoimmunity *(33,84)*. Another family of apoptosis-inhibiting proteins, the IAPs, was originally identified by their ability to substitute for p35 in protecting *Drosophila* cells from the apoptotic effects of baculovirus *(85)*. A number of mammalian IAP homologs have been identified, including (cIAP-1/HIAP/hMIHB, c-IAP-2/HIAP-1/hMIHC, X-IAP/hILP/survivin, and NIAP) *(86–90)*. These proteins all share a common structure of N-terminal tandem cysteine/histidine-rich BIR domains, as well as a C-terminal RING finger zinc-binding domain. The BIR domains of all these proteins have been demonstrated to bind directly to the effector caspases 3, 6, and 7 and inhibit their activity *(91–93)*. c-IAP1 and 2 can also be found in the TNFR2 receptor signaling complex, although the significance of this association is not known *(94)*. p35 and IAP family can inhibit Fas-mediated apoptosis, but also inhibit apoptosis caused by many stimuli, including ultraviolet (UV) light and cytotoxic chemotherapeutic agents *(91,95)*. The pleiotropic protective effects of caspase inhibitors stem from the role of effector caspases as common mediators of many forms of apoptosis.

6. LESSONS FROM ALPS: DEFECTIVE SIGNALING IN PATIENTS WITH HETEROZYGOUS Fas MUTATIONS ILLUSTRATES COOPERATIVITY IN Fas SIGNALING

An association between lymphoproliferation and autoimmune disease in humans was originally described in 1992, when two patients with a phenotype strikingly similar to mice bearing the *lpr* and *gld* mutations were identified *(96)*. These patients had a lymphoproliferative disorder associated with autoimmunity characterized by autoantibody formation and the progressive accumulation of CD4⁻CD8⁻ T cells in peripheral lymphoid tissues. The molecular defect for this syndrome was shown to be the result of mutations at the Fas gene locus *(97)*. Five patients with heterozygous Fas mutations were characterized, each with massive nonmalignant lymphadenopathy, hepatosplenomegaly, and autoimmune phenomena, including hemolytic anemia, thrombocytopenia, and glomerulonephritis. Each of the patients had significant defects in both TCR- and Fas-mediated apoptosis, attributable to a dominant interfering effect of the mutant Fas protein *(97)*. The disorder was called human autoimmune lymphoproliferative syndrome (ALPS). A number of groups have subsequently described other patients with the same phenotype along with mutations in the Fas gene *(98–100)*. The syndrome is not fully penetrant, as some relatives of affected ALPS patients carry the Fas mutations and have impaired in vitro Fas-mediated apoptosis but are clinically healthy *(97)*.

Most ALPS mutations that we have identified affect the death domain of Fas. Recently our group has demonstrated that lymphocytes from ALPS patients have defects in both FADD and caspase 8 recruitment after Fas crosslinking *(100a)*. Mutant Fas proteins that do not bind FADD in vitro dominantly interfere with Fas signaling, implying that the mutants can form complexes with wild-type Fas molecules. A further implication of this observation is that a single mutant Fas molecule out of three (i.e., two-thirds of wild-type molecules) can disrupt signaling. These results suggest that binding of FADD or caspase 8, or both, is cooperative and that subsequent enzymatic activation could depend on the quaternary architecture of the complex recruited to wild-type Fas.

7. OTHER SIGNALING PATHWAYS INFLUENCE Fas-INDUCED APOPTOSIS

While several signaling pathways have been proposed to regulate sensitivity to Fas-mediated apoptosis, how these pathways interact with Fas signaling proteins remains unknown. These signaling pathways can be divided into those that act through inducing new gene transcription (usually defined by sensitivity to cycloheximide or actinomycin D) and those that act directly on Fas signaling proteins without the requirement for *de novo* protein synthesis. In lymphocytes, stimulation through other immunomodulatory receptors has specific effects on Fas-induced apoptosis in distinct cell types.

NF-κB, one of the chief mediators of transcription triggered by inflammatory stimuli, can protect against TNF-mediated cell death. The NF-κB family of transcription factors is composed of a group of DNA-binding proteins that activate transcription as dimers. Proteins of the IκB family bind NF-κB subunits in the cytosol and inhibit their translocation to the nucleus. Signaling by multiple stimuli, including TNF, IL-1, and other mediators, triggers the phosphorylation and proteosomal degradation of IκB, which then allows nuclear NF-κB translocation and rapid transcription of inflammatory response genes. Blocking NF-κB increases the sensitivity of many cell types to apoptosis after TNF stimulation. In some cells, this abrogates the requirement to add the protein synthesis inhibitor cycloheximide to obtain significant cell death. This finding suggests that there is a short-lived inhibitor of TNF-induced apoptosis that is under the control of the NF-κB. Because TNF induces NF-κB, it may block its own apoptotic effects. Fas signaling has also been found to induce NF-κB activity in some systems, but in cell lines where Fas signaling induces apoptosis, Fas crosslinking was reported to decrease in NF-κB activity, possibly as a consequence of caspase-mediated cleavage of NF-κB p50 and p65 subunits *(101)*. Experiments in our laboratory have shown that NF-κB decreases apoptosis by Fas and that inhibiting NF-κB increases susceptibility to Fas-mediated death, both in cell lines and in primary T-cell blasts *(101a)*. One possible synthesis of these data is that the Fas receptor has a low level of constitutive NF-κB-activating ability, mediated by such adapter proteins as RIP. However, in situations in which Fas-induced caspase activation is sufficiently strong, cleavage of NF-κB components overrides this protective signal, resulting in irreversible cell death.

The c-terminal Jun kinase (JNK) pathway has been implicated in apoptosis in other systems, most notably after withdrawal of trophic factors or γ-irradiation. JNK activity is essential in the activation of the Fos/Jun heterodimers that make up the AP-1 transcriptional activator. There are a number of studies that find an increase in JNK activity after Fas crosslinking *(102,103)*. However, studies with dominant-negative JNK mutants have shown that Fas-induced apoptosis is dependent on JNK activity only in specific cell types (e.g., SHEP, L929, 293), and not in others (e.g., HeLa). Blocking apoptosis with the caspase inhibitor zVADfmk does not inhibit JNK activity, indicating that JNK can be activated by Fas independently of caspase activation. Transfection of the Daxx adapter molecule can induce JNK activation in the absence of apoptosis, whereas overexpression of FADD triggers apoptosis independent of JNK *(104)*. Thus, the JNK pathway is separate from activation of caspases through FADD, but this does not rule out a regulatory role for JNK in Fas signaling.

Members of the MAP-kinase pathway have been reported to interact directly with elements of the Fas signaling. The MAP kinase pathway is an important serine/threonine phosphorylation cascade that upregulates the ERK kinases 42 and 44 and p38/Hog1 (see other chapters in this book). ERK kinases phosphorylate the AP-1 Fos-Jun heterodimer, activating transcription of target genes. The MAPK pathway clearly induces gene transcription but may also control signaling pathways in the cytosol and even at the plasma membrane, such as Fas-mediated apoptosis *(105)*. However, these experiments employed overexpression of exogenous proteins, making it difficult to ascertain the actual role of the MAP kinase pathway in Fas-mediated apoptosis.

There may be a role for the p42/44 ERK kinases in Fas signaling as well. Pharmacological agents such as PMA potently block Fas-mediated apoptosis, and a recent study implicated ERK-activation in this effect of PMA, rather than activation of PKC *(106)*. Importantly, cycloheximide did not block the protective effect of these agents, suggesting that posttranslational modification of existing proteins was sufficient to mediate this effect. Transfection of activated Ras mutants, which strongly activate ERK through the upstream kinases RAF and MEKK1, can also protect cells against Fas-induced apoptosis. However, transfection of dominant-negative mutants of the ERK kinase MEK1 had no effect on Fas-induced apoptosis, except in one cell line in which surface levels of Fas were reduced *(103,106)*. This suggests that although a basal level of ERK activity is not necessary for Fas signaling, ERK-mediated phosphorylation can inactivate a molecule required for Fas-induced apoptosis.

8. APOPTOSIS VIA DEATH RECEPTORS: A CRITICAL MECHANISM OF IMMUNE REGULATION

It is clear that Fas-induced death plays a major role in immune cell homeostasis and the maintenance of self-tolerance. However, our understanding of the regulation of Fas signaling in cells and organs has not yet been fully explained. Fas is a primary mediator of the negative feedback death mechanism that controls the response of activated T cells to repeated antigen engagement, termed *propriocidal regulation (107)*. The first studies of T-cell response (TCR)-induced apoptosis in mice showed that apoptosis is specific for those cycling cells that have received an additional recent signal through the TCR *(108)*. This raises the question of how TCR signaling governs Fas-mediated apoptosis to ensure clonotype-specific regulation of the TCR. Although TCR stimulation leads to upregulation of FasL on the stimulated cells *(109–112)*, if this were the only mechanism of apoptosis regulation, activated bystander T cells should also be killed in *trans*, which is not the case. Mixing experiments with labeled cells showed that the basis for this specificity is the sensitization of cells through TCR signaling to the cytotoxic activity of Fas *(113)*. Furthermore, this "competency to die" signal could be triggered by altered peptide ligands for the TCR that triggered no other overt phenotypic changes *(114)*. The molecular pathway by which TCR signals modulate Fas-mediated apoptosis is currently being studied. In a hybridoma system, PMA, but not ionomycin, was able to mimic the effect of TCR stimulation *(115)*.

Another area that requires further study is the induction of B cell apoptosis by Fas. This is especially intriguing because this form of death regulates the outcome of interactions between T cells that express Fas ligand and B cells that express Fas, as B cells do not produce Fas ligand. Chronic stimulation of the antigen receptor on autoreactive B cells can sensitize them for elimination by Fas-mediated apoptosis *(116,117)*. However, acute stimulation of the B-cell antigen receptor, as would occur on exposure to a foreign antigen, protects these cells from Fas-induced apoptosis. Ligation of the co-stimulatory receptor CD40 on B cells plays a role in sensitization to Fas-induced apoptosis by upregulating Fas expression and possibly by modulating Fas signaling itself *(118)*. Moreover, the fact that B-cell killing by Fas is the result of cell:cell interactions imposes special requirements such as a need for adhesion molecules to enforce contact between cells during death induction *(119)*. The interplay of these regulatory signals in the immune system permits clonal expansion in response to foreign antigens to proceed without limitation by Fas-induced apoptosis, whereas chronic stimulation with self-antigens or repeatedly administered foreign antigens leads to elimination of reactive cells. These phenomena are crucial in producing high-zone tolerance and self-tolerance, as illustrated by the defects in Fas-deficient mice and humans. By integrating the cellular events that we observe in the intact immune system with our knowledge of the molecular actions of death receptors, we believe that a clearer understanding of critical immunological phenomena such as tolerance and autoimmunity will emerge. The relative contributions of Fas and related death receptors to apoptosis in different organ systems is also a major challenge for the future.

REFERENCES

1. Alnemri ES, Livingston DJ, Nicholson DW, Salvesen G, Thornberry NA, Wong WW, Yuan J. Human ICE/CED-3 protease nomenclature. *Cell* 1996; 87:171.
2. Salvesen GS, Dixit VM. Caspases: Intracellular signaling by proteolysis. *Cell* 1997; 91:443–446.
3. Watanabe-Fukunaga R, Brannan CI, Copeland NG, Jenkins NA, Nagata S. Lymphoproliferation disorder in mice explained by defects in Fas antigen that mediates apoptosis. *Nature* 1992; 356:314–317.
4. Rathmell JC, Townsend SE, Xu JC, Flavell RA, Goodnow CC. Expansion or elimination of B cells in vivo: Dual roles for CD40- and Fas (CD95)-ligands modulated by the B cell antigen receptor. *Cell* 1996; 87:319–329.
5. Van Parijs L, Peterson DA, Abbas AK. The Fas/Fas ligand pathway and Bcl-2 regulate T cell responses to model self and foreign antigens. *Immunity* 1998; 8:265–274.
6. Seino K, Kayagaki N, Takeda K, Fukao K, Okumura K, Yagita H. Contribution of Fas ligand to T cell-mediated hepatic injury in mice. *Gastroenterology* 1997; 113:1315–1322.
7. Mohan RR, Liang Q, Kim WJ, Helena MC, Baerveldt F, Wilson SE. Apoptosis in the cornea: further characterization of Fas/Fas ligand system. *Exp Eye Res* 1997; 65:575–589.
8. Nicholson D, Thornberry N. Caspases: Killer proteases. *TIBS* 1997; 22:299–306.
9. Kischkel FC, Hellbardt S, Behrmann I, Germer M, Pawlita M, Krammer PH, Peter ME. Cytotoxicity-dependent APO-1 (Fas/CD95)-associated proteins form a death-inducing signaling complex (DISC) with the receptor. *EMBO J* 1995; 14:5579–5588.
10. Zhang J, Winoto A. A mouse Fas-associated protein with homology to the human Mort1/FADD protein is essential for Fas-induced apoptosis. *Mol Cell Biol* 1996; 16:2756–2763.
11. Trauth BC, Klas C, Peters AM, Matzku S, Moller P, Falk W, Debatin KM, Krammer PH. Monoclonal antibody-mediated tumor regression by induction of apoptosis. *Science* 1989; 245:301–305.
12. Oehm A, Behrmann I, Falk W, Pawlita M, Maier G, Klas C, Li-Weber M, Richards S, Dhein J, Trauth BC, et al. Purification and molecular cloning of the APO-1 cell surface antigen, a member of the tumor necrosis factor/nerve growth factor receptor superfamily. Sequence identity with the Fas antigen. *J Biol Chem* 1992; 267:10,709–10,715.
13. Itoh N, Yonehara S, Ishii A, Yonehara M, Mizushima S, Sameshima M, Hase A, Seto Y, Nagata S. The polypeptide encoded by the cDNA for human cell surface antigen Fas can mediate apoptosis. *Cell* 1991; 66:233–243.
14. Orlinick JR, Vaishnaw A, Elkon KB, Chao MV. Requirement of cysteine-rich repeats of the Fas receptor for binding by the Fas ligand. *J Biol Chem* 1997; 272:28,889–28,894.
15. Tartaglia LA, Ayres TM, Wong GH, Goeddel DV. A novel domain within the 55 kd TNF receptor signals cell death. *Cell* 1993; 74:845–853.

16. Lynch DH, Watson ML, Alderson MR, Baum PR, Miller RE, Tough T, Gibson M, Davis-Smith T, Smith CA, Hunter K, et al. The mouse Fas-ligand gene is mutated in gld mice and is part of a TNF family gene cluster. *Immunity* 1994; 1:131–136.

17. Marsters SA, Sheridan JP, Donahue CJ, Pitti RM, Gray CL, Goddard AD, Bauer KD, Ashkenazi A. Apo-3, a new member of the tumor necrosis factor receptor family, contains a death domain and activates apoptosis and NF-kappa B. *Curr Biol* 1996; 6:1669–1676.

18. Chicheportiche Y, Bourdon PR, Xu H, Hsu YM, Scott H, Hession C, Garcia I, Browning JL. TWEAK, a new secreted ligand in the tumor necrosis factor family that weakly induces apoptosis. *J Biol Chem* 1997; 272:32,401–32,410.

19. Chinnaiyan AM, O'Rourke K, Yu GL, Lyons RH, Garg M, Duan DR, Xing L, Gentz R, Ni J, Dixit VM. Signal transduction by DR3, a death domain-containing receptor related to TNFR-1 and CD95. *Science* 1996; 274:990–992.

20. Chaudhary PM, Eby M, Jasmin A, Bookwalter A, Murray J, Hood L. Death receptor 5, a new member of the TNFR family, and DR4 induce FADD-dependent apoptosis and activate the NF-kappaB pathway. *Immunity* 1997; 7:821–830.

21. Marsters SA, Sheridan JP, Pitti RM, Huang A, Skubatch M, Baldwin D, Yuan J, Gurney A, Goddard AD, Godowski P, Ashkenazi A. A novel receptor for Apo2L/TRAIL contains a truncated death domain. *Curr Biol* 1997; 7:1003–1006.

22. Pan G, Ni J, Wei YF, Yu G, Gentz R, Dixit VM. An antagonist decoy receptor and a death domain-containing receptor for TRAIL. *Science* 1997; 277:815–818.

23. Screaton GR, Mongkolsapaya J, Xu XN, Cowper AE, McMichael AJ, Bell JI. TRICK2, a new alternatively spliced receptor that transduces the cytotoxic signal from TRAIL. *Curr Biol* 1997; 7:693–696.

24. Walczak H, Degli-Esposti MA, Johnson RS, Smolak PJ, Waugh JY, Boiani N, Timour MS, Gerhart MJ, Schooley KA, Smith CA, Goodwin RG, Rauch CT. TRAIL-R2: A novel apoptosis-mediating receptor for TRAIL. *EMBO J* 1997; 16:5386–5397.

25. Bodmer JL, Burns K, Schneider P, Hofmann K, Steiner V, Thome M, Bornand T, Hahne M, Schroter M, Becker K, Wilson A, French LE, Browning JL, MacDonald HR, Tschopp J. TRAMP, a novel apoptosis-mediating receptor with sequence homology to tumor necrosis factor receptor 1 and Fas(Apo-1/CD95). *Immunity* 1997; 6:79–88.

26. Golstein P. Cell death: TRAIL and its receptors. *Curr Biol* 1997; 7:R750–753.

27. Boldin MP, Varfolomeev EE, Pancer Z, Mett IL, Camonis JH, Wallach D. A novel protein that interacts with the death domain of Fas-Apo-1 contains a sequence motif related to the death doman. *J Biol Chem* 1995; 270:7795–7798.

28. Chinnaiyan AM, O'Rourke K, Tewari M, Dixit VM. FADD, a novel death domain-containing protein, interacts with the death domain of Fas and initiates apoptosis. *Cell* 1995; 81:505–512.

29. Eberstadt M, Huang B, Olejniczak ET, Fesik SW. The lymphoproliferation mutation in Fas locally unfolds the Fas death domain. *Nature Struct Biol* 1997; 4:983–985.

30. Zhang J, Cado D, Chen A, Kabra NH, Winoto A. Fas-mediated apoptosis and activation-induced T-cell proliferation are defective in mice lacking FADD/Mort1. *Nature* 1998; 392:296–300.

31. Newton K, Harris AW, Bath ML, Smith KGC, Strasser A. A dominant interfering mutant of FADD/MORT1 enhances deletion of autoreactive thymocytes and inhibits proliferation of mature T lymphocytes. *EMBO J* 1998; 17:706–718.

32. Yeh WC, Pompa JL, McCurrach ME, Shu HB, Elia AJ, Shahinian A, Ng M, Wakeham A, Khoo W, Mitchell K, El-Deiry WS, Lowe SW, Goeddel DV, Mak TW. FADD: Essential for embryo development and signaling from some, but not all, inducers of apoptosis. *Science* 1998; 279:1954–1958.

33. Walsh CM, Wen BG, Chinnaiyan AM, O'Rourke K, Dixit VM, Hedrick SM. A role for FADD in T cell activation and development. *Immunity* 1998; 8:439–449.

34. Muzio M, Chinnaiyan AM, Kischkel FC, O'Rourke K, Shevchenko A, Ni J, Scaffidi C, Bretz JD, Zhang M, Gentz R, Mann M, Krammer PH, Peter ME, Dixit VM. FLICE, a novel FADD-homologous ICE/CED-3-like protease, is recruited to the CD95 (Fas/APO-1) death-inducing signaling complex. *Cell* 1996; 85:817–827.

35. Boldin MP, Goncharov TM, Goltsev YV, Wallach D. Involvement of MACH, a novel MORT1/FADD-interacting protease, in Fas/APO-1- and TNF receptor-induced cell death. *Cell* 1996; 85:803–815.

36. Medema JP, Scaffidi C, Kischkel FC, Shevchenko A, Mann M, Krammer PH, Peter ME. FLICE is activated by association with the CD95 death-inducing signaling complex (DISC). *EMBO J* 1997; 16:2794–2804.

37. Muzio M, Stockwell BR, Stennicke HR, Salveson GS, Dixit VM. An induced proximity model for caspase-8 activation. *J Biol Chem* 1998; 273:2926–2930.

38. Martin DA, Siegel RM, Zheng L, Lenardo MJ. Membrane oligomerization and release activates the caspase 8 (FLICE/MACHα1) death signal. *J Biol Chem* 1998; 273:4345–4349.

39. Alderson MR, Armitage RJ, Maraskovsky E, Tough TW, Roux E, Schooley K, Ramsdell F, Lynch DH. Fas transduces activation signals in normal human T lymphocytes. *J Exp Med* 1993; 178:2231–2235.

40. Kelliher MA, Grimm S, Ishida Y, Kuo F, Stanger BZ, Leder P. The death domain kinase RIP mediates the TNF-induced NF-kappaB signal. *Immunity* 1998; 8:297–303.

41. Yang X, Korshravi-Far, Chang HY, Baltimore D. Daxx, a novel Fas-Binding protein activates Jnk and Apoptosis. *Cell* 1997; 89:1067–1076.

42. Sato T, Irie S, Kitada S, Reed JC. FAP-1: A protein tyrosine phosphatase that associates with Fas. *Science* 1995; 268:411–415.

43. Boddy MN, Howe K, Etkin LD, Solomon E, Freemont PS. PIC 1, a novel ubiquitin-like protein which interacts with the PML component of a multiprotein complex that is disrupted in acute promyelocytic leukaemia. *Oncogene* 1996; 13:971–982.

44. Srinivasula SM, Ahmad M, Fernandes-Alnemri T, Litwack G, Alnemri ES. Molecular ordering of the Fas-apoptotic pathway: The Fas/APO-1 protease Mch5 is a CrmA-inhibitable protease that activates multiple Ced-3/ICE-like cysteine proteases. *Proc Acad Natl Sci USA* 1996; 93:14,486–14,491.

45. Orth K, Chinnaiyan AM, Garg M, Froelich CJ, Dixit VM. The CED-3/ICE-like protease Mch2 is activated during apoptosis and cleaves the death substrate lamin A. *J Biol Chem* 1996; 271:16,443–16,446.

46. Takahashi A, Alnemri ES, Lazebnik YA, Fernandes-Alnemri T, Litwack G, Moir RD, Goldman RD, Poirier GG, Kaufmann SH, Earnshaw WC. Cleavage of lamin A by Mch2 alpha but not CPP32: Multiple interleukin 1 beta-converting enzyme-related proteases with distinct substrate recognition properties are active in apoptosis. *Proc Acad Natl Sci USA* 1996; 93:8395–8400.

47. Casciola-Rosen L, Nicholson DW, Chong T, Rowan KR, Thornberry NA, Miller DK, Rosen A. Apopain/CPP32 cleaves proteins that are essential for cellular repair: a fundamental principle of apoptotic death. *J Exp Med* 1996; 183:1957–1964.

48. Chen WD, Otterson GA, Lipkowitz S, Khleif SN, Coxon AB, Kaye FJ. Apoptosis is associated with cleavage of a 5 kDa fragment from RB which mimics dephosphorylation and modulates E2F binding. *Oncogene* 1997; 14:1243–1248.

49. Sakahira H, Enari M, Nagata S. Cleavage of CAD inhibitor in CAD activation and DNA degradation during apoptosis. *Nature* 1998; 391:96–99.

50. Enari M, Sakahira H, Yokoyama H, Okawa K, Iwamatsu A, Nagata S. A caspase-activated DNase that degrades DNA during apoptosis, and its inhibitor ICAD. *Nature* 1998; 391:43–50.

51. Srinivasula SM, Fernandes-Alnemri T, Zangrilli J, Robertson N, Armstrong RC, Wang L, Trapani JA, Tomaselli KJ, Litwack G, Alnemri ES. The Ced-3/interleukin 1beta converting

enzyme-like homolog Mch6 and the lamin-cleaving enzyme Mch2alpha are substrates for the apoptotic mediator CPP32. *J Biol Chem* 1996; 271:27,099–27,106.

52. Kluck RM, Bossy-Wetzel E, Green DR, Newmeyer DD. The release of cytochrome c from mitochondria: a primary site for Bcl-2 regulation of apoptosis. *Science* 1997; 275:1132–1136.

53. Yang J, Liu X, Bhalla K, Kim CN, Ibrado AM, Cai J, Peng TI, Jones DP, Wang X. Prevention of apoptosis by Bcl-2: Release of cytochrome c from mitochondria blocked. *Science* 1997; 275:1129–1132.

54. Hengartner MO, Horowitz HR. *C. elegans* cell survival gene ced-9 encodes a functional homolog of the mammalian proto-oncogene bcl-2. *Cell* 1994; 76:665–676.

55. Hengartner MO. Apoptosis. Death cycle and Swiss army knives. *Nature* 1998; 391:441–442.

56. Rosse T, Olivier R, Monney L, Rager M, Conus S, Fellay I, Jansen B, Borner C. Bcl-2 prolongs cell survival after Bax-induced release of cytochrome c. *Nature* 1998; 391:496–499.

57. Medema JP, Scaffidi C, Krammer PH, Peter ME. Bcl-xL acts downstream of caspase-8 activation by the CD95 death-inducing signaling complex. *J Biol Chem* 1998; 273:3388–3393.

58. Scaffidi C, Fulda S, Srinivasan A, Friesen C, Li F, Tomaselli KJ, Debatin KM, Krammer PH, Peter ME. Two CD95 (APO-1/Fas) signaling pathways. *EMBO J* 1998; 17:1675–1687.

59. Reap EA, Felix NJ, Wolthusen PA, Kotzin BL, Cohen PL, Eisenberg RA. bcl-2 transgenic Lpr mice show profound enhancement of lymphadenopathy. *J Immunol* 1995; 155:5455–5462.

60. Strasser A, Harris AW, Jacks T, Cory S. DNA damage can induce apoptosis in proliferating lymphoid cells via p53-independent mechanisms inhibitable by Bcl-2. *Cell* 1994; 79:329–339.

61. Strasser A, Harris AW, Huang DC, Krammer PH, Cory S. Bcl-2 and Fas/APO-1 regulate distinct pathways to lymphocyte apoptosis. *EMBO J* 1995; 14:6136–6147.

62. Enari M, Talanian RV, Wong WW, Nagata S. Sequential activation of ICE-like and CPP32-like proteases during Fas-mediated apoptosis. *Nature* 1996; 380:723–726.

63. Fantuzzi G, Ku G, Harding MW, Livingston DJ, Sipe JD, Kuida K, Flavell RA, Dinarello CA. Response to local inflammation of IL-1 beta-converting enzyme-deficient mice. *J Immunol* 1997; 158:1818–1824.

63a. Jiang D, Zheng L, Lenardo MJ. Caspases in T-cell receptor-induced thymocyte apoptosis. *Cell Death Differ* 1999; 6:402–411.

64. Ghayur T, Banerjee S, Hugunin M, Butler D, Herzog L, Carter A, Quintal L, Sekut L, Talanian R, Paskind M, Wong W, Kamen R, Tracey D, Allen H. Caspase-1 processes IFN-gamma-inducing factor and regulates LPS-induced IFN-gamma production. *Nature* 1997; 386:619–623.

65. Friedlander RM, Gagliardini V, Hara H, Fink KB, Li W, MacDonald G, Fishman MC, Greenberg AH, Moskowitz MA, Yuan J. Expression of a dominant negative mutant of interleukin-1 beta converting enzyme in transgenic mice prevents neuronal cell death induced by trophic factor withdrawal and ischemic brain injury. *J Exp Med* 1997; 185:933–940.

66. Friedlander RM, Gagliardini V, Rotello RJ, Yuan J. Functional role of interleukin 1 beta (IL-1 beta) in IL-1 beta- converting enzyme-mediated apoptosis. *J Exp Med* 1996; 184:717–724.

67. Gulbins E, Bissonnette R, Mahboubi A, Martin S, Nishioka W, Brunner T, Baier G, Baier-Bitterlich G, Byrd C, Lang F, et al. FAS-induced apoptosis is mediated via a ceramide-initiated RAS signaling pathway. *Immunity* 1995; 2:341–351.

68. Tepper CG, Jayadev S, Liu B, Bielawska A, Wolff R, Yonehara S, Hannum YA, Seldin MF. Role for ceramide as an endogenous mediator of Fas-induced cytotoxicity. *Proc Acad Natl Sci USA* 1995; 92:8443–8447.

69. Sillence DJ, Allan D. Evidence against an early signalling role for ceramide in Fas-mediated apoptosis. *Biochem J* 1997; 324:29–32.

70. Hsu SC, Wu CC, Luh TY, Chou CL, Han SH, Lai MZ. Apoptotic signal of Fas is not mediated by ceramide. *Blood* 1998; 91:2658–2663.

71. Oyaizu N, McCloskey TW, Than S, Hu R, Pahwa S. Mechanism of apoptosis in peripheral blood mononuclear cells of HIV-infected patients. *Adv Exp Med Biol* 1995; 374:101–114.

72. Meyaard L, Otto SA, Jonker RR, Mijnster MJ, Keet RP, Miedema F. Programmed death of T cells in HIV-1 infection. *Science* 1992; 257:217–219.

73. Estaquier J, Tanaka M, Suda T, Nagata S, Goldstein P, Ameisen JC. Fas-mediated apoptosis of CD4⁺ and CD8⁺ T cells from human immunodeficiency virus-infected persons: Differential in vitro preventive effect of cytokines and protease antagonists. *Blood* 1996; 87:4959–4966.

74. Gandhi RT, Chen BK, Straus SE, Dale JK, Lenardo MJ, Baltimore D. HIV-1 directly kills CD4⁺ T cells by a Fas-independent mechanism. *J Exp Med* 1998; 187:1113–1122.

75. Bertin J, Armstrong RC, Ottilie S, Martin DA, Wang Y, Banks S, Wang GH, Senkevich TG, Alnemri ES, Moss B, Lenardo MJ, Tomaselli KJ, Cohen JI. Death effector domain-containing herpesvirus and poxvirus proteins inhibit both Fas- and TNFR1-induced apoptosis. *Proc Natl Acad Sci USA* 1997; 94:1172–1176.

76. Thome M, Schneider P, Hofmann K, Fickenscher H, Meinl E, Neipel F, Mattmann C, Burns K, Bodmer JL, Schroter M, Scaffidi C, Krammer PH, Peter ME, Tschopp J. Viral FLICE-inhibitory proteins (FLIPs) prevent apoptosis induced by death receptors. *Nature* 1997; 386:517–521.

77. Hu S, Vincenz C, Ni J, Gentz R, Dixit VM. I-FLICE, a novel inhibitor of tumor necrosis factor receptor-1- and CD-95-induced apoptosis. *J Biol Chem* 1997; 272:17,255–17,257.

78. Han D, Chaudhary PM, Wright ME, Friedman C, Trask BJ, Riedel R, Baskin D, Schwartz SM, Hood L. MRIT, a novel death-effector domain-containing protain, interacts with caspases abd BclXl and initiates cell death. *Proc Natl Acad Sci USA* 1997; 94:11,333–11,338.

79. Shu HB, Halpin DR, Goeddel DV. Casper is a FADD- and caspase-related inducer of apoptosis. *Immunity* 1997; 6:751–763.

80. Irmler M, Thome M, Hahne M, Schneider P, Hofmann K, Steiner V, Bodmer JL, Schroter M, Burns K, Mattmann C, Rimoldi D, French LE, Tschopp J. Inhibition of death receptor signals by cellular FLIP. *Nature* 1997; 388:190–195.

81. Srinivasula SM, Ahmad M, Ottilie S, Bullrich F, Banks S, Wang Y, Fernandes-Alnemri T, Croce CM, Litwack G, Tomaselli KJ, Armstrong RC, Alnemri ES. FLAME-1, a novel FADD-like anti-apoptotic molecule that regulates Fas/TNFR1-induced apoptosis. *J Biol Chem* 1997; 272:18,542–18,545.

82. Rasper DM, Vaillancourt JP, Hadano S, Houtzager VM, Seiden I, Keen SLC, Tawa P, Xanthoudakis S, Nasir J, Martindale D, Koop BF, Peterson EP, Thornberry NA, Huang, J-Q, Black SC, Hornung F, Lenardo MJ, H, MR, Roy S, Nicholson DW. Cell death attenuation by "Usurpin," a mammalian DED-caspase homologue that precludes caspase-8 recruitment and activation by the CD-95 (Fas, APO-1) receptor complex. *Cell Death Diff* 1998; 5:271–288.

83. Zhou Q, Snipas S, Orth K, Muzio M, Dixit VM, Salvesen GS. Target protease specificity of the viral serpin CrmA. Analysis of five caspases. *J Biol Chem* 1997; 272:7797–7800.

84. Smith KG, Strasser A, Vaux DL. CrmA expression in T lymphocytes of transgenic mice inhibits CD95 (Fas/APO-1)-transduced apoptosis, but does not cause lymphadenopathy or autoimmune disease. *EMBO J* 1996; 15:5167–5176.

85. Clem RJ, Miller LK. Control of programmed cell death by the baculovirus genes p35 and iap. *Mol Cell Biol* 1994; 14:5212–5222.

86. Duckett CS, Nava VE, Gedrich RW, Clem RJ, Van Dongen JL, Gilfillan MC, Shiels H,

Hardwick JM, Thompson CB. A conserved family of cellular genes related to the baculovirus iap gene and encoding apoptosis inhibitors. *EMBO J* 1996; 15:2685–2694.

87. Hay BA, Wasserman DA, Rubin GM. Drosophila homologs of baculovirus inhibitor of apoptosis proteins function to block cell death. *Cell* 1995; 83:1253–1262.

88. Liston P, Roy N, Tamai K, Lefebvre C, Baird S, Cherton-Horvat G, Farahani R, McLean M, Ikeda JE, MacKenzie A, Korneluk RG. Suppression of apoptosis in mammalian cells by NAIP and a related family of IAP genes. *Nature* 1996; 379:349–353.

89. Ambrosini G, Adida C, Altieri DC. A novel anti-apoptosis gene, survivin, expressed in cancer and lymphoma. *Nature Med* 1997; 3:917–921.

90. Uren AG, Pakusch M, Hawkins CJ, Puls KL, Vaux DL. Cloning and expression of apoptosis inhibitory protein homologs that function to inhibit apoptosis and/or bind tumor necrosis factor receptor-associated factors. *Proc Natl Acad Sci USA* 1996; 93:4974–4978.

91. Roy N, Deveraux QL, Takahashi R, Salvesen GS, Reed JC. The c-IAP-1 and c-IAP-2 proteins are direct inhibitors of specific caspases. *EMBO J* 1997; 16:6914–6925.

92. Deveraux QL, Takahashi R, Salvesen GS, Reed JC. X-linked IAP is a direct inhibitor of cell-death proteases. *Nature* 1997; 388:300–304.

93. Deveraux QL, Roy N, Stennicke HR, Van Arsdale T, Zhou Q, Srinivasula SM, Alnemri ES, Salvesen GS, Reed JC. IAPs block apoptotic events induced by caspase-8 and cytochrome c by direct inhibition of distinct caspases. *EMBO J* 1998; 17:2215–2223.

94. Rothe M, Pan MG, Henzel WJ, Ayres TM, Goeddel DV. The TNFR2-TRAF signaling complex contains two novel proteins related to baculoviral inhibitor of apoptosis proteins. *Cell* 1995; 83:1243–1252.

95. Duckett CS, Li F, Wang Y, Tomaselli KJ, Thompson CB, Armstrong RC. Human IAP-like protein regulates programmed cell death downstream of Bcl-xL and cytochrome c. *Mol Cell Biol* 1998; 18:608–615.

96. Sneller MC, Straus SE, Jaffe ES, Jaffe JS, Fleisher TA, Stetler-Stevenson M, Strober W. A novel lymphoproliferative/autoimmune syndrome resembling murine lpr/gld disease. *J Clin Invest* 1992; 90:334–341.

97. Fisher GH, Rosenberg FJ, Straus SE, Dale JK, Middleton LA, Lin AY, Strober W, Lenardo MJ, Puck JM. Dominant interfering Fas gene mutations impair apoptosis in a human autoimmune lymphoproliferative syndrome. *Cell* 1995; 81:935–946.

98. Rieux-Laucat F, Diest FL, Roberts IA, Debatin KM, Fisher A, Villartay JP. Mutations in Fas-associated with human lymphoproliferative syndrome and autoimmunity. *Science* 1995; 268:1347–1351.

99. Drappa J, Vaishnaw AK, Sullivan KE, Chu JL, Elkon KB. Fas gene mutations in the Canale-Smith syndrome, an inherited lymphoproliferative disorder associated with autoimmunity. *N Engl J Med* 1996; 335:1643–1649.

100. Bettinardi A, Brugnoni D, Quiros-Roldan E, Malagoli A, La Grutta S, Correra A, Notarangelo LD. Missense mutations in the Fas gene resulting in autoimmune lymphoproliferative syndrome: a molecular and immunological analysis. *Blood* 1997; 89:902–909.

100a. Martin DA, Zheng L, Siegel RM, Huang B, Fisher GH, Wang J, Jackson CE, Puck JM, Dale J, Straus SE, Peter ME, Krammer PH, Fesik S, Lenardo MJ. Defective CD95/APO-1/Fas signal complex formation in the human autoimmune lymphoproliferative syndrome, type Ia. *Proc Natl Acad Sci USA* 1999; 96:4552–4557.

101. Ravi R, Bedi A, Fuchs EJ, Bedi A. CD95 (Fas)-induced caspase-mediated proteolysis of NF-kappaB. *Cancer Res* 1998; 58:882–886.

101a. Dudley E, Hornung F, Zheng L, Scherer D, Ballard D, Lenardo M. NF-kappaB regulates Fas/APO-1/CD95- and TCR-mediated apoptosis of T lymphocytes. *Eur J Immunol* 1999; 29:878–886.

102. Latinis KM, Koretzky GA. Fas ligation induces apoptosis and Jun kinase activation independently of CD45 and Lck in human T cells. *Blood* 1996; 87:871–875.

103. Goillot E, Raingeaud J, Ranger A, Tepper RI, Davis RJ, Harlow E, Sanchez I. Mitogen-activated protein kinase-mediated Fas apoptotic signaling pathway. *Proc Natl Acad Sci USA* 1997; 94:3302–3307.

104. Liu ZG, Hsu H, Goeddel DV, Karin M. Dissection of TNF receptor 1 effector functions: JNK activation is not linked to apoptosis while NF-kappaB activation prevents cell death. *Cell* 1996; 87:565–576.

105. Huang S, Jiang Y, Li Z, Nishida E, Mathias P, Lin S, Ulevitch RJ, Nemerow GR, Han J. Apoptosis signaling pathway in T cells is composed of ICE/Ced-3 family proteases and MAP kinase kinase 6b. *Immunity* 1997; 6:739–749.

106. Holmstrom TH, Chow SC, Elo I, Coffey ET, Orrenius S, Sistonen L, Eriksson JE. Suppression of Fas/APO-1-mediated apoptosis by mitogen-activated kinase signaling. *J Immunol* 1998; 160:2626–2636.

107. Lenardo MJ. The molecular regulation of lymphocyte apoptosis. *Semin Immunol.* 9:1–5.

108. Lenardo MJ. Interleukin-2 programs mouse αβ T lymphocytes for apoptosis. *Nature* 1991; 353:858–861.

109. Brunner T, Mogil RJ, LaFace D, Yoo NJ, Mahboubi A, Echeverri F, Martin SJ, Force WR, Lynch DH, Ware CF, et al. Cell-autonomous Fas (CD95)/Fas-ligand interaction mediates activation-induced apoptosis in T-cell hybridomas. *Nature* 1995; 373:441–444.

110. Ju ST, Panka DJ, Cui H, Ettinger R, el-Khatib M, Sherr DH, Stanger BZ, Marshak-Rothstein A. Fas(CD95)/FasL interactions required for programmed cell death after T-cell activation. *Nature* 1995; 373:444–448.

111. Dhein J, Walczak H, Baumler C, Debatin KM, Krammer PH. Autocrine T-cell suicide mediated by APO-1/(Fas/CD95). *Nature* 1995; 373:438–441.

112. Zheng L, Fisher G, Miller RE, Peschon J, Lynch DH, Lenardo MJ. Induction of apoptosis in mature T cells by tumour necrosis factor. *Nature* 1995; 377:348–351.

113. Hornung F, Zheng L, Lenardo MJ. Maintenance of clonotype specificity in CD95/Apo-1/Fas-mediated apoptosis of mature T lymphocytes. *J Immunol* 1997; 159:3816–3822.

114. Combadiere B, Sousa CR, Germain RN, Lenardo MJ. Selective induction of apoptosis in mature T lymphocytes by variant T cell receptor ligands. *J Exp Med* 1998; 187:349–455.

115. Wong B, Arron J, Choi Y. T cell receptor signals enhance susceptibility to Fas-mediated apoptosis. *J Exp Med* 1997; 186:1939–1944.

116. Rathmell JC, Cooke MP, Ho WY, Grein J, Townsend SE, Davis MM, Goodnow CC. CD95 (Fas)-dependent elimination of self-reactive B cells upon interaction with CD4+ T cells. *Nature* 1995; 376:181–184.

117. Francis DA, Sen R, Rothstein TL. Receptor-specific regulation of NF-kappa B, c-Myc and Fas-mediated apoptosis in primary B cells. *Curr Top Microbiol Immunol* 1997; 224:83–90.

118. Schattner EJ, Elkon KB, Yoo DH, Tumang J, Krammer PH, Crow MK, Friedman SM. CD40 ligation induces Apo-1/Fas expression on human B lymphocytes and facilitates apoptosis through the Apo-1/Fas pathway. *J Exp Med* 1995; 182:1557–1565.

119. Wang J, Taniuchi I, Maekawa Y, Howard M, Cooper MD, Watanabe T. Expression and function of Fas antigen on activated murine B cells. *Eur J Immunol* 1996; 26:92–96.

9

Signal Transduction to the Nucleus by MAP Kinase

Roger J. Davis

1. INTRODUCTION

The MAP kinases (MAPK) are a group of protein kinases that have been established to have an important function in signal transduction pathways that mediate the nuclear response of cells to changes in their environment. These enzymes are activated by pathways that have been conserved during evolution in many organisms, including plants, fungi, nematodes, insects, and mammals. This chapter reviews the current knowledge about the mechanism of nuclear signaling by MAPK.

2. THE MAP KINASE FAMILY OF SIGNALING ENZYMES

MAPK are enzymes that transfer the γ-phosphate of ATP to Ser and Thr residues in target proteins within the cell. These enzymes are activated by phosphorylation on two sites within the kinase domain. These phosphorylation sites correspond to one Thr and one Tyr residue. The atomic structure of two MAPK has been determined by X-ray crystallography *(1–3)*. These studies demonstrate that the dual phosphorylation occurs within a short segment of the primary structure that forms the activation loop located close to the kinase active site *(4)*. Conformational changes associated with the phosphorylation of the activation loop leads to MAPK activation.

The two sites of activating phosphorylation of MAPK are located within a tripeptide with the general sequence Thr-Xaa-Tyr. Different groups of MAPK are defined by the identity of the amino acid that separates the phosphorylated Thr and Tyr residues. MAPK include groups with the tripeptide dual phosphorylation motifs Thr-Glu-Tyr, Thr-Gly-Tyr, Thr-Pro-Tyr, and Thr-Asn-Tyr (Table 1). An additional group of protein kinases related to the MAPK is represented by KKIALRE and KKIAMRE, which contain the motif Thr-Asp-Tyr (Table 1).

Each of these groups of MAPK is activated by separate signal transduction pathways that are initiated by different extracellular stimuli. In addition, these groups of MAPK exhibit different substrate specificities. Thus, the response of cells to specific extracellular stimuli includes the differential activation of MAPK, and therefore the phosphorylation different groups of MAPK substrates in response to individual stimuli. This complexity in the mechanism of signal transduction by MAPK ensures that cells mount an appropriate response to extracellular stimulation.

From: Signaling Networks and Cell Cycle Control: The Molecular Basis of Cancer and Other Diseases
Edited by: J. S. Gutkind © Humana Press Inc., Totowa, NJ

Table 1
MAP Kinase-Related Proteins in Mammals, Insects, and Fungi

Dual phosphorylation motif	Mammals	Drosophila	Budding yeast
TEY	ERK1	ERKA	Fus3p
	ERK2		Kss1p
	BMK1/ERK5		Mpk1p
TGY	p38α	p38a	Hog1p
	p38β	p38b	
	p38γ		
	p38δ		
TPY	JNK1	DJNK	
	JNK2		
	JNK3		
TNY			Smk1p
TDY	KK1ALRE		
	KK1AMRE		

2.1. The ERK Group of MAP Kinases

The extracellular signal-regulated protein kinase (ERK) group of MAPK includes two mammalian enzymes (ERK1 and ERK2), the *Drosophila* MAPK ERKA, and three yeast MAPK (Fus3p, Kss1p and Mpk1p). These MAPK are characterized by the dual phosphorylation motif Thr-Glu-Tyr (Table 1).

The mammalian ERK1 and ERK2 MAPK are activated by signaling pathways that are initiated by many cell surface receptors, including seven-transmembrane spanning receptors that are linked to heterotrimeric G proteins and tyrosine kinase receptors (*see* Chapters 2 and 5). A common point of integration of these divergent upstream signals is the activation of the small G protein Ras, which functions to initiate the ERK MAPK signaling cascade (*see* Chapter 12).

Functional studies indicate that the activation of ERK1 and ERK2 provides proliferative signals that may contribute to normal growth and to the malignant transformation of fibroblasts *(5,6)*. Changes in ERK activity are also implicated in cellular differentiation processes. For example, inhibition of ERK can lead to the induction of myogenic differentiation *(7)*, whereas ERK activation may mediate growth arrest and differentiation of neurons *(6)* and megakaryocytes *(8)*. By contrast, activation of the ERK MAPK inhibits adipocyte differentiation *(9)*. Thus, the mammalian ERK MAPK are implicated in multiple physiological processes.

The proposal that the ERK MAPK play important roles in cellular differentiation is strongly supported by studies of ERK-related MAPK in genetically tractable model organisms, including nematodes and insects. Thus, the *Drosophila* ERKA MAPK is required for developmental signaling by multiple receptor tyrosine kinases *(10)*. Studies of yeast demonstrate that the ERK-related MAPK Kss1p and Fus3p participate in the pheromone-induced growth arrest and mating responses, whereas the Mpk1p MAPK

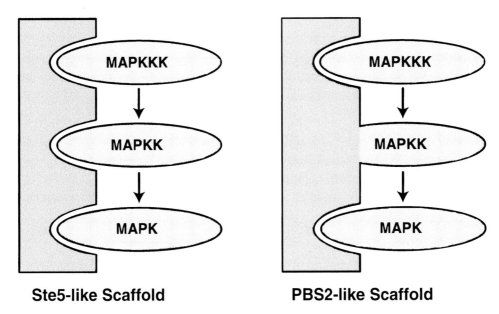

Ste5-like Scaffold   **PBS2-like Scaffold**

Fig. 1. Structure of the mammalian MAP kinase signal transduction pathways. The ERK, BMK1/ERK5, p38, and JNK signal transduction pathways are illustrated schematically. MEK1 and MEK2 are activators of the ERK subgroup of MAPK. MKK3, MKK4, and MKK6 are activators of p38 MAPK. MKK5 interacts with BMK1/ERK5. MKK7 is a specific activator of the JNK group of MAPK, whereas MKK4 activates both the p38 and JNK subgroups of MAPK. Transcription factor targets of each MAPK signaling pathway are indicated.

is required for proliferation-induced cell wall biosynthesis *(11)*. Interestingly, Kss1p and Fus3p are activated by seven-transmembrane spanning receptors through a hetero-trimeric G protein-linked signaling pathway, while Mpk1p appears to function down-stream of protein kinase C *(12)*.

2.2. The BMK Group of MAP Kinases

A distinct subgroup of ERK MAPK is represented by BMK. This group of MAPK presently includes only a single member, BMK1, also known as ERK5. Like the ERK MAPK, BMK1 is activated by phosphorylation on the motif Thr-Glu-Tyr. However, the signaling pathway that leads to BMK1 activation is distinct from the pathway that activates ERK1 and ERK2 (Fig. 1). The BMK1 activation pathway is poorly understood, and the physiological function of BMK1 is unclear. It has been proposed that BMK1 may be activated downstream of Ras or by a limited subgroup of environmental insults, including oxidation and osmotic stress *(12,13)*. Targets of the BMK1 pathway may include the transcription factors c-Myc and MEF-2C *(12,14)*. Further studies are required to establish the role of this MAPK signaling pathway. These studies would be facilitated by the identfication of BMK1 homologs in a genetically tractable model organism, such as *Caenorhabditis elegans* or *Drosophila*.

2.3. The JNK Group of MAP Kinases

The transcription factor c-Jun is phosphorylated on the N-terminal domain by a group of MAPK that are activated by exposure of cells to multiple forms of environmental stress and by treatment with cytokines. These MAPK are named the c-Jun N-terminal kinase (JNK) group of MAPK and are also known as stress-activated MAPK (SAPK) *(15)*. The JNK MAPK are characterized by the dual phosphorylation motif Thr-Pro-Tyr (Table 1).

Three genes that encode mammalian JNK protein kinases have been molecularly cloned *(16–18)*. The JNK1 and JNK2 genes are expressed ubiquitously and a total of eight JNK isoforms are created by alternative splicing *(17)*. The JNK3 gene has a more restricted pattern of expression with highest levels in brain and testis. Two forms of JNK3 are created by alternative splicing of transcripts derived from the JNK3 gene *(17)*. Homologs of JNK are not expressed by budding yeast, but this MAPK has been detected in nematodes (CJNK) and insects (DJNK) *(15)*.

The c-Jun transcription factor is a component of the AP-1 group of transcription factors *(19)*. Phosphorylation of c-Jun on the N-terminal activation domain by JNK leads to increased transcriptional activity. Targeted disruption of genes that form the JNK signal transduction pathway (MKK4 and JNK3) demonstrate that the absence of JNK signaling causes defects in stress-induced activation of AP-1 transcriptional activity *(20,21)*.

Like the ERK group of MAPK, the JNK MAPK have been demonstrated to be required for multiple biological processes. For example, studies of *Drosophila* demonstrate that DJNK is required for morphogenetic cell movements during embryogenesis *(15)*. The observation that the disruption of the MKK4 gene leads to embryonic death suggests that the JNK signaling pathway is also required for mammalian embryogenesis *(20)*. Studies of mammalian cells demonstrates that JNK is required for some forms of stress-induced neuronal apoptosis *(21,22)*. JNK is also required for inflammatory responses and for the survival and malignant transformation of certain types of cells (e.g., B cells) *(15)*. Further studies are required for full documentation of the function of the mammalian JNK signaling pathway in vivo *(15)*.

The identification of JNK in the model organism *Drosophila (23,24)* enables the genetic analysis of targets of the JNK signaling pathway *(15)*. Genetic epistasis analysis, together with the results of biochemical analysis, demonstrate that DJun, the *Drosophila* homolog of the mammalian transcription factor c-Jun, is a direct target of the JNK signaling pathway during the embryonic morphogenetic process dorsal closure *(15)*. The activation of DJun by JNK leads to the expression of the target gene *decapentaplegic*, a member of the transforming growth factor-β (TGF-β) group of growth and differentiation factors *(15)*. In mammalian cells, the transcription factors ATF2, c-Jun, Elk-1, and NFAT4 known to be regulated by the JNK signaling pathway *(15)*.

2.4. The p38 Group of MAP Kinases

The MAPK group with the dual phosphorylation motif Thr-Gly-Tyr includes four mammalian members (p38α, p38β, p38γ, and p38δ), two *Drosophila* MAPK (p38a and p38b), and the yeast MAPK Hog1p (Table 1). These MAPK are collectively named p38 MAPK and are also known as cytokine suppressive binding proteins (CSBP). This group of MAPK, like the JNK MAPK, is activated by the exposure of cells to environmental stress. Studies of *Drosophila* and mammalian p38 MAPK demonstrates that these enzymes are activated by exposure to endotoxins, including bacterial lipopolysaccharide (LPS) *(25,26)*. The mammalian p38 MAPK is also activated by treatment of cells with cytokines *(19)*.

Studies of the mammalian p38 MAPK have been facilitated by the discovery of drugs (pyridinyl imimazole derivatives) that specifically inhibit p38α and p38β MAPK. These drugs do not inhibit the p38γ and p38δ MAPK isoforms (see Chapter 27). Interestingly, these drugs have potent anti-inflammatory properties, including the inhibition of cytokine secretion by macrophages. The mechanism of inhibition appears to be mediated, in part, by translational regulation. These data indicate that the p38α and p38β MAPK contribute to inflammatory responses. However, the role of p38γ and p38δ MAPK isoforms has not been established. Further details about the role of the p38 MAPK are presented in Chapter 27.

The function of the p38 MAPK has been studied in insects and yeast. Genetic analysis of yeast indicate that the Hog1p MAPK is required for the response to osomtic stress *(11)*. This response involves the transcriptional upregulation of genes that induce the biosynthesis of the osmotic stabilizer glycerol *(11)*. In *Drosophila*, the activation of p38a and p38b by endotoxin is implicated in the downregulation of immunity gene expression *(25)*. The role of p38 MAPK to regulate gene expression in mammalian cells has been established by studies of the transcription factors ATF2, CHOP, Elk-1, MEF-2C, and SAP-1 *(27–31)*.

2.5. The Smk1p Group of MAP Kinases

The yeast MAPK Smk1p is the only MAPK that has been identified with the dual phosphorylation motif Thr-Asn-Tyr *(32)*. It is possible that homologs of Smk1p are expressed in *Drosophila* and mammals, but such enzymes have not yet been described (Table 1). The Smk1p MAPK is not expressed in vegetatively growing yeast, but the expression of Smk1p is rapidly induced during sporulation and is required for the normal completion of sporulation. This transcriptional induction of a MAPK pathway represents an interesting adaptional response to a specific stimulus. It is likely that the transcriptional induction of MAPK may account for some cell type-specific responses of differentiated mammalian cells. Further studies are required to provide evidence to support this prediction.

3. SUBSTRATE SELECTION BY MAP KINASES

Many protein kinases interact with substrates through recognition of primary sequence determinants surrounding the site(s) of phosphorylation. This type of substrate recognition is also employed by the MAPK. In general, the minimun primary sequence required for phosphorylation by MAPK is a Ser or Thr residue followed by Pro. Studies of the ERK MAPK demonstrates that the optimal primary sequence required for MAPK phosphorylation is Pro-Xaa-Ser/Thr-Pro *(33)*. The p38 and JNK MAPK also recognize Ser/Thr-Pro motifs, but they do not exhibit preference for the extended Pro-Xaa-Ser/Thr-Pro recognition sequence described for the ERK MAPK *(19)*.

While the recognition of primary sequence determinants surrounding the site(s) of phosphorylation by MAPK is important, it is clear that this does not represent the only mechanism that is employed for substrate selection by MAPK. In many, but not all, cases the MAPK appears to interact with the substrate through a binding interaction at a second site. This "docking" interaction may be required for substrate phosphorylation by MAPK in vitro and in vivo. An example is provided by the transcription factor c-Jun, which is phosphorylated by the JNK group of MAPK. A docking domain, the δ-domain, for the JNK MAPK is encoded within a small region of the N-terminal activation domain of c-Jun. Deletion of this docking domain blocks the phosphorylation of c-Jun by JNK. Similarly, peptides corresponding to the sequence of the δ-domain inhibit c-Jun phosphorylation by JNK. These data demonstrate that substrate recognition may be mediated by a two-step process in which the kinase first docks to the substrate through a binding interaction at one site leading to phosphorylation of the substrate at a second site at one or more Ser/Thr-Pro motifs. Examples of such docking interactions include the substrates ATF2 (JNK and p38) *(34,35)*, Elk-1 (ERK and JNK) *(34,35)*, MEF-2C (p38) *(30)*, NFAT4 (JNK) *(36)*. This docking interaction is likely to be an important mechanism that underlies the physical basis for the selection of high affinity substrates by MAPK in vivo.

Recent studies demonstrate that the selective interaction of MAPK with substrates may influence the physiological regulation of MAPK targets in vivo. These studies have focussed on the transcription factor Elk-1, which is phosphorylated by all three major groups of mammalian MAPK (ERK, p38, and JNK). Interestingly, the ERK and JNK MAPK interact with Elk-1 through a similar docking site *(34,35)*. By constrast, the p38 MAPK phosphorylates Elk-1 in the absence of a docking interaction *(35)*. Consistent with the hypothesis that the docking interaction facilitates high-affinity substrate interactions with MAPK, the ERK and JNK MAPK appear to mediate rapid signaling to Elk-1. However, the p38 MAPK, which does not dock to Elk-1, is a weak regulator of Elk-1 unless p38 MAPK is artificially overexpressed *(35)*.

4. THE MAP KINASE SIGNALING CASCADE

The activation of MAPK is mediated by dual phosphorylation on Thr and Tyr residues. This phosphorylation is catalyzed by a group of dual-specificity protein kinases (MAP kinase kinases; MKKs). Inactivation of MAPK requires dephosphorylation on either Thr or Tyr by a Ser/Thr or Tyr phosphatase, alternatively dephosphorylation of both Thr and Tyr residues can be mediated by a dual specificity MAPK phosphatase (*see* Chapter 10).

The mammalian MAPKK protein kinases include MEK1 and MEK2, which activate the ERK MAPK; MKK3, MKK4, and MKK6, which activate the p38 group of MAPK; MKK4 and MKK7, which activate the JNK group of MAPK; and MKK5, which interacts with the BMK1/ERK5 MAPK. Each of these MKK isoforms is specific for a particular group of MAPK, except for MKK4, which is able to activate both the JNK and p38 MAPK.

The mammalian MAPKK are activated by phosphorylation mediated by MAP kinase kinase kinases (MAPKKK). The Raf group of MAPKKK play an important role in the coupling of ERK MAPK activation to the Ras signaling pathway. A MAPKKK that is specific for the BMK1 MAPK has not been identified. The JNK signaling pathway is activated by several MAPKKK, including the MEKK group, the MLK group, TPL-2, ASK1, and TAK1. Some of these MAPKKK also lead to the activation of the stress-activated p38 MAPK signaling pathway. The large number and overlapping specificities of signaling by these MAPKKK reflects the role of MAPK signaling pathways to integrate the response of cells to multiple extracellular stimuli. It is likely that individual

MAPKKK are required for MAPK activation by specific extracellular stimuli. A detailed description of the function of MAPKKK is presented in Chapter 11.

5. STRUCTURAL ORGANIZATION OF MAP KINASE SIGNALING PATHWAYS

The MAPKKK, MAPKK, and MAPK protein kinases that form a MAPK signaling module can be reconstituted in vitro. These studies demonstrate the sequential phosphorylation and activation of each member of the protein kinase cascade. Specificity is intrinsically built into each MAPK signaling cascade because of the intrinsic substrate specificity of each component of the MAPK cascade. For example, MKK6 exclusively activates p38 MAPK, whereas MKK7 exclusively activates JNK (Fig. 1). However, it is likely that these in vitro reconstitution experiments do not faithfully represent the function of MAPK signaling pathways in vivo. It is becoming increasingly clear that MAPK can be activated within discrete signaling modules that are created by protein complexes. This paradigm of MAPK signaling requires that the interaction of MAPK signaling components is selectively organized by "scaffold" proteins. Recent studies have uncovered two types of MAPK scaffold complexes.

The first type of scaffold complex was identified through genetic analysis of the MAPK pathway that controls mating in yeast *(11)*. These MAPK are Fus3p and Kss1p (Table 1). The scaffold protein Ste5p binds to multiple components of the MAPK signaling pathway, including the MAPK-MAPKK-MAPKKK protein kinase cascade and the upstream signaling components Ste20p and heterotrimeric G protein βγ subunits. The interaction of the MAPK pathway components with the Ste5p scaffold protein acts to organize the signaling pathway. Signficantly, the absence of Ste5 leads to failure of the MAPK signaling pathway. Thus, it appears that the interaction of the MAPK pathway components in the cytoplasm is insufficient for signal transmission. The physiological function of the MAPK signaling pathway requires that the components of the MAPK module are organized through interactions with the Ste5p scaffold protein.

The second type of MAPK scaffold complex was first described for the Hog1p osmotic shock response MAPK pathway in yeast *(37,38)*. One mechanism of activation of the Hog1p MAPK involves the transmembrane protein Sho1p, which binds via an SH3 domain to a Pro-rich sequence in the MAPKK PBS2 (*see* Chapter 24, for further details about the function of SH3 domains as adapters that mediate protein–protein interactions). The recruitment of the MAPKKK Ste11p and the MAPK Hog1p does not require a separate scaffold protein. By contrast, the scaffold function is encoded within the large N-terminal domain of PBS2. The MAPK signaling module is therefore organized by one of the components of the MAPK signaling pathway.

There is substantial evidence that the normal function of MAPK signaling modules requires the organization of the MAPK pathway components within the cell. It is not established, however, that such organizational complexes are universally required. For example, it is possible that scaffold proteins may be required for targeting of MAPK signaling to some, but not all, substrates. Alternatively, some MAPK pathways may normally function in the absence of a scaffold protein in vivo. Further studies are required to identify whether scaffold complexes are involved in the physiological activation of MAPK, particularly in mammals.

6. SIGNAL TRANSMISSION TO THE NUCLEUS

MAPK signaling pathways are generally initiated at the cell surface. However, the targets of many MAPK signaling pathways include transcription factors located in the nucleus. Thus, signaling by MAPK must involve the transmission of signals from the cytoplasm to the nucleus. As MAPK pathways are composed of multiple components, the MAPK signal could be transmitted to the nucleus by any one of these components. Little is known about the mechanism of nuclear signal transmission by the JNK and p38 MAPK pathways. However, detailed studies of signaling to the nucleus have been reported for the ERK group of MAPK.

Studies of the ERK signaling pathway indicate that the activated MAPKKK c-Raf-1 is present in the plasma membrane *(39)*. The MAPKK activated by c-Raf-1, MEK1, and MEK2, are located in the cytoplasm *(40)*. This accumulation in the cytoplasm appears to be mediated by the presence of a nuclear export signal (NES) in the N-terminal region of the MAPKK *(41)*. By contrast, the ERK MAPK are located in the cytoplasm of quiescent cells and in the nucleus of activated cells *(40,42–44)*. Thus, the transmission of signals from the cytoplasm to the nucleus appears to be directly mediated by the ERK MAPK.

The mechanism that accounts for the activation-induced redistribution of ERK MAPK from the cytoplasm to the nucleus is unclear. One possible mechanism is that the ERK MAPK are sequestered in the cytoplasm by MEK1 and MEK2. This model proposes that ERK signaling pathway activation leads to MAPKK dissociation from ERK1 and ERK2, which are then able to accumulate in the nucleus. Several lines of evidence to support this model have been reported *(45)*. However, it is unclear whether the release of ERK from the MAPKK is sufficient to allow nuclear accumulation or whether additional processes are involved. In addition, the potential role of activation-induced nuclear MAPKK requires clarification *(46)*.

Further studies are required to identify the molecular mechanism of nuclear redistribution of the ERK MAPK and to establish whether similar processes are involved in the function of other MAPK signaling pathways.

7. MECHANISM OF REGULATION OF GENE EXPRESSION

It is established that the regulation of gene expression is an important function of MAPK signaling pathways *(19)*. It appears that there is no single mechanism that accounts for the regulation of gene expression by MAPK. Instead, MAPK have been reported to exert regulation at multiple pretranscriptional, transcriptional, and posttranscriptional steps. Thus, MAPK signaling pathways appear to regulate gene expression using multiple strategies. It is likely that this complexity is critical for the co-ordination of appropriate responses to a wide variety of extracellular stimuli.

Some transcription factors are sequestered in the cytoplasm in latent form before activation-induced translocation to the nucleus. Examples include the SMAD transcription factors that are activated by TGF-β and the NFAT transcription factors that are activated by calcium. Phosphorylation of SMAD1 by ERK *(47)* and phosphorylation of NFAT4 *(36)* by JNK causes cytoplasmic retention of these transcription factors and therefore inhibition of transcriptional activity. Whereas the phosphorylation of SMAD1 and NFAT4 by MAPK leads to cytoplasmic retention, it is possible that the phosphorylation of other cytoplasmic transcription factors may cause nuclear accumulation and therefore contribute to activated transcription. Further studies are required to test this hypothesis.

Regulated DNA binding activity represents a second mechanism that is employed by MAPK to control transcription factor activity. An example is provided by the Ets domain transcription factor Elk-1. Phosphorylation of Elk-1 by ERK *(48)*, JNK *(49)*, and p38 MAPK *(27)* causes increased DNA binding.

A third mechanism employed by MAPK is the regulation of transcriptional activity. For example, phosphorylation of nuclear receptors by MAPK can lead to inhibition of transcription *(9)*. By contrast, phosphorylation of other transcription factors can lead to increased transcriptional activity. For example, phosphorylation of the transcriptional activation domains of ATF2, CHOP, Elk-1, and c-Jun causes increased transcription *(29,50–53)*. Although we know little about the basic molecular mechanisms involved in the regulation of transcriptional activity by MAPK phosphorylation, detailed studies of phosphorylation-dependent transcriptional activation have been reported for the transcription factor CREB. These studies indicate that transcription factor phosphorylation can cause changes in the interaction with coactivator molecules, including CBP, p300, and Rb-family proteins which function, in part, through the regulation of histone acetylation *(54)*. Further studies are required to demonstrate that MAPK-regulated transcriptional activity is mediated by similar mechanisms.

MAPK regulation of mRNA processing and nuclear export has not been described, although these biosynthetic steps represent potential sites for intervention by MAPK. However, MAPK regulation of translation has been reported. This represents a fourth general mechanism of regulation of gene expression by MAPK. The best example is the translational regulation of cytokine expression that is observed in macrophages exposed to endotoxin. Translational regulation of the cytokine tumor necrosis factor-α (TNF-α) by p38 MAPK requires a *cis*-acting element in the mRNA. (*See* Chapter 27, for a detailed description of the mechanism of translational regulation by p38 MAPK.)

A fifth general mechanism that is employed by MAPK to regulate gene expression is the regulation of protein degradation. One example of this type of regulation is provided by the transcription factor c-Jun, which is a short-lived protein that is rapidly degraded by the ubiquitin-proteasome pathway. Phosphorylation of c-Jun by JNK inhibits the ubiquitination of c-Jun and, therefore, the rapid degradation of c-Jun. Consequently, JNK activation prolongs the half-life of c-Jun, leading to the accumulation of the c-Jun protein *(55,56)*. The regulation of protein stability by MAPK therefore contributes to the regulation of gene expression mediated by these signaling pathways.

8. CONCLUSIONS

Signal transduction mechanisms that regulate nuclear events in response to extracellular stimuli represent important regulatory processes that coordinate the physiological response of cells to their environment. In recent years, it has become clear that there is an important role for MAPK signaling pathways. Rapid progress has been achieved toward understanding mechanisms of signal transduction that lead to the nucleus, but there is much that we do not understand about the molecular mechanism of MAPK action. I predict that future studies of MAPK signaling will lead to greater understanding of cellular function and will prove to be a very exciting endeavor.

REFERENCES

1. Zhang F, Strand A, Robbins D, Cobb MH, Goldsmith EJ. Atomic structure of the MAP kinase ERK2 at 2.3 Å resolution [see comments]. *Nature* 1994; 367:704–711.
2. Wang Z, Harkins PC, Ulevitch RJ, Han J, Cobb MH, Goldsmith EJ. The structure of mitogen-activated protein kinase p38 at 2.1-A resolution. *Proc Natl Acad Sci USA* 1997; 94:2327–2332.
3. Wilson KP, Fitzgibbon MJ, Caron PR, Griffith JP, Chen W, McCaffrey PG, Chambers SP, Su MS. Crystal structure of p38 mitogen-activated protein kinase. *J Biol Chem* 1996; 271:27,696–27,700.
4. Canagarajah BJ, Khokhlatchev A, Cobb MH, Goldsmith EJ. Activation mechanism of the MAP kinase ERK2 by dual phosphorylation. *Cell* 1997; 90:859–869.
5. Mansour SJ, Matten WT, Hermann AS, Candia JM, Rong S, Fukasawa K, Vande Woude GF, Ahn NG. Transformation of mammalian cells by constitutively active MAP kinase kinase. *Science* 1994; 265:966–970.
6. Cowley S, Paterson H, Kemp P, Marshall CJ. Activation of MAP kinase kinase is necessary and sufficient for PC12 differentiation and for transformation of NIH 3T3 cells. *Cell* 1994; 77:841–852.
7. Bennett AM, Tonks NK. Regulation of distinct stages of skeletal muscle differentiation by mitogen-activated protein kinases. *Science* 1997; 278:1288–1291.
8. Whalen AM, Galasinski SC, Shapiro PS, Nahreini TS, Ahn NG. Megakaryocytic differentiation induced by constitutive activation of mitogen-activated protein kinase kinase. *Mol Cell Biol* 1997; 17:1947–1958.
9. Hu E, Kim JB, Sarraf P, Spiegelman BM. Inhibition of adipogenesis through MAP kinase-mediated phosphorylation of PPARgamma. *Science* 1996; 274:2100–2103.
10. Brunner D, Oellers N, Szabad J, Biggs WH III, Zipursky SL, Hafen E. A gain-of-function mutation in Drosophila MAP kinase activates multiple receptor tyrosine kinase signaling pathways. *Cell* 1994; 76:875–888.
11. Ammerer, G. Sex, stress and integrity: The importance of MAP kinases in yeast. *Curr Opin Genet Dev* 1994; 4:90–95.
12. English JM, Pearson G, Baer R, Cobb MH. Identification of substrates and regulators of the mitogen-activated protein kinase ERK5 using chimeric protein kinases. *J Biol Chem* 1998; 273:3854–3860.
13. Abe J, Kusuhara M, Ulevitch RJ, Berk BC, Lee JD. Big mitogen-activated protein kinase 1 (BMK1) is a redox-sensitive kinase. *J Biol Chem* 1996; 271:16,586–16,590.
14. Kato Y, Kravchenko VV, Tapping RI, Han J, Ulevitch RJ, Lee JD. BMK1/ERK5 regulates serum-induced early gene expression through transcription factor MEF2C. *EMBO J* 1997; 16:7054–7066.
15. Ip YT, Davis RJ. Signal transduction by the c-Jun N-terminal kinase (JNK)—from inflammation to development. *Curr Opin Cell Biol* 1998; 10:205–219.
16. Derijard B, Hibi M, Wu IH, Barrett T, Su B, Deng T, Karin M, Davis RJ. JNK1: A protein kinase stimulated by UV light and Ha-Ras that binds and phosphorylates the c-Jun activation domain. *Cell* 1994; 76:1025–1037.
17. Gupta S, Barrett T, Whitmarsh AJ, Cavanagh J, Sluss HK, Derijard B, Davis RJ. Selective interaction of JNK protein kinase isoforms with transcription factors. *EMBO J* 1996; 15:2760–2770.
18. Kyriakis JM, Banerjee P, Nikolakaki E, Dai T, Rubie EA, Ahmad MF, Avruch J, Woodgett

JR. The stress-activated protein kinase subfamily of c-Jun kinases. *Nature* 1994; 369: 156–160.

19. Whitmarsh AJ, Davis RJ. Transcription factor AP-1 regulation by mitogen-activated protein kinase signal transduction pathways. *J Mol Med* 1996; 74:589–607.
20. Yang D, Tournier C, Wysk M, Lu HT, Xu J, Davis RJ, Flavell RA. Targeted disruption of the MKK4 gene causes embryonic death, inhibition of c-Jun NH2-terminal kinase activation, and defects in AP-1 transcriptional activity. *Proc Natl Acad Sci USA* 1997; 94:3004–3009.
21. Yang DD, Kuan CY, Whitmarsh AJ, Rincon M, Zheng TS, Davis RJ, Rakic P, Flavell RA. Absence of excitotoxicity-induced apoptosis in the hippocampus of mice lacking the Jnk3 gene. *Nature* 1997; 389:865–870.
22. Xia Z, Dickens M, Raingeaud J, Davis RJ, Greenberg ME. Opposing effects of ERK and JNK-p38 MAP kinases on apoptosis. *Science* 1995; 270:1326–1331.
23. Sluss HK, Han Z, Barrett T, Davis RJ, Ip YT. A JNK signal transduction pathway that mediates morphogenesis and an immune response in *Drosophila*. *Genes Dev* 1996; 10:2745–2758.
24. Riesgo-Escovar JR, Jenni M, Fritz A, Hafen E. The *Drosophila* Jun-N-terminal kinase is required for cell morphogenesis but not for DJun-dependent cell fate specification in the eye. *Genes Dev* 1996; 10:2759–2768.
25. Han ZS, Enslen H, Hu X, Meng X, Wu IH, Barrett T, Davis RJ, Ip YT. A conserved p38 mitogen-activated protein kinase pathway regulates Drosophila immunity gene expression. *Mol Cell Biol* 1998; 18:3527–3539.
26. Han J, Lee JD, Bibbs L, Ulevitch RJ. A MAP kinase targeted by endotoxin and hyperosmolarity in mammalian cells. *Science* 1994; 265:808–811.
27. Whitmarsh AJ, Yang SH, Su MS, Sharrocks AD, Davis RJ. Role of p38 and JNK mitogen-activated protein kinases in the activation of ternary complex factors. *Mol Cell Biol* 1997; 17:2360–2371.
28. Raingeaud J, Whitmarsh AJ, Barrett T, Derijard B, Davis RJ. MKK3- and MKK6-regulated gene expression is mediated by the p38 mitogen-activated protein kinase signal transduction pathway. *Mol Cell Biol* 1996; 16:1247–1255.
29. Wang XZ, Ron D. Stress-induced phosphorylation and activation of the transcription factor CHOP (GADD153) by p38 MAP kinase. *Science* 1996; 272:1347–1349.
30. Han J, Jiang Y, Li Z, Kravchenko VV, Ulevitch RJ. Activation of the transcription factor MEF2C by the MAP kinase p38 in inflammation. *Nature* 1997; 386:296–299.
31. Price MA, Cruzalegui FH, Treisman R. The p38 and ERK MAP kinase pathways cooperate to activate Ternary Complex Factors and c-fos transcription in response to UV light. *EMBO J* 1996; 15:6552–6563.
32. Krisak L, Strich R, Winters RS, Hall JP, Mallory MJ, Kreitzer D, Tuan RS, Winter E. SMK1, a developmentally regulated MAP kinase, is required for spore wall assembly in Saccharomyces cerevisiae. *Genes Dev* 1994; 8:2151–2161.
33. Davis, RJ. The mitogen-activated protein kinase signal transduction pathway. *J Biol Chem* 1993; 268:14,553–14,556.
34. Yang SH, Yates PR, Whitmarsh AJ, Davis RJ, Sharrocks AD. The Elk-1 ETS-domain transcription factor contains a mitogen-activated protein kinase targeting motif. *Mol Cell Biol* 1998; 18:710–720.
35. Yang SH, Whitmarsh AJ, Davis RJ, Sharrocks AD. Differential targeting of MAP kinases to the ETS-domain transcription factor Elk-1. *EMBO J* 1998; 17:1740–1749.
36. Chow CW, Rincon M, Cavanagh J, Dickens M, Davis RJ. Nuclear accumulation of NFAT4 opposed by the JNK signal transduction pathway. *Science* 1997; 278:1638–1641.
37. Posas F, Saito H. Osmotic activation of the HOG MAPK pathway via Ste11p MAPKKK: scaffold role of Pbs2p MAPKK. *Science* 1997; 276:1702–1705.
38. Maeda T, Takekawa M, Saito H. Activation of yeast PBS2 MAPKK by MAPKKKs or by binding of an SH3- containing osmosensor. *Science* 1995; 269:554–558.

39. Leevers SJ, Paterson HF, Marshall CJ. Requirement for Ras in Raf activation is overcome by targeting Raf to the plasma membrane. *Nature* 1994; 369:411–414.

40. Lenormand P, Sardet C, Pages G, L'Allemain G, Brunet A, Pouyssegur J. Growth factors induce nuclear translocation of MAP kinases (p42mapk and p44mapk) but not of their activator MAP kinase kinase (p45mapkk) in fibroblasts. *J Cell Biol* 1993; 122:1079–1088.

41. Fukuda M, Gotoh I, Gotoh Y, Nishida E. Cytoplasmic localization of mitogen-activated protein kinase kinase directed by its NH2-terminal, leucine-rich short amino acid sequence, which acts as a nuclear export signal. *J Biol Chem* 1996; 271:20,024–20,028.

42. Seth A, Gonzalez FA, Gupta S, Raden DL, Davis RJ. Signal transduction within the nucleus by mitogen-activated protein kinase. *J Biol Chem* 1992; 267:24,796–24,804.

43. Gonzalez FA, Seth A, Raden DL, Bowman DS, Fay FS, Davis RJ. Serum-induced transloca-tion of mitogen-activated protein kinase to the cell surface ruffling membrane and the nucleus. *J Cell Biol* 1993; 122:1089–1101.

44. Chen RH, Sarnecki C, Blenis J. Nuclear localization and regulation of erk- and rsk-encoded protein kinases. *Mol Cell Biol* 1992; 12:915–927.

45. Fukuda M, Gotoh Y, Nishida E. Interaction of MAP kinase with MAP kinase kinase: Its possible role in the control of nucleocytoplasmic transport of MAP kinase. *EMBO J* 1997; 16:1901–1908.

46. Jaaro H, Rubinfeld H, Hanoch T, Seger R. Nuclear translocation of mitogen-activated protein kinase kinase (MEK1) in response to mitogenic stimulation. *Proc Natl Acad Sci USA* 1997; 94:3742–3747.

47. Kretzschmar M, Doody J, Massagué J. Opposing BMP and EGF signalling pathways converge on the TGF-beta family mediator Smad1. *Nature* 1997; 389:618–622.

48. Gille H, Sharrocks AD, Shaw PE. Phosphorylation of transcription factor p62TCF by MAP kinase stimulates ternary complex formation at c-fos promoter. *Nature* 1992; 358:414–417.

49. Whitmarsh AJ, Shore P, Sharrocks AD, Davis RJ. Integration of MAP kinase signal transduc-tion pathways at the serum response element. *Science* 1995; 269:403–407.

50. Livingstone C, Patel G, Jones N. ATF-2 contains a phosphorylation-dependent transcrip-tional activation domain. *EMBO J* 1995; 14:1785–1797.

51. Gupta S, Campbell D, Derijard B, Davis RJ. Transcription factor ATF2 regulation by the JNK signal transduction pathway. *Science* 1995; 267:389–393.

52. Pulverer BJ, Kyriakis JM, Avruch J, Nikolakaki E, Woodgett JR. Phosphorylation of c-jun mediated by MAP kinases. *Nature* 1991; 353:670–674.

53. Marais R, Wynne J, Treisman R. The SRF accessory protein Elk-1 contains a growth factor-regulated transcriptional activation domain. *Cell* 1993; 73:381–393.

54. Goldman PS, Tran VK, Goodman RH. The multifunctional role of the co-activator CBP in transcriptional regulation. *Recent Prog Horm Res* 1997; 52:103–119.

55. Fuchs SY, Dolan L, Davis RJ, Ronai Z. Phosphorylation-dependent targeting of c-Jun ubiquitination by Jun N-kinase. *Oncogene* 1996; 13:1531–1535.

56. Musti AM, Treier M, Bohmann D. Reduced ubiquitin-dependent degradation of c-Jun after phosphorylation by MAP kinases. *Science* 1997; 275:400–402.

10

The Regulation of MAP Kinase Pathways by MAP Kinase Phosphatases

Kathleen Kelly and Yanfang Chu

1. INTRODUCTION

Mitogen activated protein (MAP) kinase signal transduction pathways are evolutionary conserved protein modules that play a central role in conveying information from the extracellular environment into cytoplasmic and nuclear responses *(1,2)*. The modules consist of a three component kinase cascade (Fig. 1) (*see* Chapter 9). After its activation by an upstream component, a serine-threonine kinase (a MAP kinase kinase kinase or MEKK) phosphorylates and thereby activates a dual specificity kinase (MAP kinase kinase or MEK) which in turn phosphorylates a MAP kinase on threonine and tyrosine resulting in its activation. Dual phosphorylation of MAP kinase on the relevant threonine and tyrosine, a TXY motif in kinase subdomain VIII, is required because neither phosphorylation alone is sufficient for activity.

Various different MAP kinase modules have been described in mammalian cells (Fig. 1). The pathways can be broadly grouped as responsive to growth/differentiation signals—the ERK pathway—or responsive to environmental stresses (the JNK and p38 pathways). A variety of stimuli, such as integrin *(4)* or T-cell receptor (TCR) crosslinking *(5)*, activate both the ERK and JNK/p38 pathways. The various MAP kinases have unique and shared substrates *(6,7)*, consonant with the concept that a constellation of targets will determine the signal-specific cellular response. Among a variety of substrates, the most common defined to date include other kinases and transcription factors *(8)*.

Inactive ERK is found in the cytoplasm, apparently bound to the N-terminus of MEK *(9)*. An important concept that has developed from studies of PC12 cells is that prolonged activation of ERK results in a substantial fraction of cellular ERK translocating to the nucleus, where it can mediate phosphorylation of transcription factors and changes in gene expression programs *(10)*. Sustained ERK activation and its translocation to the nucleus are associated with neurite differentiation stimulated by NGF in PC12 cells, whereas transient ERK activation stimulated by EGF is associated with continued proliferation and no differentiative change. Although the precise timeframe of ERK activation is distinct for the various combinations of stimuli and cell types,

From: Signaling Networks and Cell Cycle Control: The Molecular Basis of Cancer and Other Diseases
Edited by: J. S. Gutkind © Humana Press Inc., Totowa, NJ

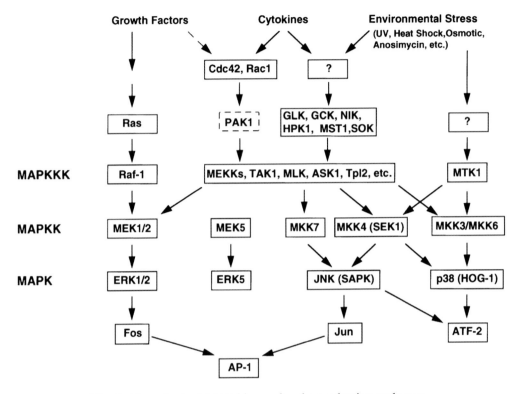

Fig. 1. Flow chart of MAP kinase signal transduction pathways.

transient ERK activation is on the order of <10 min, whereas sustained ERK activation is one-half to several hours. Sustained ERK activation is regulated and returns to nonactivated levels in a defined manner. Sustained ERK activation is distinct from constitutive ERK activation such as is seen in cells transformed by constitutively activated MEK, raf, or ras *(11)*.

This review describes a family of evolutionary conserved enzymes, the MAP kinase phosphatases, that are important in regulating the extent and timing of MAP kinase activation, in particular in response to signals that generate changes in gene expression. MAP kinase phosphatases are a family of structurally related proteins that are a subset of dual-specificity phosphatases (Table 1; Fig. 2), capable of removing phosphate from phosphothreonine, phosphoserine, and phosphotyrosine *(12)*. Importantly, there are several examples of cellular systems in which MAP kinase phosphatases are not constitutively expressed but are induced in response to the same ligands that activate MAP kinases (see specific references throughout this review). In fact, PAC-1 and MKP-1 were originally cloned based on the induction of their expression by T cell mitogens *(13)* and either oxidative stress *(14)* or serum *(15)*, respectively. Similarly, a yeast homologue (MSG5) of mammalian MAP kinase phosphatases is induced in *Saccharomyces cerevisiae* in response to pheromone *(16)*. Thus, the dual-specificity MAP kinase phosphatases are the effectors of a negative feedback loop which regulate MAP kinase activity.

Table 1
Summary of MAPK Phosphatases

Name (alterative name)	MW (kDa) (calculated)	Tissue distribution	Subcellular localization	References
VHR	20.5	Ubiquitous	?	*17*
PAC1	34.4	Hematopoietic tissues, brain	Nucleus	*13*
MKP-1 (CL100, 3CH134, ERP)	39.3	Lung, liver, placenta, skeletal muscle, pancreas, heart	Nucleus	*28,14,39*
MKP-2 (hVH2, TYP1)	42.9	Ubiquitous	Nucleus	*40,32,88*
MKP-3 (rVH6, Pyst1)	42.3	Heart, brain, spleen, lung, skeletal muscle, kidney, liver, pancreas, placenta	Cytosol	*29,42,38*
B59 (Pyst2, MKP-X)	40.5	Heart, lung, liver, brain, kidney, pancreas, skeletal muscle, placenta	?	*29,38,74*
MKP-4	41.9	Kidney, placenta	Cytosol > nucleus	*35*
hVH3 (B23)	42.1	Brain, pancreas, liver, placenta, lung, heart, kidney, skeletal muscle	Nucleus	*89,90*
M3/6 (hVH5)	68.8 (65.7)	Eye, brain, lung, heart, skeletal muscle	Nucleus and cytosol	*37,91*

2. STRUCTURAL CHARACTERISTICS

Several MAP kinase phosphatases have been described in detail, many of which were independently cloned and named by different research groups. The alternative names for single enzymes are listed in Table 1. Although no specific nomenclature has been suggested or adopted, for simplicity, this review refers to enzymes by a single name, using the MKP (MAP kinase phosphatase) nomenclature where possible. Several MAP kinase phosphatase sequences are shown in Figure 2 in addition to the dual-specificity phosphatase VHR. VHR is a robust phosphatase that is capable of dephosphorylating a variety of phosphotyrosine- and phosphothreonine/serine-containing substrates, but whose natural substrate has not been identified *(17)*. The MAP kinase phosphatases range between 34 and 69 kDa in size and contain a conserved catalytic domain of approximately 140 amino acids. Within the catalytic domain is the active site motif, HCXXGXXRS. This sequence and next 10 carboxyl amino acids are highly conserved among many dual specificity phosphatases *(18)*.

The HCXXGXXRS/T motif was first identified in enzymes that hydrolyze protein phosphotyrosine but has since been recognized as a sequence in the proper enzyme context capable of hydrolyzing phosphothreonine/serine *(12)*. Biochemically, the site

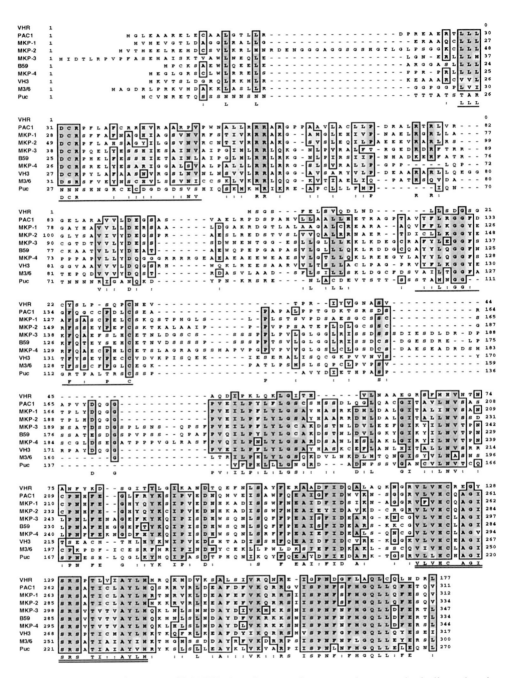

Fig. 2. Sequence alignment of MAPK phosphatases. Sequences between the indicated amino acids were aligned. The sequence alignment was generated using the MacVector™ program version 6.0.1 (Oxford Molecular Group). The signature motif of dual specific protein phosphatase is double underlined. The cdc25 homology domains are single underlined.

is characterized by sensitivity to vanadate, insensitivity to okadaic acid, a lack of dependence on metal ions, and a total loss of activity upon mutation of the active site cysteine to serine *(18)*. The catalytic mechanism for phosphotyrosine dephosphorylation by tyrosine phosphatases (PTPs) has been shown to proceed through a phosphorylcysteine intermediate *(12)*. After mutation of the active-site cysteine, the MAP kinase phosphatases lose both phosphotyrosine and phosphothreonine phosphatase activity, showing that dephosphorylation of both amino acids involves a common catalytic mechanism *(15,19,20)*.

The catalytic domains of the MAP kinase phosphatases share >80% homology (Fig. 2). A truncated recombinant version of PAC1 which contains the conserved catalytic region and approx 40 additional amino acids on the amino side dephosphorylated ERK2 but not various other tyrosine or serine/threonine phosphorylated substrates *(20)*. In addition, similarly truncated MKP-3 exhibited a turnover value similar to that of the full-length enzyme with p-nitrophenyl phosphate as a substrate *(21)*. However, recent results *(22)* from studies using MKP-3 deletions or chimeras between the catalytic and N-terminal noncatalytic domains of MKP-3 and M3/6 showed that the N-terminal domain was responsible for MKP-3 binding to ERK and that an N-terminal deleted MKP-3 required at least a 10-fold higher concentration of phosphatase for equivalent ERK dephosphorylation. Such results suggest that the sequences located outside the catalytic domain comprise a separate domain not strictly required for enzyme activity but important in fine substrate recognition.

The catalytic domains of the dual specificity phosphatases and the tyrosine phosphatases demonstrate less than 5% sequence identity *(12)*. Despite this, the solved X-ray structure of the human dual specificity phosphatase VHR *(23)* showed that its overall structural fold is very similar to the structure of the tyrosine phosphatses PTP1B *(24)* and the *Yersinia* PTP *(25)*. The tyrosine phosphatases and VHR share a five-stranded mixed β-sheet and six α-helices, with a phosphate binding loop and nearby a general acid loop that was shown for PTP1B to shift in conformation upon substrate binding. The loop between the first α-helix and the first β-strand in PTP1B is involved in the interaction with substrate; it creates a wall around the active site that only the longer phosphotyrosine can reach into *(25)*. This shortening of this region that has occurred in VHR results in a much shallower active site pocket than the PTPs, possibly permitting access for the shorter phosphothreonine and phosphoserine *(23)*. It has been speculated that the region between a1 and b1 may play a major role in substrate specificity and recognition for all PTPs; however, this possibility remains to be tested.

The noncatalytic domain sequences of the MAP kinase phosphatases show considerably less homology as a family as compared with the catalytic domains (Fig. 2). The noncatalytic domains are likely involved in fine substrate recognition and may also serve such functions in posttranslational regulation. Interestingly, many MAP kinase phosphatases contain in the amino-localized, noncatalytic domains, two short conserved stretches found in the catalytic domains of the dual-specificity cdc25 phosphatase family (Fig. 3). Although these conserved stretches are located on either side of the active site motif in cdc25, they are outside the catalytic domain region of the MAP kinase phosphatases, and therefore are not required for enzymatic activity. Cdc25 dephosphorylates an adjacent threonine and tyrosine on the cell cycle-regulated cyclin-dependent kinase, cdc2 *(26)*. It has been shown that MKP-1 does not substitute for cdc25 in

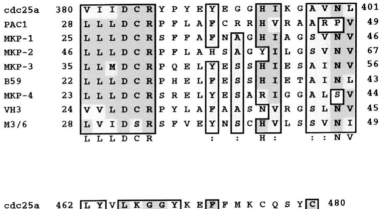

Fig. 3. Alignment of the cdc25 homology domains of MAPK phosphatases.

Xenopus extracts *(27)*, and therefore, it is unlikely that the motif functions strictly in cdc2 recognition. Although the significance of the sequences conserved between the cdc25 family and the MAP kinase phosphatases is unclear, an interesting possibility is that the sequences encode a binding site for a protein which interacts with both types of enzymes.

3. SUBSTRATE SPECIFICITY

Considerable evidence has accumulated regarding the specificity of the MAP kinase phosphatases. Studies with bacterial recombinant MKP-1 *(27,28,29)*, PAC1 *(20)*, and MKP-3 *(29)* have shown the marked preference of these enzymes for ERK1/ERK2 over a variety of other tyrosine or serine/threonine phosphorylated substrates. Since the discovery of the JNK and p38 MAP kinase families, analyses of MAP kinase phosphatase substrates have concentrated mainly on the relative specificity of the MAP kinase phosphatases for members of the MAP kinase family. As shown in Table 2, the various MAP kinase phosphatases dephosphorylate ERK, JNK, and p38 differentially as substrates. Substrate specificity for the MAP kinase phosphatases has been determined in vitro using purified, recombinant MKP-1 and MKP-3 *(28,29)*. In addition, substrate specificity has been analyzed using transient cotransfection of epitope-tagged kinases and MAP kinase phosphatases or using endogenous kinases and inducible expression of a MAP kinase phosphatase in permanent transfectants. Transfection methods assay the extent of MAP kinase activation to extracellular stimuli in the presence of an active MAP kinase phosphatase. The various methods have generated relatively similar

Table 2
Substrate Specificity of MAPK Phosphatases

	ERK	*JNK/SAPK*	*p38/HOG1*
VHR	−	?	?
PAC1	++	−	+
MKP-1	++	++	++
MKP-2	++	++	+/−
MKP-3	+++	+	+/−
B59	++	?	?
MKP-4	+++	+	+
hVH3	++	?	?
M3/6	−	+++	+++

conclusions although, not surprisingly, it appears that at high concentrations, phosphatases lose their apparent specificity.

MKP-1 may be the most general MAP kinase phosphatase, capable of dephosphorylating all three types of MAP kinases *(5,29)*, although in some systems, MKP-1 shows a preference for JNK and p38 *(30)*. PAC1 readily dephosphorylates ERK and p38, but not JNK *(5,31)*. MKP-2 shows specificity for ERK and JNK over p38 *(5,32,33)*. MKP-3 and MKP-4 have similar specificity for ERK and a lesser preference for p38 and JNK *(22,29,34,35)*. The M3/6 phosphatase dephosphorylates the stress-induced kinases, p38 and JNK, but not ERK *(34)*. *Drosophila puc* is most closely related to M3/6 and appears from genetic data to be a JNK, but not an ERK, phosphatase *(36)*. The determinants of MAP kinase phosphatase specificity are not apparent from linear sequence comparisons. It is hoped that the awaited three-dimensional structural analyses of a MAP kinase phosphatase will provide clues to the molecular basis for the substrate specificity of these enzymes. The distinct specificities of the phosphatases, coupled with differences in subcellular distribution, tissue expression, and mechanisms of induction provide a means for unique crossregulation of the various MAP kinase pathways during development and in response to various activation processes.

4. EXPRESSION CHARACTERISTICS

The various MAP kinase phosphatases have unique but overlapping tissue distributions (Table 1) when evaluated by whole tissue Northern blots. Immunohistochemical analyses to determine which cells within a tissue are expressing particular MAP kinase phosphatases have not been reported as yet. Also, because the expression of MAP kinase phosphatases is dynamic and regulated in many cell–stimulus combinations, some phosphatases may not be detectable in whole resting tissues but would be detectable after certain physiological stimuli. Some MAP kinase phosphatases, such as MKP-1, MKP-2, and MKP-3, are quite ubiquitously expressed in whole tissues, whereas others, such as PAC1, MKP-4, and M3/6, demonstrate expression in only a few tissues. It is clear from mitogen-activated T cells *(5)* and from NGF-stimulated PC12 cells *(37,38)*, that multiple MAP kinase phosphatases may be simultaneously induced in a single cell.

MAP kinase phosphatases differ in their subcellular localization. PAC1 *(13)*, MKP1 *(39)*, and MKP2 *(40)* are predominantly found in the nucleus, where they would be expected to have an effect on MAP kinase-regulated transcription factors. In fact, transient cotransfection assays have shown that PAC1 *(20)*, MKP1 *(30,41)*, and MKP-2 *(40)* reduce the level of c-fos SRE activity which is substantially dependent upon ERK activation of ELK-1. MKP-1 *(30,33)* and MKP-2 *(33)* reduce jun-dependent as well as AP-1-mediated transcription. MKP-3 and MKP-4 are cytoplasmic enzymes *(29,38,42)*. A proportion of activated ERK appears to be associated with the cytoskeleton *(43)*; several important cytoplasmic ERK substrates have been described, including cytoplasmic phospholipase A2 *(44)* and myosin light chain kinase *(45)*. Because MKP-3 is induced in many cell systems after translocation of activated ERK to the nucleus, a direct downregulation of nuclear MAP kinase by induced MKP-3 would not be expected. In addition to the MAP kinase phosphatases that appear to localize in distinct subcellular compartments, the M3/6 phosphatase has been reported to be in both the nucleus and cytoplasm.

5. MAP KINASE PHOSPHATASE ACTIVITY IN CELLS

Multiple cellular systems have been described in which MAP kinase activity correlates inversely with expression of a MAP kinase phosphatase. Several examples have demonstrated that induction of a MAP kinase phosphatase is paralleled by a decrease in the extent of MAP kinase activity. Examples include ERK inactivation and PAC1 expression in mitogen-activated T lymphocytes *(20)*, ERK downregulation, and MKP-3 induction in NGF-treated PC-12 cells *(38)*, ERK downregulation and MKP-1 expression in serum- *(15)* or EGF-stimulated 3T3 cells *(46)*, JNK inactivation after MKP-1 induction by MMS or UVC-treated HeLa cells *(47)*, ERK inactivation associated with endothelin-1 induction of MKP-1 in rat mesangial cells *(48)*, and ERK downregulation and angiotensin II induction of MKP-1 in vascular smooth muscle *(49)* or neuroblastoma cells *(50)*. Conversely, balloon injury of the rat carotid artery results in increased MAP kinase activity and a loss of detectable constitutive MKP-1 expression in arterial smooth muscle cells *(51)*.

In addition to correlative studies with endogenous MAP kinase phosphatases, expression of exogenously introduced MAP kinase phosphatase genes has been manipulated in various regulated systems. Importantly, external modulation of MAP kinase phosphatase expression results in changes in the extent and timing of MAP kinase activation. Jurkat T cells transfected with a PAC1 expression vector demonstrated accelerated kinetics of PAC1 expression following mitogen stimulation and a correlative decrease in ERK activation and IL-2 production *(20)*. Tetracycline-regulated MKP-1 in C2C12 myoblasts inhibited serum-stimulated ERK activation upon its expression and was sufficient to relieve the inhibitory effects of mitogens on muscle-specific gene expression *(52)*. Induction of MKP-1 in U937 leukemic cells by heavy metals resulted in a preferential loss of PMA-inducible p38 and JNK activity, as compared with ERK activity *(30)* and protection from UV-mediated apoptosis *(31)*.

Relatively few examples have been reported for specific loss of MAP kinase phosphatase function. The MAP kinase phosphatase Msg5p downregulates the pheromone-activated MAP kinase pathway by inactivating the Fus3p MAP kinase *(16)*. Recovery

developmental or stimulus associated crossregulation of the activities mediated by the various MAP kinase families. The specific role of individual MAP kinase phosphatases in such processes as carcinogenesis, mammalian development, animal physiology, immune responses, and nervous system function presents a challenge for the future that may be addressed at least in part with mouse genetic models.

REFERENCES

1. Herskowitz I. MAP kinase pathways in yeast: For mating and more. *Cell* 1995; 80:187–197.
2. Robinson MJ, Cobb MH. Mitogen-activated protein kinase pathways. *Cell Biology* 1997; 9:180–186.
3. Zhou G, Quin Bao Z, Dixon JE. Components of a new human protein kinase signal transduction pathway. *J Biol Chem* 1995; 270:12,655–12,669.
4. Miyamoto S, Teramoto H, Coso OA, Gutkind JS, Burbelo PD, Akiyama SK, Yamada KM. Integrin function: Molecular hierarchies of cytoskeletal and signaling molecules. *J Cell Biol* 1995; 131:791–805.
5. Chu Y, Solski PA, Khosravi-Far R, Der CJ, Kelly K. The mitogen-activated protein kinase phosphatases PAC-1, MKP-1, and MKP-2 have unique substrate specificities and reduced activity in vivo toward the ERK2 sevenmaker mutation. *J Biol Chem* 1996; 271:6497–6501.
6. Whitmarsh AJ, Shore P, Sharrocks AD, Davis RJ. Integration of MAP kinase signal transduction pathways at the serum response element. *Science* 1995; 269:403–407.
7. Ludwig S, Engel K, Hoffmeyer A, Sithanandam G, Neufeld B, Palm D, Gaestel M, Rapp UR. 3pK, a novel mitogen-activated protein (MAP) kinase-activated protein kinase, is targeted by three MAP kinase pathways. *Mol Cell Biol* 1996; 16:6687–6697.
8. Davis R. Transcriptional regulation by MAP kinases. *Mol Reprod Dev* 1995; 42:459–467.
9. Fukuda M, Gotoh Y, Nishida E. Interaction of MAP kinase with MAP kinase kinase: Its possible role in the control of nucleocytoplasmic transport of MAP kinase. *EMBO J* 1997; 16:1901–1908.
10. Marshall CJ. Specificity of receptor tyrosine kinase signaling: Transient versus sustained extracellular signal-regulated kinase activation. *Cell* 1995; 80:179–185.
11. Cowley S, Paterson H, Kemp P, Marshall CJ. Activation of MAP kinase kinase is necessary and sufficient for PC12 differentiation and for transformation of NIH 3T3 cells. *Cell* 1994; 77:841–852.
12. Denu JM, Stuckey JA, Saper MA, Dixon JE. Form and function in protein dephosphorylation. *Cell* 1996; 87:361–364.
13. Rohan PJ, Davis P, Moskaluk CA, Kearns M, Krutzsch H, Siebenlist U, Kelly K. PAC-1: A mitogen-induced nuclear protein tyrosine phosphatase. *Science* 1993; 259:1763–1766.
14. Emslie EA, Jones TA, Sheer D, Keyse SM. The CL100 gene, which encodes a dual specificity (tyr/thr) MAP kinase phosphatase, is highly conserved and maps to human chromosome 5q34. *Hum Genet* 1994; 93:513–516.
15. Sun H, Charles CH, Lau LF, Tonks NK. MKP-1 (3CH134), an immediate early gene product, is a dual specificity phosphatase that dephosphorylates MAP kinase in vivo. *Cell* 1993; 75:487–493.
16. Doi K, Gartner A, Ammerer G, Errede B, Shinkawa H, Sugimoto K, Matsumoto K. MSG5, a novel protein phosphatase promotes adaptation to pheromone response in *S. cerevisiae*. *EMBO J* 1994; 13:61–70.
17. Ishibashi T, Bottaro DP, Chan A, Miki T, Aaronson SA. Expression cloning of a human dual-specificity phosphatase. *Proc Natl Acad Sci USA* 1992; 89:12,170–12,174.
18. Fauman E, Saper M. Structure and function of the protein tyrosine phosphatases. *Trends Biochem Sci* 1996; 21:413–417.

19. Guan K, Broyles SS, Dixon JE. A tyr/ser protein phosphatase encoded by vaccinia virus. *Nature* 1991; 350:359–362.

20. Ward Y, Gupta S, Jenson P, Wartmann M, Davis RJ, Kelly K. Control of MAP kinase activation by the mitogen-induced threonine/tyrosine phosphatase PAC1. *Nature* 1994; 367:651–654.

21. Wiland AM, Denu JM, Mourey RJ, Dixon JE. Purification and kinetic characterization of the mitogen-activated protein kinase phosphatase rVH6. *J Biol Chem* 1996; 271:33,486–33,492.

22. Muda M, Theodosiou A, Gillieron C, Smith A, Chabert D, Montserrat C, Boscher U, Rodrigues N, Davies K, Ashworth A, Arkinstall S. The mitogen-activated protein kinase phosphatase-3 N-terminal noncatalytic region is responsible for tight substrate binding and enzymatic specificity. *J Biol Chem* 1998; 273:9323–9329.

23. Yuvaniyama J, Denu JM, Dixon JE, Saper MA. Crystal structure of the dual specificity protein phosphatase VHR. *Science* 1996; 272:1328–1331.

24. Barford D, Flint AJ, Tonks NK. Crystal structure of human protein tyrosine phosphatase1B. *Science* 1994; 263:1397–1404.

25. Stuckey JA, Schubert HL, Fauman EB, Zhang ZY, Dixon JE, Saper MA. Crystal structure of *Yersinia* protein tyrosine phosphatase at 2.5 Å and the complex with tungstate. *Nature* 1994; 370:571–575.

26. Coleman TR, Dunphy WG. Cdc2 regulatory factors. *Curr Opin Cell Biol* 1994; 6:877–882.

27. Alessi D, Smythe C, Keyse SM. The human CL100 gene encodes a tyr/thr-protein phosphatase which potently and specifically inactivates MAP kinase and suppresses its activation by oncogenic ras in xenopus oocyte extracts. *Oncogene* 1993; 8:2015–2020.

28. Charles CH, Sun H, Lau LF, Tonks NK. The growth factor-inducible immediate-early gene 3CH134 encodes a protein-tyrosine-phosphatase. *Proc Natl Acad Sci USA* 1993; 90:5292–5296.

29. Groom LA, Sneddon AA, Alessi DR, Dowd S, Keyse SM. Differential regulation of the MAP, SAP and RK/p38 kinases by Pyst1, a novel cytosolic dual-specificity phosphatase. *EMBO J* 1996; 15:3621–3632.

30. Franklin CC, Kraft AS. Conditional expression of the mitogen-activated protein kinase (MAPK) phosphatase MKP-1 preferentially inhibits p38 MAPK and stress-activated protein kinase in U937 cells. *J Biol Chem* 1997; 272:16,917–16,923.

31. Franklin CC, Srikanth S, Kraft AS. Conditional expression of mitogen-activated protein kinase phosphatase-1, MKP-1, is cytoprotective against UV-induced apoptosis. *Proc Natl Acad Sci USA* 1998; 95:3014–3019.

32. King AG, Ozanne BW, Smythe C, Ashworth A. Isolation and characterisation of a uniquely regulated threonine, tyrosine phosphatase (TYP 1) which inactivates ERK2 and p54jnk. *Oncogene* 1995; 11:2553–2563.

33. Hirsch DD, Stork PJS. Mitogen-activated protein kinase phosphatases inactivate stress-activated protein kinase pathways in vivo. *J Biol Chem* 1997; 272:4568–4575.

34. Muda M, Theodosiou A, Rodrigues N, Boschert U, Camps M, Gillieron C, Davies K, Ashworth A, Arkinstall S. The dual specificity phosphatases M3/6 and MKP-3 are highly selective for inactivation of distinct mitogen-activated protein kinases. *J Biol Chem* 1996; 271:27,205–27,208.

35. Muda M, Boschert U, Smith A, Antonsson B, Gillieron C, Chabert C, Camps M, Martinou I, Ashworth A, Arkinstall S. Molecular cloning and functional characterization of a novel mitogen-activated protein kinase phosphatase, MKP-4. *J Biol Chem* 1997; 272:5141–5151.

36. Martin-Blanco E, Gampel A, Ring J, Virdee K, Kirov N, Tolkovsky A, Martinez-Arias A. Puckered encodes a phosphatase that mediates a feedback loop regulating JNK activity during dorsal closure in *Drosophila*. *Genes and Dev* 1998; 12:557–570.

37. Martell KJ, Seasholtz AF, Kwak SP, Clemens KK, Dixon JE. hVH-5: A protein tyrosine phosphatase abundant in brain that inactivates mitogen-activated protein kinase. *J Neurochem* 1995; 65:1823–1833.

38. Muda M, Boschert U, Dickinson R, Martinou JC, Martinou I, Camps M, Schlegel W, Arkinstall S. MKP-3, a novel cytosolic protein-tyrosine phosphatase that exemplifies a new class of mitogen-activated protein kinase phosphatase. *J Biol Chem* 1996; 271:4319–4326.

39. Brondello JM, Brunet A, Pouyssegur J, McKenzie FR. The dual specificity mitogen-activated protein kinase phosphatase-1 and -2 are induced by the p42/p44 MAPK cascade. *J Biol Chem* 1997; 272:1368–1376.

40. Guan KL, Butch E. Isolation and characterization of a novel dual specific phosphatase, HVH2, which selectively dephosphorylates the mitogen-activated protein kinase. *J Biol Chem* 1995; 270:7197–7203.

41. Fuller SJ, Davies EL, Gillespie-Brown J, Sun H, Tonks NK. Mitogen-activated protein kinase phosphatase 1 inhibits the stimulation of gene expression by hypertrophic agonists in cardiac myocytes. *Biochem J* 1997; 323:313–319.

42. Mourey RJ, Vega QC, Campbell JS, Wenderoth MP, Hauschka SD, Krebs EG, Dixon JE. A novel cytoplasmic dual specificity protein tyrosine phosphatase implicated in muscle and neuronal differentiation. *J Biol Chem* 1996; 271:3795–3802.

43. Morishima-Kawashima M, Kosik KS. The pool of map kinase associated with microtubules is small but constitutively active. *Mol Biol Cell* 1996; 7:893–905.

44. Lin LL, Wartman M, Lin AY, Knopf JL, Seth A, Davis RJ. cPLA2 is phosphorylated and activated by MAP kinase. *Cell* 1993; 72:269–278.

45. Klemke RL, Cai S, Giannini AL, Gallagher PJ, de Lanerolle P, Cheresh DA. Regulation of cell motility by mitogen-activated protein kinase. *J Cell Biol* 1997; 137:481–492.

46. Alessi DR, Gomez N, Moorhead G, Lewis T, Keyse SM, Cohen P. Inactivation of p42 MAP kinase by protein phosphatase 2A and a protein tyrosine phosphatase, but not CL100, in various cell lines. *Curr Biol* 1995; 5:283–295.

47. Liu Y, Gorospe M, Yang C, Holbrook NJ. Role of mitogen-activated protein kinase phosphatase during the cellular response to genotoxic stress. *J Biol Chem* 1995; 270:8377–8380.

48. Foschi M, Chari S, Dunn MJ, Sorokin A. Biphasic activation of p21ras by endothelin-1 sequentially activates the ERK cascade and phosphatidylinositol 3-kinase. *EMBO J* 1997; 16:6439–6451.

49. Duff JL, Monia BP, Berk BC. Mitogen-activated protein (MAP) kinase is regulated by the MAP kinase phosphatase (MKP-1) in vascular smooth muscle cells. Effect of actinomycin D and antisense oligonucleotides. *J Biol Chem* 1995; 270:7161–7166.

50. Bedecs K, Elbaz N, Sutren M, Masson M, Susini C, Strosberg AD, Nahmias C. Angiotensin II type 2 receptors mediate inhibition of mitogen-activated protein kinase cascade and functional activation of SHP-1 tyrosine phosphatase. *Biochem J* 1997; 325:449–454.

51. Lai K, Wang H, Lee WS, Jain MK, Lee ME, Haber E. Mitogen-activated protein kinase phosphatase-1 in rat arterial smooth muscle cell proliferation. *J Clin Invest* 1996; 98:1560–1567.

52. Bennett AM, Tonks NK. Regulation of distinct stages of skeletal muscle differentiation by mitogen-activated protein kinases. *Science* 1997; 278:1288–1291.

53. Dorfman K, Carrasco D, Gruda M, Ryan C, Lira SA, Bravo R. Disruption of erp/mkp-1 gene does not affect mouse development: normal MAP kinase activity in ERP/MKP-1-deficient fibroblasts. *Oncogene* 1996; 13:925–931.

54. Gunter KC, Irving SG, Zipfel PF, Kelly K. Cyclosporin A-mediated inhibition of mitogen-induced gene transcription is specific for the mitogenic stimulus and cell type. *J Immunol* 1989; 142:3286–3291.

55. Noguchi T, Metz R, Chen L, Mattei MG, Carrasco D, Bravo R. Structure, mapping, and expression of erp, a growth factor-inducible gene encoding a nontransmembrane protein tyrosine phosphatase, and effect of ERP on growth. *Mol Cell Biol* 1993; 13:5195–5205.

56. Elion EA, Satterberg G, Kranz JE. FUS3 phosphorylates multiple components of the mating signal trasduction cascade: Evidence for STE12 and FAR1. *Mol Biol Cell* 1993; 4:495–510.

57. Grumont RJ, Rasko JE, Strasser A, Gerondakis S. Activation of the mitogen-activated

protein kinase pathway induces transcription of the PAC-1 phosphatase gene. *Mol Cell Biol* 1996; 16:2913–2921.

58. Bokemeyer D, Sorokin A, Dunn MJ. Differential regulation of the dual-specificity protein-tyrosine phosphatases CL100, B23, and PAC1 in mesangial cells. *J Am Soc Nephrol* 1997; 8:40–50.

59. Kwak SP, Hakes DJ, Martell KJ, Dixon JE. Isolation and characterization of a human dual specificity protein-tyrosine phosphatase gene. *J Biol Chem* 1994; 269:3596–3604.

60. Schliess F, Heinrich S, Haussinger D. Hyperosmotic induction of the mitogen-activated protein kinase phosphatase MKP-1 in H4IIE rat hepatoma cells. *Arch Biochem Biophys* 1998; 351:35–40.

61. Cook SJ, Beltman J, Cadwallader KA, McMahon M, McCormick F. Regulation of mitogen-activated protein kinase phosphatase-1 expression by extracellular signal-related kinase-dependent and Ca2+-dependent signal pathways in Rat-1 cells. *J Biol Chem* 1997; 272:13,309–13,319.

62. Scimeca JC, Servant MJ, Dyer JO, Meloche S. Essential role of calcium in the regulation of MAP kinase phosphatase-1 expression. *Oncogene* 1997; 15:717–725.

63. Plevin R, Malarkey K, Aidulis D, McLees A, Gould GW. Cyclic AMP inhibitors inhibits PDGF-stimulated mitogen-activated protein kinase activity in rat aortic smooth muscle cells via inactivation of c-Raf-1 kinase and induction of MAP kinase phosphatase-1. *Cell Signal* 1997; 9:323–328.

64. Kusari AB, Byon J, Bandyopadhyay D, Kenner KA, Kusari J. Insulin-induced mitogen-activated protein (MAP) kinase phosphatase-1 (MPK-1) attenuates insulin-stimulated MAP kinase activity: A mechanism for the feedback inhibition of insulin signaling. *Mol Endocrinol* 1997; 11:1532–1543.

65. Howe LR, Leevers SJ, Gomez N, Nakeilny S, Cohen P, Marshall CJ. Activation of the MAP kinase pathway by the protein kinase raf. *Cell* 1992; 71:335–342.

66. Lowy DR. Function and regulation of ras. *Annu Rev Biochem* 1993; 2:851–891.

67. Amundadottir LT, Leder P. Signal transduction pathways activated and required for mammary carcinogenesis in response to specific oncogenes. *Oncogene* 1998; 16:737–746.

68. Sivaraman VS, Wang H, Nuovo GJ, Malbon CC. Hyperexpression of mitogen-activated protein kinase in human breast cancer. *J Clin Invest* 1997; 99:1478–1483.

69. Oka H, Chatani Y, Hoshino R, Ogawa O, Kakehi Y, Terachi T, Okada Y, Kawaichi M, Kohno M, Yoshida O. Constitutive activation of mitogen-activated protein (MAP) kinases in human renal cell carcinoma. *Cancer Res* 1995; 55:4182–4187.

70. Berger DH, Jardines LA, Chang H, Ruggeri B. Activation of Raf-1 in human pancreatic adenocarcinoma. *J Surg Res* 1997; 69:199–204.

71. Towatari M, Iida H, Tanimoto M, Iwata H, Hamaguchi M, Saito H. Constitutive activation of mitogen-activated protein kinase pathway in acute leukemia cells. *Leukemia* 1997; 11:479–484.

72. Xu X, Heidenreich O, Kitajima I, McGuire K, Li Q, Su B, Nerenberg M. Constitutively activated JNK is associated with HTLV-1 mediated tumorigenesis. *Oncogene* 1996; 13:135–142.

73. Sun H, Tonks NK, Bar-Sagi D. Inhibition of ras-induced dna synthesis by expression of the phosphatase MKP-1. *Science* 1994; 266:285–288.

74. Shin DY, Ishibashi T, Choi TS, Chung E, Chung IY, Aaronson SA, Bottaro DP. A novel human ERK phosphatase regulates H-ras and v-raf signal transduction. *Oncogene* 1997; 14:2633–2639.

75. Shapiro PS, Ahn NG. Feedback regulation of Raf-1 and mitogen-activated protein kinase (MAP) kinase kinases 1 and 2 by MAP kinase phosphatase-1 (MKP-1). *J Biol Chem* 1998; 273:1788–1793.

76. Loda M, Capodieci P, Mishra R, Yao H, Corless C, Grigioni W, Wang Y, Magi-Galluzzi C, Stork PJ. Expression of mitogen-activated protein kinase phosphatase-1 in the early phases of human epithelial carcinogenesis. *Am J Pathol* 1996; 149:1553–1564.

77. Leav I, Galluzzi CM, Ziar J, Stork PJ, Ho SM, Loda M. Mitogen-activated protein kinase and mitogen-activated kinase phosphatase-1 expression in the Noble rat model of sex hormone-induced prostatic dysplasia and carcinoma. *Lab Invest* 1996; 75:361–370.

78. Magi-Galluzzi C, Mishra R, Fiorentino M, Montironi R, Yao H, Capodieci P, Wishnow K, Kaplan I, Stork PJ, Loda M. Mitogen-activated protein kinase phosphatase 1 is overexpressed in prostate cancers and is inversely related to apoptosis. *Lab Invest* 1997; 76:37–51.

79. Yokoyama A, Karasaki H, Urushibara N, Nomoto K, Imai Y, Nakamura K, Mizuno Y, Ogawa K, Kikuchi K. The characteristic gene expressions of MAPK phosphatases 1 and 2 hepatocarcinogenesis, rat ascites hepatoma cells, and regenerating rat liver. *Biochem Biophys Res Commun* 1997; 239:746–751.

80. Kelly K, Davis P, Mitsuya H, Irving S, Wright J, Grassmann R, Fleckenstein B, Wano Y, Greene W, Siebenlist U. A high proportion of early response genes are constitutively activated in T cells by HTLV-I. *Oncogene* 1992; 7:1463–1470.

81. Brunner D, Oellers N, Szabad J, Biggs WH, Zipursky SL, Hafen E. A gain-of-function mutation in *Drosophila* MAP kinase activates multiple receptor tyrosine kinase signaling pathways. *Cell* 1994; 76:875–888.

82. Wurgler-Murphy SM, Maeda T, Witten EA, Saito H. Regulation of the Saccharomyces cerevisiae HOG1 mitogen-activated protein kinase by the PTP2 and PTP3 protein tyrosine phosphatases. *Mol Cell Biol* 1997; 17:1289–1297.

83. Zhan X-L, Deschenes RJ, Guan K-L. Differential regulation of FUS3 MAP kinase by tyrosine-specific phosphatases PTP2/PTP3 and dual-specificity phosphatase MSG5 in *Saccharomyces cerevisiae*. *Genes and Dev* 1997; 11:1690–1702.

84. Millar JB, Buck V, Wilkinson MG. Pyp1 and Pyp2 PTPases dephosphorylate an osmosensing MAP kinase controlling cell size at division in fission yeast. *Genes Dev* 1995; 9:2117–2130.

85. Sarcevic B, Erikson E, Maller J. Purification and characterization of a mitogen-activated protein kinase tyrosine phosphatase from *Xenopus* eggs. *J Biol Chem* 1993; 268:25,075–25,083.

86. Braconi Quintaje SB, Church DJ, Rebsamen M, Valloton MB, Hemmings BA, Lang U. Role of protein phosphatase 2A in the regulation of mitogen-activated protein kinase activity in ventricular cardiomyocytes. *Biochem Biophys Res Commun* 1996; 221:539–547.

87. Chajry N, Martin PM, Cochet C, Berthois Y. Regulation of p42 mitogen-activated-protein kinase activity by protein phosphatase 2A under conditions of growth inhibition by epidermal growth factor in A431 cells. *Eur J Biochem* 1996; 235:97–102.

88. Misra-Press A, Rim CS, Yao H, Roberson MS, Stork PJS. A novel mitogen-activated protein kinase phosphatase. *J Biol Chem* 1995; 270:14,587–14,596.

89. Ishibashi T, Bottaro DP, Michieli P, Kelley CA, Aaronson SA. A novel dual specificity phosphatase induced by serum stimulation and heat shock. *J Biol Chem* 1994; 269:29,897–29,902.

90. Kwak SP, Dixon JE. Multiple dual specificity protein tyrosine phosphatases are expressed and regulated differentially in liver cell lines. *J Biol Chem* 1995; 270:1156–1160.

91. Theodosiou AM, Rodrigues NR, Nesbit MA, Ambrose HJ, Paterson H, McLellan-Arnold E, Boyd Y, Leversha MA, Owen N, Blake DJ, Ashworth A, Davies KE. A member of the MAP kinase phosphatase gene family in mouse containing a complex trinucleotide repeat in the coding region. *Hum Mol Genet* 1996; 5:675–684.

92. Martell KJ, Kwak S, Hakes DJ, Dixon JE, Trent JM. Chromosomal localization of four human VH1-like protein-tyrosine phosphatases. *Genomics* 1994; 22:462–464.

93. Yi H, Morton CC, Weremowicz S, McBride OW, Kelly K. Genomic organization and chromosomal localization of the DUSP2 gene, encoding a MAP kinase phosphatase, to human 2p11.2–q11. *Genomics* 1995; 28:92–96.

94. Emslie EA, Jones TA, Sheer D, Keyse SM. The CL100 gene, which encodes a dual specificity (Tyr/Thr) MAP kinase phosphatase, is highly conserved and maps to human chromosome 5q34. *Hum Genet* 1994; 93:513–516.

95. Smith A, Price C, Cullen M, Muda M, King A, Ozanne B, Arkinstall S, Ashworth A. Chromosomal localization of three human dual specificity phosphatase genes (DUSP4, DUSP6, and DUSP7). *Genomics* 1997; 42:524–527.

96. Nesbit MA, Hodges MD, Campbell L, de Meulemeester TM, Alders M, Rodrigues NR, Talbot K, Theodosiou AM, Mannens MA, Nakamura Y, Little PF, Davies KE. Genomic organization and chromosomal localization of a member of the MAP Kinase phosphatase gene family to human chromsome 11p15.5 and a pseudogene to 10q11.2. *Genomics* 1997; 42:284–294.

11

Control of MAPK Signaling by Ste20- and Ste11-Like Kinases

Gary R. Fanger, Thomas K. Schlesinger, and Gary L. Johnson

1. INTRODUCTION

Mammalian mitogen-activated protein kinases (MAPKs) were identified biochemically during the late 1980s *(1,2)*. In 1990, mammalian p44 MAPK was cloned and referred to as extracellular signal-regulated kinase (ERK) *(3)*. In parallel, MAPK pathways were being identified by genetic selection in the yeasts *Saccharomyces cerevisiae* and *Schizosaccharomyces pombe*, the fly *Drosophila melanogaster,* and the worm *Caenorhabditis elegans (4–6)*. Molecular cloning and functional characterization has defined a growing family of MAPKs in all eukaryotic organisms. MAPKs represent a family of serine/threonine kinases that are uniquely activated by dual phosphorylation of a threonine and tyrosine in a Thr-X-Tyr motif in the activation loop of the kinase domain, where X is an amino acid that varies among different MAPK family members. Eukaryotic cells express multiple MAPKs. For example, to date the number of MAPKs identified includes 12 in mammals, 6 in *S. cerevisiae*, 4 in *S. pombe*, 4 in *C. elegans*, and 3 in *D. melanogaster*. All the MAPKs characterized to date are members of a module composed of three protein kinases that form a sequential activation pathway (Fig. 1). The three component module consists of a MAPK kinase kinase (MKKK), MAPK kinase (MKK), and the MAPK. When the MKKK is activated, it phosphorylates and activates a specific MKK. The MKK, in turn, phosphorylates and activates a specific MAPK. In many instances, this three component module is regulated by a MAPK kinase kinase kinase (MKKKK). As discussed below, different MAPKs are involved in regulating specific cellular functions including mitosis, differentiation, challenge by cytokines and adaptation to stress such as nutrient starvation, osmotic imbalance, irradiation, and changes in redox state of the cell.

Activation of the three-component MAPK module occurs at the level of the MKKKs. In the few examples in which the regulation of an MKKK has been defined, they are controlled by phosphorylation, interaction with low-molecular-weight GTP-binding (LMWG) proteins such as Cdc42 or Rac, and possibly protein interaction-induced oligomerization *(7–9)*. The kinases known to phosphorylate and regulate MKKKs may

From: *Signaling Networks and Cell Cycle Control: The Molecular Basis of Cancer and Other Diseases*
Edited by: *J. S. Gutkind © Humana Press Inc., Totowa, NJ*

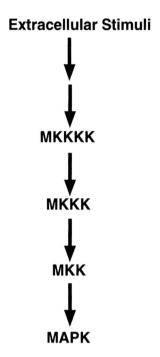

Fig. 1. Sequential protein kinase pathway controlling the regulation of mitogen-activated protein kinase (MAPK) by extracellular stimuli. MAPK activity is controlled by a MAPK kinase (MKK), which is controlled by a MAPKK kinase (MKKK), which is controlled by a MAPKKK kinase (MKKKK).

in turn bind to Cdc42 and Rac or other LMWG proteins such as Rho. The prototypical MKKK in yeast is Ste11, which functions in the pheromone regulated mating pathway. One of the upstream regulators of Ste11 may be the protein serine/threonine kinase, Ste20, which probably functions as a MKKKK. In metazoans, a prototypical MKKK is Raf1 (C-Raf), which requires interaction with Ras·GTP to become activated. Activation of Raf1 also requires phosphorylation by kinases that are still poorly characterized but may include both tyrosine and serine/threonine kinases that would be equivalent to Ste20 in the regulation of Ste11 in *S. cerevisiae*. This review attempts to define the known Ste20- and Ste11-like kinases, as well as what is known about their regulation and function in different cell types and organisms. Table 1 lists the Ste20/Ste11-like kinases that are discussed in this chapter.

2. REGULATION OF MAPK PATHWAYS IN YEAST

Both fission *(S. pombe)* and budding *(S. cerevisiae)* yeast have provided excellent genetic models with which to study MAPK regulation. Different MAPK pathways have been shown to be involved in a diverse array of regulatory functions involving the cell cycle, haploid mating, sporulation, invasive growth, and pseudohyphal development, cell wall remodeling and adaptation to changes in osmolarity *(10–12)* (Fig. 2). In each of these responses, a Ste11-like kinase is involved in regulating a MAPK module to

Table 1
Summary of Ste20- and Ste11-Like Kinases in Yeast, *Caenorhabditis elegans,*
Drosophila, **and Mammalian Cells**

Yeast	
Ste20	Sterile 20
Cla4	
Pak1	p21-activated kinase 1
YOL113w	
Mcs4	Mitotic catastrophe suppressor 4
Ste11	Sterile 11
Byr2	Bypass ras1 functions 2
Bck1	
Ssk2	
Ssk22	
Wik1	
Win1	
NRK	
Sps1	Sporulation-specific gene
Cdc15	Cell division control 15
C. elegans and *Drosophila*	
Lin-45	Lineage-45
D-raf	
Ksr	Kinase suppressor of ras
Mammalian	
Raf1, A- and B-raf	
mos	
MEKK1, 2, 3, 4	MAPK/ERK kinase kinase 1–4
MAPKKK5/ASK-1	MAP kinase kinase kinase5/apoptosis-signal regulating kinase-1
MLK1, 2, 3	Mixed lineage kinase 1–3
DLK	Dual leucine zipper-bearing kinase
TAK	TGF-β-activated kinase
TPL2	Tumor progression locus 2
KSR	Kinase suppressor of ras
PAK1, 2, 3	p21-activated kinase 1–3
GCK	Germinal center kinase
HPK1	Hematopoietic progenitor kinase 1
GLK	GCK-like kinase
KHS	Kinase homologous to Sps1/Ste20
NIK	Nck interacting kinase
MST1, 2, 3	Mammalian sterile twenty-like kinase 1–3
SOK-1	Ste20/oxidant stress response kinase-1

control the transcription of specific genes, regulate the activity of other kinases and enzymes, or alter the properties of the cytoskeleton. From the *S. cerevisiae* genome sequence, there are 10 Ste20/Ste11 family members. The Ste11 family members include Ste11, Bck1, Ssk2, and Ssk22. The Ste20 family members are Ste20, Cla4, and YOL113W. A third less defined group is the NRK/MESS family composed of NRK1, SPS1, and Cdc15 *(13)*. Although the genome sequence from *S. pombe* is not entirely

A <u>RESPONSE</u>   <u>SEQUENTIAL KINASE PATHWAY</u>

	MKKKK	MKKK	MKK	MAPK
Pheromone	Ste20	Ste11	Ste7	Fus3
Spore Formation	Sps1	?	?	Smk1
Osmolarity	Ssk1	Ssk2/22 Ste11	Pbs2	Hog1
Cell Wall	Pkc1	Bck1	Mkk1/2	Mpk1
Pseudohyphal/ Invasive Growth	Ste20	Ste11	Ste7	Kss1
Cytokinesis	Cla4	?	?	?

B <u>RESPONSE</u>   <u>SEQUENTIAL KINASE PATHWAY</u>

	MKKKK	MKKK	MKK	MAPK
Pheromone		Byr2	Byr1	Spk1
Osmolarity	Mcs4	Wik1/Win1	Wis1	Spc1
Morphology/ Cell Polarity	Pak1	?	?	?
Cell Wall	Pkc	?	?	Pmk1

Fig. 2. Sequential mitogen-activated protein kinase (MAPK) pathways that control the biological responses in yeast. Biological responses in (**A**) budding yeast *Saccharomyces cerevisiae* and (**B**) fission yeast *S. pombe*. MAPKs are regulated by MAPK kinases (MKKs), which are in turn regulated by MAPKK kinases (MKKKs), which are regulated by MAPKKK kinases (MKKKKs). ? indicate unknown identity of kinases.

determined, at least 5 Ste20/Ste11 family members have been identified. The Ste11-like kinases include Byr2, Wik1, and Win1, whereas the Ste20-like kinases include Mcs4 and Pak1. This chapter describes what is known about the function of these kinases.

2.1. Pheromone-Regulated Mating Pathway

In response to pheromone, haploid yeast undergo a mating response in which cells arrest in G1, induce the synthesis of genes required for mating and undergo morphological changes (*11,12,14*). In the budding yeast *S. cerevisiae*, genetic studies have identified genes whose disruption inhibited the mating response and were designated sterile (ste) genes. Using this approach, the pathway required for mating has been defined. The pheromone receptors are seven-transmembrane proteins coupled to a heterotrimeric G-protein. In *S. cerevisiae*, Ste2 is the pheromone receptor expressed on the a-type cell, activated by α pheromone, whereas the α-type cell expresses the Ste3 receptor, which is activated by the a pheromone. The two haploid mating subtypes of *S. pombe*, P (h⁺) or M (P⁻), express either the Mam2 or Map3 heterotrimeric G-protein-coupled receptors, respectively, and mate in response to activation of Mam2 by P factor and Map3 by M factor. A distinct difference in the early signaling for mating in budding and fission yeast is that in *S. cerevisiae*, the G protein βγ subunit complex activates the response pathway, whereas in *S. pombe* the G-protein α subunit in collaboration with Ras is involved. This is an interesting difference because both G-protein α and βγ subunits and Ras are involved in the regulation of MAPK pathways in metazoans.

As defined in *S. cerevisiae,* the βγ complex (Ste18/Ste4) activates Ste20 and interacts with the Ste5 scaffolding protein. These interactions stimulate the MAPK module containing the MKKK, Ste11, the MKK, Ste7, and the MAPK, Fus3. Activated Fus3 regulates specific transcription factors required for the expression of components of the mating pathway itself and genes required for cell cycle arrest and cell fusion. Fus3 is selectively expressed in haploid yeast and when activated phosphorylates Far1 that represses the transcription of the G1 cyclins Cln1 and Cln2, resulting in cell cycle arrest which is required for mating *(15)*. Phosphorylated Far1 also binds to and inhibits the Cdc28/Cln kinase complex further contributing to cell cycle arrest. Fus3 also phosphorylates and activates Ste12, a transcription factor involved in the regulation of the expression of Far1 and other mating response genes *(16)*.

The MAPK pathway for mating in *S. cerevisiae* is somewhat unique with the involvement of Ste5 that functions in part to segregate the Ste11/Ste7/Fus3 module in the cell. Ste5 has been shown to bind Ste11, Ste7, Fus3, and Ste4, the β subunit of the Gβγ complex *(17)*. The N-terminus of Ste5 encodes a cysteine-rich RING-H2 motif *(18,19)*. Mutation of this region of Ste5 inhibits mating, even though the mutant Ste5 protein is able to bind Ste11, Ste7, and Fus3 as efficiently as wild -ype Ste5 *(9)*. The RING-H2 Ste5 mutants no longer bind the β subunit of the βγ complex and fail to dimerize. The function of βγ in activating the mating pathway may be to induce Ste5 dimerization, as well as to activate Ste20, which in epistasis experiments has been shown to lie upstream of Ste11. Thus, activation of the Ste11/Ste7/Fus3 MAPK module involves Ste20 activity, as well as a Ste20-independent mechanism that requires Ste5 dimerization *(20)*.

In *S. pombe,* the mating pathway uses a MAPK module homologous to that in *S. cerevisiae.* The nomenclature is different for the *S. pombe* mating MAPK module because genetic selections to map the pathway were based on activating mutations that bypassed Ras1 inactivation (Byr genes were defined for bypass Ras1 functions). Byr2 is homologous to Ste11, Byr1 to Ste7, and Spk1 to Fus3 *(10)*. One role for Ras1 in *S. pombe* is to control starvation-dependent mating, whereas in *S. cerevisiae* mating is largely nutrition status independent. The function of Ras1 requires the G-protein α subunit, but the interplay of the two GTP binding proteins is not well characterized. Ras1 binds to Byr2 and has been postulated to regulate the mating pathway in part by this interaction *(21,22)*. Thus, for *S. pombe,* it seems that GTP binding proteins regulate Byr2, whereas in *S. cerevisiae* βγ regulation of Ste5 and Ste20 regulates Ste11. *S. pombe* also express a homologue of Ste20, Pak1, which binds to and is activated by Cdc42 and plays a role in morphological changes, as well as may be important in the mating response *(23)*.

2.2. Invasive Response and Pseudohyphal Development

Components of the mating response pathway are also involved in the formation of pseudohyphae and invasive growth of yeast *(12)*. Diploids starved for nitrogen undergo a developmental transition to a filamentous pseudohyphal form. Filaments elongate from the yeast colony composed of chains of elongated cells that penetrate the culture agar. Mutations in Ste20, Ste11, Ste7, or Ste12 block pseudohyphal development.

Interestingly, mutation of the pheromone receptor or G protein subunits have no effect on pseudohyphal development, indicating that they do not play a role in this response. Haploids are also capable of invasive growth and form pseudofilaments. The role of Ste20 and Ste11 as MKKKKs or MKKKs or their potential function in other pathways in the pseudohyphal/invasive growth response is poorly understood.

2.3. Spore Formation

Yeast sporulation involves meiosis leading to the packaging of haploid nuclei into spores. Sporulation is elicited by nutritional starvation in diploids. The spore forming response appears to involve a MAPK, Smk1 *(24)*. However, the MKKK and MKK have not been defined. A putative MKKKK, Sps1, appears involved in sporulation and mutations in Smk1 and Sps1 give similar phenotypes by progressing through the second meiotic division, but they are then defective in completing sporulation *(25)*.

2.4. Osmolarity Responsiveness

In response to high osmolarity, activation of the MAPK, Hog1, is required for *S. cerevisiae* cells to grow. The activity of Hog1 is regulated by the MKK, Pbs2, whose activity is controlled by two independent osmolarity-sensitive pathways, the two-component and the Sho1-dependent pathways *(26–29)*. In the two-component pathway, Pbs2 is activated by either Ssk2 or Ssk22, which are MKKKs that appear to act in a redundant manner. Ssk1 is a MKKKK that has been shown to genetically lie upstream and regulate the activity of Ssk2/Ssk22. In the two-component system, Sln1 is a cell surface-expressed histidine kinase that responds to osmolarity changes and transfers a phosphate to Ypd1, which in turn transfers the phosphate to Ssk1. During conditions of low osmolarity, Sln1 autophosphorylates and transfers a phosphate to Ypd1 suppressing Ssk1 activity. During conditions of high osmolarity, Sln1 activity is suppressed, resulting in the activation of the Hog1 pathway. In the Sho1-dependent pathway, Ste11 and not Ssk2/Ssk22 is the functional MKKK that controls the activity of Pbs2. In conditions of high osmolarity Sho1 activates Ste11, leading to stimulation of Hog1 activity.

Fission yeast also use a two-component system to regulate MAPK pathways and promote survival in response to osmolarity changes *(30–32)*. In *S. pombe*, the MAPK Spc1 is regulated by the MKK, Wis1. Wis1 can be activated by either of two MKKKs: Wik1 or Win1. Mcs4, a MKKKK homologue of the *S. cerevisiae* Ssk1, has been shown to lie genetically upstream of Wik1 and Win1. Wik1 is not essential for Hog1 activation by osmolarity changes, suggesting that Win1 is predominant in this pathway. In addition to their role in osmosensing and stress responses, Wis1 and Spc1 were identified as regulators of cell cycle progression, suggesting that they are component members of more than one signaling pathway *(33)*.

2.5. Cell Wall Integrity

In *S. cerevisiae*, cell wall integrity is controlled by a MAPK pathway composed of Bck1, Mkk1, and Mkk2 which appear to be functionally redundant, and the MAPK, Mpk1 *(34,35)*. The yeast protein kinase C (PKC1) is genetically upstream and phosphorylates Bck1 defining PKC1 as a MKKKK in this pathway *(36)*. Pmk1 is involved in the regulation of cell wall integrity in *S. pombe*, but little else is known about upstream regulators *(37,38)*.

2.6. Cytokinesis

Cla4 is a homolog of the Ste20 serine/threonine kinase in *S. cerevisiae* originally identified in a screen for mutations that cause lethality in the absence of the G1 cyclins, Cln1 and Cln2 *(39)*. Cla4 activity peaks during mitosis and cells deficient in Cla4 display a cytokinesis defect *(40)*. The GTP binding protein, Cdc42, regulates the activity of Cla4 similar to Ste20. Deletion of the Cdc42 binding region disrupts the cell cycle regulation of Cla4 kinase activity. The downstream effectors for Cla4 have not been unequivocally identified, but the cytoskeletal septin proteins are candidate Cla4 substrates. Septins localize to the bud site, consistent with Cla4 involvement in cell growth and bud site formation, in addition to cytokinesis *(41)*. Interestingly, a Cla4 mutant is viable; however, a double Cla4/Ste20 mutant cannot undergo cytokinesis. This suggests Cla4 and Ste20 have an overlapping function required for cytokinesis but the double mutant cells still are able to assemble actin, a process that requires Cdc42 and other Rho family proteins.

A third Ste20/Cla4-like kinase was defined by sequencing the yeast genome. YOL113W is a Ste20-like kinase that has all the signature domains found in Ste20 including a pleckstrin homology domain and a Cdc42/Rac interacting binding (CRIB) domain. The function of YOL113W is not understood. The NRK group of Ste20- and Ste11-like kinases are also not well characterized to date.

2.7. Ste20/Ste11-Like Kinases in C. elegans and D. melanogaster

Sequential kinase pathways that regulate MAPK modules are conserved from yeast to humans. In *C. elegans* and *D. melanogaster*, MAPK pathways have been shown to control specific aspects of development (Fig. 3). For example, Sur-1 is important for vulval development in *C. elegans*. The vulva of the hermaphrodite is an epithelial tube that extends from the uterus to the external environment and is used for egg laying *(42)*. Loss of the vulva (vulvaless phenotype; Vul) or excess vulva (multivulva phenotype; Muv) is a readily observable phenotype that has allowed for genetic screens to isolate key genes leading to this developmental event. In *Drosophila*, photoreceptor development and dorsal closure have been used to screen for genes that control these developmental events *(43,44)*. Dorsal closure involves an epithelial sheet that initially covers the ventral and lateral sides of the embryo and expands dorsally to encompass the embryo. Dorsal closure requires the activity of the MAPK, Bsk. Photoreceptor development that cues nonneuronal cone cells to differentiate into R7 photoreceptor cells relies on the appropriate regulation of the MAPK, Rolled. The regulation of these developmental pathways is controlled by Ste20/Ste11 homologs.

2.8. Caenorhabditis elegans

Appropriate vulval development in the hermaphrodite *C. elegans* is controlled by the growth factor Lin-3, which binds to and activates the cell surface tyrosine kinase receptor Let-23 *(45)*. Let-23 controls vulval development by activating the MAPK, Sur-1 (also known as Mpk-1). The Sur-1 pathway includes the MKK, Mek-2 (which

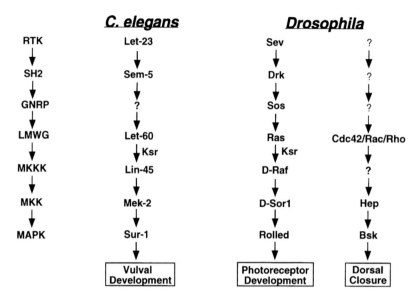

Fig. 3. Sequential MAPK pathways controlling developmental responses in *Caenorhabditis elegans* and *Drosophila*. Vulval development in *C. elegans* is controlled by the activation of the suppressor of Ras (Sur-1) mitogen-activated protein kinase (MAPK) pathway. Growth factor activates the receptor tyrosine kinase (RTK) Lethal-23 (Let-23), which activates the low-molecular-weight GTP-binding (LMWG) protein Let-60 via activation of a currently unknown guanine nucleotide releasing protein (GNRP). Sex myoblast migration defective-5 (Sem-5), a Src homology 2 (SH2) containing adapter protein, is required for activation of this pathway. Lineage-45 (Lin-45), a serine/threonine kinase, binds to, and is activated by, Let-60 and is a MAPKK kinase (MKKK) which activates the dual specificity tyrosine/threonine kinase MAP/ERK kinase-2 (Mek-2). Mek-2 is a MAPK kinase (MKK) that activates the MAPK, Sur-1. The role of kinase suppressor of Ras (Ksr), a serine/threonine kinase, in the regulation of this pathway is not well defined. In *Drosophila*, activation of the Rolled MAPK controls photoreceptor development by a pathway that is analogous to that controlling vulval development in *C. elegans*. Activation of the Sevenless (Sev) RTK activates the LMWG Ras via the GNRP son of Sevenless (Sos). The SH2 containing adapter protein Drk is required for activation of this pathway. The serine/threonine kinase D-Raf binds to and is activated by Ras which activates the MKK, D-Sor which activates the MAPK, Rolled. As in *C. elegans*, the role of Ksr in controlling the activity of this pathway is not well defined. Dorsal closure, another MAPK-regulated developmental response in *Drosophila*, is controlled by Basket (Bsk). Although this pathway is currently not well defined, the MKK Hemipterous (Hep) regulates the activity of Bsk and the LMWG proteins Cdc42, Rac and Rho are also involved.

is also referred to as Let-537), and the MKKK, Lin-45 (Fig. 3). The activity of Lin-45 is controlled by Let-60, a Ras homolog. Activation of Let-60 likely involves a guanine nucleotide releasing protein (GNRP) which stimulates GTP loading by promoting GDP dissociation, but the identity of this protein is unknown. However, Sem-5, which is a Src homology 2 (SH2) and Src homology 3 (SH3) containing protein is likely to mediate association of the GNRP with Let-23, the tyrosine kinase that mediates activation of this pathway.

2.9. Lin-45

Lin-45 was first described by a recessive mutation in a screen for extragenic suppressors of the Lin-3 mutant multivulva phenotype *(46)*. Subsequent cloning of Lin-45 indicated that it was a homolog to the human MKKK, Raf1 serine/threonine kinase, suggesting that Lin-45 was a MKKK. Overexpression of a kinase inactive, inhibitory mutant of Lin-45 interfered with vulval induction. Because mammalian Raf1 associates with, and is regulated by, Ras *(see below)*, this suggested that Lin-45 was regulated by Let-60, a prediction that was confirmed when a kinase inactive inhibitory mutant of Lin-45 was shown to suppress the multivulva phenotype induced by an activated Let-60 mutant. Thus, just as in mammalian cells, tyrosine kinase receptor-mediated MAPK activation involves a pathway in which the GTP binding protein, Ras (Let-60 in *C. elegans*), leads to activation of the MKKK (Lin-45) within the MAPK module.

2.10. KSR

Kinase suppressor of Ras-1 (Ksr-1) is a serine/threonine protein kinase that can influence the activity of the Sur-1 MAPK pathway and that displays some amino acid identity (roughly 30%) to Lin-45 *(47–49)*. Unlike Lin-45, Ksr-1 does not appear to directly phosphorylate Mek-2 and was not isolated in mutant screens for defective vulval induction. Instead, Ksr-1 was isolated as a suppressor of the activated Let-60 Muv phenotype, yet does not influence the Muv phenotype induced by a constitutively activated Lin-45, suggesting that Ksr-1 activity is important between Let-60 and Lin-45 *(47,48)*. Ksr associates with Raf1 and may directly influence Raf1 activity possibly by phosphorylation *(50)*. Thus, it is possible that Let-60 may utilize Ksr-1 to aid in activating Lin-45, suggesting that Ksr-1 may be a MKKKK. Alternatively, Let-60 may activate a pathway parallel to Lin-45 via Ksr-1, indicating that Ksr may be a MKKK for a different pathway.

2.11. Drosophila melanogaster

In *Drosophila*, activation of the MAPK, Rolled, is required for a number of different developmental events including appropriate photoreceptor development, whereas activation of the MAPK, Bsk, is necessary for dorsal closure *(4,44)*. The activity of Rolled is controlled by D-Sor1, a MKK which is a dual specificity threonine/tyrosine kinase. D-Sor1 is regulated by the serine/threonine D-Raf (a MKKK), in turn regulated by the GTP-binding protein Ras, and possibly the kinase Ksr. Sos associates with the SH2-SH3-SH2 containing protein Drk and stimulates Ras activation by promoting exchange of GDP for GTP. Sos regulation requires its receptor association via an SH2 adapter protein Drk, which brings Sos to the membrane by binding to a phosphotyrosine site on the Sev receptor. The pathway regulating Bsk is less well understood. However, the dual specificity threonine/tyrosine MKK, Hep, directly controls Bsk activity by phosphorylation. Hep is regulated by a currently unknown MKKK, that is regulated by the Rho family of GTP-binding proteins Cdc42, Rac and Rho. Recently, another MAPK family member, D-p38, has been identified, but its upstream regulators are still being defined *(51)*.

2.12. D-Raf

D-Raf was originally isolated by P-element-mediated rescue of *Drosophila*, having defects in the formation of anterior and posterior extremities and shown to act downstream of the receptor tyrosine kinase, Sev *(52,53)*. In addition, D-Raf was shown to be required for the ability of Sev to induce R7 photoreceptor development and activated D-Raf expression induced R7 photoreceptor development *(54)*. D-Raf appears to be ubiquitously expressed, is not measurably altered in expression during development and does show differences in spatial expression *(53)*. D-Raf is believed to play a primary role in controlling cell proliferation and the determination of cell fate.

2.13. KSR

In *Drosophila*, Ksr was also identified as a mutation that suppressed signaling by activated Ras, but not activated D-Raf *(49,50)*. Thus, Ksr lies either upstream or parallel to D-Raf in flies. However, in contrast to worms where Ksr deletion only results in a larval lethal effect in a low percentage of worms, Ksr deletion in *Drosophila* is recessive lethal, suggesting that there may be a redundant pathway in worms for Ksr or that Ksr has different functions in the two species.

The findings in *Drosophila* demonstrate that different receptors that mediate specific developmental cues effect these changes in part by using the same MAPK pathways *(55)*. These include Sev and Torso (tor), which can activate the rolled MAPK pathway required for photoreceptor development in the eye and terminal differentiation, respectively. In addition, the *Drosophila* epidermal growth factor receptor (Der) also uses the rolled MAPK pathway to mediate a diverse number of developmental events such as survival of specific ectodermal cells, development of the central nervous system (CNS) and germ-band retraction. This pathway is controlled by the MKKK, D-Raf. With the discovery and analysis of proteins such as Ksr, the linearity of pathways like that for Rolled are more complex than initially believed. It appears that the regulation of MAPK pathways, and in particular the Ste11/Ste20-like kinases, is one of converging, diverging and parallel regulatory events. This is even more evident in mammalian cells.

3. StE20/StE11-LIKE KINASES AND REGULATION OF MAPK PATHWAYS IN MAMMALIAN CELLS

There are 12 MAPK genes encompassing five subfamilies in mammalian cells defined by sequence homology and, to a lesser extent, by functional homology. The MAPK family members include ERK1/2, p38α,β,γ,δ, JNK1, 2, 3, ERK3, 4, and 5 *(56)*. Three of the MAPK subfamilies have been significantly characterized: ERK, JNK, and p38. ERK1 was the first mammalian MAPK to be cloned and characterized *(3)*. Two highly homologous isoforms are referred to as p42 (ERK2) and p44 (ERK1) based on their electrophoretic migration in sodium dodecyl sulfate-polyacrylamide gel electrophoresis (SDS-PAGE). ERK3 is approximately 50% homologous to ERK1/2, is nuclear localized, and is activated by mechanisms different from ERK1/2 suggesting it is likely a distinct MAPK pathway *(57,58)*. ERK4 is related to ERK3 in sequence and has been shown to be activated by NGF and EGF in a Ras-dependent manner *(59)*. Three different genes that encode c-Jun kinases (JNK) have been isolated *(60–64)*. The JNK family displays additional diversity in that each gene is alternatively spliced and the splice variants have been proposed to influence differentially the regulation of certain transcription factors *(63)*. p38 was discovered during a homology screen for kinases similar to HOG1 from yeast and, as its name denotes, it is 38 kDa in size. Other MAPKs in this group include p38β,γ,δ *(65–69)*. The identification of ERK5 indicates a fifth sequential MAPK pathway may exist *(70)*.

The MAPK family members phosphorylate and regulate the activity of a diverse set of proteins including transcription factors, other kinases, cytoskeletal proteins, and phospholipases. Many of the effects of the MAPK family members on growth and differentiation can be attributed to their ability to phosphorylate and thus control the activity of transcription factors *(71)*. Upon activation, ERK1/2 have been shown to translocate to the nucleus where they phosphorylate different transcription factors including Elk, Ets1, Sap1, c-Myc, Tal, STAT, Myb, and c-Jun. JNK1 and 2 have been shown to phosphorylate the transcription factors c-Jun, ATF-2, Elk-1, p53, DPC4, and NFAT4; p38 has been shown to phosphorylate and regulate the activity of ATF-2, Elk-1, MEF2C, Max, and CHOP/GADD. ERK1/2 have also been shown to regulate a number of kinases in the cytoplasm or at the cell membrane including the EGF receptor, Raf1, MEK, decreasing their catalytic activities in a possible feedback regulatory loop *(72)*, and S6 kinase p90^{rsk} whose phosphorylation by ERK1/2 is associated with its activation *(73)*. The microtubule associated proteins MAP-1, MAP-2, MAP-4, and Tau are phosphorylated by ERK1/2 *(73)*. ERK1/2 also phosphorylates and activates cytoplasmic phospholipase A2 affecting the release of arachidonic acid *(74)*. p38 has been shown to phosphorylate and activate the MAP kinase-activated protein (MAPKAP) kinase 2 and 3, which in turn phosphorylate small heat shock proteins, including HSP27 *(75)*. Each of the MAPKs are in separate kinase modules regulated by Ste20/Ste11-like kinases. Table 2 lists the regulatory effects of the mammalian Ste20/Ste11-like kinases on the ERK, JNK, and p38 MAPK pathways.

Seven different MKKs have been cloned, each with different specificity for a particular MAPK. The first MKKs to be cloned were MAPK/ERK kinase 1-2 (MEK1/2), which phosphorylate and activate ERK1/2 *(72)*. MKK4 (also referred to as JNK kinase or SEK-1) and MKK7 phosphorylate and activate JNK1-3, MKK3, and six specifically phosphorylate and activate p38, whereas MKK5 activates ERK5 *(72,76–78)*. The different MKKs are selectively activated by phosphorylation on serine and threonine residues by the different MKKKs. Currently 10 different groups of kinases encompassing more than 22 different genes have been defined to act upstream of the MKKs. Considerable effort is going into determining whether they are valid MKKKs; that is, they are able to phosphorylate and regulate the activity of MKKs. Several of these kinases may actually be MKKKKs; functionally, they are upstream of specific MKKKs. As the human genome project progresses, the number of Ste20/Ste11-like kinases will certainly increase. The known function of the different Ste20/Ste11-like mammalian kinases is discussed below.

3.1. Raf1, A-Raf, and B-Raf

Raf1 was first isolated on the basis of its oncogenic potential and ability to stimulate proliferation and transform cells *(79,80)*. The stimulation of G1 progression by activation of the Raf-1/MEK1/2/ERK1/2 pathway correlates with stimulation of cyclin D1 expression *(81)*. However, in some cell lines such as PC12 pheochromocytoma cells Raf1

Table 2
**Summary of Ste20- and Ste11-like Kinase-Mediated Regulation of Mitogen-
Activated Protein Kinase (MAPK) Family Members in Mammalian Cells**

	ERK	*JNK*	*p38*	*Reference*
Raf	+	−	−	*88*
Mos	+	−	−	*105*
MEKK1	+	+	−	*109*
MEKK2, 3	+	+	−	*110*
MEKK4	−	+	−	*111*
MAPKKK5/ASK-1	−	+	+	*121,122*
MLK1	?	?	?	
MLK2/MST1	−	+	+	*130*
MLK3	−	+	−	*131,132*
DLK	−	+	?	*129*
TAK	−	+	−	*135*
TPL2	+	+	?	*137,139*
PAK1, 2, 3	−	+	+	*147*
GCK	−	+	−	*157*
HPK1	?	+	?	*158*
GLK	−	+	−	*159*
KHS	−	+	−	*160*
NIK	−	+	−	*161*
MST2, 3	−	−	−	*162,163*
SOK	−	−	−	*164*

[a]Abbreviations: −, does not activate pathway; +, activates pathway; ?, activation unknown.

activation results in cell cycle arrest and differentiation *(82)*. Thus, Raf1 is capable of stimulating DNA synthesis and mitosis in some cell types and growth inhibition and differentiation in others. High sustained activity of Raf1 appears sufficient to induce cell cycle arrest via its ability to induce the expression of the G1 cell cycle regulatory protein p21[Cip1] *(83,84)*. At more modest levels of activation, Raf1 contributes to cell cycle progression. Thus, the magnitude of Raf1 activation may be a determinant in the decision for cell cycle arrest or progression leading to mitosis.

The regulation of Raf1 has been studied extensively demonstrating that subcellular localization, as well as phosphorylation are important regulatory facets in activation of this kinase. Raf1 is regulated in part by its binding to Ras·GTP. Ras·GDP has little affinity for and does not activate Raf1. In vitro, GTP loaded Ras is insufficient to activate Raf1, suggesting that there are other inputs that are important for activation such as phosphorylation. Raf1 is phosphorylated on tyrosine residues 340 and 341, as well as on serine 43, 259, 499, and 621 and threonine 269 *(85)*. There is strong evidence to indicate that the tyrosine phosphorylation is catalyzed by Src kinases and that these phosphorylations are important in Raf1 activation *(86,87)*. Serine phosphorylation of Raf1 may in part be catalyzed by protein kinase C (PKC) activity, as PKC can phospho-rylate serines 259 and 499 in vitro, phorbol esters activate Raf1 and PKCβ expression activates Raf1 in a phorbol ester-dependent manner *(85,88,89)*. GTP-bound Ras-mediated translocation of Raf1 to the plasma membrane is important for Raf1 activation presumably by mediating proximal localization to upstream activators, including Src and PKC *(90,91)*. Phosphorylation can also inhibit Raf activity. Inhibitory phosphorylation of Raf is mediated by PKA, which allows for integrated inputs from receptors that activate cyclic adenosine monophosphate (cAMP) synthesis *(73)*. ERK can also phosphorylate Raf1, which may serve as a feedback loop to inhibit pathway stimulation *(92)*.

14-3-3 proteins, a family of 30 kDa proteins that consists of eight highly homologous genes, associate with Raf1 and may play a role in regulating the activity of this kinase *(93,94)*. 14-3-3 proteins bind to Raf1 via a phosphorylated serine residue at amino acid 259 in the N-terminus of Raf1 *(95,96)*. The overall role of 14-3-3 binding to Raf1 is not well understood, as this association has been shown to activate, inactivate or not affect the relative kinase activity of Raf1 *(93,94,97–100)*. It is possible that 14-3-3 association with Raf1 prevents dephosphorylation, thus influencing activity. Alternatively, 14-3-3 proteins dimerize suggesting that 14-3-3 proteins function as scaffolds to mediate protein-protein interaction *(101)*. For example, 14-3-3 association with Raf1 may provide a means to organize signal transduction complexes contributing to signaling specificity within the cell.

Two other Raf genes have been identified—A-Raf and B-Raf—whose patterns of expression are more restricted than that for Raf1. B-Raf has two splice variants that vary in their tissue distribution. The 96 kDa B-Raf is expressed primarily in neuronal and neuroendocrine tissues and has been reported to be the primary activator of MEK in the brain *(102)*. The 68-kDa B-Raf is expressed in fibroblasts and many other cell types. Both the 96- and 68-kDa forms of B-Raf are activated by Ras·GTP. A unique function for B-Raf is its regulation by the GTP-binding protein, Rap1a *(92)*. Rap1a in the GTP-bound form activates 96 kDa, but not 68 kDa, B-Raf. Rap1a is phosphorylated near its C-terminus by PKA *(103)*, which enhances exchange of GDP for GTP. Thus, in cells expressing the 96 kDa B-Raf, cAMP will activate the ERK1/2 pathway. Less is known about the regulation of A-Raf, but its activation requires Ras GTP and additional inputs such as phosphorylation by Src. A-Raf is activated by growth factor and cytokine stimulation of cells such as endothelin-1 stimulation of cardiac monocytes *(104)*. Neither Raf1 nor A-Raf is activated by Rap1a.

3.2. Mos

Mos is a 39-kDa serine/threonine kinase with homology to Raf1 that can activate ERK by directly phosphorylating and activating MEK1/2 *(105,106)*. Mos, like Raf1, is capable of inducing cellular transformation by driving the ERK1/2 pathway when ectopically expressed in somatic cells. However, Mos expression is restricted to germ cells and plays an important role in meiotic maturation and arrest of cells at metaphase II of the meiotic cell cycle *(107,108)*. One function of Mos activation of the ERK1/2 pathway in germ cells is to stabilize M-phase promoting factor (MPF), a cell cycle switch whose activity leads to cell cycle arrest at the second meiotic metaphase.

3.3. MEKK1, 2, 3, and 4

The MAPK/ERK kinase kinases (MEKKs) were cloned based on homology of their kinase domains to the Ste11 and Byr2. Their ability to phosphorylate and activate specific MKKs, MEK1/2, and MKK4, categorize the MEKK family members as legitimate MKKKs *(109–111)*. MEKK1–4 are highly conserved within their C-terminally located kinase domains, roughly 50% homologous at the amino acid level, whereas the N-terminal regulatory domains are quite different from each other *(8)*. The sizes of the MEKK family members range from MEKK1, which is a 196-kDa, and MEKK4, which is 180 kDa, to MEKK2 and MEKK3, which are approx 80 kDa. When overexpressed in cells MEKK1, 2, and 3, but not MEKK4, are able to activate ERK1/2, whereas all the MEKKs activate JNK. However, MEKK1–4 do not significantly activate p38. MEKK2 and MEKK3 contain putative bipartate nuclear localization sequences but have no other signature domains indicative of specific regulatory functions. MEKK1 and 4 contain putative pleckstrin homology (PH) domains in their N-terminus. MEKK4 contains a modified Cdc42/Rac interactive binding (CRIB) motif and associates with Cdc42 and Rac in both GDP and GTP bound states *(112)*. MEKK1 does not contain an identifiable CRIB domain, yet binds to Cdc42/Rac in a strongly GTP-dependent manner. Unlike MEKK2 and 3, which do not bind to Cdc42/Rac, MEKK1 and 4 appear to be required for JNK activation by Cdc42/Rac. In addition, MEKK1 also binds to Ras in a GTP dependent manner and Ras activity is required for EGF-mediated stimulation of MEKK1 activity *(113,114)*. MEKK family members also show binding specificity for 14-3-3 proteins and MEKK1, 2 and 3, but not MEKK4 selectively interact with 14-3-3 proteins *(115)*. Although 14-3-3 association does not appear to dramatically effect MEKK1, 2, and 3 activity, 14-3-3 proteins may mediate interaction of specific MEKKs with other regulatory proteins and be important for controlling subcellular localization of these kinases.

Studies from our laboratory indicate that the activity of the MEKK family members are controlled by a variety of extracellular cues making them "sensor" kinases that respond to environmental stimuli frequently involving stress challenges. MEKK1 is the best studied with regard to regulation by extracellular cues and is activated by stimuli ranging from growth and survival promoting factors to cytotoxic drugs and irradiation that can induce apoptosis. For example, factors that bind to and activate cell surface receptors, such as epidermal growth factor (EGF), tumor necrosis factor-α (TNF-α), and antigen challenge of mast cells stimulate MEKK1 activation, which is critical for effecting changes in ERK1/2 and JNK activities, as well as the activation of NFκB. Functional downstream responses involving MEKK1 activation include specific cytokine expression. Evidence from embryonic stem cells with targeted deletion of both MEKK1 alleles suggest that MEKK1 also plays an important role in cell survival as loss of expression potentiates the induction of apoptosis by stress stimuli *(116)*. MEKK1 but not the other MEKKs is a substrate for caspase-3. Stimuli such as irradiation and genotoxic agents activate MEKK1 and induce a caspase-mediated cleavage releasing a 91-kDa C-terminal fragment of MEKK1 that is no longer tethered to membranes *(115,117,118)*. MEKK1 cleavage contributes to the apoptotic response by amplifying caspase activation and effectively establishing a MEKK1-caspase amplification loop that accelerates apoptosis. Furthermore, MEKK1 activity has been shown to induce expression of Fas (CD95) and Fas ligand which may also contribute to the apoptotic response characteristic of MEKK1 overexpression and activation *(119)*. Thus, MEKK1 is truly a "sensor" for a wide variety of environmental inputs contributing to the control of cell fate.

Recent experiments indicate that 196 kDa MEKK1 is likely an important regulator of the G2/M interface of the cell cycle (G.R. Fanger and G.L. Johnson, unpublished observations). For example, overexpression of 196 kDa MEKK1 leads to disregulated cell cycle control and an increase in accumulation of cells in the G2/M stage of the cell cycle, as well as a multinucleated phenotype. The 196-kDa MEKK1 protein levels, as well as activity, are low at G1/S but accumulate at G2/M. Disruption of microtubules by nocodazole leads to a very rapid activation of 196 kDa MEKK1 protein indicating that 196 kDa MEKK1 is regulated by the tubulin cytoskeleton. Thus, it is postulated that changes in microtubule organization at G2/M activates 196 kDa MEKK1 which has accumulated at this stage of the cell cycle and it is possible that 196-kDa MEKK1 may be required for cytokinesis to occur or to block cell cycle progression in a checkpoint function at G2/M. However, it is becoming evident that MEKK1, like a number of other Ste11/Ste20-like kinases that include Cla4, PAK, Raf1, and Mos, play a critical role in cell cycle control. Utilizing kinases whose activity is controlled by a wide range of environmental cues that are integrated into cell cycle and cytoskeletal control is an efficient mechanism of cell fate control.

3.4. MAP Three Kinase 1 (MTK-1)

Map Three Kinase-1 (MTK-1) is a 1607-amino acid protein that is the human homologue to MEKK4 *(120)*. When overexpressed, MTK-1 was reported to activate the JNK and p38, but not ERK. It was suggested that MTK-1 (hMEKK4) could play a role in p38 activation by cellular stresses such as osmotic shock, UV, and anisomycin. Interestingly, MTK-1 is not required for p38 activation by TNF-α and the low molecular weight GTP-binding proteins Cdc42 and Rac could not be shown to regulate MTK-1. MTK-1 was originally cloned using a functional complementation assay in yeast for osmosensitivity and both homology and function make it a human homolog to the yeast Ssk2/Ssk22 MKKKs. The ability to phosphorylate the MKKs MKK4, MKK3 and MKK6, but not MEK1 makes MEKK4/MTK-1 a MKKK. Because the mouse MEKK4 was cloned before its human homolog MTK-1, it should be referred to as hMEKK4.

3.5. MKKK5/ASK-1

Similar to the isolation of MEKK1-4, mitogen-activated protein kinase kinase kinase 5 (MKKK5) was isolated in a PCR screen using degenerate oligonucleotide primers corresponding to conserved regions in the kinase domains of yeast Ste11 and Byr2 *(121)*. The same kinase, apoptosis signal related kinase 1 (ASK-1), was also isolated based on its ability to complement Ssk2/Ssk22/Sho1 deficiency in *S. cerevisiae (122)*. The catalytic domain of MKKK5/ASK-1 is roughly 40% identical to MEKK1-3, as well as Ste11 and Byr2 of yeast. However, unlike these proteins, the kinase domain of MAPKKK5/ASK-1 is not at the C-terminus and is located within the middle of the 154-kDa protein. A putative FK506-binding protein (FKBP)-type peptidyl-prolyl *cis-trans*-isomerase is located in the N-terminal portion of MAPKKK5/ASK-1. MAPKKK5/ASK-1 activates JNK and p38 but not ERK1/2 activity when overexpressed in cells and induces apoptosis. Consistent with its role as a MKKK in the JNK pathway, MKKK5/ASK-1 phosphorylates MKK4 when immunoprecipitated from cells. MKKK5/ASK-1 is activated in response to TNF-α and inactive forms are able to inhibit apoptosis induced by TNF-α. Thus, MKKK5/ASK-1 is a TNF-α-regulated kinase that is important in controlling p38 and JNK activation in response to a cytokines.

3.6. MLK1, 2, 3 and DLK

The mixed lineage kinases (MLKs) consist of a family of at least four different proteins, MLK-1, MLK-2 (MST), MLK-3 (SPRK/PTK-1), and dual leucine zipper bearing kinase (DLK; also known as ZPK/MUK) *(23,123–129)*. Although their catalytic domains have features of both tyrosine and serine/threonine protein kinases, only serine/threonine kinase activity has been demonstrated. MLK-2 (also referred to as MST1) was originally reported not to activate any of the MAPK pathways but recent findings indicate that MLK-2 can activate JNK and p38 when overexpressed in cells *(130)*. Expression of MLK-3 activates the JNK pathway, but poorly activates the ERK and p38 pathways *(131,132)*. DLK can activate the JNK pathway *(129)*. Although it has been suggested that MLK-3 mediates activation of the JNK pathway by a downstream MEKK, MLK-3 can phosphorylate and activate MKK4, indicating that activation of the MKK4/JNK pathway is direct and most likely MLK-3 is a true MKKK *(131,132)*. With regard to regulation of the JNK pathway, MLK-3 and DLK contain a modified CRIB domain at their N-terminus which may mediate interaction with Cdc42 and Rac *(131,133)*. However, DLK does not appear to bind Cdc42 and Rac and association of MLK-3 with these GTP binding proteins is weak compared to that of PAK *(131,134)* or MEKK1 and 4 *(112)*. The kinase domain of MLK-3 is flanked by an SH3 domain located at the N-terminus and two leucine zipper motifs, as well as a proline rich region at the C-terminus, suggesting that MLK-3 may dimerize and interact with proteins other than Cdc42/Rac *(8)*.

3.7. TAK

Transforming growth factor-β (TGF-β)-activated kinase (TAK1), which was identified and cloned by its ability to rescue Ste11 mutants in *S. cerevisiae*, is able to activate JNK but not ERK when overexpressed in cells *(135)*. TAK1 is activated by TGF-β and appears required for signaling by TGF-β. However, TGF-β only modestly activates JNK and the major TAK1 regulated pathway may not be MKK4/JNK. The kinase domain of the 64-kDa TAK1 is located at the N-terminus of the protein which is approx 30% identical to the kinase domains of both Raf1 and MEKK1. Although the C-terminal domain of TAK1 has no signature sequences for identified regulatory domains, two-hybrid analysis identified TAK1 binding protein (TAB) which binds to this region, stimulates TAK kinase activity and also plays a role in TGF-β signaling, presumably via its ability to regulate TAK1 activity *(136)*.

3.8. TPL-2

The tumor progression locus 2 (TPL-2) gene was originally identified as a protooncogene involved in the progression of T-lymphomas by Moloney murine leukemia virus *(137)*. At the amino acid level, the 54 kDa TPL-2 protein is roughly 90% identical to the product of the human cancer Osaka thyroid (COT) protooncogene indicating that TPL-2 is likely the rat homologue to the human gene *(138)*. Ste11 and MEKK1 are most closely related to TPL-2 and the amino acid sequence of the kinase domains of these proteins are approx 32% identical. When overexpressed, ERK and JNK but not p38 are activated by TPL-2 *(137,139)*. Activation of the ERK and JNK pathways appears to be a direct result of MEK1 and MKK4 activation, as TPL-2 is able to phosphorylate MEK1 and MKK4 in vitro. The mechanisms of TPL-2 regulation are not well understood. It was first reported that inactive forms of TPL-2 could block ERK activation by Ras and Raf1 and that inactive forms of Ras and Raf1 could block ERK activation by TPL-2, suggesting that TPL-2 was acting in concert with Ras and Raf1 *(137)*. However, alternative studies have indicated that the activation of ERK by TPL-2 is Ras and Raf1-independent *(139)*.

3.9. KSR

The discovery of KSR in *C. elegans* and *Drosophila* directly led to identification of the mammalian form of this kinase *(140)*. Comparison of the mouse KSR to Raf1 demonstrated some interesting similarities including a 61% amino acid similarity in the C-terminal catalytic domain, as well as an N-terminally located cysteine-rich motif which is also conserved. These similarities between KSR and Raf1 are suggestive of KSR being a MKKK. Characterization of KSR in *Xenopus* oocytes and Balb/3T3 cells supports the notion that KSR cooperates with Ras to effect activation of the ERK1/2 pathway and to augment functions associated with ERK1/2 activation including transformation and oocyte maturation *(50)*. KSR does not bind Ras but appears to associate with Raf1 in a Ras-dependent manner at the plasma membrane indicating that KSR forms a membrane-bound kinase signaling complex with Ras GTP and Raf1. However, KSR does not phosphorylate Raf1 and so there is little evidence that KSR might function as a MKKKK. KSR was reported to be activated in by ceramide and in cells by ceramide-inducing factors such as TNF-α, resulting in phosphorylation of Raf1 *(141)*. However, other labs have been unable to demonstrate that TNF-α can activate KSR, that KSR is activated by ceramide or that KSR phosphorylates Raf1. To add complexity to the mechanisms by which KSR influences ERK1/2 activity, KSR has been shown to associate with MEK1 and ERK1/2 and, in contrast to earlier observations, that overexpression of KSR inhibits ERK activation *(142,143)*. Although KSR binds to MEK1, no MEK1 phosphorylation was observed. Thus, it is possible that KSR is a MKKK with unknown substrate specificity. KSR does not phosphorylate, MKK-3 or MKK-4. Alternatively, KSR could be acting as a "scaffolding-like" protein that stabilizes the Raf1/MEK1/ERK signaling module or facilitates presentation of MEK1 to Raf1. Therefore, KSR may represent a kinase having a novel mechanism of MAPK pathway regulation in mammalian cells.

3.10. PAK1, 2, and 3

The p21-activated kinase (PAK) family of approx 65-kDa proteins were first cloned based on their ability to bind Cdc42 and Rac in a GTP-dependent manner. As a result of sequence homology with Ste20, PAKs were classified as Ste20-like kinases *(144–146)*. It was later shown that PAK contains a CRIB motif that contributes to binding of PAK to Cdc42/Rac. Unlike Raf1, which requires another input in addition to Ras GTP for its activation, PAK activity is stimulated directly by physical interaction with Cdc42 GTP or Rac GTP. PAK is activated by cell surface receptors, such as IL-1, the platelet-derived growth factor (PDGF) receptor, insulin receptor and heterotrimeric G-protein coupled receptors *(147–149)*. PAK1 also binds to Nck, an adapter protein containing one SH2 and three SH3 domains, via the second SH3 domain of Nck and the first proline-rich SH3 binding motif near the N-terminus of PAK1. Thus, Pak1 could bind to activated growth factor receptor tyrosine kinases via its Nck interaction site and be regulated and/or recruited to the cytoplasmic surface of autophosphorylated growth factor receptors. Therefore, PAK may be coordinately regulated by both Cdc42/ Rac and Nck adapter protein interactions in order to effect activation of downstream pathways. PAK overexpression has been demonstrated to activate the JNK and p38 pathways, but not the ERK1/2 pathway. However, unlike other bona fide MKKKs such as MEKK1-4, PAK has not been shown to phosphorylate and activate MKK4 directly in the JNK pathway or MKK3 or 6 in the p38 pathway. The homology of PAK to Ste20 and its ability to regulate the JNK and p38 pathways when overexpressed suggests its function as either an MKKKK or MKKK but the unequivocal biochemical proof is not currently available.

As with MEKKs, the biological roles of the PAK family members appears to be quite diverse. In addition to regulating MAPK pathways, PAKs are strongly implicated in controlling cytoskeletal events, the stimulation of NADPH oxidase in neutrophils, and cellular transformation. With regard to cytoskeletal regulation and control of membrane morphology, overexpression of PAK elicits changes in actin organization and has been shown to colocalize with cortical actin during growth factor stimulated morphology changes *(150,151)*. Furthermore, expression of membrane-localized PAK induces neurite outgrowth of PC12 cells *(152)*. Stimulation of caspase activity by Fas receptor stimulation cleaves PAK2 which regulates morphological changes associated with an apoptotic phenotype *(153)*. However, using mutant forms of Cdc42 and Rac which do not bind PAK, morphological and cytoskeletal changes remain normal indicating that either PAK is not necessary for cytoskeletal changes brought about by Cdc42/Rac or other Rac/Cdc42 binding proteins can compensate for loss of PAK activation *(134,154)*. Although experiments using inhibitory forms of PAK indicate its requirement in transformation, mutants of Cdc42 and Rac do not support the notion that PAK is important for the transforming potential of these GTP binding proteins *(134,154,155)*. Cloning and identification of a *Xenopus* PAK gene indicates that the activity of PAK is important for G2/prophase arrest and prevention of apoptosis, suggesting that in oocytes PAK may have several different regulatory roles.

3.11. GCK

Germinal center kinase (GCK) was originally discovered as a 97-kDa serine/threonine kinase preferentially expressed in B lymphocytes of the germinal center region of lymphoid follicles that develop in response to stimulation with thymus-dependent antigens *(156)*. Sequence analysis of GCK indicated that its closest homolog was Ste20. However, GCK is also expressed in tissues other than B cells in germinal centers and one function that has been ascribed to this kinase is as a regulator of MAPK pathways *(157)*. Overexpression of GCK does not affect ERK and p38 activity but leads to an increase in JNK activation. However, as with PAK, activation of MKK4 may not be direct because GCK has not been demonstrated to phosphorylate MKK4 in biochemical studies. Thus, it is possible that a Ste11-like protein may mediate the effects of GCK on the JNK pathway. It is presently unclear if a Ste11 homolog is a substrate for GCK. Relatively little is known about the regulation of GCK activity by upstream effector pathways, but it appears that TNF-α is capable of mediating its activation. Thus, GCK has sequence homology in its kinase domain to Ste20/Ste11 kinases but its placement in MAPK pathways is not clear.

3.12. HPK1

Hematopoietic progenitor kinase 1 (HPK1) was identified as a 90-kDa serine/threonine kinase that was distantly related to Ste20 and PAK and predominantly expressed in hematopoietic cells *(158)*. Overexpression of HPK1 leads to JNK activation, whether HPK1 can induce ERK or p38 activation remains to be determined. MEKK1 was reported to associate with and can be phosphorylated by HPK1. Because an inactive form of MEKK1 can inhibit JNK activation by HPK1, it is possible that HPK1 functions as a MKKKK in the JNK pathway. In contrast to PAK, HPK1 does not bind to nor is activated by Cdc42 and Rac and at present little is known about HPK1 regulation.

3.13. GLK

Degenerate oligonucleotide primers to conserved regions of serine/threonine kinases were used to isolate GCK-like kinase (GLK), a protein with close homology to GCK and HPK1 *(159)*. GLK is a 97-kDa serine/threonine kinase that is activated by stress such as ultraviolet radiation and the proinflammatory cytokine TNF-α. In addition, overexpression of GLK activates the JNK but not the ERK or p38 pathways. Since inhibitory forms of MEKK1 and MKK4 block JNK activation by GLK, it is a candidate MKKKK in the JNK pathway. GLK was shown to phosphorylate a recombinant form of a MEKK1 fragment providing further evidence that GLK may lie upstream of MEKK1. Thus, evidence supports the notion that GLK may reside upstream of MEKK1 in stress response pathways leading to JNK regulation.

3.14. KHS

Kinase homologous to Sps1/Ste20 (KHS) is a 95 kDa serine/threonine kinase with greatest similarity to GCK (approx 74% within the kinase domain) *(160)*. The catalytic domain is located at the extreme N-terminus. Overexpression of KHS leads to JNK activation but not ERK and p38. Virtually nothing is known about the regulation of KHS except that its overexpression can activate the JNK pathway. The role of KHS in stress response pathways remains to be defined. Its sequence homology to Ste20 kinase domain suggests that it could be a MKKKK.

3.15. NIK

Nck interacting kinase (NIK) was isolated in a screen for proteins that interact with the SH3 domain of Nck *(161)*. Sequence analysis indicated that it displayed homology to Ste20-like kinases. Although NIK overexpression did not activate ERK or p38, it did induce activation of JNK, which was inhibited by an inactive form of MEKK1. Because NIK associates with MEKK1, it is possible that NIK like HPK1 and GLK is a MAPKKKK and used MEKK1 to effect JNK activation. Like HPK1 and GLK, NIK does not associate with Cdc42 and Rac, and little is known with regard to how NIK activity is regulated.

3.16. MST1, 2, and 3

Mammalian sterile twenty-like (MST) 1, 2, and 3 kinases are a family of serine/threonine kinases that display homology to the Ste20-like kinases. They are regulated by stress responses but were believed not to effect activation of MAPK pathways. More recently, MST1 (also known as MLK-2) was shown to activate the JNK pathway and to modestly activate the p38 pathway *(130)*. MST1 and 2 were originally cloned in a PCR screen with degenerate oligonucleotides to the serine/threonine kinase region *(23,128)*. Subsequent to this isolation, MST1 and 2 were also cloned as kinase regulated by stress (KRS)-1 (MST2) and KRS-2 (MST1), which were identified as a 63-kDa band that became highly phosphorylated in cell lysates after exposure to various stresses such as arsenite, okadaic acid and staurosporine *(162)*. A third MST family member has been isolated, MST-3, yet no effective activator of its kinase activity has been found *(163)*. It is predicted that the MST family members are Ste20/Ste11-like kinases that impart function to regulate MAPK pathways. Similar to PAK2 and MEKK1, MST1 was recently shown to be a caspase-3 substrate and to contribute to apoptotic responses *(130)*.

3.17. SOK

Using degenerate primers to conserved regions of subdomains II and VI to protein kinase domains, Ste20/oxidant stress response kinase-1 (SOK1) was isolated and sequence analysis indicated that it was most closely related to Ste20-like kinases *(163)*. However, unlike other Ste20-like kinases, such as GCK and PAK, SOK-1 was unable to activate the MAPK pathways. Even though SOK-1 could not activate stress response pathways associated with the MAPK family members, SOK-1 activity was activated by oxidant stress suggesting that other unique stress-activated pathways are regulated by SOK-1.

4. CONCLUSIONS

Newly identified kinases that have sequence homology to Ste20 and Ste11 have added to the obvious complexity of regulatory networks controlled by this family of kinases. In *S. cerevisiae* alone, there are ten Ste20/Ste11 family members. The number in mammalian cells will be much greater than this. Why have so many Ste20/Ste11 kinases? It is highly probable that each Ste20/Ste11-like kinase is integrated into specific pathways for responsiveness to different upstream inputs. These inputs are diverse, as the cell has the ability to sense exposure to cytokines, hormones, toxic agents, cell shape, cell cycle progression, and so on. Regulation often appears to involve GTP-binding proteins, phosphorylation, and relocalization in the cell. In addition, it is likely that many of these kinases can serve in more than one pathway, like is the case for Ste11, which is important for the pheromone-regulated mating response, osmosensing and pseudohyphal invasion. Some Ste20/Ste11-like kinases appear to regulate a single MAPK pathway while others are capable of regulating two or even three MAPK pathways. Thus, the regulation of different Ste20/Ste11 kinases allows for differential integration of MAPK pathways. Many of the Ste20/Ste11-like kinases also have functions independent of MAPK pathways. For example, the actin cytoskeleton regulatory functions attributed to PAK are probably largely independent of MAPK pathways.

The genome projects will define the total number of Ste20/Ste11 kinases in different organisms. The challenge facing investigators in the field is to define the expression pattern of each of these kinases, the upstream inputs that control their activity and the bona fide downstream substrates. This has been an enormous task in yeast where genetic selection is so powerful. Similar genetic strategies are not straightforward in mammalian cells and transfection experiments using overexpression and dominant-negative mutants have been elucidating but also confusing and probably frequently incorrectly interpreted. Targeted disruption of the Ste20/Ste11-like kinases is a daunting challenge, but one that will probably be required for elucidating function in addition to strong biochemistry. Another property of Ste20/Ste11-like kinases that is becoming apparent is that they are differentially localized in the cell. This indicates that subcellular location is important for their function and normal regulatory properties. Transfection studies do not always mimic the proper localization of the Ste20/Ste11-like kinases. It will be necessary to define how and why Ste20/Ste11-like kinases are located in different subcellular locales and this will undoubtedly help define their regulation. Our present understanding would assign a function for Ste20/Ste11-like kinases as localized sensors to control cell responses at the level of gene expression, metabolism, and the cytoskeleton.

REFERENCES

1. Ray LB, Sturgill TW. Insulin-stimulated microtubule-associated protein kinase is phosphorylated on tyrosine and threonine in vivo. *Proc Natl Acad Sci USA* 1988; 85:3753–3757.
2. Rossomando AJ, Payne DM, Weber MJ, Sturgill TW. Evidence that pp42, a major tyrosine kinase target protein, is a mitogen-activated serine/threonine protein kinase. *Proc Natl Acad Sci USA* 1989; 86:6940–6943.
3. Boulton TG, Yancopoulos GD, Gregory JS, Slaughter C, Moomaw C, Hsu J, Cobb MH. An insulin-stimulated protein kinase similar to yeast kinases involved in cell cycle control. *Science* 1990; 249:64–67.
4. Biggs WHI, Lipursky SL. Primary structure, expression, and signal-dependent tyrosine phosphorylation of a *Drosophila* homolog of extracellular signal-regulated kinase. *Proc Natl Acad Sci USA* 1994; 89:6295–6299.
5. Neiman AM, Stevenson BJ, Xu HP, Sprague GF, Herskowitz I, Wigler M, Marcus S. Functional homology of protein kinases required for sexual differentiation *in Schizosaccharomyces pombe* and *Saccharomyces cerevisiae* suggests a conserved signal transduction module in eukaryotic organsims. *Mol Cell Biol* 1993; 4:107–120.
6. Wu J, Han M. Suppression of activated Let-60 ras protein defines a role *of Caenorhabditis elegans* Sur-1 MAP kinase in vulval differentiation. *Genes Dev* 1994; 8:147–159.
7. Herskowitz I, Park HO, Sanders S, Valtz N, Peter M. Programming of cell polarity in budding yeast by endogenous and exogenous signals. *Cold Spring Harbor Symposia Quant Biol* 1995; 60:717–727.
8. Fanger GR, Gerwins P, Widmann C, Jarpe MB, Johnson GL. MEKKs, GCKs, MLKs, PAKs, TAKs, and Tpls: Upstream regulators of the c-jun amino-terminal kinases. *Curr Op Gen Dev* 1997; 7:67–74.
9. Inouye C, Dhillon N, Thorner J. Ste5 RING-H2 domain: Role in Ste4-promoted oligomerization for yeast pheromone signaling. *Science* 1997; 278:103–106.
10. Errede B, Levin DA. A conserved kinase cascade for MAPK kinase activation in yeast. *Curr Opin Cell Biol* 1993; 5:254–260.
11. Schultz J, Furguson B, Sprague GF. Signal transduction and growth control in yeast. *Curr Opin Gen Dev* 1995; 5:31–37.
12. Herskowitz I. MAP kinase pathways in yeast: For mating and more. *Cell* 1995; 80:187–197.
13. Hunter T. The protein kinases of budding yeast: Six score and more. *Tr. Biochem. Sci.* 1997; 18–22.
14. Bardwell L, Cook JG, Inouye CJ, Thorner J. Signal propagation and regulation in the mating phermone response pathway of the yeast *Saccharomyces cerevisiae. Dev. Biol.* 1994; 166:363–379.

15. Peter M, Gartner A, Horecka J, Ammerer G, Herskowitz I. FAR1 links the signal transduction pathway to the cell cycle machinery in yeast. *Cell* 1993; 73:747–769.

16. Elion EA, Satterberg B, Kranz JE. FUS3 phosphorylates multiple components of the mating signal transduction cascade: Evidence for STE12 and FAR1. *Mol Biol Cell* 1993; 4.

17. Whiteway MS, Wu C, Leeuw T, Clark K, Fourest-Lieuvin A, Thomas DY, Leberer E. Association of the yeast pheromone response G protein beta gamma subunits with the MAP kinase scaffold Ste5p. *Science* 1995; 269:1572–1575.

18. Bienstock RJ, Darden T, Wiseman R, Pedersen L, Barrett JC. Molecular modeling of the amino-terminal zinc RING domain of BRCA1. *Cancer Res* 1996; 56:2539–2545.

19. Borden KL, Freemont PS. The RING finger domain: A recent example of a sequence-structure family. *Curr Opin Struct Biol* 1996; 6:395–401.

20. Feng Y, Song LY, Kincaid E, Mahanty SK, Elion EA. Functional binding between Gβ and the LIM domain of Ste5 is required for activate the MEKK Ste11. *Curr Biol* 1998; 8:267–278.

21. Aelst LV, Barr M, Marcus S, Polverino A, Wigler M. Complex formation between Ras and Raf and other protein kinases. *Proc Natl Acad Sci USA* 1993; 90:6213–6217.

22. Chang EC, Barr M, Wang Y, Jung V, Xu HP, Wigler MH. Cooperative interaction of *S. pombe* proteins required for mating and morphogenesis. *Cell* 1994; 79:131–141.

23. Ottilie S, Miller PJ, Johnson DI, Creasy CL, Sells MA, Bagrodia S, Forsburg SL, Chernoff J. Fission yeast pak1+ encodes a protein kinase that interacts with Cdc42p and is involved in the control of cell polarity and mating. *EMBO J* 1995; 14:5908–5919.

24. Krisak L, Strich R, Winters RS, Hall JP, Mallory MJ, Kreitzer D, Tuan RS, Winter W. SMK1, a developmentally regulated MAP kinase, is required for spore wall assembly in *Saccharomyces cerevisiae*. *Genes Dev* 1994; 8:2151–2161.

25. Friesen H, Lunz R, Doyle S, Segall J. Mutation of the SPS1-encoded protein kinase of *Saccharomyces cerevisiae* leads to defects in transcription and morphology during spore formation. *Genes Dev* 1994; 8:2162–2175.

26. Brewster JL, Valoir T, Dwyer ND, Winter E, Gustin MC. An osmosensing signal transduction pathway in yeast. *Science* 1993; 259:1760–1763.

27. Maeda T, Takekawa M, Saito H. Activation of yeast PBS2 MAPKK by MAPKKKs or by binding of a SH3-containing osmosensor. *Science* 1995; 269:554–558.

28. Posas F, Wurgler-Murphy SM, Maeda T, Witten EA, Thai TC, Saito H. Yeast HOG1 MAP kinase cascade is regulated by a multistep phosphorelay mechanism in the SLN1-YPD1-SSK1 "Two-component" osmosensor. *Cell* 1996; 86:865–875.

29. Posas F, Saito H. Osmotic activation of the HOG MAPK pathway via Ste11p MAPKKK: scaffold role of Pbs2p MAPKK. *Science* 1997; 276:1702–1705.

30. Samejima I, Makie S, Fantes PA. Multiple modes of activation of the stress-responsive MAP kinase pathway in fission yeast. *EMBO J* 1997; 16:6162–6170.

31. Shioazaki K, Shiozaki M, Russel P. Mcs4 mitotic catastrophe suppressor regulates the fission yeast cell cycle through the Wik1-Wis1-Spc1 kinase cascade. *Mol Biol Cell* 1997; 8:409–419.

32. Shieh J, Wilkinson MG, Buck V, Morgan BA, Makino K, Millar JBA. The Mcs4 response regulator coordinately controls the stress-activated Wak1-Wis1-Sty1 MAPK kinase pathway and fission yeast cell cycle. *Genes Dev* 1997; 11:1008–1022.

33. Warbrick E, Fantes PA. The wis1 protein kinase is a dosage-dependent regulator of mitosis in *Schizosaccharomyces pombe*. *EMBO J* 1991; 10:4291–4299.

34. Irie K, Gotoh Y, Yashar BM, Errede B, Nishida E, Matsumoto K. MKK1 and MKK2, which encode *Saccharomyces cerevisiae* mitogen-activated protein kinase-kinase homologs, funcion in the pathway mediated by protein kinase C. *Mol Cell Biol* 1993; 13:3076–3083.

35. Lee KS, Irie K, Gotoh Y, Watanabe Y, Araki H, Nishida E, Matsumoto K, Levin DE. A yeast mitogen-activated protein kinase homolog (Mpk1p) mediates signalling by protein kinase C. *Mol Cell Biol* 1993; 13:3067–3075.

36. Levin DE, Bartlett-Heubusch E. Mutants in the *S. cerevisiae* PKC1 gene display a cell cycle-specific stability defect. *J Cell Biol* 1992; 116:1221–1229.

37. Toda T, Dhut S, Superti-Furga G, Gotoh Y, Nishida E, Sugiura R, Kuno T. The fission yeast pmk1⁺ gene encodes a novel mitogen-activated protein kinase homolog which regulates cell integrity and functions coordinately with the protein kinase C pathway. *Mol Cell Biol* 1996; 16:6752–6764.

38. Zaitsevskaya-Carter T, Cooper JA. Spm1, a stress-activated MAPK kinase that regulates morphogenesis in *S. pombe*. *EMBO J* 1997; 16:1318–1331.

39. Cvrckova F, DeVirgilio C, Manser E, Pringle JR, Nasmyth K. Ste20-like protein kinases are required for normal localization of cell growth and for cytokinesis in budding yeast. *Genes Dev* 1995; 1818–1830.

40. Benton BK, Tinkelenberg A, Gonzalez I, Cross FR. Cla4p, a *Saccharomyces cerevisiae* Cdc42p-activated kinase involved in cytokinesis, is activated at mitosis. *Mol Cell Biol* 1997; 17:5067–5076.

41. Leberer E, Thomas DY, Whiteway M. Pheromone signalling and polarized morphogenesis in yeast. *Curr Op Genet Dev* 1997; 7:59–66.

42. Kornfeld K. Vulval development in *Caenorhabditis elegans*. *Trends Genet* 1997; 13:55–61.

43. Rubin GM. Signal transduction and the fate of the R7 photoreceptor in *Drosophila*. *Trends Genet* 1991; 7:372–377.

44. Knust E. *Drosophila* morphogenesis: Movements behind the edge. *Curr Biol* 1997; 7:R558–R561.

45. Sundaram M, Han M. Control and integration of cell signaling pathways during *C. elegans* vulval development. *BioEssays* 1996; 18:473–480.

46. Han M, Golden A, Han Y, Sternberg PW. *C. elegans* lin-45 raf gene participates in let-60 ras-stimulated vulval differentiation. *Nature* 1993; 363:133–140.

47. Sundaram M, Han M. The *C. elegans* ksr-1 gene encodes a novel Raf-related kinase involved in Ras-mediated signal transduction. *Cell* 1995; 83:889–901.

48. Kornfeld K, Hom DB, Horvitz HR. The ksr-1 gene encodes a novel protein kinase involved in Ras-mediated signaling in *C. elegans*. *Cell* 1995; 83:909–913.

49. Downward J. KSR: A novel player in the Ras pathway. *Cell* 1995; 83:831–834.

50. Therrien M, Michaud NR, Rubin GM, Morrison DK. KSR modulates signal propagation within the MAPK cascade. *Genes Dev* 1996; 10:2684–2695.

51. Han J, Choi KY, Brey PT, Lee WJ. Molecular cloning and characterization of a *Drosophila* p38 mitogen-activated protein kinase. *J Biol Chem* 1998; 273:369–374.

52. Nishida Y, Hata M, Ayaki T, Ryo H, Yamagata M, Shimizu K, Nishizuka Y. Proliferation of both somatic and germ cells is affected in the *Drosophila* mutants of raf proto-oncogene. *EMBO J* 1988; 7:775–781.

53. Ambrosio L, Mahowald AP, Perrimon N. Requirement of the *Drosophila* raf homologue for torso function. *Nature* 1989; 342:288–291.

54. Dickson B, Sprenger F, Morrison D, Hafen E. Raf functions downstream of Ras1 in the sevenless signal transduction pathway. *Nature* 1992; 360:600–603.

55. Perrimon N. Signalling pathways initiated by receptor protein tyrosine kinases in *Drosophila*. *Curr Biol* 1994; 6:260–266.

56. Robinson MJ, Cobb MH. Mitogen-activated protein kinase pathways. *Curr Opin Cell Biol* 1997; 9:180–186.

57. Boulton TG, Nye SH, Robbins DJ, Nye I, Radziejeska E, Morgenbesser SD, DePinho RA, Panayatatos N, Cobb MH, Yancopoulos GD. ERKs: A family of protein-serine/threonine kinases that are activated and tyrosine phosphorylated in response to insulin and NGF. *Cell* 1991; 65:663–675.

58. Cheng M, Boulton TG, Cobb MH. ERK3 is a constitutively nuclear protein kinase. *J Biol Chem* 1996; 271:8951–8958.

59. Peng X, Angelastro JM, Greene LA. Tyrosine phosphorylation of extracellular signal-

regulated protein kinase 4 in response to growth factors. *J Neurochem* 1996; 66:1191–1197.

60. Derijard B, Hibi M, Wu I, Barrett T, Su B, Deng R, Karin M, Davis RJ. JNK1: A protein kinase stimulated by UV light and Ha-Ras that binds and phosphorylates the c-Jun activation domain. *Cell* 1994; 76:1025–1037.

61. Kyriakis JM, Banerjee P, Nikolakaki E, Dai T, Rubie EA, Ahmad MF, Avruch J, Woodgett JR. The stress-activated protein kinase subfamily of c-jun kinases. *Nature* 1994; 369:156–160.

62. Kallunki T, Su B, Tsigelny I, Sluss HK, Derijard B, Moore G, Davis RJ, Karin M. JNK2 contains a specificity-determining region responsible for efficient c-Jun binding and phosphorylation. *Genes Dev* 1994; 8:2996–3007.

63. Gupta S, Barrett T, Whitmarsh AJ, Cavanagh J, Sluss HK, Derijard B, Davis RJ. Selective interaction of JNK protein kinase isoforms with transcription factors. *EMBO J* 1996; 15:2760–2770.

64. Mertens S, Craxton M, Goedert M. SAP kinase-3, a new member of the family of mammalian stress-activated protein kinases. *FEBS Lett* 1996; 383:273–276.

65. Zervos AS, Faccio L, Gatto JP, Kyriakis JM, Brent R. Mxi2, a mitogen-activated protein kinase that recognizes and phosphorylates Max protein. *Proc Natl Acad Sci USA* 1995; 92:10,531–10,534.

66. Jiang Y, Chen C, Li Z, Guo W, Gegner JA, Lin S, Han J. Characterization of the structure and function of a new mitogen-activated protein kinase (p38β). *J Biol Chem* 1996; 271:17,920–17,926.

67. Lechner N, Zahalka MA, Giot J, Moller NPH, Ullrich A. ERK6, a mitogen-activated protein kinase involved in C2C12 myoblast differentiation. *Proc Natl Acad Sci USA* 1996; 93:4355–4359.

68. Stein B, Yang MX, Young DB, Janknech R, Hunter T, Murray BW, Barbosa MS. p38–2, a novel mitogen-activated protein kinase with distinct properties. *J Biol Chem* 1997; 272:19,509–19,517.

69. Jiang Y, Gram H, Zhao M, New L, Gu J, Feng L, Dipadova F, Ulevitch RJ, Han J. Characterization of the structure and function of the fourth member of p38 group mitogen-activated protein kinases. *J Biol Chem* 1997; 272:30,122–30,128.

70. Zhou G, Qin BZ, Dixon JE. Components of a new human protein kinase signal transduction pathway. *J Biol Chem* 1995; 270:12,665–12,669.

71. Treisman R. Regulation of transcription by MAP kinase cascades. *Curr Opin Cell Biol* 1996; 8:205–215.

72. Whitmarsh AJ, Davis RJ. Transcription factor AP-1 regulation by mitogen-activated protein kinase signal transduction pathways. *J Mol Med* 1996; 74:589–607.

73. Seger R, Krebs EG. The MAPK signaling cascade. *FASEB J* 1995; 9:726–735.

74. Lin LL, Wartmann M, Lin AY, Knopf JL, Seth A, Davis RJ. cPLA₂ is phosphorylated and activated by MAP kinase. *Cell* 1993; 72:269–278.

75. Rouse J, Cohen P, Trigon S, Morange M, Alonso-Llamazares A, Zamanillo D, Hunt T, Nebreda AR. A novel kinase cascade triggered by stress and heast shock that stimulates MAPKAP kinase-2 and phosphorylation of the small heat shock proteins. *Cell* 1993; 78:1027–1037.

76. Sanchez I, Hughes RT, Mayer BJ, Yee K, Woodgett JR, Avruch J, Kyriakis JM, Zon LI. Role of SAPK/ERK kinase-1 in the stress-activated pathway regulating transcription factor c-Jun. *Nature* 1994; 372:794–798.

77. Moriguchi T, Toyoshima F, Gotoh Y, Iwamatsu A, Irie K, Mori E, Kuroyanagi N, Hagiwara M, Matsumoto K, Nishida E. Purification and identification of a major activator for p38 from osmotically shocked cells. Activation of mitogen-activated protein kinase kinase 6 by osmotic shock, tumor necrosis factor-alpha, and H_2O_2. *J Biol Chem* 1996; 271:26,981–26,988.

78. Tournier C, Whitmarsh AJ, Cavanagh J, Barrett T, Davis RJ. Mitogen-activated protein kinase kinase 7 is an activator of the c-Jun NH$_2$-terminal kinase. *Proc Natl Acad Sci USA* 1997; 94:7337–7342.

79. Beck EW, Huleihel M, Gunnell M, Bonner TI, Rapp UR. The complete coding sequence of the human A-raf-1 oncogene and transformming activity of a human A-raf carrying retrovirus. *Nucleic Acid Res* 1987; 15:595–609.

80. Jansen HW, Ruckert B, Lurz R, Bister K. Two unrelated cell-derived sequences in the genome of avian leukemia and carcinoma inducing retrovirus MH2. *EMBO J* 1983; 2:1969–1975.

81. Lavoie JN, L'Allemain G, Brunet A, Muller R, Pouyssegur J. Cyclin D1 expression is regulated positively by the p42/p44MAPK and negatively by the p38/HOGMAPK pathway. *J Biol Chem* 1996; 271:20,608–20,616.

82. Wood KW, Qi H, D'Arcangelo G, Armstrong RC, Roberts TM, Halegoua S. The cytoplasmic raf oncogene induces a neuronal phenotype in PC12 cells: A potential role for cellular raf kinases in neuronal growth factor signal transduction. *Proc Natl Acad Sci USA* 1993; 90:5016–5020.

83. Woods D, Parry D, Cherwinski H, Bosch E, Lees E, McMahon M. Raf-induced proliferation of cell cycle arrest is determined by the level of Raf activity with arrest mediated by p21^{Cip1}. *Mol Cell Biol* 1997; 17:5598–5611.

84. Sewing A, Wiseman B, Llyod AC, Land H. High-intensity Raf signal causes cell cycle arrest mediated by p21^{Cip1}. *Mol Cell Biol* 1997; 17:5588–5597.

85. Kolch W, Heidecker G, Lloyd P, Rapp UR. Raf-1 protein kinase is required for growth of NIH/3T3 cells. *Nature* 1991; 349:426–428.

86. Jelinek T, Dent P, Sturgill TW, Weber MJ. Ras-induced activation of Raf-1 is dependent on tyrosine phosphorylation. *Mol Cell Biol* 1996; 16:1027–1034.

87. Marais R, Light Y, Paterson HF, Mason CS, Marshall CJ. Differential regulation of Raf-1, A-Raf and B-Raf by oncogenic Ras and tyrosine kinases. *J Biol Chem* 1997; 272:4378–4383.

88. Howe LR, Levers SJ, Gomez N, Nakielny S, Cohen P, Marshall CJ. Activation of the MAP kinase pathway by the protein kinase raf. *Cell* 1992; 71:335–342.

89. Marquardt B, Frith D, Stabel S. Signalling from TPA to MAP kinase requires protein kinase C, raf and MEK: Reconstitution of the signalling pathway *in vitro*. *Oncogene* 1994; 9:3213–3218.

90. Hancock JF, Cadwallader K, Paterson H, Marshall CJ. CAAX or a CAAL motif and a second signal are sufficient for plasma membrane targeting of ras proteins. *EMBO J* 1991; 10:4033–4039.

91. Leevers SJ, Paterson HF, Marshall CJ. Requirement for Ras in Raf activation is overcome by targetting Raf to the plasma membrane. *Nature* 1994; 369:411–414.

92. Vossler MR, Yao H, York RD, Pan MG, Rim CS, Stork PJ. cAMP activates MAP kinase and Elk-1 through a B-Raf-and Rap1-dependent pathway. *Cell* 1997; 89:73–82.

93. Freed E, Symons M, Macdonald SG, McCormick F, Ruggieri R. Binding of 14-3-3 proteins to the protein kinase Raf and effects on its activation. *Science* 1994; 265:1713–1715.

94. Fu H, Xia K, Pallas DC, Cui C, Conroy K, Narsimhan RP, Mamon H, Collier RJ, Roberts TM. Interaction of the protein kinase Raf-1 with 14-3-3 proteins. *Science* 1994; 266:126–128.

95. Muslin AJ, Tanner JW, Allen PM, Shaw AS. Interaction of 14-3-3 with signaling proteins is mediated by the recognition of phosphoserine. *Cell* 1996; 84:889–897.

96. Yaffe MB, Rittinger K, Vollinia S, Caron PR, Aitken A, Leffers H, Gamblin SJ, Smerdon SJ, Cantley LC. The structural basis for 14-3-3: Phosphopeptide binding specificity. *Cell* 1997; 91:961–971.

97. Fantl WJ, Muslin AJ, Kikuchi A, Martin JA, MacNicol AM, Gross RW, Williams LT. Activation of Raf-1 by 14-3-3 proteins. *Nature* 1994; 371:612–614.

98. Irie K, Gotoh Y, Yashar BM, Errede B, Nishida E, Matsumoto K. Stimulatory effects of yeast and mammalian 14-3-3 proteins on the Raf protein kinase. *Science* 1994; 265:1716–1719.

99. Clark GJ, Drugan JK, Rossman KL, Carpenter JW, Rogers-Graham K, Fu H, Der CJ, Campbell SL. 14-3-3ζ negatively regulates Raf-1 activity by interactions with the Raf-1 cysteine-rich domain. *J Biol Chem* 1997; 272:20,990–20,993.

100. Morrison DK, Cutler RE. The complexity of Raf-1 regulation. *Curr Op Cell Biol* 1997; 9:174–179.

101. Xiao B, Smerdon SJ, Jones DH, Dodson GG, Soneji Y, Aitken A, Gamblin SJ. Structure of a 14-3-3 protein and implications for coordination of multiple signalling pathways. *Nature* 1995; 376:188–191.

102. Catling AD, Reuter CW, Cox ME, Parsons SJ, Weber MJ. Partial purification of a mitogen-activated protein kinase kinase activator from bovine brain. Identification as B-Raf or a B-Raf-associated activity. *J Biol Chem* 1994; 269:30,014–30,021.

103. Lerosey I, Pizon B, Tavitian A, Gunzburg Jd. The cAMP-dependent protein kinase phosphorylates the rap1 protein in vitro as well as in intact fibroblasts, but not the closely related rap2 protein. *Bichem Biophys Res Comm* 1991; 175:430–436.

104. Bogoyevitch MA, Marshall CJ, Sugden PH. Hypertrophic agonists stimulate the activities of the protein kinases c-Raf and A-Raf in cultured ventricular myocytes. *J Biol Chem* 1995; 270:26,303–26,310.

105. Posada J, Yew N, Ahn NG, Woude, G. F. V. and Cooper JA. Mos stimulates MAPK kinase in Xenopus Oocytes and activates a MAPK kinase kinase in vitro. *Mol Cell Biol* 1993; 13:2546–2553.

106. Resing KA, Mansour SJ, Hermann AS, Johnson RS, Candia JM, Fukasawa K, Woude, G. F. V. and Ahn NG. Determination of v-Mos-catalyzed phosphorylation sites and autophosphorylation sites on MAPK kinase kinase by ESI/MS. *Biochemistry* 1995; 34:2610–2620.

107. Gebauer F, Richter JD. Synthesis and function of Mos: The control switch of vertebrate oocyte meiosis. *BioEssays* 1997; 19:23–28.

108. Sagata N. What does Mos do in oocytes and somatic cells? *BioEssays* 1997; 19:13–21.

109. Lange-Carter CA, Pleiman CM, Gardner AM, Blumer KJ, Johnson GL. A divergence in the MAP kinase regulatory network defined by MEK kinase and raf. *Science* 260:315–319.

110. Blank JL, Gerwins P, Elliott EM, Sather S, Johnson GL. Molecular cloning of mitogen-activated protein/ERK kinases (MEKK) 2 and 3. *J Biol Chem* 1996; 271:5361–5368.

111. Gerwins P, Blank JL, Johnson GL. Cloning of a novel mitogen-activated protein kinase kinase kinase MEKK4, that selectively regulates the c-Jun amino terminal kinase pathway. *J Biol Chem* 1997; 272:8288–8295.

112. Fanger GR, Johnson NL, Johnson GL. MEK kinases are regulated by EGF and selectively interact with Rac/Cdc42. *EMBO J* 1997; 16:4961–4972.

113. Russell M, Lange-Carter CA, Johnson GL. Direct interaction between Ras and the kinase domain of mitogen-activated protein kinase kinase kinase (MEKK1). *J Biol Chem* 1995; 270:11,757–11,760.

114. Lange-Carter CA, Johnson GL. Ras-dependent growth factor regulation of MEK kinase in PC12 cells. *Science* 1994; 265:1458–1461.

115. Fanger GR, Widmann C, Porter AC, Sather S, Johnson GL, Vaillancourt RR. 14-3-3 proteins interact with specific MEK kinases. *J Biol Chem* 1998; 273:3476–3483.

116. Yujiri T, Sather S, Johnson GL. Targeted disruption of the MEK kinase 1 gene defines its function as a dual MAPK kinase kinase for the selective activation of MAPK[jnk] and MAPK[erk] in response to specific stress stimuli and the mitogen lysophosphatidic acid. *submitted*

117. Cardone MH, Salvesen GS, Widmann C, Johnson GL, Frisch SM. The regulation of anoikis: MEKK-1 activation requires cleavage by caspases. *Cell* 1997; 90:315–323.

118. Widmann C, Gerwins P, Johnson NL, Jarpe MB, Johnson GL. MEKK1, a substrate for DEVD-directed caspases, is involved in genotoxin-induced apoptosis. *Mol Cell Biol* 1998; 18:2416–2429.
119. Faris M, Kokot N, Latinis K, Kasibhatla S, Green DR, Koretzky GA, Nel A. The c-Jun N-terminal kinase cascade plays a role in stress-induced apoptosis in Jurkat cells by up-regulating Fas ligand expression. *J Immunol* 1998; 160:134–144.
120. Takekawa M, Posas F, Saito H. A human homolog of yeast Ssk2/Ssk22 MAP kinase kinase kinases, MTK1, mediates stress-induced activation of the p38 and JNK pathways. *EMBO J* 1997; 16:4973–4982.
121. Wang XS, Diener K, Jannuzzi D, Trollinger D, Tan T, Lichenstein H, Zukowsi M, Yao Z. Molecular cloning and characterization of a novel protein kinase with a catalytic domain homologous to mitogen-activated protein kinase kinase kinase. *J Biol Chem* 1996; 271:31,607–31,611.
122. Ichijo H, Nishida E, Irie K, Dijke P, Saitoh M, Moriguchi T, Takagi M, Matsumoto K, Miyanzono K, Gotoh Y. Induction of apoptosis by ASK1, a mammalian MAPKKK that activates SAPK/JNK and p38 singaling pathways. *Science* 1997; 275:90–94.
123. Dorow DS, Devereux L, Dietzsch E, Kretser T. Identification of a new family of human epithelial protein kinases containing two leucin/isoleucine-zipper domains. *Eur J Biochem* 1993; 213:701–710.
124. Ezoe K, Lee S, Strunk KM, Spritz RA. PTK1, a novel protein kinase required for proliferation of human melanocytes. *Oncogene* 1994; 9:935–938.
125. Gallo KA, Mark MR, Scadden DT, Wang Z, Gu Q, Godowski PJ. Identification and characterization of SPRK, a novel src-homology 3 domain-containing proline-rich kinase with serine/threonine kinase activity. *J Biol Chem* 1994; 269:15,092–15,100.
126. Holzman LB, Merritt SE, Fan B. Identification, molecular cloning, and characterization of dual leucine zipper bearing kinase. *J Biol Chem* 1994; 269:30,808–30,817.
127. Reddy UR, Pleasure D. Cloning of a novel putative protein kinase having a leucine zipper domain from human brain. *Biochem Biophys Res Comm* 1994; 202:613–620.
128. Katoh M, Hirai M, Sugimura T, Terada M. Cloning and characterization of MST, a novel (putative) serine/threonine kinase with SH3 domain. *Oncogene* 1995; 10:1447–1451.
129. Hirai S, Izawa M, Osada S, Spyrou G, Ohno S. Activation of the JNK pathway by distantly related protein kinases, MEKK and MUK. *Oncogene* 1996; 12:641–650.
130. Graves JD, Gotoh Y, Draves KE, Ambrose D, Han, D. K. M., Wright M, Chernoff J, Clark EA, Krebs EG. Caspase-mediated activation and induction of apoptosis by the mammalian Ste20-like kinase Mst1. *EMBO J* 1998; 17:2224–2234.
131. Teramoto H, Coso OA, Miyata H, Igishi T, Miki T, Gutkind JS. Signaling from the small GTP-binding proteins Rac1 and Cdc42 to the c-Jun N-terminal kinase/stress-activated protein kinase pathway. *J Biol Chem* 1996; 271:27,225–27,228.
132. Rana A, Gallo K, Godowski P, Hirai S, Ohno S, Zon L, Kyriakis JM, Avruch J. The mixed lineage kinase SPRK phosphorylates and activates the stress-activated protein kinase activator, SEK-1. *J Biol Chem* 1996; 271:19,025–19,028.
133. Burbelo PD, Drechsel D, Hall A. A conserved binding motif defines numerous candidate target proteins for both Cdc42 and Rac GTPases. *J Biol Chem* 1995; 270:29,071–29,074.
134. Lamarche N, Tapon N, Stowers L, Burbelo PD, Aspenstrom P, Bridges P, Chant J, Hall A. Rac and Cdc42 induce actin polymerization and G1 cell cycle progression independently of p65PAK and the JNK/SAPK MAP kinase cascade. *Cell* 1996; 87:519–529.
135. Yamaguchi K, Shirakabe K, Shibuya H, Irie K, Oishi I, Ueno N, Taniguch T, Nishida E, Matsumoto K. Identification of a member of the MAPKKK family as a potiential mediator of TGF-β signal transduction. *Science* 1995; 270:2008–2011.
136. Shibuya H, Yamaguchi K, Shirakabe K, Tonegawa A, Gotoh Y, Ueno N, Irie K, Nishida E, Matsumoto K. TAB1: An activator of the TAK1 MAPKKK in TGF-β signal transduction. *Science* 1996; 272:1179–1182.

137. Patriotis C, Makris A, Chernoff J, Tsichlis PN. Tpl-2 acts in conert with Ras and Raf-1 to activate mitogen-activated protein kinase. *Proc Natl Acad Sci USA* 1994; 91:9755–9759.

138. Miyoshi J, Higashi T, Mukai H, Ohuchi T, Kakunaga T. Structure and transforming potential of the human cot oncogene encoding a putative protein kinase. *Mol Cell Biol* 1991; 11:4088–4096.

139. Salmeron A, Ahmad TB, Carlile GW, Pappin D, Narsimhan RP, Ley SC. Activation of MEK-1 and SEK-1 by Tpl-2 protooncoprotein, a novel MAP kinase kinase kinase. *EMBO J* 1996; 15:817–826.

140. Therrien M, Chang HC, Solomon NM, Karim FD, Wassarman DA, Rubin GM. KSR, a novel protein kinase required for RAS signal transduction. *Cell* 1995; 83:879–888.

141. Zhang Y, Yao B, Delikat S, Bayoumy S, Lichenstein H, Kolesnick R. Kinase suppressor of Ras is Ceramide-Activated Protein Kinase. *Cell* 1997; 89:63–72.

142. Denouel-Galy A, Douville EM, Warne PH, Papin C, Laugier D, Calothy G, Downward J, Eychene A. Murine Ksr interacts with MEK and inhibits Ras-induced transformation. *Curr Biol* 1997; 8:46–55.

143. Yu W, Fantl WJ, Harrowe G, Williams LT. Regulation of the MAP kinase pathway by mammalian Ksr through direct interaction with MEK and ERK. *Curr Biol* 1997; 8:56–64.

144. Manser E, Leung T, Salihuddin H, Zhao Z, Lim L. A brain serine/threonine protein kinase acivated by Cdc42 and Rac1. *Nature* 1994; 367:40–46.

145. Teo M, Manser E, Lim L. Identification and molecular cloning of a p21$^{cdc42/rac1}$-activated serine/threonine kinase that is rapidly activated by thrombin in platelets. *J Biol Chem* 1995; 270:26,690–26,697.

146. Martin GA, Bollag G, McCormick F, Aboe A. A novel serine kinase activated by rac1/CDC42Hs-dependent autophosphorylation is related to PAK65 and STE20. *EMBO J* 1995; 14:1970–1978.

147. Zhang S, Han J, Sells MA, Chernoff J, Knaus UG, Ulevitch RJ, Bokoch GM. Rho family GTPases regulated p38 mitogen-activated protein kinase through the downstream mediator Pak1. *J Biol Chem* 1995; 270:23,934–2,3936.

148. Bokoch GM, Wang Y, Bohl BP, Sells MA, Quilliam LA, Knaus UG. Interaction of the Nck adapter protein with p21-activated kinase (PAK1). *J Biol Chem* 1996; 271:25,746–25,749.

149. Tsakiridis T, Taha C, Grinstein S, Klip A. Insulin activates a p21-activated kinase in muscle cells via phosphatidylinositol 3-kinase. *J Biol Chem* 1996; 271:19,664–19,667.

150. Sells MA, Knaus UG, Bagrodia S, Ambrose DM, Bokoch GM, Chernoff J. Human p21-activated kianse (Pak1) regulates actin organization in mammalian cells. *Curr Biol* 1997; 7:202–210.

151. Manser E, Huang H, Loo T, Chen X, Dong J, Leung T, Lim L. Expression of constitutively active α-PAK reveals effects of the kinase on actin and focal complexes. *Mol Cell Biol* 1997; 17:1129–1143.

152. Daniels RH, Hall PS, Bokoch GM. Membrane targeting of p21-activated kinase 1 (PAK1) induces neurite outgrowth from PC12 cells. *EMBO J* 1998; 17:754–764.

153. Rudel T, Bokoch GM. Membrane and morphological changes in apoptotic cells regulated by caspase-mediated activation of PAK2. *Science* 1997; 276:1571–1574.

154. Westwick JK, Lambert QT, Clark GJ, Symons M, Aelst LV, Pestell RG, Der CJ. Rac regulation of transformation, gene expression, and actin organization by multiple, PAK-independent pathways. *Mol Cell Biol* 1997; 17:1324–1335.

155. Tang Y, Chen Z, Ambrose D, Liu J, Gibbs JB, Chernoff J, Field J. Kinase-deficient Pak1 mutants inhibit Ras transformation of Rat-1 fibroblasts. *Mol Cell Biol* 1997; 17:4454–4464.

156. Katz P, Whalen G, Kehrl JH. Differential expression of a novel protein kinase in human B lymphocytes. *J Biol Chem* 1994; 269:16,802–16,809.

157. Pombo CM, Kehrl JH, Sanchez I, Katz P, Avruch J, Zon LI, Woodgett JR, Force T, Kyriakis JM. Activation of the SAPK pathway by the human STE20 homologue germinal centre kinase. *Nature* 1995; 377:750–754.

158. Hu MC, Qiu WR, Wang X, Meyer CF, Tan T. Human HPK1, a novel human hematopoietic progenitor kinase that activates the JNK/SAPK kinase cascade. *Genes Dev* 1996; 10:2251–2264.

159. Diener K, Wang XS, Chen C, Meyer CF, Keesler G, Zukowski M, Tan T, Yao Z. Activation of the c-Jun N-terminal kinase pathway by a novel protein kinase related to human germinal center kinase. *Proc Natl Acad Sci USA* 1997; 94:9687–9692.

160. Tung RM, Blenis J. A novel human SPS1/STE20 homologue, KHS, activates Jun N-terminal kinase. *Oncogene* 1997; 14:653–659.

161. Su Y, Han J, Xu S, Cobb M, Skolnik EY. NIK is a new Ste20-related kinase that binds NCK and MEKK1 and activates the SAPK/JNK cascade via a conserved regulatory domain. *EMBO J* 1997; 16:1279–1290.

162. Taylor LK, Wang HR, Erickson RL. Newly identified stress-responsive protein kinases, Krs-1 and Krs-2. *Proc Natl Acad Sci USA* 1996; 93:10099–10104.

163. Schinkmann K, Blenis J. Cloning and characterization of a human STE20-like protein kinase with unusual cofactor requirements. *J Biol Chem* 1997; 272:28,695–28,703.

164.

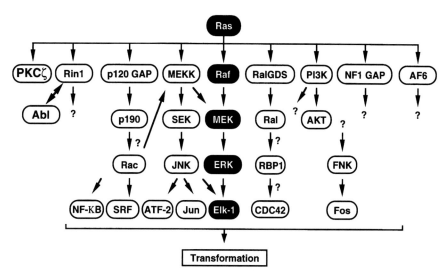

Fig. 2. RAS activates multiple, effector-mediated signaling pathways. Although substantial evidence implicates Raf kinases as key effectors of Ras function, it is clear that Ras mediates its actions by activation of Raf-independent signaling pathways. Candidate effectors of Ras include RalGDS family proteins (RasGDS, RGL, and Rlf/RGL2), P13K family proteins, Ras GAPs, MEKK1, AF6, Rin1, and PKC ζ. Some aspects of signaling via these effectors are indicated. The ability to block Ras transformation by selective intervention at many points downstream of Ras argues that many of these signaling pathways are important for mediating full Ras transformation. For example, inhibition of the Fos, Jun, or NF–κB nuclear transcription factors can impair Ras transformation.

Integrins regulate the interaction of cells with extracellular matrix (ECM) proteins such as collagen, fibronectin, and laminin. The interplay between cells and ECM has biochemical ramifications on the growth properties of cells and indeed may affect the ability of cells to respond to growth factors *(29)*. Recent insights in integrin signaling have uncovered a number of pathways leading to Ras activation *(30)*. As with immuno-receptors, these different pathways represent a variation on the common theme illustrated by RTKs. Although integrins lack intrinsic tyrosine kinase activity, integrin activation leads to an increase in the tyrosine phosphorylation of numerous cellular proteins *(31)*. Analysis of the biochemical events triggered by integrin engagement has uncovered a number of mechanisms for integrin signaling. A subset of integrins activate Ras through direct binding of Shc to tyrosine phosphorylation sites on the b subunits *(32)*. Shc, in turn, becomes phosphorylated and subsequently binds the Grb2–Sos complex. Another subset of integrins activate Shc, and therefore Ras, through an as yet unknown mecha-nism. This appears to be directed in part by sequences in the extracellular domain of the integrins and possibly involves interaction of Shc and integrins with caveolae and/ or other proteins localized within these cellular structures *(33)*. Other integrins can bypass Shc through activation of the focal adhesion kinase (FAK), which can recruit Grb2 directly *(34)*. Although integrin engagement leads to ERK activation, there is some evidence suggesting a Ras-independent component in ERK activation by integrins *(35)*.

G protein-coupled receptors (GPCRs) represent a large family of cell surface receptors that respond to a diverse array of extracellular signals (36). These receptors are linked to a heterotrimeric complex consisting of a GTPase α subunit (Gα) and a βγ heterodimer (Gβγ) that negatively regulates Gα. The inactive GDP-bound Gα subunit is complexed with the Gβγ heterodimer. After ligand activation occurs, the activated GPCR causes GDP/GTP exchange to form the active GTP-complexed Gα subunit and to promote the release of the Gβγ subunits.

Mounting evidence suggests that both Gα and Gβγ perform important signaling functions one of which involves activation of ERKs (36,37). The activation of ERKs by Gα subunits can be either Ras-dependent or Ras-independent depending on the Gα subtype. By contrast, Gβγ appears to activate Ras through a mechanism similar to RTKs. Gβγ expression induces tyrosine phosphorylation of Shc through Src family tyrosine kinases, leading to the formation of a Shc–Grb2–Sos complex, activating Ras. GPCR signaling, however, is further complicated by the discovery of crosstalk with RTKs (38). Activation of some GPCRs, such as the angiotensin II or the lysophosphatidic acid receptors, leads to a ligand-independent activation of RTKs such EGFR and platelet-derived growth factor (PDGF) βR receptor. These findings suggest that GPCRs may activate Ras either directly, most likely through Gβγ, or indirectly through RTK activation.

3.3. Other Adaptors That Link to Ras

The formation of a Shc–Grb2–Sos signaling complex is not the only means by which ligand-stimulated receptors activate Ras proteins. Grb2 can link with activated receptors through alternative means such as binding Shp2 phosphatase, the insulin receptor substrates (IRS-1 and -2), as well as other adaptor proteins that include Lnk and APS (39,40). Other adaptor proteins exist which can also link with Sos as well as additional GEFs. The Nck adaptor protein, which consists of three SH3 domains, followed by a C-terminal SH2 domain, has been shown to activate Sos (41). However, Nck also interacts with additional components implicated in the regulation of Rho family proteins. These Nck interacting proteins include, but are not limited to, the Wiskott-Aldrich syndrome protein (WASP) (42), p21 activated kinase (PAK) (43), and PKN-related kinase (PRK2) (44). The identification of additional Nck-interacting proteins such as caesin kinase 1 (45) and Nap-1 (Nck-associated protein 1) (46) illustrate the diversity of signals emanating from this protein and suggests that Nck may regulate signaling cascades separate from or in addition to Ras (47). Thus, Nck may regulate both Ras and Rho signaling cascades (47). Crk and CrkL are two closely related adaptors that also link to GEFs. Although these proteins can also bind Sos, their predominant function likely involves the interaction with additional exchange factors such as C3G. C3G is most highly related to the Ras GEFs Sos and GRF, and indeed expression of the C3G catalytic domain, can rescue loss of CDC25 function in yeast (48). However, in vitro analysis of exchange activities suggests that C3G is a regulator of Rap1A function (49).

This discussion has focused primarily on the activation of Ras family proteins through activation of GEFs. However, one must keep in mind that another means of activating Ras proteins is to downregulate Ras GAP function. For example, p120 Ras GAP, which has been shown to be a target of RTKs (50). p120 Ras GAP may also be an effector for Ras suggesting a dual function for this protein. Furthermore, the mechanisms of activation of the brain-specific Ras GEFs (RasGRF/CDC25) are distinct from those that lead to activation of SOS. New Ras GEFs exists, such as the hematopoietic cell-specific CXR (R. Kay, unpublished observations), where formation of diacylglycerol or calcium, rather than via Grb2, may lead to its activation.

Finally, regulation of phosphatase activity is also important in regulation of signal cascades as illustrated from signaling by the TCR. Interaction of Shp-1 or -2 with the TCR complex appears to inactivate tyrosine kinases such as ZAP-70, as well as Shc proteins *(51,52)*. The above findings illustrate the complex network of protein–protein interactions which exist to regulate a multitude of signaling cascades, one of which is Ras activation. The relative activation and duration of each of these signals is likely the source of diversity in cellular responses. Additional complexity is derived from the plethora of putative targets of Ras proteins or Ras "effectors."

4. THE Raf/MEK/ERK CASCADE

The process of signal transduction involves the passage of information along a chain or pathway of proteins. Ras proteins exert control over not one but a host of signal transduction pathways whose components and relationships are currently the subject of intense scrutiny. The best characterized Ras signal transduction pathway is the Raf/MEK/ERK MAPK cascade. Critical evidence connecting this kinase cascade with Ras was the observation was that active Ras-GTP, but not inactive Ras-GDP, forms a high-affinity complex with Raf-1 *(53–57)*. This leads to the recruitment of Raf-1 from the cytosol to the plasma membrane. The ability of membrane-targeted forms of Raf-1 to cause transformation argued that the biochemical function of Ras was simply to regulate Raf-1 membrane association *(58,59)*. However, the role of Ras in Raf-1 activation has turned out to be much more intricate than originally hypothesized *(60)*.

Ras was first shown to bind to the N-terminus of Raf-1 at a single site (Raf-1 residues 50–131), designated Ras-binding site 1 (RBS1) *(57)*. However, it has now been determined that Ras actually binds to two sites on Raf-1 *(61–65)*. Ras interaction with RBS1 is essential for plasma membrane localization. Ras then interacts with a second binding site that is localized in the cysteine-rich domain (Raf-CRD) of Raf-1. The Ras–Raf-CRD interaction appears to be dispensable for membrane localization, and instead, is essential for facilitating full activation of Raf-1 *(66,67)*. Our mutagenesis analyses of Raf-CRD support a model where Ras interaction with RBS1 unmasks the normally cryptic Raf-CRD site. Ras interaction with Raf-CRD further stabilizes the association with the plasma membrane, promotes phospholipid interactions with Raf-CRD, which in turn disrupt Raf-CRD interaction with 14-3-3 proteins. In turn the removal of the negative regulatory action of 14-3-3 leads to additional events that promote full activation of Raf-1 *(68)*. The involvement of other protein kinases, heat shock proteins, KSR and other components has been described, but their precise contribution to Raf-1 activation remains to be fully appreciated. Therefore, although not fully understood by any means, the action of Ras on Raf-1 is slowly being revealed and is clearly much more complex than was originally thought. The formation of a signaling complex as a consequence of Ras:Raf interaction is likely to be duplicated in the interaction of Ras with other effectors.

5. Ras ACTIVATION OF Raf-INDEPENDENT SIGNALING PATHWAYS

Although initial studies suggested that the main or even only function of Ras was to activate Raf-1, it is now clear that this is not the case. First, it has been shown that Raf can only activate a subset of the signal transduction pathways that are activated by Ras. For example, Ras activation of the Jun N-terminal kinases (JNKs, also called SAPKs) or p38 MAPKs occurs via a Raf-independent pathway *(69,70)*. Second, activated forms of Raf cannot substitute for Ras in a variety of biological assays. We have observed that activated Ras, but not Raf, can cause transformation of a variety of epithelial cells *(71,72)*. Third, Ras effector domain mutants, that are impaired in Raf-1 interaction, retain transforming activity *(73,74)*. Therefore, non-Raf effector-mediated pathways are very important in mediating many of the biological effects of Ras. Finally, neither R-Ras nor TC21/R-Ras2 are activators of the Raf/ERK pathway *(75,76)*. Therefore, the ability of constitutively activated mutants of these two Ras-related to cause tumorigenic transformation provides further support for the contribution of Raf-independent pathways in promoting Ras transformation.

The realization that Raf kinases are not the sole targets of Ras paralleled the discovery of other proteins that could interact with Ras in the same way as Raf-1. Like Raf, their association with Ras requires an intact Ras effector domain. Mutagenesis of the Ras effector domain (residues 25–45) leads to concomitant loss of effector binding and transforming activity *(1,77)*. Moreover, they also show preferential binding to active Ras-GTP. The precise contribution of these candidate effectors remains to be determined. In contrast to Raf, no clear genetic validation of any non-Raf mammalian effectors has been described. The genetic, biochemical, and biological activity of Raf-1 has been sufficiently overt that its validation as a Ras effector, and defining the signaling pathways emanating from it, has been a relatively simple task. The actions of other potential Ras effectors are more subtle, and consequently, elucidating their contributions to Ras function, and defining their signaling pathways, is proving more elusive. However, progress has been made with some effectors and more are likely to be found.

5.1. More Ras Effectors?

Although p120 GAP and NF1/neurofibromin clearly serve as negative regulators of Ras function *(15)*, there is also evidence that they may also serve a second role as Ras effectors. For example, Tocque and colleagues found that an antibody directed against the SH3 domain of p120 GAP blocked Ras-induced germinal vesicle breakdown, but not ERK activation, when assayed in *Xenopus* oocytes *(78)*. Similarly, coexpression of an N-terminal fragment of p120 GAP was shown to block oncogenic H-Ras, but not Raf, transforming activity *(79)*. Evidence for NF1 as a Ras effector is less compelling and is based largely on a detection of NF1 function beyond its role as a Ras GTPase stimulator. For example, no elevation in Ras-GTP was seen in a number of NF1-deficient tumors *(80–82)*, yet introduction of full length NF1 into these cells resulted in severe reductions in growth *(83)*. These observations suggest that a loss of NF1 function, other than as a Ras GTPase stimulator, contributes to the development of these tumors.

Strong support has been seen for PI3K family proteins as important effectors of Ras. PI3K is a lipid kinase that phosphorylates phosphoinositides at the 3′ position of the inositol ring and leads to the formation of the second messenger phosphatidylinositol 3,4,5-triphosphate *(84)*. PI3K is composed of a p110 catalytic and a p85 regulator subunit and both are members of a family of related proteins. Recombinant p110 (α and β) showed high-affinity interaction with the GTP-bound form of recombinant Ras through the Ras effector domain *(85,86)*. Activated Ras, but not Raf, overexpression in COS cells resulted in a significant induction of inositol phosphates demonstrating the convergence of Raf and PI3K pathways at the level of Ras. Taken together, these observations strongly suggest the involvement of PI3K as a downstream effector of Ras function *(85)*. R-Ras, but not Rap1A, has also been shown to bind to and activate PI3K *(87)*.

One downstream target of activated PI3K is protein kinase B (PKB; also Akt) *(87–89)*. A recent study using Ras effector domain mutants implicated the PI3K/PKB in oncogenic Ras suppression of Myc-induced apoptosis in Rat-1 fibroblasts, whereas Ras activation of the Raf>MEK>ERK pathway was found to promote the Myc apoptotic response *(90)*. Since oncogenic Ras also potentiated the apoptotic response, the Raf-mediated pathway may be dominant over the PI3K pathway.

The Ral guanine nucleotide exchange factor (RalGDS) and two closely related proteins (RGL and RGL2/Rlf) represent intriguing candidate effectors of Ras that may link Ras with other Ras-related proteins. Members of this family have been identified repeatedly by yeast two-hybrid library screening searches for candidate effectors of Ras and Ras-related proteins (Rap, R-Ras, and TC21/R-Ras2) *(91–95)*. Ras association with RalGDS has also been observed when overexpressed in COS cells *(96)*. Transient expression assays in COS cells showed that Ras, but not Rap1A or R-Ras, enhanced the Ral GEF activity of RalGDS *(12)*. Although constitutively activated Ral alone does not cause transformed foci, one study reported that its coexpression enhanced Ras transformation, whereas dominant negative Ral impaired Ras focus-forming activity *(12)*. Coexpression of RalGDS cooperated synergistically with activated Raf-1 to induce transformation of NIH 3T3 cells *(97)*. In summary, there is intriguing, but very limited, evidence for RalGDS function as a Ras effector.

AF-6 shows high degree of sequence similarity to *Drosophila* Canoe, which is assumed to function in signaling pathways downstream from the Notch receptor, acting as a regulator of cellular differentiation *(98)*. The p180 AF-6 protein was also identified independently as a fusion partner of the MLL protein associated with chromosome translocation events in human leukemias *(99)*. The MLL/AF-6 chimeric protein is the gene product of a reciprocal translocation t(6;11)(q27;q23) associated with a subset of human acute lymphoblastic leukemias *(99–101)*. In vitro analyses showed that the N-terminal domains of AF-6 and Canoe interacted specifically with GTP-bound form of Ras and this interaction interferes the binding of Ras with Raf *(102)*. AF-6 appears to be expressed in a variety of tissues. Presently, a function for AF-6 has not been determined. However, limited sequence homology was observed between AF-6 and proteins that may be involved in signal transduction at special cell–cell junctions.

Rin1 was initially identified as a Ras-interfering protein in a genetic screen in yeast and found to exhibit properties of a Ras effector *(103)*. Although Rin1 can complex with Ras-GTP in mammalian cells, a role for Rin1 in Ras function remains to be determined *(104)*. Subsequent studies showed that Rin1 could interact with Abl and BCR-Abl through a domain distinct from the Ras-binding domain *(104,105)*. Thus, Rin1 may coordinate signals from Ras and Abl.

Other candidate Ras effectors include MEKK1, which activates the SEK/JNK MAPK cascade. The ζ isoform of protein kinase C (PKCζ) has also been implicated as a Ras effector. First, PKCζ was required for Ras-induced maturation in *Xenopus* oocytes *(106)* and serum-stimulated mitogenic signaling in mammalian cells *(107)*. Second, the regulatory N-terminal fragment of PKCζ showed preferential binding to Ras-GTP in vitro and a peptide corresponding to Ras residues 17–44 blocked this interaction *(108)*.

In summary, although Raf remains the key effector of Ras function, the contributions of other effectors are beginning to emerge. In addition to defining their contributions to Ras function, other key questions remain to be answered. For example, how is interaction of Ras with multiple effectors regulated? Do Ras-related proteins use effectors shared with Ras? Will effector utilization be distinct in different cell types? Answers to some of these questions are certain to be approached in the coming years.

6. LINKING Ras TO Rho FAMILY PROTEINS

While it is clear that Ras must utilize effectors other than Raf, the precise nature of these Raf-independent pathways remains to be fully delineated *(1,77)*. However, several lines of evidence have implicated specific Rho family proteins as key downstream mediators of Ras transformation. The Rho family of small GTPases constitute a major branch of the Ras superfamily of proteins. To date, at least 14 mammalian members have been identified, with RhoA, Rac1, and CDC42 being the most heavily studied *(109–111)*. Their important roles in regulating actin cytoskeletal organization, gene expression, and cell cycle progression argue that their contributions to oncogenic Ras transformation will be significant. This section summarizes the evidence for a Ras connection with Rho family proteins and discusses our current understanding of how they may contribute to oncogenic Ras-mediated transformation.

Key evidence for the involvement of Rho family members in mediating oncogenic Ras function came from microinjection studies in Swiss 3T3 cells by Hall and colleagues *(112,113)*. These studies demonstrated that oncogenic Ras activated Rac1, which in turn activated RhoA, as measured by changes in actin cytoskeletal organization. Activated Rac stimulated the formation of lamellipodia to cause membrane ruffling and to stimulate RhoA function. Activated RhoA, in turn, controls the formation of actin stress fibers and focal adhesions. Thus, in addition to the activation of kinase cascades, oncogenic Ras also activates a cascade of small GTPases. Further evidence of a connection between Ras and Rho family proteins was also provided by genetic studies of Ras function in *S. pombe (114)*.

The function of five mammalian Rho family proteins has been shown to be important for oncogenic Ras transforming activity. Three experimental approaches have been applied to support key contributions of RhoA, RhoB, Rac1, Cdc42, and RhoG to Ras transformation *(115–121)*. First, coexpression of dominant negative mutants [equivalent to the Ras(17N) mutant] of each Rho family protein caused a significant, although incomplete, reduction in oncogenic Ras focus-forming activity when analyzed in rodent fibroblasts. Second, co-expression of constitutively activated versions of each Rho family GTPase with activated Raf-1 mutants showed cooperative and synergistic focus-forming activity. Finally, as described above, constitutively activated mutants caused growth transformation of NIH 3T3 or Rat1 rodent fibroblasts. Taken together, these observations support a model in which oncogenic Ras causes constitutive activation of specific Rho family proteins, which in turn activate a spectrum of functions that contribute to full Ras transforming activity. However, it should be emphasized that a demonstration that Ras-transformed cells exhibit constitutively elevated GTP-bound levels of a specific Rho family protein has not been determined. Thus, which, if any, of the known Rho family proteins are clearly targeted by oncogenic Ras remains to be established.

The effectors by which Ras feeds into Rho family proteins still defies full definition. Indeed, multiple effectors may promote independent links with each Rho family protein. One possible connection is via p120 GAP association with a Rho GAP, p190 Rho GAP. A second potential connection is via PI3K. PI3K products can regulate Vav and Sos *(122,123)*, both members of the Dbl family of Rho GEFs *(124)*. It seems likely that there may be other unidentified Ras effectors that lead to Rho signaling. In *S. pombe*, the homolog of Ras binds directly to an exchange factor for a Dbl family protein, Scd1, that then serves to activate the yeast CDC42 homolog. Whether such a mammalian counterpart for Scd1 exists remains to be identified. Finally, a RalGDS connection with Ral, which then regulates a Ral-GTP binding protein that exhibits GAP activity for CDC42 and Rac (RalBP1/RLIP1/RIP1) provides yet another possible link between small GTPases *(125)*. Since prevailing evidence suggests that Ras linkage with each Rho family protein may be distinct, rather than through a GTPase cascade, multiple effectors are likely to be involved.

7. CONCLUSIONS AND FUTURE QUESTIONS

In closing, our understanding of the role of Ras in cellular biology has evolved from the simplistic assumption that Ras is merely a plasma membrane escort for Raf-1 to the realization that Ras proteins act at a signal transduction node. Multiple signals feed into Ras and multiple signals feed out. These signaling pathways are not isolated but are capable of cooperating with each other such that the net biological function of Ras reflects the sum of the synergies of all the diverse pathways activated. We are clearly in the early days of fully appreciating the complexities of Ras signaling pathways. Further complexity is certain to be demonstrated and a process of revising or discarding our current notions will probably follow.

Targeting components of the Ras signaling pathways has been proposed as one approach for the development of anti-Ras drugs for cancer treatment *(126)*. The realization that our comprehension of the complexities of Ras signaling is quite limited, and simple-minded, may discourage any serious consideration that this is a fruitful direction for drug discovery at this time. Thus, there are some who are of the opinion that such efforts are premature and must await a complete knowledge of this signaling circuitry. However, evidence that intervention of Ras signaling at multiple points can significantly impact the ability of Ras to cause cellular transformation argues that a full unveiling of all the complexities of Ras signaling will not be required before successful targeting of Ras signaling pathways for drug discovery can be achieved. Ongoing development of drugs that target specific downstream components of Ras signaling (e.g., MEK inhibitors) may determine whether this optimistic outlook will prevail.

ACKNOWLEDGMENTS

We thank Jennifer Parrish for excellent assistance in the preparation of the text, references, and figures. Our studies are supported by grants from the National Institutes of Health (CA72644) (to G.J.C.), (CA76570) (to J.P.O.), and (CA42978, CA52072, CA55008 and CA67771) (to C.J.D.). G.J.C. is the recipient of DOD Career Development Award DAMD17-97-1-7050.

REFERENCES

1. Khosravi-Far R, Campbell S, Rossman KL, Der CJ. Increasing complexity of Ras signal transduction: Involvement of Rho family proteins. *Adv Cancer Res* 1998; 72:57–107.
2. Matsumoto K, Asano T, Endo T. Novel small GTPase M-Ras participates in reorganization of actin cytoskeleton. *Oncogene* 1997; 15:2409–2418.
3. Kimmelman A, Tolkacheva T, Lorinzi MV, Osada M, Chan AM-L. Identification and characterization of R-*ras*3: A novel member of the *RAS* gene family with a non-ubiquitous pattern of tissue distribution. *Oncogene* 1997; 15:2675–2686.
4. Barbacid M. *ras* genes. *Annu Rev Biochem* 1987; 56:779–827.
5. Bos JL. *ras* oncogenes in human cancer: A review. *Cancer Res* 1989; 49:4682–4689.
6. Clark GJ, Der CJ, Dickey BF, Birnbaumer L, editors. GTPases, in *Biology* Vol I, 18: *Oncogenic Activation of* Ras *Proteins*. Springer-Verlag, Berlin, 1993; pp. 259–288.
7. Graham SM, Cox AD, Drivas G, Rush MR, D'Eustachio P, Der CJ. Aberrant function of the Ras-related TC21/R-Ras2 protein triggers malignant transformation. *Mol Cell Biol* 1994; 14:4108–4115.
8. Cox AD, Brtva TR, Lowe DG, Der CJ. R-Ras induces malignant, but not morphologic, transformation of NIH3T3 cells. *Oncogene* 1994; 9:3281–3288.
9. Chan AM-L, Miki T, Meyers KA, Aaronson SA. A human oncogene of the *ras* superfamily unmasked by expression cDNA cloning. *Proc Natl Acad Sci USA* 1994; 91:7558–7562.
10. Saez R, Chan AM-L, Miki T, Aaronson SA. Oncogenic activation of human R-*ras* by point mutations analogous to those of prototype H-*ras* oncogenes. *Oncogene* 1994; 9:2977–2982.
11. Kitayama H, Sugimoto Y, Matsuzaki T, Ikawa Y, Noda M. A *ras*-related gene with transformation suppressor activity. *Cell* 1989; 56:77–84.
12. Urano T, Emkey R, Feig LA. Ral-GTPases mediate a distinct downstream signaling pathway from Ras that facilitates cellular transformation. *EMBO J* 1996; 15:810–816.
13. Egan SE, Weinberg RA. The pathway to signal achievement. *Nature* 1993; 365:781–783.
14. Bourne HR, Sanders DA, McCormick F. The GTPase superfamily: Conserved structure and molecular mechanism. *Nature* 1990; 349:117–126.
15. Boguski MS, McCormick F. Proteins regulating Ras and its relatives. *Nature* 1993; 366:643–654.
16. Quilliam LA, Khosravi-Far R, Huff SY, Der CJ. Activators of Ras superfamily proteins. *BioEssays* 1995; 17:395–404.
17. Tong L, de Vos AM, Milburn MV, Jancarik J, Noguchi S, Nishimura S, Miura K, Ohtsuka E, Kim S-H. Structural differences between a RAS oncogene protein and the normal protein. *Nature* 1989; 337:90–93.
18. Milburn MV, Tong L, DeVos AM, Brunger A, Yamaizumi Z, Nishimura S, Kim S-H.

Molecular switch for signal transduction: Structural differences between active and inactive forms of protooncogenic *ras* proteins. *Science* 1990; 247:939–945.

19. Krengel U, Schlichting L, Scherer A, Schumann R, Frech M, John J, Kabsch W, Pai EF, Wittinghofer A. Three-dimensional structures of H-*ras* p21 mutants: Molecular basis for their inability to function as signal switch molecules. *Cell* 1990; 62:539–548.

20. Khosravi-Far R, Der CJ. The Ras signal transduction pathway. *Cancer Metastasis Rev* 1994; 13:67–89.

21. Pawson T. Protein modules and signalling networks. *Nature* 1995; 373:573–580.

22. Bonfini L, Migliaccio E, Pelicci G, Lanfrancone L, Pelicci PG. Not all Shc's roads lead to Ras. *Trends Biochem Sci* 1996; 21:259–261.

23. Gotoh N, Tojo A, Muroya K, Hashimoto Y, Hattori S, Nakamura S, Takenawa T, Yazaki Y, Shibuya M. Epidermal growth factor-receptor mutant lacking the autophosphorylation sites induces phosphorylation of Shc protein and Shc-Grb2/ASH association and retains mitogenic activity. *Proc Natl Acad Sci USA* 1994; 91:167–171.

24. Li N, Schlessinger J, Margolis B. Autophosphorylation mutants of the EGF-receptor signal through auxiliary mechanisms involving SH2 domain proteins. *Oncogene* 1997; 9:3457–3465.

25. Meyer S, LaBudda K, McGlade J, Hayman MJ. Analysis of the role of the Shc and Grb2 proteins in signal transduction by the v-ErbB protein. *Mol Cell Biol* 1994; 14:3253–3263.

26. Soler C, Alvarez CV, Beguinot L, Carpenter G. Potent SHC tyrosine phosphorylation by epidermal growth factor at low receptor density or in the absence of receptor autophosphorylation sites. *Oncogene* 1994; 9:2207–2215.

27. Alberola-Ila J, Takaki S, Kerner JD, Perlmutter RM. Differential signaling by lymphocyte antigen receptors. *Ann Rev Immunol* 1997; 15:125–154.

28. Weiss A. T cell antigen receptor signal transduction: A tale of tails and cytoplasmic protein-tyrosine kinases. *Cell* 1993; 73:209–212.

29. Mainiero F, Murgia C, Wary KK, Curatola AM, Pepe A, Blumemberg M, Westwick JK, Der CJ, Giancotti FG. The coupling of alpha6beta4 integrin to Ras-MAP kinase pathways mediated by Shc controls keratinocyte proliferation. *EMBO J* 1997; 16:2365–2375.

30. Aplin AE, Howe A, Alahari SK, Juliano RL. Signal transduction and signal modulation by cell adhesion receptors: The role of integrin, cadherin, Ig-CAMs and selectins. *Pharm Rev* 1998; (in press).

31. Clark EA, Brugge JS. Integrins and signal transduction pathways: The road taken. *Science* 1995; 268:233–239.

32. Mainiero F, Pepe A, Wary KK, Spinardi L, Mohammadi M, Schlessinger J, Giancotti FG. Signal transduction by the 6 4 integrin: Distinct 4 subunit sites mediate recruitment of Shc/Grb2 and association with the cytoskeleton of hermidesmosomes. *EMBO J* 1995; 14:4470–4481.

33. Wary KK, Mainiero F, Isakoff SJ, Marcantonio EE, Giancotti FG. The adaptor protein Shc couples a class of integrins to the control of cell cycle progression. *Cell* 1996; 87:733–743.

34. Hanks SK, Polte TR. Signaling through focal adhesion kinase. *BioEssays* 1997; 19:137–145.

35. Chen Q, Lin TH, Der CJ, Juliano RL. Integrin-mediated activation of MEK and mitogen-activated protein kinase is independent of Ras. *J Biol Chem* 1996; 271:18,122–18,127.

36. Gutkind JS. The pathways connecting G protein-coupled receptors to the nucleus through divergent mitogen-activated protein kinase cascades. *J Biol Chem* 1998; 273:1839–1842.

37. van Biesen T, Luttrell LM, Hawes BE, Lefkowitz RJ. Mitogenic signaling via G protein-coupled receptors. *Endocrine Rev* 1996; 17:698–714.

38. Daub H, Weiss FU, Wallasch C, Ullrich A. Role of transactivation of the EGF receptor in signaling by G-protein-coupled receptors. *Nature* 1996; 557–560.

39. Huang X, Li Y, Tanaka K, Moore G, Hayashi JI. Cloning and characterization of Lnk, a signal transduction protein that linked T-cell receptor activation signal to phospholipase

Cgamma$_1$, Grb2 and phosphatidylinositol 3-kinase. *Proc Natl Acad Sci USA* 1995; 92:11,618–11,622.

40. Yokouchi M, Suzuki R, Masuhara M, Komiya S, Inoue A, Yoshimura A. Cloning and characterization of APS, as adaptor molecule containing PH and SH2 domains that is tyrosine phosphorylated upon B-cell receptor stimulation. *Oncogene* 1997; 15:7–15.

41. Hu Q, Milfay D, Williams LT. Binding of NCK to SOS and activation of *ras*-dependent gene expression. *Mol Cell Biol* 1995; 15:1169–1174.

42. Rivero-Lezcano OM, Marcilla A, Sameshima JH, Robbins KC. Wiskott-Aldrich Syndrome protein physically associates with Nck through Src homology 3 domains. *Mol Cell Biol* 1995; 15:5725–5731.

43. Sells MA, Knaus UG, Bagrodia S, Ambrose DM, Bokoch GM, Chernoff J. Human p21-activated kinase (Pak1) regulates actin organization in mammalian cells. *Curr Biol* 1997; 7:202–210.

44. Quilliam LA, Lambert QT, Westwick JK, Mickelson-Young LA, Sparks AB, Kay BK, Jenkins NA, Gilbert DJ, Copeland NG, Der CJ. Isolation of a NCK-associated kinase, PRK2, and SH3-binding protein and potential effector of Rho protein signaling. *J Biol Chem* 1996; 271:28,772–28,776.

45. Lussier G, Larose L. A casein kinase I activity is constitutively associated with Nck. *J Biol Chem* 1997; 272:2688–2694.

46. Kitamura T, Kitamura Y, Yonezawa K, Totty NF, Gout I, Hara K, Waterfield MD, Sakaue M, Ogawa W, Kasuga M. Molecular cloning of p125Nap1, a protein that associates with an SH3 domain of Nck. *Biochem Biophys Res Commun* 1996; 219:509–514.

47. Birge RB, Knudsen BS, Besser D, Hanafusa H. SH2 and SH3-containing adaptor proteins: Redundant of independent mediators of intracellular signal transduction. *Genes Cells* 1996; 1:595–613.

48. Tanaka S, Morishita T, Hashimoto Y, Hattori S, Nakamura S, Shibuya M, Matuoka K, Takenawa T, Kurata T, Nagashima K, Matsuda M. C3G, a guanine nucleotide-releasing protein expressed ubiquitously, binds to the Src homology 3 domains of CRK and GRB2/ ASH proteins. *Proc Natl Acad Sci USA* 1994; 91:3443–3447.

49. Gotoh T, Hattori S, Nakamura S, Kitayama H, Noda M, Takai Y, Kaibuchi K, Matsui H, Hatase O, Takahashi H, Kurata T, Matsuda M. Identification of Rap1 as a target for the Crk SH3 domain-binding guanine nucleotide-releasing factor C3G. *Mol Cell Biol* 1995; 15:6746–6753.

50. Kazlauskas A, Ellis C, Pawson T, Cooper JA. Binding of GAP to activated PDGF receptors. *Science* 1990; 247:1578–1581.

51. Plas DR, Johnson R, Pingel JT, Matthews RJ, Dalton M, Roy G, Chan SC, Thomas ML. Direct regulation of ZAP-70 by Shp-1 in T cell antigen receptor signaling. *Science* 1996; 272:1173–1176.

52. Marengére LEM, Waterhouse P, Duncan GS, Mittrücker H-W, Feng G-S, Mak TW. Regulation of T cell receptor signaling by tyrosine phosphatase SYP association with CTLA-4. *Science* 1996; 272:1170–1173.

53. Van Aelst L, Barr M, Marcus S, Polverino A, Wigler M. Complex formation between RAS and RAF and other protein kinases. *Proc Natl Acad Sci USA* 1993; 90:6213–6217.

54. Moodie SA, Willumsen BM, Weber MJ, Wolfman A. Complexes of Ras-GTP with Raf-1 and mitogen-activated protein kinase kinase. *Science* 1993; 260:1658–1661.

55. Zhang X, Settleman J, Kyriakis JM, Takeuchi-Suzuki E, Elledge SJ, Marshall MS, Bruder JT, Rapp UR, Avruch J. Normal and oncogenic p21^{ras} proteins bind to the amino-terminal regulatory domain of c-Raf-1. *Nature* 1993; 364:308–313.

56. Warne PH, Viciana PR, Downward J. Direct interaction of Ras and the amino-terminal region of Raf-1 *in vitro. Nature* 1993; 364:352–355.

57. Vojtek AB, Hollenberg SM, Cooper JA. Mammalian Ras interacts directly with the serine/ threonine kinase Raf. *Cell* 1993; 74:205–214.

58. Leevers SJ, Paterson HF, Marshall CJ. Requirement for Ras in Raf activation is overcome by targeting Raf to the plasma membrane. *Nature* 1994; 369:411–414.

59. Stokoe D, Macdonald SG, Cadwallader K, Symons M, Hancock JF. Activation of Raf as a result of recruitment to the plasma membrane. *Science* 1994; 264:1463–1467.

60. Hirsch DD, Stork PJS. Mitogen-activated protein kinase phosphatases inactivate stress-activated protein kinase pathways in vivo. *J Biol Chem* 1997; 272:4568–4575.

61. Brtva TR, Drugan JK, Ghosh S, Terrell RS, Campbell-Burk S, Bell RM, Der CJ. Two distinct Raf domains mediate interaction with Ras. *J Biol Chem* 1995; 270:9809–9812.

62. Drugan JK, Khosravi-Far R, White MA, Der CJ, Sung Y-J, Huang Y-W, Campbell SL. Ras interaction with two distinct binding domains in Raf-1 may be required for Ras transformation. *J Biol Chem* 1996; 271:233–237.

63. Clark GJ, Drugan JK, Terrell RS, Bradham C, Der CJ, Bell RM, Campbell-Burk S. Peptides containing a consensus Ras binding sequence from Raf-1 and NF1-GAP inhibit Ras function. *Proc Natl Acad Sci USA* 1995; 93:1577–1581.

64. Luo Z, Diaz B, Marshall MS, Avruch J. An intact Raf zinc finger is required for optimal binding to processed Ras and for Ras-dependent Raf activation in situ. *Mol Cell Biol* 1997; 17:46–53.

65. Hu C, Kariya K, Tamada M, Akasaka K, Shirouzu M, Yokoyama S, Kataoka T. Cysteine-rich region of Raf-1 interacts with activator domain of post-translationally modified Ha-Ras. *J Biol Chem* 1995; 270:30,274–30,277.

66. Roy S, Lane A, Yan J, McPherson R, Hancock JF. Activity of plasma membrane-recruited Raf-1 is regulated by Ras via the Raf zinc finger. *J Biol Chem* 1997; 272:20,139–20,145.

67. Mineo C, Anderson RGW, White MA. Physical association with Ras enhances activation of membrane-bound Raf (RafCAAX). *J Biol Chem* 1997; 272:10,345–10,348.

68. Clark GJ, Drugan JK, Rossman KL, Carpenter JW, Rogers-Graham K, Fu H, Der CJ, Campbell SL. 14-3-3 zeta negatively regulates Raf-1 activity by interactions with the Raf-1 cysteine-rich domain. *J Biol Chem* 1997; 272:20,990–20,993.

69. Minden A, Lin A, McMahon M, Lange-Carter C, Derijard B, Davis RJ, Johnson GL, Karin M. Differential activation of ERK and JNK mitogen-activated protein kinases by Raf-1 and MEKK. *Science* 1994; 266:1719–1723.

70. Olson MF, Ashworth A, Hall A. An essential role for Rho, Rac and Cdc42 GTPases in cell cycle progression through G_1. *Science* 1995; 269:1270–1272.

71. Oldham SM, Clark GJ, Gangarosa LM, Coffey RJ Jr, Der CJ. Activation of the Raf-1/MAP kinase cascade is not sufficient for Ras transformation of RIE-1 epithelial cells. *Proc Natl Acad Sci USA* 1996; 93:6924–6928.

72. Gangarosa LM, Sizemore N, Graves-Deal R, Oldham SM, Der CJ, Coffey RJ. A Raf-independent epidermal growth factor receptor autocrine loop is necessary for Ras transformation of rat intestinal epithelial cells. *J Biol Chem* 1997; 272:18,926–18,931.

73. White MA, Nicolette C, Minden A, Polverino A, Van Aelst L, Karin M, Wigler MH. Multiple Ras functions can contribute to mammalian cell transformation. *Cell* 1995; 80:533–541.

74. Khosravi-Far R, White MA, Westwick JK, Solski PA, Chrzanowska-Wodnicka M, Van Aelst L, Wigler MH, Der CJ. Oncogenic Ras activation of Raf/MAP kinase-independent pathways is sufficient to cause tumorigenic transformation. *Mol Cell Biol* 1996; 16:3923–3933.

75. Graham SM, Vojtek AB, Huff SY, Cox AD, Clark GJ, Cooper JA, Der CJ. TC21 causes transformation by Raf-independent signaling pathways. *Mol Cell Biol* 1996; 16:6132–6140.

76. Huff SY, Quilliam LA, Cox AD, Der CJ. R-Ras is regulated by activators and effectors distinct from those that control Ras function. *Oncogene* 1997; 14:133–143.

77. Marshall CJ. Ras effectors. *Curr Opin Cell Biol* 1996; 8:197–204.

78. Pomerance M, Thang MN, Tocque B, Pierre M. The Ras-GTPase-activating protein SH3 domain is required for Cdc2 activation and mos induction by oncogenic Ras in *Xenopus*

oocytes independently of mitogen-activated protein kinase activation. *Mol Cell Biol* 1996; 16:3179–3186.

79. Clark GJ, Quilliam LA, Hisaka MM, Der CJ. Differential antagonism of Ras biological activity by catalytic and Src homology domains of Ras GTPase activation protein. *Proc Natl Acad Sci USA* 1993; 90:4887–4891.

80. Andersen LB, Fountain JW, Gutmann DH, Tarlé SA, Glover TW, Dracopoli NC, Housman DE, Collins FS. Mutations in the neurofibromatosis 1 gene in sporadic malignant melanoma cell lines. *Nature Genet* 1993; 3:118–126.

81. The I, Murthy AE, Hannigan GE, Jacoby LB, Menon AG, Gusella JF, Bernards A. Neurofibromatosis type 1 gene mutations in neuroblastoma. *Nature Genet* 1993; 3:62–66.

82. Johnson MR, Look AT, DeClue JE, Valentine MB, Lowy DR. Inactivation of the *NF1* gene in human melanoma and neuroblastoma cell lines without impaired regulation of GTP-Ras. *Proc Natl Acad Sci USA* 1993; 90:5539–5543.

83. Johnson MR, DeClue JE, Felzmann S, Vass WC, Xu G, White R, Lowy DR. Neurofibromin can inhibit Ras-dependent growth by a mechanism independent of its GTPase-accelerating function. *Mol Cell Biol* 1994; 14:641–645.

84. Carpenter CL, Cantley LC. Phosphoinositide kinases. *Curr Opin Cell Biol* 1996; 8:153–158.

85. Rodriguez-Viciana P, Warne PH, Dhand R, Vanhaesebroeck B, Gout I, Fry MJ, Waterfield MD, Downward J. Phosphatidylinositol-3-OH kinase as a direct target of Ras. *Nature* 1994; 370:527–532.

86. Rodriguez-Viciana P, Warne PH, Vanhaesebroeck B, Waterfield MD, Downward J. Activation of phosphoinositide 3-kinase by interaction with Ras and by point mutation. *EMBO J* 1996; 15:2442–2451.

87. Marte BM, Rodriguez-Viciana P, Wennström S, Warne PH, Downward J. R-Ras can activate the phosphoinositide 3-kinase but not the MAP kinase arm of the Ras effector pathways. *Curr Biol* 1996; 7:63–70.

88. Franke TF, Ynag S-I, Chan TO, Datta K, Kazlauskas A, Morrison DK, Kaplan DR, Tsichlis PN. The protein kinase encoded by the *Akt* proto-oncogene is a target of the PDGF-activated phosphatidylinositol 3-kinase. *Cell* 1995; 81:727–736.

89. Klippel A, Reinhard C, Kavanaugh M, Apell G, Escobedo M-A, Williams LT. Membrane localization phosphatidylinositol 3-kinase is sufficient to activate multiple signal-transducing kinase pathways. *Mol Cell Biol* 1996; 16:4117–4127.

90. Kauffmann-Zeh A, Rodriguez-Viciana P, Ulrich E, Gilbert C, Coffer P, Downward J, Evan G. Suppression of c-Myc-induced apoptosis by Ras signalling through PI(3)K and PKB. *Nature* 1997; 385:544–548.

91. Kikuchi A, Demo SD, Ye Z-H, Chen Y-W, Williams LT. ralGDS family members interact with the effector loop of *ras* p21. *Mol Cell Biol* 1994; 14:7483–7491.

92. Hofer F, Fields S, Schneider C, Martin GS. Activated Ras interacts with the Ral guanine nucleotide dissociation stimulator. *Proc Natl Acad Sci USA* 1994; 91:11,089–11,093.

93. Spaargaren M, Bischoff JR. Identification of the guanine nucleotide dissociation stimulator for Ral as a putative effector molecule of R-ras, H-ras, K-ras and Rap. *Proc Natl Acad Sci USA* 1994; 91:12,609–12,613.

94. Peterson SN, Trabalzini L, Brtva TR, Fischer T, Altschuler DL, Martelli P, Lapetina EG, Der CJ, White II GC. Identification of a novel RalGDS-related protein as a candidate effector for Ras and Rap1. *J Biol Chem* 1996; 271:29,903–29,908.

95. López-Barahona M, Bustelo XR, Barbacid M. The TC21 oncoprotein interacts with the Ral guanosine nucleotide dissociation factor. *Oncogene* 1996; 12:463–470.

96. Kikuchi A, Williams LT. Regulation of interaction of *ras* p21 with RalGDS and Raf-1 by cyclic AMP-dependent protein kinase. *J Biol Chem* 1996; 271:588–594.

97. White MA, Vale T, Camonis JH, Schaefer E, Wigler MH. A role for the Ral guanine

nucleotide dissociation stimulator in mediating Ras-induced transformation. *J Biol Chem* 1996; 271:16,439–16,442.

98. Hunter T. Oncoprotein networks. *Cell* 1997; 88:333–346.
99. Prasad R, Gu Y, Alder H, Nakamura T, Canaani O, Saito H, Huebner K, Gale RP, Nowell PC, Kuriyama K, Miyazaki Y, Croce CM, Canaani E. Cloning of the *ALL-1* fusion partner, the *AF-6* gene, involved in acute myeloid leukemias with the t(6;11) chromosome translocation. *Cancer Res* 1993; 53:5624–5628.
100. Tanabe S, Zeleznik-Le NJ, Kobayashi H, Vignon C, Espinosa RI, LeBeau MM, Thirman MJ, Rowley JD. Analysis of the t(6;11)(q27;q23) in leukemia shows a consistent breakpoint in *AF6* in three patients and in the ML-2 cell line. *Genes Chromosom Cancer* 1996; 15:206–216.
101. Taki T, Hayashi Y, Taniwaki M, Seto M, Ueda R, Hanada R, Suzukawa K, Yokota J, Morishita K. Fusion of the *MLL* gene with two different genes, *AF*-6 and *AF*-5, by a complex translocation involving chromosomes 5, 6, 8 and 11 in infant leukemia. *Oncogene* 1996; 13:2121–2130.
102. Kuriyama M, Harada N, Kuroda S, Yamamoto T, Nakafuku M, Iwamatsu A, Yamamoto D, Prasad R, Croce C, Canaani E, Kaibuchi K. Identification of AF-6 and Canoe as putative targets for Ras. *J Biol Chem* 1996; 271:607–610.
103. Han L, Colicelli J. A human protein selected for interference with Ras function interacts directly with Ras and competes with Raf1. *Mol Cell Biol* 1995; 15:1318–1323.
104. Han L, Wong D, Dhaka A, Afar D, White M, Xie W, Herschman H, Witte O, Colicelli J. Protein binding and signaling properties of RIN1 suggest a unique effector function. *Proc Natl Acad Sci USA* 1997; 94:4954–4959.
105. Afar DE, Han L, McLaughlin J, Wong S, Dhada A, Parmar K, Rosenberg N, Witte ON, Colicelli J. *Immunity* 1997; 6:773–782.
106. Dominguez I, Diaz-Meco MT, Municio MM, Berra E, Garcìa de Herreros A, Cornet ME, Sanz L, Moscat J. Evidence for a role of protein kinase C zeta subspecies in maturation of *Xenopus laevis* oocytes. *Mol Cell Biol* 1992; 12:3776–3783.
107. Berra E, Diaz-Meco MT, Dominguez I, Municio MM, Sanz L, Lozano J, Chapkin RS, Moscat J. Protein kinase C zeta isoform is critical for mitogenic signal transduction. *Cell* 1993; 74:555–563.
108. Diaz-Meco MT, Lozano J, Municio MM, Berra E, Frutos S, S., Sanz L, Moscat J. Evidence for the *in vitro* and *in vivo* interaction of Ras with protein kinase Cζ. *J Biol Chem* 1994; 269:31,706–31,710.
109. Van Aelst L, D'Souza-Schorey C. Rho GTPases and signaling networks. *Genes Dev* 1997; 11:2295–2322.
110. Hall A. Rho GTPases and the actin cytoskeleton. *Science* 1998; 279:509–514.
111. Zohn IE, Campbell S, Khosravi-Far R, Rossman K, Der CJ. Rho family proteins and Ras transfomation: The RHOad least traveled gets congested. *Oncogene* 1998; (in press).
112. Ridley AJ, Paterson HF, Johnston CL, Diekmann D, Hall A. The small GTP-binding protein rac regulates growth factor-induced membrane ruffling. *Cell* 1992; 70:401–410.
113. Ridley AJ, Hall A. The small GTP-binding protein rho regulates the assembly of focal adhesions and actin stress fibers in response to growth factors. *Cell* 1992; 70:389–399.
114. Chang EC, Barr M, Wang Y, Jung V, Xu, H.-P., Wigler MH. Cooperative interaction of *S. pombe* proteins required for mating and morphogenesis. *Cell* 1994; 79:131–141.
115. Qiu R-G, Chen J, Kirn D, McCormick F, Symons M. An essential role for Rac in Ras transformation. *Nature* 1995; 374:457–459.
116. Khosravi-Far R, Solski PA, Kinch MS, Burridge K, Der CJ. Activation of Rac and Rho, and mitogen activated protein kinases, are required for Ras transformation. *Mol Cell Biol* 1995; 15:6443–6453.
117. Prendergast GC, Khosravi-Far R, Solski PA, Kurzawa H, Lebowitz PF, Der CJ. Critical role of RhoB in cell transformation by oncogenic Ras. *Oncogene* 1995; 10:2289–2296.

118. Qiu R-G, Chen J, McCormick F, Symons M. A role for Rho in Ras transformation. *Proc Natl Acad Sci USA* 1995; 92:11,781–11,785.

119. Qiu R-G, Abo A, McCormick F, Symons M. Cdc42 regulates anchorage-independent growth and is necessary for Ras transformation. *Mol Cell Biol* 1997; 17:3449–3458.

120. Roux P, Gauthier-Rouvière C, Doucet-Brutin S, Fort P. The small GTPases Cdc42Hs, Rac1 and RhoG delineate Raf-independent pathways that cooperate to transform NIH3T3 cells. *Curr Biol* 1997; 7:629–637.

121. Lebowitz PF, Du W, Prendergast GC. Prenylation of RhoB is required for its cell transforming function but not its ability to activate serum response element-dependent transcription. *J Biol Chem* 1997; 272:16,093–16,095.

122. Nimnual AS, Yatsula BA, Bar-Sagi D. Coupling of Ras and Rac guanosine triphosphatases through the Ras exchanger Sos. *Science* 1998; 279:560–563.

123. Han J, Luby-Phelps K, Das B, Shu X, Xia Y, Mosteller RD, Krishna UM, Falck JR, White MA, Broek D. Role of substrates and products of PI 3-kinase in regulating activation of Rac-related guanosine triphosphatases by Vav. *Science* 1998; 279:558–560.

124. Whitehead IP, Campbell S, Rossman KL, Der CJ. Dbl family proteins. *Biochim Biophys Acta* 1997; 1332:F1-F23.

125. Feig LA, Urano T, Cantor S. Evidence for a Ras/Ral signaling cascade. *Trends Biochem Sci* 1996; 21:438–441.

126. Cox AD, Der CJ. Farnesyltransferase inhibitors and cancer treatment: Targeting simply Ras? *Biochim Biophys Acta* 1997; 1333:F51-F71.

13

Signaling Pathways Controlled by Rho Family GTP-Binding Proteins

Marc Symons, PhD

1. INTRODUCTION

The current Rho family picture contains 11 mammalian members, which can be subdivided into five groups on the basis of sequence and functional differences: (1) RhoA, RhoB, and RhoC; (2) Rac1, Rac2, and RhoG; (3) Cdc42 and TC10; (4) RhoD; and (5) RhoE and TTF *(1,2)*. In addition, homologs of several of these GTPases have been identified and functionally characterized in lower organisms ranging from yeast to the fruit fly *(1)*.

Until recently, studies of Rho proteins have focused on their role in the regulation of the actin cytoskeleton. Over the past few years, it has become apparent that Rho proteins also play crucial roles in several other important cellular activities, which include gene transcription, lipid metabolism, and vesicle trafficking. This chapter summarizes the current understanding of the regulatory mechanisms that govern the activity of Rho family members and reviews the major functions of these proteins and the signaling pathways that mediate these functions. An attempt is made to place these GTPases within the context of the complex regulatory networks that control cell proliferation and motile behavior. The current explosion in research on Rho GTPases has made it impossible to cover all the relevant recent contributions to the field in the limited amount of space allotted for these overviews. The reader is referred to several excellent and detailed recent reviews *(2–5)*.

2. REGULATORS OF Rho PROTEINS

Like all proteins belonging to the Ras family of GTPases, Rho family members act as switches: they are on in the GTP-bound state and off in the GDP-bound state (Fig. 1). The level of active protein is controlled by three types of regulatory proteins. The guanine nucleotide exchange factors (GEFs) activate Rho proteins by catalyzing the release of GDP. The Rho GEFs constitute the Dbl family, most of which have been discovered as transforming genes in focus formation assays *(6)*. Hallmarks of Dbl proteins are a Dbl homology (DH) domain, which is responsible for the catalytic activity of the protein, and a pleckstrin homology (PH) domain, a protein– and lipid–interaction

From: Signaling Networks and Cell Cycle Control: The Molecular Basis of Cancer and Other Diseases
Edited by: J. S. Gutkind © Humana Press Inc., Totowa, NJ

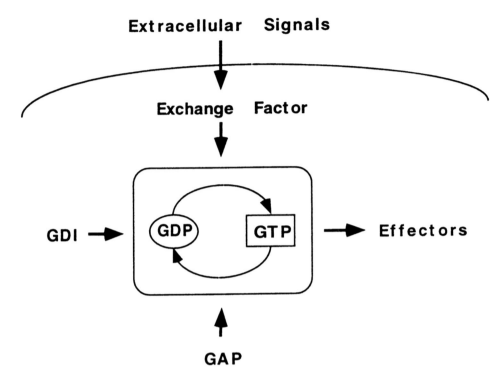

Fig. 1. Rho family members act like binary switches. Extracellular stimuli can activate Rho proteins by modulating the activities of Rho GEFs or GAPs. Rho proteins, in turn, relay these extracellular signals to effectors that initiate distinct downstream pathways. Cellular functions regulated by Rho proteins include regulation of the actin cytoskeleton, adhesion, and motility and cell proliferation.

domain *(7)* that is invariably juxtaposed C-terminal to the DH domain. More than 15 distinct Rho GEFs have thus far been identified *(6)*. The existence of that large a family probably reflects both the tissue specificity of most of these enzymes and the multiple roles played by the various GTPases.

The second class of regulatory proteins consists of Rho GAPs, which accelerate the intrinsic GTPase activity of the Rho proteins and therefore act as negative regulators *(3,8)*. Interestingly, N-chimerin, which exhibits GAP activity toward Rac, has been shown to induce Rac-dependent cytoskeletal changes *(9)*. This activity is not mediated by its GAP domain, however.

The third set of accessory proteins consists of the Rho GDP-dissociation inhibitory factors (GDIs) *(3,8,10)*. In addition to inhibiting guanine nucleotide dissociation, Rho GDI has been shown to inhibit both the intrinsic and GAP-stimulated GTP hydrolysis of Rho GTPases *(11)*. Rho GDI also controls Rho behavior by functioning as a shuttle between different cellular compartments *(10)*. Recently, Rho GDI activity was shown to be inhibited by members of the ERM (ezrin, radixin, moesin) family, providing the first indication that the activity of Rho GDI can be regulated *(12)*. ERM proteins bind both filamentous actin (F-actin) and CD44, a membrane-spanning protein, and in this way can attach the actin cytoskeleton to the plasma membrane. In addition, ERM proteins play an essential role in the formation of cytoskeletal structures controlled by

Rac and Rho *(13)*. Thus, these two novel functions of ERMs may both contribute to restrict the activity of Rho proteins to their appropriate sites of action.

3. TOOLS FOR STUDYING Rho PROTEIN FUNCTION

The availability of dominant negative mutants has provided the field with powerful tools to dissect the signaling pathways controlled by the various Rho proteins. These dominant negative versions display decreased GTP binding and increased binding to GEFs and therefore inhibit the activation of their endogenous counterparts. The action of these dominant negatives is surprisingly specific, taking into account the observations that several GEFs display pleiotropic activities in vitro *(6)*. It is therefore possible that in vivo, the intracellular localization of these GEFs and/or the existence of still unidentified accessory factors provide additional specificity. Extensive use has also been made of mutants that have impaired GTP hydrolysis and hence are constitutively active.

The fast intrinsic hydrolysis rate characteristic of Rho family members, and the current lack of immunoprecipitating antibodies that clamp the nucleotide state of Rho GTPases, have thus far made it difficult to evaluate the activation state of Rho proteins in vivo, although several successful measurements have been described *(14–16)*. Another fruitful avenue consists of the use of recombinant Rho effectors that serve to coprecipitate the activated Rho protein out of cell lysates. A similar method has been used to measure cellular levels of activated Ras and Rap *(17,18)*. This paradigm has recently been extended successfully to determine the activation of Rac by the exchange factor PIX *(19)*.

An additional tool for the study of small GTPase functions has been provided by the characterization of Effector Domain mutants. These constitutively active mutants carry an additional mutation in regions that interact with effectors. These partially crippled GTPases can only interact with a subset of the multitude of effectors and therefore only transduce a subset of the normal array of functions. Thus, the panels of Effector Domain mutants established for Ras, Rac, and Cdc42 have been very useful for the dissection of the signaling cascades activated by these GTPases *(20–25)*.

4. SIGNALING PATHWAYS CONTROLLING THE ACTIVATION OF Rho PROTEINS

Numerous studies have shown that the three prominent Rho family members, Cdc42, Rac, and Rho, can be selectively stimulated by growth factors and neurotransmitters *(26–30)*. In addition, Cdc42, Rac, and Rho have been shown in some conditions to be able to act in a cascade-like fashion to organize the cytoskeleton *(31)*, suggesting that these GTPases participate in a complex network of signaling interactions. To date, however, very little is known about the details of the upstream signaling pathways that regulate the activity of Rho family members. This situation is mainly caused by the technical limitations concerning the measurement of the in vivo activation state of these proteins. Still, one early study demonstrated that Rac activation by PDGF is largely mediated by activation of guanine nucleotide exchange, rather than by inhibition of GAP activity *(14)*.

In several instances, plasma membrane localization has been shown to be essential for the in vivo activity of Dbl proteins. Deletion of the PH domain of the Dbl family members Dbs and Lfc has been shown to cause a loss of transformation potential, which could be restored by addition of the plasma membrane targeting domain of N-Ras *(6,32)*, indicating a role for the PH domain in GEF localization. Several reports have demonstrated an important function for phosphatidylinositol lipids in the activation of Rho proteins *(14,33)*, suggesting the possibility that it is the lipid-binding activity of PH domains *(7)* that is important for membrane interaction. For Tiam1, a Rac-specific GEF *(34)*, the N-terminal PH domain, in conjunction with a flanking putative protein–protein interaction domain, is also essential for plasma membrane localization *(35)*. GEF phosphorylation may present an additional control mechanism. For instance, tyrosine phosphorylation by Lck has been shown to activate both the in vitro and in vivo exchange activity of Vav *(15)*.

5. REGULATION OF THE ACTIN CYTOSKELETON BY Rho PROTEINS

In fibroblasts, the three best characterized members of the Rho family, Rho, Rac, and Cdc42, have been shown to play crucial roles in the reorganization of the actin cytoskeleton caused by growth factors: lysophosphatidic acid-induced stress fiber formation is governed by Rho, lamellipodia extension stimulated by growth factors acting on tyrosine kinase receptors is regulated by Rac, and the activity of filipodia is controlled by Cdc42 *(4)*.

The actin cytoskeleton is made up of polymerized actin (F-actin), which is in equilibrium with a pool of monomeric actin (G-actin). The turnover between these two states is governed by various classes of actin binding proteins *(36)*. In concert with contractile proteins, other types of actin binding proteins (ABP), such as crosslinking and bundling proteins, in turn assemble F-actin into distinct structures, such as the various types of actin bundles that make up stress fibers and filipodia.

The identification of various isoforms of the serine/threonine kinase ROK (also termed p160ROCK or Rho kinase) as Rho effectors has provided an important step toward the understanding of the molecular mechanisms of Rho function. Studies employing dominant negative and constitutively active forms of ROK have indicated that this effector is a crucial mediator of stress fiber formation *(37–40)*. ROK has been shown to phosphorylate the myosin-binding subunit (MBS) of myosin light chain (MLC) phosphatase in vitro, leading to inhibition of its phosphatase activity *(41)*. In addition, MLC itself is a good substrate for phosphorylation by ROK *(38)*, indicating that ROK may induce MLC phosphorylation and thereby activate myosin contractile activity, by a dual mechanism. These findings are consistent with observations showing that Rho-mediated stress fiber formation can occur in the absence of de novo assembly of G-actin and that the MLC kinase inhibitor KT5926 causes loss of stress fiber formation *(42–44)*. Interestingly, the Na^+-H^+ exchanger NHE1 has recently been identified as another substrate of ROK *(44a)*, and increased NHE1 activity is necessary for Rho-mediated stress fiber formation, but not for Rac-induced lamellipodia *(45)*, adding yet another layer of complexity to the regulation of stress fiber assembly.

Although de novo actin polymerization is not necessary for stress fiber formation, expression of constitutively active Rho leads to an increase in F-actin, even in the presence of dominant negative ROK *(39)*. In line with this finding, recent studies have identified formin family proteins as binding partners for Rho in the control of actin polymerization. Members of this family are important regulators of cell structure and polarity and are characterized by two formin homology domains: FH1 and FH2 *(46)*. The former, proline-rich domain binds to the G-actin binding protein profilin, an ABP that can decrease the critical concentration for actin polymerization *(47)*. One formin family member, p140mDia, the mammalian homolog of *Drosophila* diaphenous, has been demonstrated to bind both activated Rho and profilin *(48)*. Furthermore, profilin colocalizes with p140mDia and Rho to ruffling membranes, and overexpression of p140mDia increases actin polymerization *(48)*. In *Saccharomyces cerevisiae*, two formin family members, Bni1 and Bnr1, have been identified as effectors of Rho1 and Rho4, respectively *(49)*. Also in this system, these formins are likely to regulate the actin cytoskeleton through their interaction with profilin *(49)*.

In contrast with Rho-induced stress fiber formation, the extension of lamellipodia induced by Rac is likely to be coupled to actin polymerization *(42)*. Studies using permeabilized platelets support a model in which activated Rac causes actin polymerization by stimulating phosphatidylinositol(4,5)bisphosphate (PIP$_2$) synthesis, which in turn induces the release of actin filament capping proteins *(50)*. As growth factor-induced ruffling is abolished in fibroblasts derived from gelsolin-null mice, this PIP$_2$-regulated capping protein is an excellent candidate to mediate the effect of Rac on actin polymerization *(51,52)*.

Progress has also been made toward the dissection of the mechanisms employed by Cdc42 to control actin dynamics. Cdc42 has been shown to bind to WASP-family proteins, named for the protein implicated in the Wiskott-Aldrich immunodeficiency syndrome *(53)*. Whereas overexpression of the hematopoietically specific WASP causes ectopic actin polymerization in a Cdc42-dependent fashion *(54)*, the ubiquitously expressed N-WASP strongly enhances Cdc42-induced filipodia formation *(55)*. A role for WASP in actin polymerization also is supported by observations showing that the WASP homolog Bee1 is essential for cortical actin assembly in *S. cerevisiae (56)*. The effect of WASP on the actin cytoskeleton might be mediated by WIP, a binding partner of WASP that has distinct binding sites for both profilin and actin *(57)*. The recently identified Cdc42 effector MRCK and its *Drosophila* homolog Gek also have been shown to be necessary for the formation of Cdc42-controlled cytoskeletal structures, providing an additional link between Cdc42 and the actin cytoskeleton *(58,59)*.

A large number of reports support the notion that Rho proteins also play a prominent role in the control of cell–substrate adhesion. In fibroblasts, constitutive activation of distinct Rho family members induce the formation of specialized adhesion structures, indicating that the Rho GTPases may be important elements in signaling pathways that control "inside-out" signaling *(60)*. Rho induces the classical focal adhesions that anchor stress fibers to the extracellular matrix, whereas both Cdc42 and Rac elicit the formation of smaller focal complexes localized to the cell periphery *(31)*. In addition, recent data support the idea that the activity of Rho proteins is essential for "outside-in" signaling initiated at the level of integrins through interaction with components of the extracellular matrix. Thus, the activity of all three prominent Rho family members—Cdc42, Rac, and Rho—was shown to be important for fibroblast spreading on fibronectin *(61,62)*.

Rho proteins also modulate the function of intercellular junctions of polarized epithelial cells. A role for Rac in the assembly of adherens junctions and the actin belts that associate with these junctions was first identified in *Drosophila (63)* and subsequently extended to mammalian cell lines *(64–67)*. Although inhibition of Rho function by introduction of the *Clostridium botulinum* C3 ADP-ribosyltransferase also affects adherens junctions, several studies concur, suggesting that Rho may preferentially regulate the formation of tight junctions that define the permeability properties of epithelial monolayers *(65,68)*.

6. CONTROL OF CELL PROLIFERATION BY Rho PROTEINS

A series of reports have demonstrated that the activities of Rac, Rho, Cdc42 and RhoG are essential for Ras transformation *(69–74)*. Conversely, expression of constitutively active versions of Rac and Cdc42, and to a lesser extent Rho, were shown to be sufficient for the malignant transformation of fibroblasts *(69–73,75,76)*. Further support for a role for Rho in cell proliferation comes from observations that indicate that RhoB may be a critical element for the reversion of Ras transformation by farnesyl-tranferase inhibitors *(77)*. In addition, Cdc42, Rac, and Rho have been shown to be necessary and sufficient for the stimulation of DNA synthesis *(78)*. These observations are consistent with the strong oncogenic activity of most members of the Dbl family *(6)* and indicate an important function for Rho family members in the control of cell proliferation.

It is important to point out that although Rho GTPases can function in a cascade-like fashion to organize the actin cytoskeleton *(31)*, recent studies have indicated that, with respect to cell proliferation, at least some of these GTPases may function independent from each other *(73,74)*. For example, whereas expression of constitutively active Cdc42 induces cytoskeletal changes that are abolished by coexpression of dominant negative Rac *(28,31)*, anchorage-independent growth caused by Cdc42 appears to be Rac independent *(73)*. The Rho-controlled pathways also appear to act largely independent of the ERK pathway *(79–81)*, although some degree of crosstalk may exist *(82)*. The existence of multiple separate pathways that are necessary for transformation by oncogenic Ras suggests that these pathways may mediate different aspects of the transformed phenotype. Detailed examination of the proliferation properties of fibroblasts coexpressing dominant negative versions of Rho proteins with the Ras or Abl oncogenes indicates that this may indeed be the case: Cdc42 was shown to control anchorage-independent growth differentially, whereas Rac is predominantly responsible for the growth in low serum *(73,83)*. Furthermore, both Cdc42 and Rho are necessary for the maintenance of the morphological phenotype of Ras-transformed cells, whereas Rac is not *(72,73)*.

A likely mechanism for the control of cell proliferation by Rho proteins consists of transcriptional activation. In line with this possibility, Rho family members have been shown to activate nuclear transcription factor-κB (NF-κB), serum response factor (SRF) and the Ets protein PEA3 *(81,84–86)*.

The signaling pathways that mediate transcriptional activation by Rho GTPases remain largely uncharted. In the budding yeast *S. cerevisiae*, genetic evidence indicates that Rho and Cdc42 can control transcription by activation of a mitogen-activated protein kinase (MAPK) module. Rho controls cell wall integrity through activation of PKC1 and subsequent activation of the MPK1 cascade, and Cdc42 mediates pheromone-induced cell cycle arrest by activation of Ste20 and the KSS1/FUS3 cascade *(87)*.

Several studies using mammalian cell lines have shown that Rho family members can activate the Jun N-terminal kinase (JNK) and p38 pathways *(79,80)*. Interestingly, the details of these effects may depend on the cell types used. Whereas in most cell lines tested thus far, Cdc42 and Rac, but not Rho, were found to activate the JNK pathway, in the human kidney epithelial cell line, 293T, Cdc42, and Rho activate JNK, but Rac does not *(88)*. Different elements have been proposed to link the GTPases to the JNK and p38 modules. The p21-activated kinase (PAK) was the first candidate for this function, since PAK binds to and is activated by Cdc42 and Rac *(89)*, and some constitutively active forms of PAK have been shown to activate JNK and p38 *(90,91)*. Recent studies, however, have identified an effector domain mutant of Rac that is a potent activator of JNK but that fails to bind to PAK, indicating that PAK is dispensable for JNK activation by Rac *(25)*. MLK3, a member of the mixed lineage kinase family, provides another possible connection, as it was shown to be able to associate with Cdc42 and Rac and in turn to activate JNK *(92,93)*. In addition, two members of the MAP/ERK kinase kinase (MEKK) family—MEKK 1 and 4—both of which activate JNK, were shown to form a complex with Cdc42 and Rac *(94)*. Thus, exactly how Cdc42 and Rac stimulate the JNK and p38 cascades remains to be resolved. The use of sufficiently large panels of effector domain mutants of Rho proteins may prove very helpful in this task.

Because of the key roles played by Rho GTPases in controlling cytoskeletal dynamics, modulation of Rho protein activity has been thought to underly the alterations in cell morphology that typically accompany malignant transformation. As mentioned above, studies in fibroblasts showed that both Cdc42 and Rho, but not Rac, contribute to the characteristic spindle-shaped morphology of Ras-transformed cells. Surprisingly, these roles of Cdc42 and Rho are likely to be distinct from the direct effect exerted by these GTPases to assemble actin cytoskeletal structures *(72,73)*. This is illustrated most strikingly in the case of stress fibers, which are disassembled upon oncogenic transformation by Ras, whereas coexpression with dominant negative Rho restores stress fiber formation *(72)*. It is therefore possible that Cdc42 and Rho control the production of autocrine factors that regulate morphological transformation.

7. OTHER FUNCTIONS MEDIATED BY Rho PROTEINS

Evidence has been accumulating for a critical role for Rho family members in cell motility, in line with the involvement of these GTPases in cell spreading and the organization of the actin cytoskeleton. Earlier work had already indicated a role for Rho in cell locomotion *(10)*. More recent studies in a variety of different systems have substantiated a role for Rac in the control of cell migration. Dominant negative Rac was shown both to inhibit epithelial cell scattering by hepatocyte growth factor and fibroblast motility stimulated by platelet-derived growth factor (PDGF) and lysophosphatidic acid *(95–97)*. In both systems, it is likely that PI3K mediates growth-factor activation of Rac *(14,97,98)*. Rac1 was also found to be essential for the migration of border cells during *Drosophila* oogenesis *(99)*. In addition, dominant-negative mutants of either Rac or Cdc42 were shown to impair dorsal closure in *Drosophila (100,101)*. Dorsal closure involves the elongation and coordinated movement of the dorsalmost cells of the lateral epidermis during embryonic development. Interestingly, the *Drosophila* homologs of JNK (DJNK) and its activating kinase *hemipterous* are also necessary for dorsal closure; also implicated in this process *(102)* is *puckered*, the expression of which is activated by DJNK. These observations further underline a theme, played out from yeast to mammals, in which Rho proteins stimulate a MAPK module, that in turn leads to transcriptional activation, in this case of genes involved in motile behavior.

Several studies have also implicated Rho family members in invasive behavior. The first indication of a role for Rac in invasion came from the identification of Tiam1, a Rac GEF, in a screen for genes that induce invasion in T lymphoma *(103)*. Subsequent studies on mammary epithelial cells showed that constitutive activation of either Cdc42 or Rac confers invasive potential to these cells *(66)*. Rac was also found necessary for the invasion of breast carcinoma cells induced by expression of the $\alpha6\beta4$ integrin *(104)*. As is the case for growth factor-induced activation of Rac, this study also placed PI3K upstream of Rac in the integrin-stimulated pathway. Importantly, recent studies have indicated that constitutive activation of Rho and Rac is also sufficient for metastatic spreading of fibroblasts *(105)*.

Evidence also has been accumulating for a role of Rho GTPases in various functions relating to membrane trafficking. These include phagocytosis *(106,107)*, endocytosis *(108)*, and exocytosis *(109,110)*, *(see* ref. *3* for a detailed review). The molecular mechanisms underlying these Rho functions remain to be elucidated. Because of the involvement of polyphosphoinositides in vesicle trafficking, a possible mechanism could involve the control of phosphoinositide (PI) metabolism by Rho family members. Indeed, both Rac and Rho have been shown to regulate PI 5-kinase activity *(50,111)*, and Cdc42, Rac, and Rho can all bind PI 3-kinase *(112–114)*.

8. ELEMENTS OF Rho SIGNALING PATHWAYS AS DRUG TARGETS

The important role of Rho family members in cell proliferation and motility suggests that the elements of Rho-controlled pathways may constitute a vast and expanding array of drug targets for use in cancer therapy *(2,115)* and other hyperproliferative diseases, including cardiovascular pathologies. Rho proteins are also involved in other biological functions that are clinically important. Thus, Rac has been implicated in the activation of the NADPH oxidase in phagocytic cells *(116,117)*, suggesting that it may play a critical function in inflammatory conditions, and Cdc42 and Rho have been shown to be involved in the internalization of pathogenic bacteria into their target cells *(106,107)*.

The discovery of the Rho effector ROK as the site of action of Y-27632, a compound found in a drug screen that assayed for inhibition of smooth muscle contraction, has added hypertension to the list of pathological processes mediated by Rho proteins *(118)*. Another relevant drug, SCH 51344, was initially identified in a screen that monitored the activity of the α-actin promoter, a transcriptional readout that is sensitive to Ras transformation *(119)*. Recently, this compound has been shown to inhibit anchorage-independent growth and ruffling activity induced by constitutively active Rac, but not Rac-induced JNK activity *(120)*. Thus, the development of drugs that interfere with Rho protein-regulated functions may not only be clinically important, but may also provide powerful tools for the further dissection the signaling pathways controlled by these GTPases.

9. CONCLUSIONS AND PERSPECTIVES

Research during the past few years has demonstrated a multitude of diverse functions that are controlled by members of the Rho family. Whereas substantial inroads have been made toward the identification of the signaling elements that function downstream of Rho proteins in the regulation of actin cytoskeletal structures, the elements that mediate other functions, such as cell proliferation, motile behavior, and metabolic control, remain largely unknown. Substantial progress has been made both in the genetic analysis of Rho protein function in *S. cerevisiae* and the identification and characterization of a plethora of effectors for these proteins in mammals. This work has led to the realization that the pathways that mediate the multitude of functions governed by Rho proteins, branch out at the level of the GTPases themselves *(4,25,121)*. These findings also suggest that Rho family members can regulate downstream pathways in a coordinate fashion, a crucial feature for the orchestration of essential biological functions such as cell proliferation and motility.

REFERENCES

1. Ridley AJ. Rho: Theme and variations. *Cur Biol* 1996; 6:1256–1264.
2. Khosravi-Far R, Campbell S, Rossman KL, Der CJ. Increasing complexity of Ras signal transduction: Involvement of Rho family proteins. *Adv Cancer Res* 1998; 72:57–107.
3. Van Aelst L, D'Souza-Schorey C. Rho GTPases and signaling networks. *Genes Dev* 1997; 11:2295–2322.
4. Hall A. Rho GTPases and the actin cytoskeleton. *Science* 1998; 279:509–514.
5. Tanaka K, Takai Y. Control of reorganization of the actin cytoskeleton by Rho family small GTP-binding proteins in yeast. *Curr Opin Cell Biol* 1998; 10:112–116.
6. Whitehead IP, Campbell S, Rossman KL, Der CJ. Dbl family proteins. *Biochim Biophys Acta* 1997; 1332:F1–F23.
7. Shaw G. The pleckstrin homology domain: An intriguing multifunctional protein module. *BioEssays* 1996; 18:35–46.
8. Boguski MS, McCormick F. Proteins regulating Ras and its relatives. *Nature* 1993; 366:643–654.
9. Kozma R, Ahmed S, Best A, Lim L. The GTPase-activating protein n-chimaerin cooperates with Rac1 and Cdc42Hs to induce the formation of lamellipodia and filopodia. *Mol Cell Biol* 1996; 16:5069–5080.
10. Takai Y, Sasaki T, Tanaka K, Nakanishi H. Rho as a regulator of the cytoskeleton. *TIBS* 1995; 20:227–231.
11. Hart MJ, Maru Y, Leonard D, Witte ON, Evans T, Cerione RA. *Science* 1992; 258:812–815.
12. Takahashi K, Sasaki T, Mammoto A, Takaishi K, Kameyama T, Tsukita S, Takai Y. Direct interaction of the Rho GDP dissociation inhibitor with ezrin/radixin/moesin initiates the activation of the Rho small G protein. *J Biol Chem* 1997; 272:23,371–23,375.
13. Mackay DJ, Esch F, Furthmayr H, Hall A. Rho- and rac-dependent assembly of focal adhesion complexes and actin filaments in permeabilized fibroblasts: An essential role for ezrin/radixin/moesin proteins. *J Cell Biol* 1997; 138:927–938.
14. Hawkins PT, Eguinoa A, Qiu R-Q, Stokoe D, Cooke F, Walters R, Wennstrom S, Claesson-Welsh L, Evans T, Symons M, Stephens L. PDGF stimulates an increase in GTP-Rac via activation of phosphoinositide 3-kinase. *Curr Biol* 1995; 5:393–403.
15. Crespo P, et al. Phosphotyrosine-dependent activation of Rac1 GDP/GTP exchange by the Vav proto-oncogene product. *Nature* 1997; 385:169–172.
16. Laudanna C, Campbell JJ, Butcher EC. Role of Rho in chemoattractant-activated leukocyte adhesion through integrins. *Science* 1996; 271:981–983.

17. Taylor S, Shalloway D. Cell cycle-dependent activation of Ras. *Curr Biol* 1996; 6:1621–1627.

18. Franke B, Akkerman JW, Bos JL. Rapid Ca^{2+}-mediated activation of Rap1 in human platelets. *EMBO J* 1997; 16:252–259.

19. Manser E, Loo T-H, Koh C-G, Zhao Z-S, Chen X-Q, Tan L, Tan I, Leung T, Lim L. PAK Kinases Are Directly Coupled to the PIX Family of Nucleotide Exchange Factors. *Mol Cell* 1998; 1:183–192.

20. White MA, Nicolette C, Minden A, Polverino A, Van Aelst L, Karin M, Wigler MH. Multiple Ras functions can contribute to mammalian cell transformation. *Cell* 1995; 80:533–541.

21. Rodriguez-Viciana P, Warne PH, Khwaja A, Marte BM, Pappin D, Das P, Waterfield MD, Ridley A, Downward J. Role of phosphoinositide 3-OH kinase in cell transformation and control of the actin cytoskeleton by Ras. *Cell* 1997; 89:457–467.

22. Freeman JL, Abo A, Lambeth JD. Rac "insert region" is a novel effector region that is implicated in the activation of NADPH oxidase, but not PAK65. *J Biol Chem* 1996; 271:19,794–19,801.

23. Lamarche N, Tapon N, Stowers L, Burbelo PD, Aspenström P, Bridges T, Chant J, Hall A. Rac and Cdc42 induce actin polymerization and G1 cell cycle progression independently of p65PAK and the JNK/SAPK MAP kinase cascade. *Cell* 1996; 87:519–529.

24. Joneson T, McDonough M, Bar-Sagi D, Van Aelst L. Rac regulation of actin polymerization by a pathway distinct from jun kinase. *Science* 1996; 274:1374–1376.

25. Westwick JK, Lambert QT, Clark GJ, Symons M, Aelst LV, Pestell RG, Der CJ. Rac regulation of transformation, gene expression and actin organization by multiple, PAK-independent pathways. *Mol Cell Biol* 1997; 17:1324–1335.

26. Ridley AJ, Paterson HF, Johnston CL, Diekman D, Hall A. The small GTP-binding protein rac regulates growth factor-induced membrane ruffling. *Cell* 1992; 70:401–410.

27. Ridley AJ, Hall A. The small GTP-binding protein rho regulates the assembly of focal adhesions and actin stress fibers in response to growth factors. *Cell* 1992; 70:389–399.

28. Kozma R, Ahmed S, Best A, Lim L. The Ras-related protein Cdc42Hs and bradykinin promote formation of peripheral actin microspikes and filopodia in Swiss 3T3 fibroblasts. *Mol Cell Biol* 1995; 15:1942–1952.

29. Hooley R, Yu C-Y, Symons M, Barber DL. Ga13 stimulates Na^+-H^+ exchange through distinct Cdc42-dependent and RhoA-dependent pathways. *J Biol Chem* 1996; 271:6152–6156.

30. Coso OA, Teramoto H, Simonds WF, Gutkind JS. Signaling from G protein-coupled receptors to c-Jun kinase involves beta gamma subunits of heterotrimeric G proteins acting on a Ras and Rac1-dependent pathway. *J Biol Chem* 1996; 271:3963–3966.

31. Nobes CD, Hall A. Rho, Rac, and Cdc42 GTPases regulate the assembly of multimolecular focal complexes associated with actin stress fibers, lamellipodia and filopodia. *Cell* 1995; 81:53–62.

32. Whitehead I, Kirk H, Tognon C, Trigo-Gonzalez G, Kay R. Expression cloning of lfc, a novel oncogene with structural similarities to guanine nucleotide exchange factors and to the regulatory region of protein kinase C. *J Biol Chem* 1995; 270:18,388–18,395.

33. Schmidt A, Bickle M, Beck T, Hall M. The yeast phosphatidylinositol kinase homolog TOR2 activates RHO1 and RHO2 via the exchange factor ROM2. *Cell* 1997; 88:531–542.

34. Michiels F, Habets, G.G.M., Stam JC, van der Kammen RA, Collard JG. A role for Rac in Tiam1-induced membrane ruffling and invasion. *Nature* 1995; 375:338–340.

35. Stam JC, Sander EE, Michiels F, van Leeuwen FN, Kain HE, van der Kammen RA, Collard JG. Targeting of Tiam1 to the plasma membrane requires the cooperative function of the N-terminal pleckstrin homology domain and an adjacent protein interaction domain. *J Biol Chem* 1997; 272:28,447–28,454.

36. Kreis T, Vale R. 1998. Oxford University Press, Oxford, UK.
37. Leung T, Chen X-Q, Manser E, Lim L. The p160 RhoA-binding kinase ROKa is a member of a kinase family and is involved in the reorganization of the cytoskeleton. *Mol Cell Biol* 1996; 16:5313–5327.
38. Amano M, Chihara K, Kimura K, Fukata Y, Nakamura N, Matsuura Y, Kaibuchi K. Formation of actin stress fibers and focal adhesions enhanced by Rho-kinase. *Science* 1997; 275:1308–1311.
39. Ishizaki T, Naito M, Fujisawa K, Maekawa M, Watanabe N, Saito Y, Narumiya S. p160ROCK, a Rho-associated coiled-coil forming protein kinase, works downstream of Rho and induces focal adhesions. *FEBS Lett* 1997; 404:118–124.
40. Narumiya S, Ishizaki T, Watanabe N. Rho effectors and reorganization of actin cytoskeleton. *FEBS Lett* 1997; 410:68–72.
41. Kimura K, Ito M, Amano M, Chihara K, Fukata Y, Nakafuku M, Yamamori B, Feng J, Nakano T, Okawa K, Iwamatsu A, Kaibuchi K. Regulation of myosin phosphatase by rho and Rho-associated kinase (Rho-kinase). *Science* 1996; 273:245–248.
42. Machesky LM, Hall A. Role of actin polymerization and adhesion to extracellular matrix in Rac- and Rho-induced cytoskeletal reorganization. *J Cell Biol* 1997; 138:913–926.
43. Chrzanowska-Wodnicka M, Burridge K. Rho-stimulated contractility drives the formation of stress fibers and focal adhesions. *J Cell Biol* 1996; 133:1403–1415.
44. Burridge K, Chrzanowska-Wodnicka M, Zhong C. Focal adhesion assembly. *Trends Cell Biol* 1997; 7:342–347.
44a. Tominaga T, Ishizaki T, Narumiya S, Barber D. p160ROCK mediates RhoA activation of Na-H exchange. *EMBO J* 1998; 17:4712–4722.
45. Vexler SZ, Symons M, Barber DL. Activation of Na^+-H^+ exchange is necessary for RhoA-induced stress fiber formation. *J Biol Chem* 1996; 271:22,281–22,284.
46. Frazier JA, Field CM. Actin cytoskeleton: Are FH proteins local organizers? *Curr Biol* 1997; 7:R414–7.
47. Theriot JA, Mitchison TJ. Three faces of profilin. *Cell* 1993; 75:835–838.
48. Watanabe N, Madaule P, Reid T, Ishizaki T, Watanabe G, Kakizuka A, Saito Y, Nakao K, Jockusch BM, Narumiya S. p140mDia, a mammalian homolog of *Drosophila* diaphanous, is a target protein for Rho small GTPase and is ligand for profilin. *EMBO J* 1997; 16:3044–3056.
49. Imamura H, Tanaka K, Hihara T, Umikawa M, Kamei T, Takahashi K, Sasaki T, Takai Y. Bni1p and Bnr1p: Downstream targets of the Rho family small G-proteins which interact with profilin and regulate actin cytoskeleton in *Saccharomyces cerevisiae*. *EMBO J* 1997; 16:2745–2755.
50. Hartwig JH, Bokoch GM, Carpenter CL, Janmey PA, Taylor LA, Toker A, Stossel TP. Thrombin receptor ligation and activated Rac uncap actin filament barbed ends through phosphoinositide synthesis in permeabilized human platelets. *Cell* 1995; 82:643–653.
51. Arcaro A. The small GTP-binding protein rac promotes the dissociation of gelsolin from actin filaments in neutrophils. *J Biol Chem* 1998; 273:805–813.
52. Azuma T, Witke W, Stossel TP, Hartwig JH, Kwiatkowski DJ. Gelsolin is a downstream effector of Rac for fibroblast motility. *EMBO J* 1998; 17:1362–1370.
53. Kirchhausen T, Rosen FS. Unravelling Wiskott-Aldrich syndrome. *Curr Biol* 1996; 6:676–678.
54. Symons M, Derry JMJ, Karlak B, Jiang S, Lemahieu V, McCormick F, Francke U, Abo A. Wiskott-Aldrich Syndrome protein, a novel effector for the GTPase Cdc42Hs, is implicated in actin polymerization. *Cell* 1996; 84:723–734.
55. Miki H, Sasaki T, Takai Y, Takenawa T. Induction of filopodium formation by a WASP-related actin-depolymerizing protein N-WASP. *Nature* 1998; 391:93–96.
56. Li R. Bee1, a yeast protein with homology to Wiscott-Aldrich syndrome protein, is critical for the assembly of cortical actin cytoskeleton. *J Cell Biol* 1997; 136:649–658.

57. Ramesh N, Anton IM, Hartwig JH, Geha RS. WIP, a protein associated with Wiskott-Aldrich syndrome protein, induces actin polymerization and redistribution in lymphoid cells. *Proc Natl Acad Sci USA* 1997; 94:14,671–14,676.

58. Leung T, Chen XQ, Tan I, Manser E, Lim L. Myotonic dystrophy kinase-related Cdc42-binding kinase acts as a Cdc42 effector in promoting cytoskeletal reorganization. *Mol Cell Biol* 1998; 18:130–140.

59. Luo L, Lee T, Tsai L, Tang G, Jan LY, Jan YN. Genghis Khan (Gek) as a putative effector for *Drosophila* Cdc42 and regulator of actin polymerization. *Proc Natl Acad Sci USA* 1997; 94:12,963–12,968.

60. Dedhar S, Hannigan GE. Integrin cytoplasmic interactions and bidirectional transmembrane signalling. *Curr Opin Cell Biol* 1996; 8:657–669.

61. Schwartz MA. Integrins, oncogenes, and anchorage independence. *J Cell Biol* 1997; 139: 575–578.

62. Clark EA, Hynes RO. 1997 keystone symposium on signal transduction by cell adhesion receptors. *Biochim Biophys Acta* 1997; 1333:R9–16.

63. Eaton S, Auvinen P, Luo L, Jan YN, Simons K. CDC42 and Rac1 control different actin-dependent processes in the *Drosophila* wing disc epithelium. *J Cell Biol* 1993; 131:151–164.

64. Braga VM, Machesky LM, Hall A, Hotchin NA. The small GTPases Rho and Rac are required for the establishment of cadherin-dependent cell-cell contacts. *J Cell Biol* 1997; 137:1421–1431.

65. Takaishi K, Sasaki T, Kotani H, Nishioka H, Takai Y. Regulation of cell-cell adhesion by rac and rho small G proteins in MDCK cells. *J Cell Biol* 1997; 139:1047–1059.

66. Keely PJ, Westwick JK, Whitehead IP, Der CJ, Parise LV. Cdc42 and Rac1 induce integrin-mediated cell motility and invasiveness through PI(3)K. *Nature* 1997; 390:632–636.

67. Hordijk PL, ten Klooster JP, van der Kammen RA, Michiels F, Oomen LC, Collard JG. Inhibition of invasion of epithelial cells by Tiam1-Rac signaling. *Science* 1997; 278:1464–1466.

68. Nusrat A, Giry M, Turner JR, Colgan SP, Parkos CA, Carnes D, Lemichez E, Boquet P, Madara JL. Rho protein regulates tight junctions and perijunctional actin organization in polarized epithelia. *Proc Natl Acad Sci USA* 1995; 92:5027–5031.

69. Qiu R-G, Chen J, Kirn D, McCormick F, Symons M. An essential role for Rac in Ras transformation. *Nature* 1995; 374:457–459.

70. Prendergast GC, Khosravi-Far R, Solski PA, Kurzawa H, Lebowitz PF, Der CJ. Critical role for Rho in cell transformation by oncogenic Ras. *Oncogene* 1995; 10:2289–2296.

71. Khosravi-Far R, Solski PA, Clark GJ, Kinch MS, Der CJ. Activation of Rac1 and RhoA, and mitogen activated protein kinases, is required for Ras transformation. *Mol Cell Biol* 1995; 15:6443–6453.

72. Qiu R-G, Chen J, McCormick F, Symons M. A role for Rho in Ras transformation. *Proc Natl Acad Sci USA* 1995; 92:11,781–11,785.

73. Qiu R-G, Abo A, McCormick F, Symons M. Cdc42 regulates anchorage-independent growth and is necessary for Ras transformation. *Mol Cell Biol* 1997; 17:3449–3458.

74. Roux P, Gauthier-Rouviere C, Doucet-Brutin S, Fort P. The small GTPases Cdc42Hs, Rac1 and RhoG delineate Raf-independent pathways that cooperate to transform NIH 3T3 cells. *Curr Biol* 1997; 7:629–637.

75. Perona R, Esteve P, Jimenez B, Ballestro RP, Ramon y Cajal S, Lacal JC. Tumorigenic activity of *rho* genes from *Aplysia californica*. *Oncogene* 1993; 8:1285–1292.

76. Lin R, Bagrodia S, Cerione R, Manor D. A novel Cdc42Hs mutant induces cellular transformation. *Curr Biol* 1997; 7:794–797.

77. Lebowitz P, Casey P, Prendergast G, Thissen J. Farnesyltransferase inhibitors alter the prenylation and growth-stimulating function of RhoB. *J Biol Chem* 1997; 272:15,591–15,594.

78. Olson MF, Ashworth A, Hall A. An essential role for Rho, Rac, and Cdc42 GTPases in cell cycle progression through G1. *Science* 1995; 269:1270–1272.
79. Coso OA, Chiariello M, Yu J-C, Teramoto H, Crespo P, Xu N, Miki T, Gutkind JS. The small GTP-binding proteins Rac1 and Cdc42 regulate the activity of the JNK/SAPK signalling pathway. *Cell* 1995; 81:1137–1146.
80. Minden A, Lin A, Claret F-X, Abo A, Karin M. Selective activation of the JNK signalling pathway and c-Jun transcriptional activity by the small GTPases Rac and Cdc42Hs. *Cell* 1995; 81:1147–1157.
81. O'Hagan RC, Tozer RG, Symons M, McCormick F, Hassell JA. The activity of the Ets transcription factor PEA3 is regulated by two distinct MAPK cascades. *Oncogene* 1996; 13:1323–1333.
82. Frost JA, Steen H, Shapiro P, Lewis T, Ahn N, Shaw PE, Cobb MH. Cross-cascade activation of ERKs and ternary complex factors by Rho family proteins. *EMBO J* 1997; 16:6426–6438.
83. Renshaw MW, Lea-Chou E, Wang JYJ. Rac is required for v-Abl tyrosine kinase to activate mitogenesis. *Curr Biol* 1996; 6:76–83.
84. Sulciner DJ, Irani K, Yu ZX, Ferrans VJ, Goldschmidt-Clermont P, Finkel T. rac1 regulates a cytokine-stimulated, redox-dependent pathway necessary for NF-kappaB activation. *Mol Cell Biol* 1996; 16:7115–7121.
85. Perona R, Montaner S, Saniger L, Sanchez-Perez I, Bravo R, Lacal JC. Activation of the nuclear factor-kappaB by Rho, CDC42, and Rac-1 proteins. *Genes Dev* 1997; 11:463–475.
86. Hill CS, Wynne J, Treisman R. The Rho family GTPases RhoA, Rac1 and CDC42hs regulate transcriptional activation by SRF. *Cell* 1995; 81:1159–1170.
87. Treisman R. Regulation of transcription by MAP kinase cascades. *Curr Opin Cell Biol* 1996; 8:205–215.
88. Teramoto H, Crespo P, Coso OA, Igishi T, Xu N, Gutkind JS. The small GTP-binding protein rho activates c-Jun N-terminal kinases/stress-activated protein kinases in human kidney 293T cells. Evidence for a Pak-independent signaling pathway. *J Biol Chem* 1996; 271:25,731–25,734.
89. Manser E, Leung T, Salihuddin H, Zhao Z-S, Lim L. A brain serine/threonine protein kinase activated by Cdc42 and Rac1. *Nature* 1994; 367:40–46.
90. Bagrodia S, Derijard B, Davis RJ, Cerione RA. Cdc42 and PAK-mediated signaling leads to Jun kinase and p38 mitogen-activated protein kinase activation. *J Biol Chem* 1995; 270:27,995–27,998.
91. Zhang S, Han J, Sells MA, Chernoff J, Knaus UG, Ulevitch RJ, Bokoch GM. Rho family GTPases regulate p38 mitogen-activated protein kinase through the downstream mediator Pak1. *J Biol Chem* 1995; 270:23,934–23,936.
92. Teramoto H, Coso OA, Miyata H, Igishi T, Miki T, Gutkind JS. Signaling from the small GTP-binding proteins Rac1 and Cdc42 to the c-Jun N-terminal kinase/stress-activated protein kinase pathway. A role for mixed lineage kinase 3/protein-tyrosine kinase 1, a novel member of the mixed lineage kinase family. *J Biol Chem* 1996; 271:27,225–27,228.
93. Tibbles LA, Ing YL, Kiefer F, Chan J, Iscove N, Woodgett JR, Lassam NJ. MLK-3 activates the SAPK/JNK and p38/RK pathways via SEK1 and MKK3/6. *EMBO J* 1996; 15:7026–7035.
94. Fanger GR, Johnson NL, Johnson GL. MEK kinases are regulated by EGF and selectively interact with Rac/Cdc42. *EMBO J* 1997; 16:4961–4972.
95. Ridley AJ, Comoglio PM, Hall A. Regulation of scatter factor/hepatocyte growth factor responses by Ras, Rac and Rho in MDCK cells. *Mol Cell Biol* 1995; 15:1110–1122.
96. Anand-Apte B, Zetter BR, Viswanathan A, Qiu RG, Chen J, Ruggieri R, Symons M. Platelet-derived growth factor and fibronectin-stimulated migration are differentially regulated by the rac and extracellular signal-regulated kinase pathways. *J Biol Chem* 1997; 272:30,688–30,692.

97. Hooshmand-Rad R, Claesson-Welsh L, Wennstrom S, Yokote K, Siegbahn A, Heldin CH. Involvement of phosphatidylinositide 3′-kinase and Rac in platelet-derived growth factor-induced actin reorganization and chemotaxis. *Exp Cell Res* 1997; 234:434–441.

98. Royal I, Park M. Hepatocyte growth factor-induced scatter of Madin-Darby canine kidney cells requires phosphatidylinositol 3-kinase. *J Biol Chem* 1995; 270:27,780–27,787.

99. Murphy A, Montell D. Cell type-specific roles for Cdc42, Rac, and RhoL in *Drosophila* oogenesis. *J Cell Biol* 1996; 133:617–630.

100. Harden N, Loh HY, Chia W, Lim L. A dominant inhibitory version of the small GTP-binding protein Rac disrupts cytoskeletal structures and inhibits developmental cell shape changes in *Drosophila. Devlopment* 1995; 121:903–914.

101. Riesgo-Escovar J, Jenni M, Fritz A, Hafen E. The *Drosophila* Jun-N-terminal kinase is required for cell morphogenesis but not for DJun-dependent cell fate specification in the eye. *Genes Dev* 1996; 10:2759–2768.

102. Knust E. *Drosophila* morphogenesis: Follow-my-leader in epithelia. *Curr Biol* 1996; 6:379–381.

103. Habets GGM, Scholtes EHM, Zuydgeest D, van der Kammen RA, Stam JC, Berns A, Collard JG. Identification of an invasion-inducing gene Tiam-1, that encodes a protein with homology to GDP-GTP exchangers for Rho-like proteins. *Cell* 1994; 77:537–549.

104. Shaw LM, Rabinovitz I, Wang HH, Toker A, Mercurio AM. Activation of phosphoinositide 3-OH kinase by the alpha6beta4 integrin promotes carcinoma invasion. *Cell* 1997; 91: 949–960.

105. del Peso L, Hernandez-Alcoceba R, Embade N, Carnero A, Esteve P, Paje C, Lacal JC. Rho proteins induce metastatic properties in vivo. *Oncogene* 1997; 15:3047–3057.

106. Adam T, Giry M, Boquet P, Sansonetti P. Rho-dependent membrane folding causes *Shigella* entry into epithelial cells. *EMBO J* 1996; 15:3315–3321.

107. Chen L-M, Hobbie S, Galan JE. Requirement of CDC42 for *Salmonella*-induced cytoskeletal and nuclear responses. *Science* 1996; 274:2115–2118.

108. Lamaze C, Chuang T-H, Terlecky L, Bokoch GM, L SS. Regulation of receptor-mediated endocytosis by Rho and Rac. *Nature* 1996; 382:177–179.

109. Norman JC, Price LS, Ridley AJ, Koffer A. The small GTP-binding proteins, Rac and Rho, regulate cytoskeletal reorganization and exocytosis in mast cells by parallel pathways. *Mol Biol Cell* 1996; 7:1429–1442.

110. Mariot P, O'Sullivan AJ, Brown AM, Tatham PER. Rho guanine nucleotide dissociation inhibitor protein (RhoGDI) inhibits exocytosis in mast cells. *EMBO J* 1996; 15:6476–6482.

111. Chong LD, Traynor-Kaplan A, Bokoch GM, Schwartz MA. The small GTP-binding protein Rho regulates a phosphatidylinositol 4-phosphate 5-kinase in mammalian cells. *Cell* 1994; 79:507–513.

112. Zhang Z-F, Settleman J, Kyriakis JM, Takeuchi-Suzuki E, Elledge SJ, Marshall MS, Bruder JT, Rapp UR, Avruch J. Normal and oncogenic p21Ras proteins bind to the amino-terminal regulatory domain of c-Raf-1. *Nature* 1993; 364:308–313.

113. Zheng Y, Bagrodia S, Cerione RA. Activation of phosphoinositide-3-kinase activity by Cdc42Hs binding to p85. *J Biol Chem* 1994; 269:18,727–18,730.

114. Tolias KF, Cantley LC, Carpenter CL. Rho family GTPases bind to phosphoinositide kinases. *J Biol Chem* 1995; 270:17,656–17,659.

115. Symons M. The Rac and Rho pathways as a source of drug targets for Ras-mediated malignancies. *Curr Opin Biotechnol* 1995; 6:668–674.

116. Abo A et al. Activation of the NADPH oxidase involves the small GTP-binding protein p21rac1. *Nature* 1991; 353:668–669.

117. Voncken JW, van Schaick H, Kaartinen V, Deemer K, Coates T, Landing B, Pattengale P, Dorseuil O, Bokoch GM, Groffen J, et al. Increased neutrophil respiratory burst in bcr-null mutants. *Cell* 1995; 80:719–728.

118. Uehata M, Ishizaki T, Satoh H, Ono T, Kawahara T, Morishita T, Tamakawa H, Yamagami

K, Inui J, Maekawa M, Narumiya S. Calcium sensitization of smooth muscle mediated by a Rho-associated protein kinase in hypertension [see comments]. *Nature* 1997; 389: 990–994.

119. Kumar CC, Kim JH, Bushel P, Armstrong L, Catino JJ. Activation of smooth muscle alpha-actin promoter in ras-transformed cells by treatments with antimitotic agents: Correlation with stimulation of SRF:SRE mediated gene transcription. *J Biochem (Tokyo)* 1995; 118:1285–1292.

120. Walsh AB, Dhanasekaran M, Bar-Sagi D, Kumar CC. SCH 51344-induced reversal of RAS-transformation is accompanied by the specific inhibition of the RAS and RAC-dependent cell morphology pathway. *Oncogene* 1997; 15:2553–2560.

121. Symons M. Rho family GTPases: The cytoskeleton and beyond. *Trends Biol Sci* 1996; 21:178–181.

14

PI3-Kinases

Role in Signal Transduction

David A. Fruman, PhD and Lewis C. Cantley, PhD

1. INTRODUCTION

The membrane lipid phosphatidylinositol (PtdIns) possesses a head group with five free hydroxyl groups (Fig. 1A). Reversible phosphorylation of the hydroxyl moieties generates a family of PtdIns derivatives known as phosphoinositides. The PI3K family of enzymes phosphorylates the 3′ hydroxyl group of PtdIns, PtdIns 4-phosphate (PtdIns-4-P) and PtdIns 4,5-bisphosphate (PtdIns-4,5-P_2), resulting in the formation of PtdIns 3-phosphate (PtdIns-3-P), PtdIns 3,4-bisphosphate (PtdIns-3,4-P_2), and PtdIns 3,4,5-trisphosphate (PtdIns-3,4,5-P_3), respectively. Three PI3K classes have been defined on the basis of substrate preference and sequence homology *(1)*. Class I PI3Ks appear to be selective for PtdIns-4,5-P_2 in vivo, but can also use PtdIns-4-P and PtdIns in vitro. Class II PI3Ks preferentially phosphorylate PtdIns and PtdIns-4-P, whereas Class III enzymes use only PtdIns. PtdIns-3-P can also be phosphorylated further by another group of enzymes, the PtdInsP kinases, to produce PtdIns-3,4-P_2 and PtdIns-3,5-P_2 *(2,3)*. Thus, PI3Ks are either directly or indirectly involved in the production of four phosphoinositides: PtdIns-3-P, PtdIns-3,4-P_2, PtdIns-3,5-P_2, and PtdIns-3,4,5-P_3. Yeast contain only the class III enzyme (vps34), whereas higher eukaryotes express all three classes of PI3K.

The lipid products of PI3Ks are termed D-3 phosphoinositides. These lipids apparently are not direct precursors of soluble inositol phosphates (InsPs), as they are resistant to hydrolysis by the known phospholipase C (PLC) isozymes *(4)*. Rather, D-3 phosphoinositides are themselves second messengers that recruit cytoplasmic proteins to the membrane and, in some cases, alter their activity. This chapter focuses on the proteins known to interact directly with these lipids. We also review genetic data supporting a role for PI3Ks in various physiological functions. Although the structure and regulation of PI3Ks has been reviewed elsewhere in detail *(5–7)*, we will begin with a brief overview of how these enzymes are activated in cells.

2. ACTIVATION

Class I PI3Ks are heterodimeric enzymes that consist of a catalytic subunit of approx 110 kDa (p110) and an adapter (also termed regulatory) subunit *(8–14)* (Fig. 1B).

From: Signaling Networks and Cell Cycle Control: The Molecular Basis of Cancer and Other Diseases
Edited by: J. S. Gutkind © Humana Press Inc., Totowa, NJ

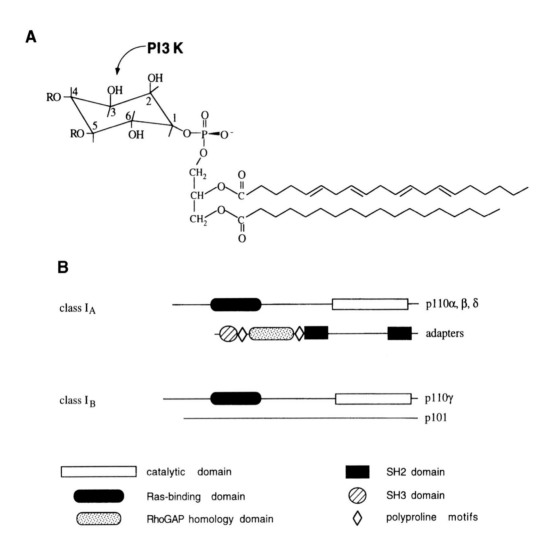

Fig. 1. (A) Structure of PI3K substrates. In phosphatidylinositol (PtdIns), both R groups represent hydrogen atoms. In PtdIns-4-P and PtdIns-4,5-P$_2$, one or both R groups represent phosphate groups. **(B)** Domain structure of class I PI3Ks. There are several forms of class I$_A$ adapter proteins. Two of these, p85α and p85β, have the structure shown, whereas p55α, p50α, and p55γ are shorter proteins lacking the SH3 domain, RhoGAP-homology domain and first polyproline motif.

These enzymes have been further subdivided into class I$_A$ and class I$_B$ based on the type of adapter subunit. The adapters for class I$_A$ enzymes contain two Src-homology 2 (SH2) domains that mediate interaction with phosphotyrosine (pTyr) residues within specific sequence contexts *(15)* (Fig. 1B). Many of these pTyr motifs are found in membrane-associated signaling proteins, including activated growth factor receptors and oncoproteins. The SH2-pTyr interaction increases lipid kinase activity of the catalytic subunit by two- to three-fold *(16,17)* and also serves to concentrate the enzyme near membranes in proximity to its substrates. Some class I$_A$ adapters possess additional sequence motifs (Src-homology 3 [SH3] domain, rhoGAP-homology domain, polyproline motifs; Fig. 1B) that may mediate activation by pTyr-independent mechanisms (9–11,18). Class I_B enzymes possess an adapter subunit termed p101 whose sequence lacks motifs with recognizable homology to other signaling proteins (14) (Fig. 1B).

G proteins can directly activate class I PI3Ks. The small G protein Ras, a central component of many signaling pathways, binds to the p110 subunit of class I_A enzymes in a GTP-dependent manner (19) (Fig. 1B). There is considerable evidence that this interaction increases PI3K activity and that PI3Ks are critical downstream effectors of Ras (20). Full activation of the lipid kinase may require concurrent association of the catalytic subunit with Ras, and the adapter subunit with a pTyr-containing protein (21).

The βγ subunits of heterotrimeric G proteins activate class I_B enzymes (13,22,23). One group found that the p101 adapter is required for Gβγ activation (14), but others have found the adapter subunit to be dispensable (13). Gβγ subunits may also increase the activity of one class I_A isoform, p110β, but only in the presence of pTyr peptides that bind to the adapter subunit (24). Conversely, Ras may regulate class I_B enzymes (25), which retain a region of homology to the Ras binding site on class I_A enzymes. Little is known about the regulation of class II and III enzymes. There is some evidence for regulated tyrosine phosphorylation of class II PI3Ks (26). The class III enzyme forms a heterodimer with a serine/threonine kinase in both yeast (vps15p) and mammals (p150) (27,28).

3. FUNCTION

3.1. Downstream Targets

In most resting cells, PtdIns-4-P and PtdIns-4,5-P_2 represent >90% of the total phosphoinositides. PtdIns-3-P represents about 3–5% of the total, whereas PtdIns-3,4-P_2 and PtdIns-3,4,5-P_3 are nominally absent. Agonists that stimulate class I PI3Ks cause the levels of PtdIns-3,4-P_2 and PtdIns-3,4,5-P_3 to increase rapidly and transiently (29,30), consistent with their roles as regulated second messengers. Yet, even after cell stimulation, PtdIns-4-P and PtdIns-4,5-P_2 are still present in significant molar excess at the whole cell level. Therefore, only those proteins that bind with strong selectivity to D-3 phosphoinositides are likely to be relevant downstream targets of PI3K. Table 1 lists the proteins currently known to bind selectively to D-3 phosphoinositides in vitro. The function of many of these proteins in vivo has been shown to require PI3K activation, and in some cases this requirement can be bypassed by attaching a constitutive membrane-targeting signal to the protein. These putative PI3K downstream targets can be divided into several classes discussed in the following sections.

3.1.1. PH Domains

Pleckstrin-homology (PH) domains are stretches of about 100 amino acids found in many cytoplasmic proteins (31). Although they share limited sequence homology, PH domains exhibit similar three-dimensional folds. Different PH domains selectively bind to different phosphoinositides and soluble inositol phosphates (32). PH domains may also be involved in protein–protein interactions (33).

A well-characterized target of D-3 phosphoinositides is the PH domain of Akt (sometimes termed protein kinase B or Rac-PK), a serine/threonine kinase. Akt was

Table 1
Targets of D-3 Phosphoinositides

| Binding domain | Protein | | Selectivity[a] |
	Name	Activity	
PH domain	**Akt**[b]	Ser/Thr kinase	PtdIns-3,4-P_2 = PtdIns-3,4,5-P_3[c]
	PDK1	Ser/Thr kinase	PtdIns-3,4,5-P_3 • PtdIns-3,4-P_2
	Btk/Itk	Tyr kinase	PtdIns-3,4,5-P_3 >> PtdIns-3,4-P_2
	Grp-1	Arf exchange factor	PtdIns-3,4,5-P_3 >> PtdIns-3,4-P_2
	Gab-1	Adaptor protein	PtdIns-3,4,5-P_3 >> PtdIns-3,4-P_2
	Sos	Rac/Cdc42 exchange factor	PtdIns-3,4,5-P_3 > PtdIns-3,4-P_2
	TIAM-1	Rac/Cdc42 exchange factor	PtdIns-3,4,5-P_3 > PtdIns-3,4-P_2
	Vav	Rac/Cdc42 exchange factor	N.D.[d]
	Centaurin-α	Arf-GTPase activating protein	PtdIns-3,4,5-P_3 > PtdIns-3,4-P_2
SH2 domain	PI3K p85	Adapter	PtdIns-3,4,5-P_3 >> PtdIns-3,4-P_2
	Src	Tyr kinase	PtdIns-3,4,5-P_3 >> PtdIns-3,4-P_2
	PLCγ	Phospholipase	PtdIns-3,4,5-P_3 >> PtdIns-3,4-P_2
Unknown	PKC-δ,ε, η	Ser/Thr kinase	PtdIns-3,4-P_2 = PtdIns-3,4,5-P_3
	AP-2	Clathrin adapter	PtdIns-3-P > PtdIns-3,4-P_2
Basic sequence motif	AP-3	Clathrin adapter	PtdIns-3,4,5-P_3 > PtdIns-3,4-P_2
(In N-terminus)			
(In C2 domain)	Synaptotagmin	Synaptic vesicle function	PtdIns-3,4,5-P_3 > PtdIns-4,5-P_2 reversed with increased calcium
(Around Arg-88)	Profilin	Actin regulatory	PtdIns-3,4-P_2 = PtdIns-3,4,5-P_3
Two sites	Gelsolin	Actin uncapping	N.D.

[a]Determined by in vitro binding experiments.

[b]Proteins in bold type have highest affinity for D-3 phosphoinositides and best evidence for binding in vivo.

[c]Although both lipids bind with comparable affinity, only PtdIns-3,4-P_2 appears to increase basal Akt kinase activity *(37,119)*.

[d]Not determined.

first shown to function downstream of PI3K by transfection experiments and by the use of wortmannin, a pharmacological PI3K inhibitor *(34,35)*. PI3K-dependent activation was found to require the N-terminal PH domain of Akt *(34,36)*. Direct binding experiments have established that the PH domain of Akt binds to PtdIns-3,4-P_2 with high affinity ($K_d = 5$ μM) *(37)*. This interaction is structurally specific because PtdIns-4,5-P_2 binds much more weakly. Full activation of Akt kinase requires phosphorylation of threonine-308 (T308) and serine-473 (S473) in the protein *(38)*. It has been proposed that PtdIns-3,4-P$_2$ and/or PtdIns-3,4,5-P$_3$ recruits Akt to the membrane, relieving an intramolecular inhibitory effect of the PH domain and inducing a transiently activated state. Subsequently, other membrane-associated kinases phosphorylate Akt and lock it in its high activity conformation *(39)*.

A kinase that phosphorylates Akt at T308 has been isolated *(40,41)* and cloned *(42,43)*. Termed phosphoinositide-dependent kinase-1 (PDK1), the ability of this kinase to phosphorylate Akt is potentiated by both PtdIns-3,4-P$_2$ and PtdIns-3,4,5-P$_3$ *(40,41)*. PDK1 contains a C-terminal PH domain that binds tightly to PtdIns-3,4,5-P$_3$ and may mediate membrane recruitment in a PI3K-dependent manner *(43)*. However, it appears that PDK1 is a constitutively active kinase; only its access to substrates is regulated by phosphoinositides. Thus, the role of PtdIns-3,4-P$_2$ and PtdIns-3,4,5-P$_3$ seems to be to recruit both Akt and PDK1 to the membrane, unmasking the T308 site on Akt in the process. This model fits with observations that artificial membrane targeting of Akt confers constitutive activation even without PI3K activation *(35,44,45)*, and that wortmannin treatment does not inhibit PDK1 kinase activity *(46)*. Phosphorylation of S473 on Akt may be mediated by yet another phosphoinositide-dependent kinase(s) *(40,41)*.

An important physiological function of PI3K-dependent Akt activation is to transmit a cellular survival signal *(39,47)*. Activated forms of both PI3Ks and Akt have been shown to protect from apoptosis induced by withdrawal of growth and survival factors *(48–50)*, expression of c-*myc* *(51)*, and detachment from extracellular matrix *(52)*. The pro-apoptotic protein BAD is a substrate of Akt *(53,54)*. Phosphorylation of BAD induces its association with the phosphoserine-binding protein 14-3-3, sequestering BAD and relieving its pro-apoptotic function. It is worth investigating whether other Akt substrates associate with 14-3-3, which recognizes phosphoserine only within specific sequence contexts *(55)*.

PDK-1 has important signaling functions in addition to helping activate Akt. Recent experiments indicate that PDK-1 can phosphorylate and activate p70^{S6K} *(46,56)*, a kinase that was shown to be downstream of PI3K in growth factor-dependent mitogenic signaling *(57)*. Phosphorylation of threonine-229 of p70^{S6K} by PDK1 in vitro occurs in the absence of D-3 phosphoinositides *(56)*. However, p70^{S6K} is only a good substrate for PDK1 if serine-389 has been converted to an acidic amino acid, mimicking a phosphorylation step that is known to be wortmannin sensitive *(46,56)*. Thus, PI3K indirectly regulates the efficiency of PDK-1 phosphorylation of both p70^{S6K} and Akt.

The PH domain of Bruton's tyrosine kinase (Btk) binds to PtdIns-3,4,5-P$_3$ with a K_d value of 0.8 μM; its affinities for soluble inositol 1,3,4,5-tetrakisphosphate (InsP$_4$), PtdIns-3,4-P$_2$ and PtdIns-4,5-P$_2$ are 10- to 100-fold lower *(32)*. Mutations in the B lymphocyte-specific Btk are linked to immunodeficiencies both in humans and in mice; importantly, some of these point mutations map to the PH domain and abolish PtdIns-3,4,5-P$_3$ binding *(32,58,59)*. Activation of PI3K correlates with increased tyrosine phosphorylation of both Btk and an important Btk substrate, PLCγ *(60,61)*. Btk can be phosphorylated and activated by Src family kinases. As for the phosphorylation of Akt by PDK-1, phosphorylation of Btk by Src kinases may be facilitated in vivo by phosphoinositide-dependent membrane recruitment of the substrate *(60,61)*. Such a paradigm is supported by studies of Itk, a T-cell-specific kinase highly related to Btk.

Itk is recruited to the membrane by an interaction of its PH domain with PtdIns-3,4,5-P_3, leading to phosphorylation by membrane bound Src *(62)*. Another member of the Btk kinase subfamily, Tec, is likely to be regulated by D-3 phosphoinositides as well *(61)*. Interestingly, overexpression of Btk increases cellular levels of PtdIns-3,4,5-P_3 by a mechanism that requires a functional PH domain, but not kinase activity, suggesting that the Btk PH domain may protect PtdIns-3,4,5-P_3 from degradation in vivo *(61)*.

Other PH domain-containing proteins that bind selectively to PtdIns-3,4,5-P_3 include certain guanine nucleotide exchange factors (GEF) (Table 1). This class of enzymes triggers activation of small G proteins by facilitating exchange of GDP for GTP. Because most small G proteins are constitutively membrane-associated as a result of farnesylation or myristoylation, or both, efficient nucleotide exchange requires movement of the cytoplasmic exchange factors to the membrane. This membrane localization appears to be mediated in part by PH domains that are found in all known GEFs for small G proteins *(63)*.

The PH domain of Sos, the best-studied Ras exchange factor, binds to both PtdIns-4,5-P_2 and PtdIns-3,4,5-P_3 in vitro. Using synthetic water-soluble lipids with short fatty acyl chains, it was demonstrated that Sos binds about threefold better to PtdIns-3,4,5-P_3 than to PtdIns-4,5-P_2 *(32)*. This relatively small difference may be sufficient to alter the localization of Sos after activation of PI3K, since the isolated PH domain of Sos was found to associate with cellular membranes only after serum stimulation *(64)*. However, Sos recruitment is also greatly facilitated by the binding of its proline-rich regions to SH3 domains of the adapter protein Grb2, which itself is brought to the membrane by an interaction of its SH2 domain with pTyr residues in growth factor receptors *(65)*. The function of the PH domain of Sos is further complicated by the recent discovery that the adjacent Dbl-homology domain of Sos can act as an exchange factor for Rac *(see below)*. PtdIns-3,4,5-P_3 may serve to direct Sos to particular regions of the membrane, or to stabilize its membrane attachment. Such an influence of PtdIns-3,4,5-P_3 on Sos localization could reconcile the seemingly contradictory findings that Ras is both downstream *(66)* and upstream *(21)* of PI3K. Ras may be downstream of PI3K because of PtdIns-3,4,5-P_3-mediated membrane recruitment of Sos, and upstream because Ras binds to and directly activates class I PI3K catalytic subunits. It is conceivable that this coupling of Ras and PI3K creates feedback amplification of a signaling cascade.

A similar mechanism could be involved in the regulation of Rac and Cdc42, two members of the Rho family of small G proteins that are involved in cytoskeletal responses to growth factors. Rac and Cdc42 have been reported to lie both upstream and downstream of PI3K in different systems. For example, several studies suggest that class I PI3Ks act upstream of Rac in a pathway leading to membrane ruffling and chemotaxis (67 and references therein). Conversely, activated forms of Rac and Cdc42 act upstream of PI3K to increase cellular motility and invasiveness *(68)*. As mentioned above, the Dbl domain of SOS has exchange activity for Rac *(69)*, so PtdIns-3,4,5-P_3-dependent recruitment of SOS to the membrane could facilitate Rac activation. The Rac-specific exchange factor TIAM-1 contains an N-terminal PH domain which, like the Sos PH domain, selectively binds PtdIns-3,4,5-P_3 *(32)*. Thus, PI3K products may recruit multiple Rac-GEFs to the membrane. On the other hand, both Rac and Cdc42, when bound to GTP, can interact with class I PI3K adapter subunits *(70,71)*. Although these interactions do not stimulate PI3K significantly in vitro, they may result in membrane recruitment in vivo.

Recent evidence points to a direct effect of lipid binding on exchange factor activity. Rho-GEF activity of the oncoprotein Vav is stimulated about twofold in vitro by a PI3K product, PtdIns-3,4,5-P_3, and greatly inhibited by a PI3K substrate, PtdIns-4,5-P_2 *(72)*. The PH domain of Vav is required for the effect of lipids. This suggests that PI3K may activate Vav by changing the phosphoinositide to which the PH domain is bound, not by altering its localization. A similar mechanism may exist for regulation of the Rac-GEF activity of Sos. Interestingly, Rac activation by the Dbl-homology domain of Sos appears to be suppressed by the adjacent PH domain under conditions where PI3K is inactive *(69)*. These results suggest a model to explain the previous findings that activated Ras induces membrane ruffling through PI3K and Rac *(73,74)*. Specifically, Ras activates PI3K leading to the production of D-3 phosphoinositides locally; these lipids then bind to the PH domain of Sos, unmasking the Rac-GEF activity of the adjacent domain.

The Arf family of small G proteins regulates vesicle sorting. Recently, GEF activity for Arf proteins has been associated with protein domains homologous to the yeast Sec7 protein *(75)*. Three members of this Sec7-containing protein family, termed ARNO, cytohesin-1 and Grp-1, also contain PH domains *(75–77)*. The PH domain of Grp-1 binds PtdIns-3,4,5-P_3 more than 10-fold better than PtdIns-4,5-P_2 *(77,78)*. In addition, PtdIns-3,4,5-P_3 binding increases the Arf exchange activity of Grp-1 in lipid micelles *(78)*. It is unknown whether the lipid has a direct effect on GEF activity of Grp-1 or an indirect effect via membrane recruitment. Studies of ARNO indicate that the primary purpose of the PH domain/lipid interaction is to target the exchange factor to membranes where Arf resides *(79)*. It is noteworthy that centaurin-α *(80)*, a brain-specific protein with homology to Arf-GAPs (GTPase-activating protein), contains a PH domain that interacts selectively with PtdIns-3,4,5-P_3. This finding indicates that PI3K lipid products may have both positive and negative effects on Arf function.

PI3K may also influence vesicle trafficking at the level of membrane fusion. The Rab family of small G proteins regulates membrane fusion of vesicles. Experiments with wortmannin and dominant-negative forms of PI3K have suggested that PI3K activation is required for endosome fusion mediated by Rab5 *(81)*. It is possible that PI3K lipid products interact with exchange factors for Rab G proteins, as they do with the PH domains in GEFs for Ras, Rac/Cdc42 and Arf. Further experiments are required to test this hypothesis.

Some PH domains bind soluble InsPs with high affinity *(32)*. This suggests that accumulation of high levels of InsPs may favor binding and release of PH domains from the membrane. This may be a key mechanism for turning off signaling cascades involving PH domains. Dephosphorylation of phosphoinositides by specific phosphatases probably contributes to attenuation of signaling as well.

3.1.2. SH2 Domains

PtdIns-3,4,5-P_3 interacts specifically with certain SH2 domains, including those in Src kinases, PLCγ, and adapter subunits of class I PI3Ks *(82,83)*. In the case of Src-SH2, lipid binding is competed by pTyr peptides and by phenylphosphate, suggesting that the lipid and peptide binding pockets overlap *(82)*. However, mutations in the Src SH2 domain that abolish pTyr peptide binding do not reduce lipid binding, suggesting that there is some difference in the modes of binding.

Clues to the functional significance of SH2-lipid association have begun to emerge. Binding of PtdIns-3,4,5-P_3 to the PLCγ1 SH2 domains increases enzyme activity *(83)*, which may explain why wortmannin treatment inhibits IP_3 generation and calcium responses in some cells *(84,85)*. Interestingly, another group found that the PH domain of PLCγ1 contributed to PtdIns-3,4,5-P_3-dependent activation of PLCγ1 *(86)*. Association of PtdIns-3,4,5-P_3 with the SH2 domains of Src family kinases may drive the conversion from the closed inactive conformation to an open active conformation. This mechanism has been proposed to explain the activation of a tyrosine kinase activity downstream of the PI3K isoform p110γ *(87)*. PtdIns-3,4,5-P_3 may also influence SH2-containing proteins by membrane localization. For PI3K adapter subunits, this may be a mechanism to keep the catalytic subunit near its substrates even after the enzyme dissociates from membrane-bound proteins.

3.1.3. Protein Kinase C

Another group of signaling proteins affected directly by D-3 phosphoinositides are protein kinase C (PKC) enzymes. PKCs are classified as conventional, novel, or atypical based on their cofactor requirements and domain structure *(88)*. Conventional and novel PKCs contain a C1 domain that mediates binding to diacylglyerol (DAG) and phorbol esters, and a C2 domain that confers binding to acidic phospholipids. The interaction of phosphatidylserine (PS) with the C2 domains of conventional PKCs, but not novel PKCs, is greatly enhanced by Ca^{2+} *(88)*. Three novel PKCs (PKC-δ, PKC-ε and PKC-η) are activated in vitro by synthetic versions of PtdIns-3,4-P_2 and PtdIns-3,4,5-P_3 in the presence of PS *(89)*. PtdIns-4,5-P_2 is less potent at activating these kinases, and Ins-1,3,4-P_3 and Ins-1,3,4,5-P_4 fail to activate. Thus, the interaction is both stereospecific and dependent on the esterified glycerol moiety. Activation of PI3K is sufficient to induce membrane recruitment and activation of PKC-ε and ζ in fibroblasts *(90,120)*.

The domain of novel PKCs that interacts with D-3 phosphoinositides has not been mapped. These kinases may be regulated by phosphoinositides by the C1 domains, in a manner analogous to the activation by DAG. However, the C2 domain may also contribute to D-3 lipid binding. In this regard, a C2-like domain in the synaptic vesicle membrane protein synaptotagmin binds strongly to PtdIns-3,4-P_2 and PtdIns-3,4,5-P_3 *(91)*. Like the C2 domain of conventional PKCs, lipid binding to the synaptotagmin C2 domain is regulated by calcium ions. In this case, the effect of Ca^{2+} is to shift binding selectivity toward PtdIns-4,5-P_2, perhaps releasing synaptotagmin from D-3 phosphoinositides *(91)*. It is interesting that class II PI3Ks possess C2 domains that bind acidic phospholipids. For the C2 domain of the *Drosophila* class II enzyme, phospholipid binding is Ca^{2+} independent *(92)*. Although the function of these C2 domains is not yet established, it is conceivable that they could interact with the lipid products of the class II enzyme, much the same as the class I adapter subunit SH2 domains interact with PtdIns-3,4,5-P_3.

The regulation of atypical PKCs is poorly understood. These isozymes possess a C1-related domain that does not bind DAG *(88)*. They lack a C2 domain, yet their activity is stimulated by PS *(88)*. There is disagreement about whether the activity of the atypical PKC-ζ is enhanced by D-3 phosphoinositides in vitro *(89,93)*. In vivo, the atypical PKC-λ has been reported to function downstream of PI3K in fibroblasts stimulated with the growth factors EGF or PDGF *(94)*. The PKC-related kinase PRK1, which is regulated directly by the small G protein Rho, has also been found to be activated in vitro by both PtdIns-3,4,5-P_3 and PtdIns-4,5-P_2 *(95)*.

It is likely that one result of D-3 lipid-dependent PKC activation is to couple PI3Ks to the raf/MEK/MAP kinase cascade. Conventional and novel PKCs can phosphorylate and activate raf in vitro *(96* and references therein), and treatment of cells with PKC-activating phorbol esters leads to potent raf phosphorylation *(97)*. In addition, wortmannin can inhibit the activation of raf and/or MAPK triggered by certain stimuli *(98)*. For growth factor-dependent MAPK activation, this pathway may be especially important when amounts of the growth factor or its receptor are limiting *(99)*. Another PKC substrate whose phosphorylation is wortmannin-sensitive is pleckstrin. In permeabilized platelets, the addition of synthetic PtdIns-3,4-P_2 or PtdIns-3,4,5-P_3 induces pleckstrin phosphorylation *(30)*.

3.1.4. Clathrin Adapter Proteins

Two proteins involved in clathrin coated pit assembly have been reported to interact with D-3 phosphoinositides. The AP-2 adapter complex binds to endocytic sorting signals in proteins destined for clathrin-mediated internalization. This interaction was found to be strengthened by D-3 phosphoinositides *(100)*. Interestingly, PtdIns-3-P functioned better than PtdIns-3,4-P_2 or PtdIns-3,4,5-P_3 within this context. The synapse-specific clathrin assembly protein AP-3 was shown to interact with phosphoinositides with the order of preference PtdIns-3,4,5-P_3>PtdIns-3,4-P_2>PtdIns-4,5-P_2 *(101)*. The binding of PtdIns-3-P was not addressed in this study. The presence of the fatty acids and glycerol backbone was essential in studies of both AP-2 and AP-3. Together with the involvement of PI3K in the function of Arf and Rab G proteins, these findings may lead to a better understanding of the previously suggested role of PI3K in vesicle trafficking *(102)*.

3.1.5. Actin Regulatory Proteins

PI3K regulates cytoskeletal changes partly through its influence on the Rho family G proteins Rac and Cdc42. In addition, D-3 phosphoinositides affect actin assembly by directly binding to actin regulatory proteins. Both gelsolin and profilin contain basic stretches of amino acids that interact with negatively charged phosphoinositides in vitro *(103,104)*. Profilin, which suppresses actin polymerization, binds to PtdIns-3,4,5-P_3 and PtdIns-3,4-P_2 with affinities 2- and 10-fold higher, respectively, than PtdIns-4,5-P_2 *(105)*. Spectroscopic data indicate that lipid binding induces a conformational change in profilin *(105)*. The affinity of lipid binding correlates with the ability to block the inhibitory effect of profilin on actin assembly. D-3 phosphoinositides also inhibit the actin-severing activity of gelsolin *(106)*, and induce actin uncapping in permeabilized platelets *(107)*. It has also been reported that profilin and gelsolin increase the catalytic activity of a class I PI3K in vitro, perhaps via an interaction with the adapter subunit *(108)*.

3.2. Genetic Studies

Genetic experiments have provided dramatic evidence of the importance of PI 3-kinases in vivo. In general, increased expression of PI3Ks correlates with dysregulated cell growth. Overproduction of the *Drosophila* class I_A PI3K in imaginal disks causes an increase in size of the corresponding adult tissue *(109)*. The transforming avian retrovirus ASV16 expresses a p110α-related gene (v-p3k) with PI3K activity *(110)*. Overexpression of v-p3k in chick embryo fibroblasts causes cellular transformation. In mouse fibroblasts, constitutively active forms of PI3K possess weak transforming activity that can synergize with other proto-oncogenes, such as v-raf *(74,111)*. It will be interesting to determine which downstream targets of PI3K are required for maintenance of the transformed phenotype. One clear candidate is the anti-apoptotic kinase Akt, itself a proto-oncogene with a transforming viral counterpart *(112)*. Akt activity is increased in the transformed chicken fibroblasts *(110)*. In mouse fibroblasts, transformation by constitutively active PI3K requires Rac function *(74,111)*.

Gene disruption studies have been performed in several species. Mouse embryos lacking a functional p110α gene die at around d 10 *(121)*. Disruption of the class I_A PI3K gene (age-1/daf-23) in *Caenorhabditis elegans* results in two interesting phenotypes depending on the genotype of the mother *(113)*. Homozygous mutant offspring of homozygous mutant mothers display a constitutive dauer phenotype. Because normal worm larvae enter the developmentally arrested dauer stage only when food is scarce, this result indicates that the PI3K gene product may function in a pathway that senses nutrients. As PI3K is activated by insulin when glucose is abundant in mammals, perhaps an insulin-like regulatory system exists in worms. A different phenotype is observed in mutant offspring of heterozygous mothers, who presumably supply some age-1/daf-23 protein to the embryo. These worms develop to adulthood without entering dauer but live two to three times longer than normal. It is unclear how this phenotype correlates with the known functions of PI3Ks in mammalian cells. Nevertheless, this observation has fostered much speculation about a role for PI3Ks in longevity.

The slime mold *Dictyostelium discoideum* carries two class I_A PI3K genes and one class I_B gene. Single disruption of each gene does not cause a detectable phenotype, suggesting that the gene products have redundant functions *(114)*. However, removal of the two class I_A genes together causes defects in both growth and development, and disruption of either of these genes with the class I_B gene is lethal.

Disruption of the yeast class III PI3K gene *VPS34* causes a defect in vacuolar protein sorting *(115)*. Specifically, *VPS34* mutants fail to transport newly synthesized proteins from the Golgi to the vacuole. Genetic and biochemical studies have shown that the protein product of this gene interacts with a serine/threonine kinase that is the product of the *VPS15* gene in yeast *(27)*. As its name implies, this kinase is also required for vacuolar protein sorting. A related kinase has been found to be associated with the mammalian homolog of *VPS34 (28)*. Originally, class III PI3Ks were thought to fulfill a housekeeping function in mammalian cells, because PI-3-P levels do not generally change upon stimulation. However, recent work on integrin-stimulated platelets indicates that formation of PtdIns-3,4-P_2 and subsequent activation of Akt occurs through a PtdIns-3-P intermediate that is wortmannin-sensitive *(116)*.

Organisms and cell lines lacking particular PI3K genes will be useful for testing hypotheses about downstream targets of PI3Ks. In particular, one could ask whether overexpression of suspected targets of PI3Ks can complement mutant phenotypes. It may be especially informative to express modified forms of these proteins that are constitutively membrane targeted. Such genetic studies will provide a powerful means to sort out which of the interactions summarized in Table 1 are physiologically relevant.

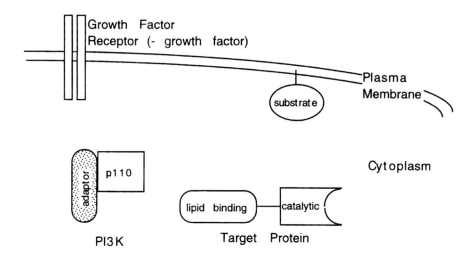

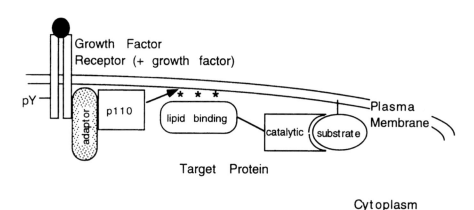

Fig. 2. General model for signaling mediated by PI3K lipid products. In the absence of growth factor, both PI3K and target proteins are in the cytoplasm. Upon growth factor binding, receptors are phosphorylated on tyrosine, leading to the recruitment and activation of PI3K. PI3K activation is also enhanced by activated Ras (not shown). The formation of D-3 phosphoinositides then recruits target proteins via their lipid binding domains, concentrating their catalytic domains near membrane-bound substrates.

4. PERSPECTIVES

During the past few years, a great deal has been learned about the protein targets of PI3K lipid products. These advances have been mainly driven by the availability of recombinant proteins and pure synthetic forms of the lipids. In some cases (e.g., Grp-1), the target was cloned based on its affinity for D-3 phosphoinositides. This approach will probably continue to reveal novel targets of phosphoinositides.

A common paradigm has emerged as the targets of D-3 phosphoinositides have been studied (Fig. 2). Most of these proteins are found in the cytoplasm in resting cells.

Upon activation of PI3Ks, lipids are produced that selectively bind to small domains in the target proteins. These proteins, now concentrated at the membrane, contain enzymatic domains (e.g., exchange factors) whose relevant substrates are also membrane-bound (e.g., G proteins). In the case of protein kinase C isozymes, whose substrate preference is relatively broad in vitro, targeting to particular regions of the membrane may play a crucial role in guiding substrate recognition in vivo.

As protein targets are discovered, new questions arise. For example, which target(s) is relevant for the function of PI3K in different cellular responses? The myriad functions blocked by wortmannin can probably be attributed to specific subsets of proteins that interact with D-3 phosphoinositides. It will also be important to determine which class and isoform of PI3K generate the lipids that recruit particular target proteins. For responses involving PtdIns-3,4,5-P_3, class I PI3Ks are apparently responsible. However, production of PtdIns-3,4-P_2 and subsequent activation of Akt may involve either class I or class II enzymes. PtdIns-3,4-P_2 may also be produced by the action of a PtdInsP kinase on PtdIns-3-P, or of a 5-phosphatase on PtdIns-3,4,5-P_3. PtdIns-3-P, which plays a role in clathrin coated pit assembly and probably other protein trafficking events, is formed primarily by class III PI3Ks, with class II enzymes and phosphoinositide phosphatases perhaps also involved. Another challenge will be to define the subcellular distribution of PI3Ks, their lipid products, and their protein targets. By constructing green fluorescent protein fusion proteins of isolated protein domains, it should be possible to obtain precise information about where and when PI3K-mediated signaling occurs, as was recently investigated with other signaling proteins *(117,118)*. These efforts should continue to shed light on the role of PI3Ks in signal transduction.

NOTE ADDED IN PROOF

Since the original submission of this review, many advances have been made in the field of PI3-kinase signaling. We will mention some of the most important ones in this note and refer the reader to recent reviews of these areas. First, the mechanism of activation of PKCs by PI3K has become more clear. Many PKCs are themselves regulated by PDK-1-mediated phosphorylation of the activation loop within their kinase domains *(122)*. Thus, as for activation of Akt, the activation of certain PKCs by D-3 phophoinositides involves PDK-1 in addition to direct lipid binding. Second, a novel class of lipid binding domain has been described. Termed the FYVE domain, this module selectively binds PtdIns-3-P and is present in many proteins involved in vesicle trafficking in yeast and in mammals *(123,124)*. PI3K-dependent activation of Rab5 is probably mediated by EEA1, a Rab5-interacting protein with a FYVE domain. Third, the tumor suppressor PTEN was determined to be a lipid phosphatase that removes the 3-phosphate from PtdIns-3,4,5-P3 and attenuates PI3K-mediated activation of Akt *(125)*. Finally, additional mouse knockouts of PI3K genes have been reported. Mice lacking p85α are viable but hypoglycemic *(126)*. Mice lacking p85α, p55α, and p50α die before adulthood, show hepatocellular necrosis and chylous ascites, and are also hypoglycemic (DA Fruman, LC Cantley, et al., submitted). Both strains of mice show defects in B cell development and activation that are quite similar to the defects observed in mice lacking Btk function *(127,128)*. These findings suggest that individual PI3K isoforms have nonredundant functions and that the relevant downstream effectors of PI3K signaling vary in different cell types.

ACKNOWLEDGMENT

D.A.F. is supported by a fellowship from the Cancer Research Fund of the Damon Runyon-Walter Winchell Foundation.

REFERENCES

1. Domin J, Waterfield MD. Using structure to define the function of phosphoinositide 3-kinase family members. *FEBS Lett* 1997; 410:91–95.
2. Zhang X, Loijens JC, Boronenkov IV, Parker GJ, Norris FA, Chen J, Thum O, Prestwich GD, Majerus PW, Anderson RA. Phosphatidylinositol-4-phosphate 5-kinase isozymes catalyze the synthesis of 3-phosphate-containing phosphatidylinositol signaling molecules. *J Biol Chem* 1997; 272:17,756–17,761.
3. Rameh L, Tolias K, Duckworth B, Cantley L. A novel pathway for synthesis of PtdIns-4,5-bisphosphate. *Nature* 1997; 390:192–196.
4. Serunian LA, Haber MT, Fukui T, Kim JW, Rhee SG, Lowenstein JM, Cantley LC. Polyphosphoinositides produced by phosphatidylinositol 3-kinase are poor substrates for phospholipases C from rat liver and bovine brain. *J Biol Chem* 1989; 264:17,809–17,815.
5. Duckworth BC, Cantley LC. PI 3-kinase and receptor-linked signal transduction, in *Handbook of Lipid Research: Lipid Second Messengers* (Bell RM, Exton JH, eds). Plenum Press, New York, pp 125–175.
6. Vanhaesebroeck B, Leevers SJ, Panayotou G, Waterfield MD. Phosphoinositide 3-kinases: A conserved family of signal transducers. *Trends Biochem Sci* 1997; 22:267–272.
7. Fruman DA, Meyers RE, Cantley LC. Phosphoinositide kinases. *Annu Rev Biochem* 1998; 67:481–507.
8. Carpenter CL, Duckworth BC, Auger KR, Cohen B, Schaffhausen BS, Cantley LC. Purification and characterization of phosphoinositide 3-kinase from rat liver. *J Biol Chem* 1990; 265:19,704–19,711.
9. Otsu M, Hiles I, Gout I, Fry MJ, Ruiz-Larrea F, Panayotou G, Thompson A, Dhand R, Hsuan J, Totty N, Smith AD, Morgan SJ, Courtneidge SA, Parker PJ, Waterfield MJ. Characterization of two 85 kd proteins that associate with receptor tyrosine kinases, middle T/pp60c-src complexes, and PI 3-kinase. *Cell* 1991; 65:91–104.
10. Escobedo JA, Navankasattusas S, Kavanaugh WM, Milfay D, Fried VA, Williams LT. cDNA cloning of a novel 85 kd protein that has SH2 domains and regulates binding of PI3-kinase to the PDGF beta-receptor. *Cell* 1991; 65:75–82.
11. Skolnik EY, Margolis B, Mohammadi M, Lowenstein E, Fischer R, Drepps A, Ullrich A, Schlessinger J. Cloning of PI3 kinase-associated p85 utilizing a novel method for expression/cloning of target proteins for receptor tyrosine kinases. *Cell* 1991; 65:83–90.
12. Hiles ID, Otsu M, Volinia S, Fry MJ, Gout I, Dhand R, Panayotou G, Ruiz LF, Thompson A, Totty NF, et al. Phosphatidylinositol 3-kinase: Structure and expression of the 110 kd catalytic subunit. *Cell* 1992; 70:419–429.
13. Stoyanov B, Volinia S, Hanck T, Rubio I, Loubtchenkov M, Malek D, Stoyanova S, Vanhaesebroeck B, Dhand R, Nurnberg B, et al. Cloning and characterization of a G protein-activated human phosphoinositide-3 kinase. *Science* 1995; 269:690–693.

14. Stephens LR, Eguinoa A, Erdjument-Bromage H, Lui M, Cooke F, Coadwell J, Smrcka AS, Thelen M, Cadwallader K, Tempst P, Hawkins PT. The G beta gamma sensitivity of a PI3K is dependent upon a tightly associated adaptor, p101. *Cell* 1997; 89:105–114.

15. Zhou S, Shoelson SE, Chaudhuri M, Gish G, Pawson T, Haser WG, King F, Roberts T, Ratnofsky S, Lechleider RJ, et al. SH2 domains recognize specific phosphopeptide sequences. *Cell* 1993; 72:767–778.

16. Backer JM, Myers MJ, Shoelson SE, Chin DJ, Sun XJ, Miralpeix M, Hu P, Margolis B, Skolnik EY, Schlessinger J, et al. Phosphatidylinositol 3′-kinase is activated by association with IRS-1 during insulin stimulation. *EMBO J* 1992; 11:3469–3479.

17. Carpenter CL, Auger KR, Chanudhuri M, Yoakim M, Schaffhausen B, Shoelson S, Cantley LC. Phosphoinositide 3-kinase is activated by phosphopeptides that bind to the SH2 domains of the 85-kDa subunit. *J Biol Chem* 1993; 268:9478–9483.

18. Pleiman CM, Hertz WM, Cambier JC. Activation of phosphatidylinositol-3′ kinase by Src-family kinase SH3 binding to the p85 subunit. *Science* 1994; 63:1609–1612.

19. Rodriguez VP, Warne PH, Dhand R, Vanhaesebroeck B, Gout I, Fry MJ, Waterfield MD, Downward J. Phosphatidylinositol-3-OH kinase as a direct target of Ras. *Nature* 1994; 370:527–532.

20. Rodriguez-Viciana P, Warne PH, Vanhaesebroeck B, Waterfield MD, Downward J. Activation of phosphoinositide 3-kinase by interaction with Ras and by point mutation. *EMBO J* 1996; 15:2442–2451.

21. Rodriguez-Viciana P, Marte BM, Warne PH, Downward J. Phosphatidylinositol 3′ kinase: One of the effectors of Ras. *Philos Trans R Soc Lond Biol Sci* 1996; 351:225–231.

22. Stephens L, Smrcka A, Cooke FT, Jackson TR, Sternweis PC, Hawkins PT. A novel phosphoinositide 3 kinase activity in myeloid-derived cells is activated by G protein beta gamma subunits. *Cell* 1994; 77:83–93.

23. Tang X, Downes CP. Purification and characterization of Gbetagamma-responsive phosphoinositide 3-kinases from pig platelet cytosol. *J Biol Chem* 1997; 272:14,193–14,199.

24. Kurosu H, Maehama T, Okada T, Yamamoto T, Hoshino S, Fukui Y, Ui M, Hazeki O, Katada T. Heterodimeric phosphoinositide 3-kinase consisting of p85 and p110beta is synergistically activated by the betagamma subunits of G proteins and phosphotyrosyl peptide. *J Biol Chem* 1997; 272:24,252–24,256.

25. Rubio I, Rodriguez-Viciana P, Downward J, Wetzker R. Interaction of Ras with phosphoinositide 3-kinase gamma. *Biochem J* 1997; 326:891–895.

26. Molz L, Chen Y-W, Hirano M, Williams LT. Cpk is a novel class of *Drosophila* PtdIns 3-kinase containing a C2 domain. *J Biol Chem* 1996; 271:13,892–13,899.

27. Stack JH, Herman PK, Schu PV, Emr SD. A membrane-associated complex containing the Vps15 protein kinase and the Vps34 PI 3-kinase is essential for protein sorting to the yeast lysosome-like vacuole. *EMBO J* 1993; 12:2195–2204.

28. Panaretou C, Domin J, Cockcroft S, Waterfield MD. Characterization of p150, an adaptor protein for the human phosphatidylinositol (PtdIns) 3-kinase. Substrate presentation by phosphatidylinositol transfer protein to the p150.Ptdins 3-kinase complex. *J Biol Chem* 1997; 272:2477–2485.

29. Stephens LR, Hughes KT, Irvine RF. Pathway of phosphatidylinositol(3,4,5)-trisphosphate synthesis in activated neutrophils. *Nature* 1991; 351:33–39.

30. Toker A, Bachelot C, Chen C-S, Falck JR, Hartwig JH, Cantley LC, Kovacsovics T. Phosphorylation of the p47 platelet phosphoprotein is mediated by the lipid products of phosphoinositide 3-kinase. *J Biol Chem* 1995; 270:29,525–29,531.

31. Lemmon MA, Ferguson KM, Schlessinger J. PH domains: Diverse sequences with a common fold recruit signaling molecules to the cell surface. *Cell* 1996; 85:621–624.

32. Rameh LE, Arvidsson A, Carraway KLR, Couvillon AD, Rathbun G, Crompton A, VanRenterghem B, Czech MP, Ravichandran KS, Burakoff SJ, Wang DS, Chen CS, Cantley

LC. A comparative analysis of the phosphoinositide binding specificity of pleckstrin homology domains. *J Biol Chem* 1997; 272:22,059–22,066.

33. Touhara K, Inglese J, Pitcher JA, Shaw G, Lefkowitz RJ. Binding of G protein beta gamma-subunits to pleckstrin homology domains. *J Biol Chem* 1994; 269:10,217–10,220.

34. Franke TF, Yang SI, Chan TO, Datta K, Kazlauskas A, Morrison DK, Kaplan DR, Tsichlis PN. The protein kinase encoded by the Akt proto-oncogene is a target of the PDGF-activated phosphatidylinositol 3-kinase. *Cell* 1995; 81:727–736.

35. Burgering BM, Coffer PJ. Protein kinase B (c-Akt) in phosphatidylinositol-3-OH kinase signal transduction. *Nature* 1995; 376:599–602.

36. Klippel A, Reinhard C, Kavanaugh WM, Apell G, Escobedo MA, Williams LT. Membrane localization of phosphatidylinositol 3-kinase is sufficient to activate multiple signal-transducing kinase pathways. *Mol Cell Biol* 1996; 16:4117–4127.

37. Franke TF, Kaplan DR, Cantley LC, Toker A. Direct regulation of the Akt proto-oncogene product by phosphatidylinositol-3,4-bisphosphate. *Science* 1997; 275:665–668.

38. Alessi DR, Andjelkovic M, Caudwell B, Cron P, Morrice N, Cohen P, Hemmings BA. Mechanism of activation of protein kinase B by insulin and IGF-1. *EMBO J* 1996; 15:6541–6551.

39. Franke TF, Kaplan DR, Cantley LC. PI3K: Downstream AKTion blocks apoptosis. *Cell* 1997; 88:435–437.

40. Alessi DR, James SR, Downes CP, Holmes AB, Gaffney PR, Reese CB, Cohen P. Characterization of a 3-phosphoinositide-dependent protein kinase which phosphorylates and activates protein kinase Balpha. *Curr Biol* 1997; 7:261–269.

41. Stokoe D, Stephens LR, Copeland T, Gaffney PR, Reese CB, Painter GF, Holmes AB, McCormick F, Hawkins PT. Dual role of phosphatidylinositol-3,4,5-trisphosphate in the activation of protein kinase B. *Science* 1997; 277:567–570.

42. Alessi DR, Deak M, Casamayor A, Caudwell FB, Morrice N, Norman DG, Gaffney P, Reese CB, MacDougall CN, Harbison D, Ashworth A, Bownes M. 3-phosphoinositide-dependent protein kinase-1 (PDK1): structural and functional homology with the *Drosophila* DSTPK61 kinase. *Curr Biol* 1997; 7:776–789.

43. Stephens L, Anderson K, Stokoe D, Erdjument-Bromage H, Painter GF, Holmes AB, Gaffney P R J, Reese CB, McCormick F, Tempst P, Coadwell J, Hawkins PT. Protein kinase B kinases that mediate phosphatidylinositol 3,4,5-trisphosphate-dependent activation of protein kinase B. *Science* 1998; 279:710–714.

44. Kohn AD, Takeuchi F, Roth RA. Akt, a pleckstrin homology domain containing kinase, is activated primarily by phosphorylation. *J Biol Chem* 1996; 271:21,920–21,926.

45. Andjelkovic M, Alessi DR, Meier R, Fernandez A, Lamb NJ, Frech M, Cron P, Cohen P, Lucocq JM, Hemmings BA. Role of translocation in the activation and function of protein kinase B. *J Biol Chem* 1997; 272:31,515–31,524.

46. Pullen N, Dennis PB, Andjelkovic M, Dufner A, Kozma SC, Hemmings BA, Thomas G. Phosphorylation and activation of p70s6k by PDK1. *Science* 1998; 279:707–710.

47. Marte BM, Downward J. PKB/Akt: connecting phosphoinositide 3-kinase to cell survival and beyond. *Trends Biochem Sci* 1997; 22:355–358.

48. Kulik G, Klippel A, Weber MJ. Antiapoptotic signalling by the insulin-like growth factor I receptor, phosphatidylinositol 3-kinase, and Akt. *Mol Cell Biol* 1997; 17:1595–1606.

49. Ahmed NN, Grimes HL, Bellacosa A, Chan TO, Tsichlis PN. Transduction of interleukin-2 antiapoptotic and proliferative signals via Akt protein kinase. *Proc Natl Acad Sci USA* 1997; 94:3627–3632.

50. Kennedy SG, Wagner AJ, Conzen SD, Jordan J, Bellacosa A, Tsichlis PN, Hay N. The PI 3-kinase/Akt signaling pathway delivers an anti-apoptotic signal. *Genes Dev* 1997; 11:701–713.

51. Kauffmann-Zeh A, Rodriguez-Viciana P, Ulrich E, Gilbert C, Coffer P, Downward J,

Evan G. Suppression of c-Myc-induced apoptosis by Ras signalling through PI(3)K and PKB. *Nature* 1997; 385:544–548.

52. Khwaja A, Rodriguez-Viciana P, Wennstrom S, Warne PH, Downward J. Matrix adhesion and Ras transformation both activate a phosphoinositide 3-OH kinase and protein kinase B/Akt cellular survival pathway. *EMBO J* 1997; 16:2783–2793.

53. Datta SR, Dudek H, Tao X, Masters S, Fu H, Gotoh Y, Greenberg ME. Akt phosphorylation of BAD couples survival signals to the cell—Intrinsic death machinery. *Cell* 1997; 91:231–241.

54. del Peso L, Gonzalez-Garcia M, Page C, Herrera R, Nunez G. Interleukin-3-induced phosphorylation of BAD through the protein kinase Akt. *Science* 1997; 278:687–689.

55. Yaffe MB, Rittinger K, Volinia S, Caron PR, Aitken A, Leffers H, Gamblin SJ, Smerdon SJ, Cantley LC. The structural basis for 14-3-3: Phosphopeptide binding specificity. *Cell* 1997; 91:961–971.

56. Alessi DR, Kozlowski MT, Weng QP, Morrice N, Avruch J. 3-Phosphoinositide-dependent protein kinase 1 (PDK1) phosphorylates and activates the p70 S6 kinase in vivo and in vitro. *Curr Biol* 1998; 8:69–81.

57. Chung J, Grammer TC, Lemon KP, Kazlauskas A, Blenis J. PDGF- and insulin-dependent pp70S6k activation mediated by phosphatidylinositol-3-OH kinase. *Nature* 1994; 370: 71–75.

58. Salim K, Bottomley MJ, Querfurth E, Zvelebil MJ, Gout I, Scaife R, Margolis RL, Gigg R, Smith CI, Driscoll PC, Waterfield MD, Panayotou G. Distinct specificity in the recognition of phosphoinositides by the pleckstrin homology domains of dynamin and Bruton's tyrosine kinase. *EMBO J* 1996; 15:6241–6250.

59. Fukuda M, Kojima T, Kabayama H, Mikoshiba K. Mutation of the pleckstrin homology domain of Bruton's tyrosine kinase in immunodeficiency impaired inositol 1,3,4,5-tetrakis-phosphate binding capacity. *J Biol Chem* 1996; 271:30,303–30,306.

60. Li Z, Wahl MI, Eguinoa A, Stephens LR, Hawkins PT, Witte ON. Phosphatidylinositol 3-kinase-gamma activates Bruton's tyrosine kinase in concert with Src family kinases. *Proc Natl Acad Sci USA* 1997; 94:13,820–13,825.

61. Scharenberg AM, El-Hillal O, Fruman DA, Beitz LO, Li Z, Lin S, Gout I, Cantley LC, Rawlings DJ, Kinet J-P. Phosphatidylinositol-3,4,5-trisphosphate (PtdIns-3,4,5-P_3)/ Tec kinase-dependent calcium signaling pathway: A target for SHIP-mediated inhibitory signals. *EMBO J* 1998; 17:1961–1972.

62. August A, Sadra A, Dupont B, Hanafusa H. Src-induced activation of inducible T cell kinase (ITK) requires phosphatidylinositol 3-kinase activity and the Pleckstrin homology domain of inducible T cell kinase. *Proc Natl Acad Sci USA* 1997; 94:11,227–11,232.

63. Hall A. Rho GTPases and the actin cytoskeleton. *Science* 1998; 279:509–514.

64. Chen RH, Corbalan-Garcia S, Bar-Sagi D. The role of the PH domain in the signal-dependent membrane targeting of Sos. *EMBO J* 1997; 16:1351–1359.

65. Olivier JP, Raabe T, Henkemeyer M, Dickson B, Mbamalu G, Margolis B, Schlessinger J, Hafen E, Pawson T. A *Drosophila* SH2-SH3 adaptor protein implicated in coupling the sevenless tyrosine kinase to an activator of Ras guanine nucleotide exchange, Sos. *Cell* 1993; 73:179–191.

66. Hu P, Margolis B, Skolnik EY, Lammers R, Ullrich A, Schlessinger AJ. Interaction of phosphatidylinositol 3-kinase-associated p85 with epidermal growth factor and platelet-derived growth factor receptors. *Mol Cell Biol* 1992; 12:981–990.

67. Reif K, Nobes CD, Thomas G, Hall A, Cantrell DA. Phosphatidylinositol 3-kinase signals activate a selective subset of Rac/Rho-dependent effector pathways. *Curr Biol* 1996; 6:1445–1455.

68. Keely PJ, Westwick JK, Whitehead IP, Der CJ, Parise LV. Cdc42 and Rac1 induce integrin-mediated cell motility and invasiveness through PI(3)K. *Nature* 1997; 390:632–636.

69. Nimnual AS, Yatsula BA, Bar-Sagi D. Coupling of Ras and Rac guanosine triphosphatases through the Ras exchanger Sos. *Science* 1998; 279:560–563.

70. Zheng Y, Bagrodia S, Cerione RA. Activation of phosphoinositide 3-kinase activity by Cdc42Hs binding to p85. *J Biol Chem* 1994; 269:18,727–18,730.

71. Tolias KF, Cantley LC, Carpenter CL. Rho family GTPases bind to phosphoinositide kinases. *J Biol Chem* 1995; 270:17,656–17,659.

72. Han J, Luby-Phelps K, Das B, Shu X, Xia Y, Mosteller RD, Krishna UM, Falck JR, White MA, Broek D. Role of substrates and products of PI 3-kinase in regulating activation of Rac-related guanosine triphosphatases by Vav. *Science* 1998; 279:558–560.

73. Ridley AJ, Paterson HF, Johnston CL, Diekmann D, Hall A. The small GTP-binding protein rac regulates growth factor-induced membrane ruffling. *Cell* 1992; 70:401–410.

74. Rodriguez-Viciana P, Warne PH, Khwaja A, Marte BM, Pappin D, Das P, Waterfield MD, Ridley A, Downward J. Role of phosphoinositide 3-OH kinase in cell transformation and control of the actin cytoskeleton by Ras. *Cell* 1997; 89:457–467.

75. Chardin P, Paris S, Antonny B, Robineau S, Beraud-Dufour S, Jackson CL, Chabre M. A human exchange factor for ARF contains Sec7- and pleckstrin-homology domains. *Nature* 1996; 384:481–484.

76. Kolanus W, Nagel W, Schiller B, Zeitlmann L, Godar S, Stockinger H, Seed B. Alpha L beta 2 integrin/LFA-1 binding to ICAM-1 induced by cytohesin-1, a cytoplasmic regulatory molecule. *Cell* 1996; 86:233–242.

77. Klarlund JK, Guilherme A, Holik JJ, Virbasius JV, Chawla A, Czech MP. Signaling by phosphoinositide-3,4,5-trisphosphate through proteins containing pleckstrin and Sec7 homology domains. *Science* 1997; 275:1927–1930.

78. Klarlund JK, Rameh LE, Cantley LC, Buxton JM, Holik JJ, Sakelis C, Patki V, Corvera S, Czech MP. Regulation of GRP1-catalyzed ADP ribosylation factor guanine nucleotide exchange by phosphatidylinositol 3,4,5-trisphosphate. *J Biol Chem* 1998; 273:1859–1862.

79. Paris S, Beraud-Dufour S, Robineau S, Bigay J, Antonny B, Chabre M, Chardin P. Role of protein-phospholipid interactions in the activation of ARF1 by the guanine nucleotide exchange factor Arno. *J Biol Chem* 1997; 272:22,221–22,226.

80. Hammonds-Odie LP, Jackson TR, Profit AA, Blader IJ, Turck CW, Prestwich GD, Theibert AB. Identification and cloning of centaurin-alpha. A novel phosphatidylinositol 3,4,5-trisphosphate-binding protein from rat brain. *J Biol Chem* 1996; 271:18,859–18,868.

81. Li G, D'Souza-Schorey C, Barbieri MA, Roberts RL, Klippel A, Williams LT, Stahl PD. Evidence for phosphatidylinositol 3-kinase as a regulator of endocytosis via activation of Rab5. *Proc Natl Acad Sci USA* 1995; 92:10,207–10,211.

82. Rameh LE, Chen C-S, Cantley LC. Phosphatidylinositol-3,4,5-P_3 interacts with SH2 domains and modulates phosphoinositide 3-kinase association with tyrosine-phosphorylated proteins. *Cell* 1995; 83:1–20.

83. Bae YS, Cantley LG, Chen C-S, Kim S-R, Kwon K-S, Rhee SG. Activation of phospholipase C-γ by phosphatidylinositol 3,4,5-trisphosphate. *J Biol Chem* 1998; 273:4465–4469.

84. Barker SA, Caldwell KK, Hall A, Martinez AM, Pfeiffer JR, Oliver JM, Wilson BS. Wortmannin blocks lipid and protein kinase activities associated with PI 3-kinase and inhibits a subset of responses induced by Fc epsilon R1 cross-linking. *Mol Biol Cell* 1995; 6:1145–1158.

85. Vossebeld PJ, Homburg CH, Schweizer RC, Ibarrola I, Kessler J, Koenderman L, Roos D, Verhoeven AJ. Tyrosine phosphorylation-dependent activation of phosphatidylinositide 3-kinase occurs upstream of Ca^{2+}-signalling induced by Fcgamma receptor cross-linking in human neutrophils. *Biochem J* 1997; 323:87–94.

86. Falasca M, Logan SK, Lehto VP, Baccante G, Lemmon MA, Schlessinger J. Activation of phospholipase Cgamma by PI 3-kinase-induced PH domain-mediated membrane targeting. *EMBO J* 17:414–422.

87. Lopez-Ilasaca M, Crespo P, Pellici PG, Gutkind JS, Wetzker R. Linkage of G protein-coupled receptors to the MAPK signaling pathway through PI 3-kinase gamma. *Science* 1997; 275:394–397.

88. Newton AC. Regulation of protein kinase C. *Curr Opin Cell Biol* 1997; 9:161–167.
89. Toker A, Meyer M, Reddy KK, Falck JR, Aneja R, Aneja S, Parra A, Burns DJ, Ballas LM, Cantley LC. Activation of protein kinase C family members by the novel polyphospho-inositides PtdIns-3,4-P2 and PtdIns-3,4,5-P3. *J Biol Chem* 1994; 269:32,358–32,367.
90. Moriya S, Kazlauskas A, Akimoto K, Hirai S, Mizuno K, Takenawa T, Fukui Y, Watanabe Y, Ozaki S, Ohno S. Platelet-derived growth factor activates protein kinase C epsilon through redundant and independent signaling pathways involving phospholipase C gamma or phosphatidylinositol 3-kinase. *Proc Natl Acad Sci USA* 1996; 93:151–155.
91. Schiavo G, Gu QM, Prestwich GD, Sollner TH, Rothman JE. Calcium-dependent switching of the specificity of phosphoinositide binding to synaptotagmin. *Proc Natl Acad Sci USA* 1996; 93:13,327–13,332.
92. MacDougall LK, Domin J, Waterfield MD. A family of phosphoinositide 3-kinases in *Drosophila* identifies a new mediator of signal transduction. *Curr Biol* 1995; 5:1404–1415.
93. Nakanishi H, Brewer KA, Exton JH. Activation of the zeta isozyme of protein kinase C by phosphatidylinositol 3,4,5-trisphosphate. *J Biol Chem* 1993; 268:13–16.
94. Akimoto K, Takahashi R, Moriya S, Nishioka N, Takayanagi J, Kimura K, Fukui Y, Osada S, Mizuno K, Hirai S, Kazlauskas A, Ohno S. EGF or PDGF receptors activate atypical PKClambda through phosphatidylinositol 3-kinase. *EMBO J* 1996; 15:788–798.
95. Palmer RH, Dekker LV, Woscholski R, Le Good JA, Gigg R, Parker P. Activation of PRK1 by phosphatidylinositol 4,5-bisphosphate and phosphatidylinositol 3,4,5-trisphosphate. *J Biol Chem* 1995; 270:22,412–22,416.
96. Schonwasser DC, Marais RM, Marshall CJ, Parker PJ. Activation of the mitogen-activated protein kinase/extracellular signal-regulated kinase pathway by conventional, novel, and atypical protein kinase C isotypes. *Mol Cell Biol* 1998; 18:790–798.
97. Morrison DK, Kaplan DR, Rapp U, Roberts TM. Signal transduction from membrane to cytoplasm: growth factors and membrane-bound oncogene products increase Raf-1 phosphorylation and associated protein kinase activity. *Proc Natl Acad Sci USA* 1988; 85:8855–8859.
98. Cross DA, Alessi DR, Vandenheede JR, McDowell HE, Hundal HS, Cohen P. The inhibition of glycogen synthase kinase-3 by insulin or insulin-like growth factor 1 in the rat skeletal muscle cell line L6 is blocked by wortmannin, but not by rapamycin: Evidence that wortmannin blocks activation of the mitogen-activated protein kinase pathway in L6 cells between Ras and Raf. *Biochem J* 1994; 303:21–26.
99. Duckworth BC, Cantley LC. Conditional inhibition of the mitogen-activated protein kinase cascade by wortmannin. Dependence on signal strength. *J Biol Chem* 1997; 272:27,665–27,670.
100. Rapoport I, Miyazaki M, Boll W, Duckworth B, Cantley LC, Shoelson S, Kirchhausen T. Regulatory interactions in the recognition of endocytic sorting signals by AP-2 complexes. *EMBO J* 1997; 16:2240–2250.
101. Hao W, Tan Z, Prasad K, Reddy KK, Chen J, Prestwich GD, Falck JR, Shears SB, Lafer EM. Regulation of AP-3 function by inositides. Identification of phosphatidylinositol 3,4,5-trisphosphate as a potent ligand. *J Biol Chem* 1997; 272:6393–6398.
102. Joly M, Kazlauskas A, Fay FS, Corvera S. Disruption of PDGF receptor trafficking by mutation of its PI-3 kinase binding sites. *Science* 1994; 263:684–687.
103. Yu FX, Sun HQ, Janmey PA, Yin HL. Identification of a polyphosphoinositide-binding sequence in an actin monomer-binding domain of gelsolin. *J Biol Chem* 1992; 267:14,616–14,621.
104. Sohn RH, Chen J, Koblan KS, Bray PF, Goldschmidt-Clermont PJ. Localisation of a binding site for phosphatidylinositol-4,5-bisphosphate on human profilin. *J Biol Chem* 1995; 270:21,114–21,120.
105. Lu PJ, Shieh WR, Rhee SG, Yin HL, Chen CS. Lipid products of phosphoinositide 3-kinase bind human profilin with high affinity. *Biochemistry* 1996; 35:14,027–14,034.

cell for rapamycin is the activated T lymphocyte, which undergoes G_1-to-S phase progression in response to IL-2 or T-cell growth-promoting cytokines. IL-2-stimulated T cells accumulate in the mid/late G_1 phase of the cell cycle in the presence of ≤ 10 n*M* rapamycin *(134,135)*. The growth-arrested T cells are characterized by the presence of fully assembled, but catalytically-inactive cyclin E-Cdk2 complexes *(135)*. This drug-induced disruption of G_1 cyclin-Cdk2 activation is due to the failure of the cells to downregulate the Cdk inhibitor, p27[Kip1] *(54,146)*. In the absence of rapamycin, IL-2 normally triggers the ubiquitination and proteosome-mediated degradation of p27[Kip1] as the cells progress through early G_1 phase. The failure to induce p27[Kip1] proteolysis explains the defective activation of cyclin E–Cdk2 complexes in rapamycin-treated T cells. Commensurate with the loss of cyclin E–Cdk2 activity, rapamycin-treated T cells fail to phosphorylate the retinoblastoma protein, and, hence, do not pass through the so-called "restriction point," after which the cells are committed to enter S phase. Although these results support an attractive model to explain the G_1-phase growth arrest state induced by rapamycin, it seems likely that inhibition of p27[Kip1] degradation is not the sole mechanism whereby this drug blocks the activation of G_1 cyclin–Cdk complexes in mammalian cells. The variable correlation between p27[Kip1] expression and rapamycin-induced growth inhibition in other cell types is probably explained, in part, by the fact that the suppression of G_1 cyclin-Cdk activities is a relatively distal consequence of the suppression of mTOR-dependent signaling by the FKBP12–rapamycin complex.

3.5. Role of mTOR in p70 S6 Kinase Activation

The search for more proximal biochemical responses to rapamycin treatment led to the identification of two proteins whose phosphorylation state is regulated by mTOR. The first target protein is p70 S6 kinase (p70[S6K]), a serine-threonine kinase that is activated in response to a broad range of mitogenic stimuli. Rapamycin blocks both the phosphorylation and activation of p70[S6K] in all mammalian cell types examined to date. The second end point for the mTOR-dependent phosphorylation pathway is the translational-repressor protein, PHAS-I (also termed 4E-BP1). It is striking that both p70[S6K] and PHAS-I participate in the regulation of protein synthesis in cells stimulated with mitogens or certain hormones, including insulin.

The regulation of p70[S6K] by upstream protein kinases is exceedingly complex, and the reader is referred to specialized reviews for details concerning this topic *(162,164)*. However, it is clear that treatment with rapamycin quickly and efficiently inhibits the *de novo* phosphorylation of p70[S6K] induced by hormonal stimuli, as well as the phosphorylation of previously activated p70[S6K]. The predicted epistatic relationship between mTOR and p70[S6K] was confirmed in cell transfection experiments, which demonstrated that introduction of a rapamycin-resistant mTOR mutant (*see* Section 2.1.) into Jurkat T cells rendered p70[S6K] activation correspondingly resistant to rapamycin *(22)*. The only documented physiologic substrate for p70[S6K] is the 40S ribosomal protein S6, although recent data suggest that this protein kinase may also phosphorylate two translation initiation factors: eIF-4G and eIF-4B *(187)*. The overall effect of these phosphorylation events is to increase the rate of protein synthesis, which, as discussed earlier, is especially important as cells pass through G_1 phase.

Mitogenic stimuli induce the phosphorylation of p70[S6K] on at least 10 serine and threonine residues. Both the Ras- and PI3K-dependent signaling pathways participate in p70^{S6K} phosphorylation in response to many growth factors, although other types of stimuli almost certainly activate p70^{S6K} via different protein kinase cascades. Of the identified phosphorylation sites, only three (Thr^{229}, Thr^{389}, and Ser^{404}) are phosphorylated in a rapamycin-sensitive fashion *(45,137,157,164)*. Phosphorylation of Thr^{389} appears to be particularly crucial for p70^{S6K} activation, because substitution of this residue with Ala blocks activation of the kinase domain, whereas a Thr^{389}→Glu substitution yields a partially activated and rapamycin-resistant form of p70^{S6K}. Indeed, a recent report provided evidence that the Thr^{389} site in p70^{S6K} may be directly phosphorylated by mTOR in an immune complex kinase assay *(28)*. Whether mTOR actually phosphorylates full-length p70^{S6K} at Thr^{389} (or any other site) in intact cells remains unresolved, and somewhat controversial. An alternative possibility that has not received sufficient attention is that mTOR activation represses a protein serine-threonine phosphatase that dephosphorylates the rapamycin-sensitive sites in p70^{S6K}. The derepression of this phosphatase by the binding of the FKBP12–rapamycin complex to mTOR explains the rapid dephosphorylation of p70^{S6K} when cells are exposed to the drug after insulin or growth factor treatment. Studies in both yeast and mammalian cells indicate that the activity of a PP2A-like phosphatase may be controlled by the TOR-dependent signaling pathway *(46,140)*.

3.6. Regulation of the Translational Repressor Function of PHAS-I by mTOR

The rate-limiting step in the translation of most eukaryotic mRNAs is initiation, a process that includes the binding of the 43S ribosomal preinitiation complex to the 5′-terminus of the mRNA, and the 5′→3′ translocation of this complex as it scans the 5′-UTR for an AUG initiation codon *(149,163,187)*. Both the ribosome binding and scanning steps are facilitated by the eukaryotic initiation factor (eIF)-4F complex, which itself binds to the cap structure (m^{7}GpppN, where N is any nucleotide) found at the extreme 5′-terminus of nearly all eukaryotic mRNAs. The eIF-4F complex contains eIF-4G, a large scaffolding protein, eIF-4A, an ATP-dependent RNA helicase (when partnered with an additional initiation factor, eIF-4B), and eIF-4E, the mRNA cap-binding subunit (Fig. 2). An exciting realization over the past several years is that rates of translation initiation are controlled by extracellular stimuli, including growth factors, cytokines, and insulin. Moreover, this regulatory mechanism is highly discriminant. In mitogen-stimulated cells, translation of some mRNAs increases dramatically (>30-fold), whereas the overall increase in protein synthesis is quite modest (1.5 to 2-fold).

The major determinants of eIF-4F dependence reside within the 5′-UTRs of translatable mRNAs. In quiescent cells, mRNAs bearing 5′-UTRs with extensive secondary structure and/or multiple upstream open reading frames tend to be translated very inefficiently as a result of impaired initiation. Interestingly, a number of growth-regulatory proteins (e.g., c-Myc, cyclin D$_1$, and ornithine decarboxylase) are encoded by mRNAs that contain such structural complexity in their 5′-UTRs. Mitogenic stimuli increase the translational efficiencies of these mRNAs by stimulating eIF-4F binding and function, often through the phosphorylation of specific components of this complex *(125,167,168)*. Collectively, this activated eIF-4F increases both ribosome binding to the mRNA, and simplifies the structure of the 5′-UTR via the RNA-unwinding activity of eIF-4A, acting in concert with eIF-4B. The positive regulatory effect of mitogens on eIF-4F function therefore provides a mechanism by which the expression of certain growth-related genes can be controlled at the translational level. The importance of

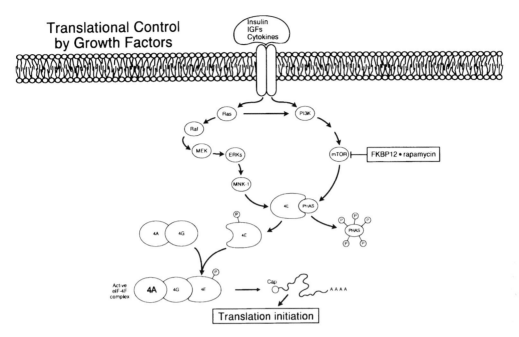

Fig. 2. Regulation of translation initiation by extracellular stimuli. Stimulation of insulin or growth factor receptors triggers the phosphorylation of the PHAS-I protein, which leads in turn to the release of free eIF-4E. The eIF-4E binds directly to eIF-4G, resulting in the formation of the eIF-4F complex. The assembly of the eIF-4F complex at the 5′-cap structure of mRNA increases the efficiency with which the ribosomal 43S preinitiation complex locates the AUG initiation codon for translation initiation. A second signaling pathway initiated by the activation of Ras also increases the function of eIF-4E. This pathway leads to the activation of the MNK1 kinase by MAP/Erk kinases *(61,201)*. Recent evidence suggests that MNK1 phosphorylates eIF-4E at Ser[209], which results an increase in the binding of eIF-4E to the mRNA cap structure.

the eIF-4F complex in cell growth control is underscored by the observation that overexpression of eIF-4E, the limiting component of this complex, is sufficient to transform NIH 3T3 fibroblasts *(105,106)*.

The cap-binding eIF-4E subunit is a target for multiple intracellular signaling pathways, including the pathway governed by mTOR. The interaction of eIF-4E with the remaining components of the eIF-4F complex is competitively inhibited by the formation of complexes with 4E-binding proteins (4E-BPs) *(104,117,156)*. These eIF-4E interactors are also termed phosphorylated heat and acid-stable (PHAS) proteins *(117)*. For historical reasons, the latter terminology is used for the remainder of this discussion. The most well-studied member of this family of eIF-4E inhibitors is PHAS-I. In quiescent cells, PHAS-I is not phosphorylated, and is tightly bound to eIF-4E. Under these conditions, eIF-4F function, and therefore translation initiation, is repressed. Exposure of these cells to growth factors or insulin results in the rapid phosphorylation of PHAS-I at 5 serine or threonine residues, and a consequent decrease in the binding affinity of PHAS-I for eIF-4E. Thus, the multisite phosphorylation of PHAS-I removes a significant obstacle to eIF-4E-dependent translation initiation, and facilitates the synthesis of proteins needed for G_1-phase progression.

The protein kinase(s) responsible for the phosphorylation of PHAS-I quickly became a topic of considerable interest. Although the original studies implicated a MAP/Erk kinase *(117)*, subsequent work clearly separated MAP/Erk kinase activation from PHAS-I phosphorylation in insulin-treated cells. A seminal observation was that this response was effectively blocked by rapamycin, which strongly hinted that mTOR served as an upstream kinase in the PHAS-I phosphorylation pathway *(14,67,118,197)*. In a somewhat unexpected turn of events, it was recently shown that mTOR itself phosphorylates PHAS-I, at least under in vitro kinase assay conditions *(25)*. The physiologic relevance of these findings is supported by the findings that the 5 sites phosphorylated by mTOR in vitro are identical to the sites of PHAS-I phosphorylation during insulin stimulation of intact cells *(24,52)*. The same serine and threonine residues are rapidly dephosphorylated after addition of rapamycin to these cells. Finally, the in vitro phosphorylation of PHAS-I by mTOR effectively inhibits the binding of PHAS-I to eIF-4E. Collectively, these findings argue that mTOR may be directly responsible for the phosphorylation of PHAS-I and subsequent activation of eIF-4E induced by insulin and other mitogenic factors.

It is important to recognize that the model outlined above carries several uncertainties. First, the available results do not rule out the possibility that an mTOR-activated kinase actually mediates inducible PHAS-I phosphorylation in intact cells. Second, the picture is complicated by the fact that all five phosphorylation sites in PHAS-I contain a Pro residue at the +1 position. Hence, these sites may be also be targeted for phosphorylation by one or more members of the large family of low-molecular mass, proline-directed kinases. Indeed, a plausible scenario is that PHAS-I phosphorylation is processive in vivo; that is, the phosphorylation of one or two sites in PHAS-I by mTOR primes the protein for subsequent phosphorylation by a separate proline-directed kinase(s). Finally, many investigators in the field continue to speculate that mTOR actually functions as an inhibitor of a protein serine-threonine phosphatase whose function is to dephosphorylate PHAS-I and p70^{S6K} when conditions are not appropriate for G_1-phase progression. Derepression of an mTOR-linked protein phosphatase by rapamycin treatment offers an attractive explanation for the rapid reversal of the phosphorylation of both proteins when rapamycin is added to cells after hormonal stimuli. Studies in budding yeast suggest that the TOR signaling pathway regulates the activity of a PP2A-like phosphatase in these cells *(46,140)*. Ongoing studies will undoubtedly resolve these lingering questions concerning the relationship between mTOR and its downstream targets over the next few years.

An important area for ongoing studies concerns the pathways through which mTOR is regulated in response to extracellular stimuli. Signals emanating from activated PI3K have been implicated in the stimulation of protein synthesis for some time (Fig. 3). More recent evidence suggests that both PI3K and its downstream serine-threonine kinase, AKT, participate in mTOR activation by insulin and other polypeptide hormones *(65,178)*. Interestingly, the C-terminal region of mTOR contains at least two consensus sites for phosphorylation by AKT; indirect evidence suggests that these sites are, in fact, phosphorylated in an AKT-dependent fashion in intact cells *(178)*. Emerging results suggest that mTOR may also be regulated by a more fundamental signaling pathway with obvious parallels to TOR protein signaling in yeast cells. These findings

substitution are unknown, but effects on substrate selection and/or the kinetics of phosphate transfer are possible. A potentially related observation is that ATR catalytic activity is significantly more resistant to wortmannin (IC_{50}, 2 μM) than are the activities of DNA-PK or mTOR (IC_{50}, 0.15–0.3 μM) *(26,73,161,174)*.

5.2. Cellular Functions of ATR

The lack of $ATR^{-/-}$ model systems or a suitably specific pharmacologic ATR inhibitor has seriously hampered efforts to elucidate the signaling functions of this protein in mammalian cells. The initial insights into ATR functions came from studies of meiotic events in developing spermatocytes. The ATR protein was specifically localized to asynapsed regions of meiotically paired chromosomes during zygonema *(92)*. This pattern is physically, as well as temporally, distinct from the localization pattern of ATM, which associates with meiotic chromosomes only after synapsis has occurred *(92)*. Although the specific function of ATR during meiosis is purely conjectural at this time, the localization pattern suggests that ATR may be involved in either the recognition or response to regions of sequence homology that eventually lead to meiotic recombination *(92)*.

The obvious structural similarity between ATR and ATM, Rad3, and Mec1p implied that ATR functions as a component of checkpoint control pathways activated by DNA replication blocks and/or DNA strand breaks. In an effort to create a genetic model system for the study of ATR function, Friend and colleagues engineered a SV40-transformed human fibroblast cell line that inducibly expressed a catalytically inactive ATR mutant protein (ATR^{kd}). In agreement with the predicted cell cycle checkpoint functions of ATR, overexpression of ATR^{kd} compromised the radiation-induced G_2 checkpoint and decreased cell survival in response to γ-radiation, methyl methane-sulfonate, *cis*-platinum, and HU. Hypersensitivity to HU was accompanied by micro-tubule abnormalities that suggest an uncoupling of the completion of DNA replica-tion from entry into mitosis. The requirement for ATR in the cellular response to HU and MMS represents a functional divergence from ATM, because A-T cells dis-play normal sensitivity to these agents. However, functional overlap between ATM and ATR has also been documented. Overexpression of ATR^{kd} confers a mild RDS phenotype on human fibroblasts and, remarkably, overexpression of wild-type ATR almost completely complements the RDS defect of A-T cells *(40)*. Therefore, over-expressed ATR assumes at least some ATM-dependent cellular functions in the absence of ATM.

The use of SV40-transformed fibroblasts in the above study precluded the investiga-tion of whether ATR functions in the p53-dependent G_1 checkpoint. However, given its structural and functional relatedness to ATM, a role for ATR in p53 regulation and G_1 checkpoint activation is plausible. Several observations support the notion that ATM-independent pathways leading to p53 activation exist. First, as discussed earlier, the p53 induction defects observed in A-T cells *(30,122)*, and *ATM*-null mice *(204)* are not absolute. In most A-T cell lines examined, the γ-radiation-induced accumulation of p53 is delayed, but not entirely absent, and the induction of p53 in response to other DNA damaging agents, such as the topoisomerase I inhibitor, camptothecin, is nearly normal *(30)*. The radiation-induced phosphorylation of p53 at Ser^{15}, which may be a key step in its stabilization and/or transcriptional activation *(182,184)*, is defective in

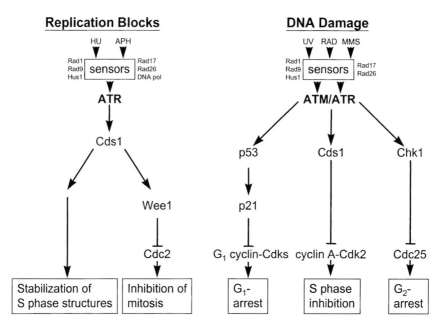

Fig. 4. Potential ATM- and ATR-dependent checkpoint signaling pathways. (Left) Activation of an ATR-dependent DNA replication checkpoint in response to inhibitors of DNA synthesis, including hydroxyurea (HU) and aphidicolin (APH). In this model, HU/APH cause the formation of abnormal DNA replication structures that may be detected by human homologs of *Saccharomyces pombe* Rad genes, or DNA polymerases *(see text)*. After interaction with the sensor complex, ATR becomes catalytically activated, and initiates two Cds1-dependent kinase signaling cascades that are based on analogous pathways in *S. pombe* *(see* Section 4.2.). The end results of Cds1 activation are the stabilization of DNA replication structures, which is essential for maintenance of viability, and inhibition of mitosis. (Right) DNA damaging agents, including ultraviolet light (UV), radiation (RAD), or alkylating agents (MMS), activate ATM- and ATR-dependent signaling pathways that result in G_1 arrest, slowed progression through S phase, and G_2 arrest. Differential activation of ATM and ATR by distinct combinations of DNA damage and DNA damage sensor proteins is not depicted, but may occur.

some *(184)*, but not all (C. Prives, personal communication) A-T cell lines, indicating that ATM may not be solely responsible for Ser^{15} phosphorylation in vivo. In light of the finding that ATR also phosphorylates p53 at Ser^{15}, the potential role of ATR in the regulation of p53 accumulation and function merits further investigation.

5.3. Roles of ATR and ATM in Checkpoint-Mediated Signaling

The information currently available supports the formulation of only a very preliminary working model for ATM and ATR functions in cell cycle checkpoint signaling pathways (Fig. 4). In this model, ATM and ATR perform distinct, as well as partially redundant checkpoint functions. The two proteins are envisioned as independent signaling molecules, although the possibilities that they may act within the same multimeric complex, or in the same checkpoint pathway, cannot be excluded. As described in the previous section, ATM, and possibly ATR, function in the p53-dependent G_1/S checkpoint pathway that leads to p21 induction and G_1 arrest. The functions of ATM and ATR in the DNA replication, S-phase damage, and G_2/M damage pathways are modeled after their apparent analogs in *S. pombe (31)*. Despite the fact that the human counterpart of yeast Cds1 has not been identified to date, the mammalian DNA replication checkpoint likely resembles the Rad3-Cds1 pathway of *S. pombe* (*see* Section 4.2.). This pathway is depicted as exclusively ATR-dependent, because A-T cells are not hypersensitive to DNA replication inhibitors. Because, Cds1 also controls the S-phase DNA damage checkpoint in *S. pombe*, human Cds1 may act downstream of both ATM and ATR in a signaling pathway that slows S-phase progression. With respect to the G_2/M checkpoint, functional ATM and ATR both appear to be required for its activation. Whether both proteins function upstream of human Chk1 remains to be determined, but it is formally possible that either ATM or ATR also regulate the G_2/M checkpoint independently of Chk1.

The mechanisms whereby ATM and ATR sense damage to the genome remain elusive. Once again, however, the yeast checkpoint pathways provide a framework upon to construct a working model. In both *S. cerevisiae* and *S. pombe*, a set of checkpoint Rad genes with putative DNA damaging sensing and/or DNA damage processing functions are located upstream of Mec1p and Rad3 in the checkpoint pathways. In *S. cerevisiae*, DNA polymerase ε serves a sensory function for activation of the DNA replication checkpoint *(144)*, and Rad9p, Rad24p, and Rad17p may execute both sensory and processing functions in the DNA damage checkpoints *(50,124)*. Rad1, Rad9 (not to be confused with *S. cerevisiae* Rad9p), Rad26, and Hus1 appear to perform similar functions in *S. pombe (31)*. Human orthologs of these yeast Rad proteins are rapidly being identified *(98,116)*. It is likely that the type of genetic lesion (e.g., DSB vs stalled DNA replication fork) determines which combinatorial arrangement of Rad proteins assembles at the damaged site, and, in turn, may dictate whether ATM or ATR, or both PIKKs, are recruited to this site. After the recognition of a genetic abnormality, the catalytic activities of ATR and ATM may be stimulated via the dissociation of inhibitor proteins or phosphorylation by upstream kinases. Obviously, understanding the regulatory controls that impinge on the ATR and ATM kinase domains represents a fertile area for future studies.

5.4. Roles of ATM and ATR in Cancer Development

Loss of ATM is clearly associated with susceptibility to cancer development in humans. A-T patients have a >100-fold increased risk of developing lymphoma relative to the general population *(194)*, and loss of heterozygosity at the *ATM* locus has been observed in T-prolymphocytic leukemia *(190)*. Recent evidence suggests that abnormalities in ATR may also contribute to cancer via a somewhat surprising mechanism. ATR is localized to a region of human chromosome 3 *(39)* that is amplified or otherwise altered in several human malignancies *(57,113,188)*. During genetic screens for loci that can suppress the differentiation of C2C12 murine myoblast cells, a fragment of chromosome 3q (i3q) was isolated that, when overexpressed in C2C12 cells inhibits differentiation, eliminates the G_1 checkpoint, and causes aneuploidy *(186)*. The i(3q) chromosome fragment contains the *ATR* gene locus, and the phenotype of i(3q)-transfected C2C12 cells is at least partially explained by the overexpression of ATR, as overexpression of a wild-type ATR cDNA construct in these cells also induces aneuploidy and inhibits differentiation. The cellular abnormalities resulting from i(3q) overexpression are remarkably similar to those found in p53-null cells *(47)*, which raises the unexpected possibility that amplification of *ATR* or loss of p53 may be similar predisposing events in the progression toward malignancy.

6. DNA-DEPENDENT PROTEIN KINASE

6.1. Structure and Catalytic Activity

Several excellent reviews pertaining to the cellular and biochemical functions of DNA-PK have been published *(3,84,114)*. Consequently, this section provides only a brief synopsis of recent advances in this field. DNA-PK was originally identified as a double-stranded DNA (dsDNA)-inducible protein kinase activity in rabbit reticulocyte lysates and HeLa cells *(32,198)*. Subsequently, DNA-PK was biochemically purified and was identified as a heterotrimer composed of the 70- and 86-kDa Ku autoantigens *(128,129)* and of a very large catalytic subunit, DNA-PK$_{cs}$ *(66)*. The molecular cloning of the DNA-PK$_{cs}$ cDNA revealed that it encoded a 465 kDa polypeptide bearing the PI3K-related catalytic domain *(73)*. The deduced amino acid sequence of this cDNA indicated that DNA-PK$_{cs}$ was the single member of a distinct subfamily of PIKKs. The N-terminus of DNA-PK$_{cs}$ is extended by approx 1000 amino acids relative to other PIKK family members, and lacks sequence elements common to the ATM/ATR or TOR subfamilies. The N-terminus of DNA-PK$_{cs}$ does not contain any recognizable sequence motifs with the possible exception of a leucine zipper region that may mediate interactions with Ku *(3)*. Ku represents the major dsDNA end-binding activity in mammalian cells *(38,128)*. It performs a DNA targeting-function for DNA-PK$_{cs}$ *(66)*. Other DNA binding proteins, including RPA and HSF1, may also target DNA-PK$_{cs}$ to DNA *(27,159)*. Although DNA-PK$_{cs}$ may also interact directly with dsDNA in the absence of targeting subunits *(70,213)*, the indirect interaction mediated by the Ku subunits stimulates DNA-PK$_{cs}$ activity by at least 10-fold *(70)*, suggesting that Ku is probably an important contributor to DNA-PK$_{cs}$ activation in vivo.

Of all the PIKK family members, DNA-PK$_{cs}$ is the most well-characterized biochemically. DNA-PK$_{cs}$ exhibits a strong, if not absolute, preference for phosphorylating serine or threonine residues, followed by glutamine at the +1 position *(3)*. Among the more than two dozen known substrates for DNA-PK$_{cs}$ activity in vitro *(3)* are nuclear proteins that function in transcription, including p53, c-Jun, c-Fos, Oct1, Sp1, c-Myc, and the CTD domain of RNA polymerase II. Other notable substrates include SV40 T antigen *(32,110)*, hsp90 *(32,109)*, both subunits of the Ku heterodimer *(110)*, the p34 subunit of RPA *(27,151)*, and DNA-PK$_{cs}$ itself *(32,110)*. With the exception of autophosphorylation, which inhibits DNA-PK$_{cs}$ catalytic activity *(34)*, the physiologic relevance of these modifications remains largely undetermined. Similarly, DNA-PK$_{cs}$ phosphorylates p53 at the DNA damage-inducible site, Ser[15], which is also phosphorylated by ATM and ATR *(111)*. However, unlike *ATM*-null cells, radiation-induced p53 protein induction and p53-dependent G$_1$ checkpoint function appear normal in DNA-PK$_{cs}$-deficient cell lines *(60,165)*. Thus, if DNA-PK$_{cs}$ plays any role in the regulation of p53 function in vivo, it seems that other protein kinases, such as ATM or ATR, fully compensate for this activity in cells that lack DNA-PK$_{cs}$.

6.2. Cellular Functions of DNA-PK

Studies of cells from mice with severe combined immunodeficiency (*scid*), which contain germline mutations that inactivate DNA-PK$_{cs}$, have documented an essential function for DNA-PK$_{cs}$ in DNA repair and recombination *(17,18,44,86)*. Cells from *scid* mice are exquisitely radiosensitive *(15,62)*, and lymphoid development in these mice is arrested as a result of defects in V(D)J recombination *(20,115)*. The radiosensitivity and V(D)J recombination abnormalities observed in *scid* mice are the results of an underlying inability to rejoin dsDNA ends accurately *(17)*. In stark contrast to *ATM*-null mice, cell cycle checkpoint activation in response to DNA damage is normal in *scid* mice *(60,165)*, indicating that checkpoint defects do not contribute to the *scid* phenotype.

The precise function of DNA-PK$_{cs}$ in DSB repair is currently unknown. On the basis of fine structure analysis of V(D)J recombination intermediates in *scid* versus normal lymphocytes, models for DNA-PK heterotrimer function in V(D)J recombination and DNA repair have been proposed *(38,84,85)*. According to these models, DNA-PK$_{cs}$ performs protective and/or alignment functions when bound to free DNA ends via interactions with the Ku proteins. The juxtaposition and association of two DNA-bound DNA-PK$_{cs}$ proteins, which may involve motifs in their extended N-terminal domains, may drive the alignment of the free DNA ends for rejoining. The XRCC4 gene product, which binds to DNA-PK$_{cs}$ in vitro, may assist during this process *(107)*. Once the DNA ends are aligned, DNA-PK$_{cs}$ phosphorylates Ku and activates an intrinsic helicase activity that unwinds DNA and permits the hybridization of complementary sequences on the two opposing DNA ends (homology-dependent repair). Alternatively, the aligned DNA ends are filled-in and ligated directly (homology-independent repair). DNA-PK$_{cs}$ probably fulfills other roles in DNA repair as well. Its large size is compatible with the recruitment of other proteins involved in DNA repair and, by phosphorylating these proteins, DNA-PK$_{cs}$ may coordinate the multi-step repair process. To summarize, the essential function of DNA-PK appears to revolve around the orchestration of the DNA repair process itself, rather than the damage-sensor and cell cycle arrest functions attributed to ATR and ATM. The potential interplay between the checkpoint kinases, ATR and ATM, and the "repair" kinase, DNA-PK$_{cs}$, during the DNA damage response is obviously an important area for future investigation.

7. CONCLUSIONS AND PERSPECTIVES

During the past decade, it has become apparent that the machinery that drives the cell cycle, i.e., the cyclins and their associated Cdks, has been remarkably conserved during the evolution of eukaryotic cells. The conservation of biochemical pathways that surround the fundamental processes of DNA replication and cell division is further reinforced by the functional characterizations of cellular responses to mitogenic signals, environmental stress, and genetic damage in yeast, flies, and mammalian cells. The members of the PIKK family represent key components of signaling cascades that coordinate the activity of the intrinsic cell cycle machinery with the availability of growth factors, nutrient supply, and the integrity of the genome during cellular proliferation. Functional characterizations of the PIKKs in mammalian cells are already yielding exciting insights into the molecular bases of cell growth control and cell cycle checkpoint function. Undoubtedly, some entirely novel signaling cascades—at least with respect to mammalian cells—will be uncovered along the way—a relevant example being the apparent stimulatory effect of amino acids on mTOR function in G_1-phase cells. Nonetheless, what attracts the attention of many cell biologists is the notion that amplified or deficient PIKK function contributes to the stepwise progression toward malignancy in humans. Understanding the normal functions of these kinases will certainly help flesh out the roles of genome surveillance mechanisms in cancer prevention. Furthermore, it is quite plausible that constitutive activation of the mTOR signaling pathway contributes to the abnormal growth and survival characteristics of certain tumor cells.

Studies of the mammalian PIKKs have also opened new arenas for anticancer drug development. The mTOR inhibitor, rapamycin, is already in the clinic as an immunosuppressive agent, and will soon be tested in patients with brain tumors and other neoplasms. A second agent, wortmannin, has little clinical potential but has permitted proof-of-principle testing of the concept that an inhibitor of ATM, ATR, or DNA-PK might sensitize tumor cells to ionizing radiation or DNA-damaging chemotherapeutic agents. Indeed, wortmannin exerts striking radiosensitizing effects in lung cancer cells at drug concentrations that block the protein kinase activities of ATM and DNA-PK$_{cs}$ *(73,174)*. If ATR amplification or overexpression in cancer cells actually evokes a cancer-susceptible phenotype resembling that induced by loss of p53, ATR may well become the most appealing target of all the PIKKs for anticancer drug development. The progression of knowledge from yeast to mammals to new drug discovery is a paradigm that can certainly be applied to the PIKK family members and, as indicated by the other chapters in this volume, many other signaling proteins as well.

ACKNOWLEDGMENTS

Research performed in R.T. Abraham's laboratory is funded by grants from the National Institutes of Health (CA76143 and CA52495). R.S.T. is a Leukemia Society of America Fellow.

REFERENCES

1. Abraham RT, Wiederrecht GJ. Immunopharmacology of rapamycin. *Annu Rev Immunol* 1996; 14:483–510.
2. Allen JB, Zhou Z, Siede W, Friedberg EC, Elledge SJ. The SAD1/RAD53 protein kinase controls multiple checkpoints and DNA damage-induced transcription in yeast. *Genes Dev* 1994; 8:2401–2415.
3. Anderson CW, Carter TH. The DNA-activated protein kinase—DNA-PK. *Curr Top Microbiol Immunol* 1996; 217:91–111.
4. Araki H, Leem SH, Phongdara A, Sugino A. Dpb11, which interacts with DNA polymerase II(epsilon) in *Saccharomyces cerevisiae,* has a dual role in S-phase progression and at a cell cycle checkpoint. *Proc Natl Acad Sci USA* 1995; 92:11,791–11,795.
5. Artuso M, Esteve A, Bresil H, Vuillaume M, Hall J. The role of the Ataxia telangiectasia gene in the p53, WAF1/CIP1(p21)- and GADD45-mediated response to DNA damage produced by ionising radiation. *Oncogene* 1995; 11:1427–1435.
6. Barbet NC, Schneider U, Helliwell SB, Stansfield I, Tuite MF, Hall MN. TOR controls translation initiation and early G1 progression in yeast. *Mol Biol Cell* 1996; 7:25–42.

7. Barlow C, Brown KD, Deng CX, Tagle DA, Wynshaw-Boris A. Atm selectively regulates distinct p53-dependent cell-cycle checkpoint and apoptotic pathways. *Nature Genet* 1997; 17:453–456.

8. Barlow C, Hirotsune S, Paylor R, Liyanage M, Eckhaus M, Collins F, Shiloh Y, Crawley JN, Ried T, Tagle D, Wynshaw-Boris A. Atm-deficient mice: A paradigm of ataxia telangiectasia. *Cell* 1996; 86:159–171.

9. Baskaran R, Wood LD, Whitaker LL, Canman CE, Morgan SE, Xu Y, Barlow C, Baltimore D, Wynshaw-Boris A, Kastan MB, Wang JYJ. Ataxia telangiectasia mutant protein activates c-Abl tyrosine kinase in response to ionizing radiation. *Nature* 1997; 387:516–519.

10. Beamish H, Khanna KK, Lavin MF. Ionizing radiation and cell cycle progression in ataxia telangiectasia. *Radiat Res* 1994; 138:S130–3.

11. Beamish H, Lavin MF. Radiosensitivity in ataxia-telangiectasia: Anomalies in radiation-induced cell cycle delay. *Int J Radiat Biol* 1994; 65:175–184.

12. Beamish H, Williams R, Chen P, Lavin MF. Defect in multiple cell cycle checkpoints in ataxia-telangiectasia postirradiation. *J Biol Chem* 1996; 271:20,486–20,493.

13. Bentley NJ, Holtzman DA, Flaggs G, Keegan KS, DeMaggio A, Ford JC, Hoekstra M, Carr AM. The *Schizosaccharomyces pombe* rad3 checkpoint gene. *EMBO J* 1996; 15:6641–6651.

14. Beretta L, Gingras AC, Svitkin YV, Hall MN, Sonenberg N. Rapamycin blocks the phosphorylation of 4E-BP1 and inhibits cap-dependent initiation of translation. *EMBO J* 1996; 15:658–664.

15. Biedermann KA, Sun JR, Giaccia AJ, Tosto LM, Brown JM. *scid* mutation in mice confers hypersensitivity to ionizing radiation and a deficiency in DNA double-strand break repair. *Proc Natl Acad Sci USA* 1991; 88:1394–1397.

16. Blocher D, Sigut D, Hannan MA. Fibroblasts from ataxia telangiectasia (AT) and AT heterozygotes show an enhanced level of residual DNA double-strand breaks after low dose-rate gamma-irradiation as assayed by pulsed field gel electrophoresis. *Int J Radiat Biol* 1991; 60:791–802.

17. Blunt T, Finnie NJ, Taccioli GE, Smith GC, Demengeot J, Gottlieb TM, Mizuta R, Varghese AJ, Alt FW, Jeggo PA, Jackson SP. Defective DNA-dependent protein kinase activity is linked to V(D)J recombination and DNA repair defects associated with the murine scid mutation. *Cell* 1995; 80:813–823.

18. Blunt T, Gell D, Fox M, Taccioli GE, Lehmann AR, Jackson SP, Jeggo PA. Identification of a nonsense mutation in the carboxyl-terminal region of DNA-dependent protein kinase catalytic subunit in the scid mouse. *Proc Natl Acad Sci USA* 1996; 93:10,285–10,290.

19. Boddy MN, Furnari B, Mondesert O, Russell P. Replication checkpoint enforced by kinases Cds1 and Chk1. *Science* 1998; 280:909–912.

20. Bosma MJ, Carroll AM. The SCID mouse mutant: Definition, characterization, and potential uses. *Annu Rev Immunol* 1991; 9:323–350.

21. Brown EJ, Albers MW, Shin TB, Ichikawa K, Keith CT, Lane WS, Schreiber SL. A mammalian protein targeted by G1-arresting rapamycin-receptor complex. Nature 1994; 369:756–758.

22. Brown EJ, Beal PA, Keith CT, Chen J, Shin TB, Schreiber SL. Control of p70 s6 kinase by kinase activity of FRAP in vivo. *Nature* 1995; 377:441–446.

23. Brown KD, Ziv Y, Sadanandan SN, Chessa L, Collins FS, Shiloh Y, Tagle DA. The ataxia-telangiectasia gene product, a constitutively expressed nuclear protein that is not up-regulated following genome damage. *Proc Natl Acad Sci USA* 1997; 94:1840–1845.

24. Brunn GJ, Fadden P, Haystead TAJ, Lawrence JC Jr. The mammalian target of rapamycin phosphorylates sites having a (Ser/Thr)-Pro motif and is activated by antibodies to a region near its COOH terminus. *J Biol Chem* 1997; 272:32,547–32,550.

25. Brunn GJ, Hudson CC, Sekulic A, Williams JM, Hosoi J, Houghton PJ, Lawrence JC,

Abraham RT. Phosphorylation of the translational repressor PHAS-I by the mammalian target of rapamycin. *Science* 1997a; 277:99–101.

26. Brunn GJ, Williams J, Sabers C, Wiederrecht G, Lawrence JC Jr, Abraham RT. Direct inhibition of the signaling functions of the mammalian target of rapamycin by the phospho-inositide 3-kinase inhibitors, wortmannin and LY294002. *EMBO J* 1996; 15:5256–5267.

27. Brush GS, Anderson CW, Kelly TJ. The DNA-activated protein kinase is required for the phosphorylation of replication protein A during simian virus 40 DNA replication. *Proc Natl Acad Sci USA* 1995; 91:12,520–12,524.

28. Burnett PE, Barrow RK, Cohen NA, Snyder SH, Sabatini DM. RAFT1 phosphorylation of the translational regulators p70 S6 kinase and 4E-BP1. *Proc Natl Acad Sci USA* 1998; 95:1432–1437.

29. Cafferkey R, Young PR, McLaughlin MM, Bergsma DJ, Koltin Y, Sathe GM, Faucette L, Eng WK, Johnson RK, Livi GP. Dominant missense mutations in a novel yeast protein related to mammalian phosphatidylinositol 3-kinase and VPS34 abrogate rapamycin cyto-toxicity. *Mol Cell Biol* 1993; 13:6012–6023.

30. Canman CE, Wolff AC, Chen CY, Fornace AJ Jr, Kastan MB. The p53-dependent G1 cell cycle checkpoint pathway and ataxia-telangiectasia. *Cancer Res* 1994; 54:5054–5058.

31. Carr AM. Analysis of fission yeast DNA structure checkpoints. *Microbiology* 1998; 144:5–11.

32. Carter T, Vancurova I, Sun I, Lou W, DeLeon S. A DNA-activated protein kinase from HeLa cell nuclei. *Mol Cell Biol* 1990; 10:6460–6471.

33. Carty MP, Zernik-Kobak M, McGrath S, Dixon K. UV light-induced DNA synthesis arrest in HeLa cells is associated with changes in phosphorylation of human single-stranded DNA-binding protein. *EMBO J* 1994; 13:2114–2123.

34. Chan DW, Lees-Miller SP. The DNA-dependent protein kinase is inactivated by autopho-sphorylation of the catalytic subunit. *J Biol Chem* 1996; 271:8936–8941.

35. Chen J, Zheng XF, Brown EJ, Schreiber SL. Identification of an 11-kDa FKBP12-rapa-mycin-binding domain within the 289-kDa FKBP12-rapamycin-associated protein and characterization of a critical serine residue. *Proc Natl Acad Sci USA* 1995; 92:4947–4951.

36. Chen X, Ko LJ, Jayaraman L, Prives C. p53 levels, functional domains, and DNA damage determine the extent of the apoptotic response of tumor cells. *Genes Dev* 1996; 10:2438–2451.

37. Chiu MI, Katz H, Berlin V. RAPT1, a mammalian homolog of yeast Tor, interacts with the FKBP12/rapamycin complex. *Proc Natl Acad Sci USA* 1994; 91:12,574–12,578.

38. Chu G. Role of the Ku autoantigen in V(D)J recombination and double-strand break repair. *Curr Top Microbiol Immunol* 1996; 217:113–132.

39. Cimprich KA, Shin TB, Keith CT, Schreiber SL. cDNA cloning and gene mapping of a candidate human cell cycle checkpoint protein. *Proc Natl Acad Sci USA* 1996; 93:2850–2855.

40. Cliby WA, Roberts CJ, Cimprich KA, Stringer CM, Lamb JR, Schreiber SL, Friend SH. Overexpression of a kinase-inactive ATR protein causes sensitivity to DNA-damaging agents and defects in cell cycle checkpoints. *EMBO J* 1998; 17:159–169.

41. Cohen MM, Levy HP. Chromosome instability syndromes. *Adv Hum Genet* 1936; 18:43–149.

42. Cornforth MN, Bedford JS. On the nature of a defect in cells from individuals with ataxia-telangiectasia. *Science* 1985; 227:1589–1591.

43. Coverley D, Kenny MK, Munn M, Rupp WD, Lane DP, Wood RD. Requirement for the replication protein SSB in human DNA excision repair. *Nature* 1991; 349:538–541.

44. Danska JS, Holland DP, Mariathasan S, Williams KM, Guidos CJ. Biochemical and genetic defects in the DNA-dependent protein kinase in murine scid lymphocytes. *Mol Cell Biol* 1996; 16:5507–5517.

45. Dennis PB, Pullen N, Kozma SC, Thomas G. The principal rapamycin-sensitive p70(s6k)

phosphorylation sites, T-229 and T-389, are differentially regulated by rapamycin-insensitive kinase kinases. *Mol Cell Biol* 1996; 16:6242–6251.

46. Di Como CJ, Arndt KT. Nutrients, via the Tor proteins, stimulate the association of Tap42 with type 2A phosphatases. *Genes Dev* 1996; 10:1904–1916.

47. Donehower LA, Harvey M, Slagle BL, McArthur MJ, Montgomery CAJ, Butel JS, Bradley A. Mice deficient for p53 are developmentally normal but susceptible to spontaneous tumours. *Nature* 1992; 356:215–221.

48. el-Deiry WS, Harper JW, O'Connor PM, Velculescu VE, Canman CE, Jackman J, Pietenpol JA, Burrell M, Hill DE, Wang Y. WAF1/CIP1 is induced in p53-mediated G1 arrest and apoptosis. *Cancer Res* 1994; 54:1169–1174.

49. el-Deiry WS, Tokino T, Velculescu VE, Levy DB, Parsons R, Trent JM, Lin D, Mercer WE, Kinzler KW, Vogelstein B. WAF1, a potential mediator of p53 tumor suppression. *Cell* 1993; 75:817–825.

50. Elledge SJ. Cell cycle checkpoints: Preventing an identity crisis. *Science* 1996; 274:1664–1672.

51. Elledge SJ, Harper JW. Cdk inhibitors: On the threshold of checkpoints and development. *Curr Opin Cell Biol* 1994; 6:847–852.

52. Fadden P, Haystead TA, Lawrence JC Jr. Identification of phosphorylation sites in the translational regulator, PHAS-I, that are controlled by insulin and rapamycin in rat adipocytes. *J Biol Chem* 1997; 272:10,240–10,247.

53. Fairman MP, Stillman B. Cellular factors required for multiple stages of SV40 DNA replication in vitro. *EMBO J* 1988; 7:1211–1218.

54. Firpo EJ, Koff A, Solomon MJ, Roberts JM. Inactivation of a Cdk2 inhibitor during interleukin 2-induced proliferation of human T lymphocytes. *Mol Cell Biol* 1994; 14:4889–4901.

55. Ford MD, Martin L, Lavin MF. The effects of ionizing radiation on cell cycle progression in ataxia telangiectasia. *Mutat Res* 1984; 125:115–122.

56. Fornace AJJ, Little JB. Normal repair of DNA single-strand breaks in patients with ataxia telangiectasia. *Biochim Biophys Acta* 1980; 607:432–437.

57. Forozan F, Karhu R, Kononen J, Kallioniemi A, Kallioniemi OP. Genome screening by comparative genomic hybridization. *Trends Genet* 1997; 13:405–409.

58. Francesconi S, Grenon M, Bouvier D, Baldacci G. p56(chk1) protein kinase is required for the DNA replication checkpoint at 37 degrees C in fission yeast. *EMBO J* 1997; 16:1332–1341.

59. Freeman K, Livi GP. Missense mutations at the FKBP12-rapamycin-binding site of TOR1. *Gene* 1996; 172:143–147.

60. Fried LM, Koumenis C, Peterson SR, Green SL, van Zijl P, Allalunis-Turner J, Chen DJ, Fishel R, Giaccia AJ, Brown JM, Kirchgessner CU. The DNA damage response in DNA-dependent protein kinase-deficient SCID mouse cells: Replication protein A hyperphosphorylation and p53 induction. *Proc Natl Acad Sci USA* 1996; 93:13,825–13,830.

61. Fukunaga R, Hunter T. MNK1, a new MAP kinase-activated protein kinase, isolated by a novel expression screening method for identifying protein kinase substrates. *EMBO J* 1997; 16:1921–1933.

62. Fulop GM, Phillips RA. The scid mutation in mice causes a general defect in DNA repair. *Nature* 1990; 347:479–482.

63. Furnari B, Rhind N, Russell P. Cdc25 mitotic inducer targeted by chk1 DNA damage checkpoint kinase. *Science* 1997; 277:1495–1497.

64. Gatti RA, Boder E, Vinters HV, Sparkes RS, Norman A, Lange K. Ataxia-telangiectasia: An interdisciplinary approach to pathogenesis. *Medicine* 1991; 70:99–117.

65. Gingras AC, Kennedy SG, O'Leary MA, Sonenberg N, Hay N. 4E-BP1, a repressor of mRNA translation, is phosphorylated and inactivated by the Akt(PKB) signaling pathway. *Genes Dev* 1998; 12:502–513.

66. Gottlieb TM, Jackson SP. The DNA-dependent protein kinase: Requirement for DNA ends and association with Ku antigen. *Cell* 1993; 72:131–142.

67. Graves LM, Bornfeldt KE, Argast GM, Krebs EG, Kong X, Lin TA, Lawrence JC Jr. cAMP- and rapamycin-sensitive regulation of the association of eukaryotic initiation factor 4E and the translational regulator PHAS-I in aortic smooth muscle cells. *Proc Natl Acad Sci USA* 1995; 92:7222–7226.

68. Greenwell PW, Kronmal SL, Porter SE, Gassenhuber J, Obermaier B, Petes TD. TEL1, a gene involved in controlling telomere length in S. cerevisiae, is homologous to the human ataxia telangiectasia gene. *Cell* 1995; 82:823–829.

69. Hall MN. The TOR signalling pathway and growth control in yeast. *Biochem Soc Trans* 1996; 24:234–239.

70. Hammarsten O, Chu G. DNA-dependent protein kinase: DNA binding and activation in the absence of Ku. *Proc Natl Acad Sci USA* 1998; 95:525–530.

71. Hara K, Yonezawa K, Weng QP, Kozlowski MT, Belham C, Avruch J. Amino acid sufficiency and mTOR regulate p70 S6 kinase and eIF-4E BP1 through a common effector mechanism. *J Biol Chem* 1998; 273:14,484–14,494.

72. Harper JW, Adami GR, Wei N, Keyomarsi K, Elledge SJ. The p21 Cdk-interacting protein Cip1 is a potent inhibitor of G1 cyclin-dependent kinases. *Cell* 1993; 75:805–816.

73. Hartley KO, Gell D, Smith GC, Zhang H, Divecha N, Connelly MA, Admon A, Lees-Miller SP, Anderson CW, Jackson SP. DNA-dependent protein kinase catalytic subunit: A relative of phosphatidylinositol 3-kinase and the ataxia telangiectasia gene product. *Cell* 1995; 82:849–856.

74. Hartwell LH, Kastan MB. Cell cycle control and cancer. *Science* 1994; 266:1821–1828.

75. Hartwell LH, Weinert TA. Checkpoints: Controls that ensure the order of cell cycle events. *Science* 1989; 246:629–634.

76. Haupt Y, Maya R, Kazaz A, Oren M. Mdm2 promotes the rapid degradation of p53. *Nature* 1997; 387:296–299.

77. Hawley RS, Tartof KD. The effect of mei-41 on rDNA redundancy in *Drosophila melanogaster*. *Genetics* 1983; 104:63–80.

78. Heinz-Herzog K, Chong MJ, Kapsetaki M, Morgan JI, Mckinnon PJ. Requirement for Atm ionizing radiation-induced cell death in the developing nervous system. *Science* 1998; 280:1089–1091.

79. Heitman J, Movva NR, Hall MN. Targets for cell cycle arrest by the immunosuppressant rapamycin in yeast. *Science* 1991; 253:905–909.

80. Helliwell SB, Howald I, Barbet N, Hall MN. TOR2 is part of two related signaling pathways coordinating cell growth in *Saccharomyces cerevisiae*. *Genetics* 1998; 148:99–112.

81. Helliwell SB, Wagner P, Kunz J, Deuter-Reinhard M, Henriquez R, Hall MN. TOR1 and TOR2 are structurally and functionally similar but not identical phosphatidylinositol kinase homologues in yeast. *Mol Biol Cell* 1994; 5:105–118.

82. Henricksen LA, Wold MS. Replication protein A mutants lacking phosphorylation sites for p34cdc2 kinase support DNA replication. *J Biol Chem* 1994; 269:24,203–24,208.

83. Hunter T. When is a lipid kinase not a lipid kinase? When it is a protein kinase. *Cell* 1995; 83:1–4.

84. Jackson SP. DNA damage detection by DNA dependent protein kinase and related enzymes. *Cancer Surv* 1996; 28:261–279.

85. Jackson SP. The recognition of DNA damage. *Curr Opin Genet Dev* 1996; 6:19–25.

86. Jhappan C, Morse HC, Fleischmann RD, Gottesman MM, Merlino G. DNA-PKcs: A T-cell tumour suppressor encoded at the mouse scid locus. *Nature Genet* 1997; 17:483–486.

87. Jimenez G, Yucel J, Rowley R, Subramani S. The rad3+ gene of *Schizosaccharomyces pombe* is involved in multiple checkpoint functions and in DNA repair. *Proc Natl Acad Sci USA* 1992; 89:4952–4956.

88. Jin P, Gu Y, Morgan DO. Role of inhibitory CDC2 phosphorylation in radiation-induced G2 arrest in human cells. *J Cell Biol* 1996; 134:963–970.
89. Jung M, Kondratyev A, Lee SA, Dimtchev A, Dritschilo A. ATM gene product phosphorylates I kappa B-alpha. *Cancer Res* 1997; 57:24–27.
90. Kastan MB, Zhan Q, el-Deiry WS, Carrier F, Jacks T, Walsh WV, Plunkett BS, Vogelstein B, Fornace AJ Jr. A mammalian cell cycle checkpoint pathway utilizing p53 and GADD45 is defective in ataxia-telangiectasia. *Cell* 1992; 71:587–597.
91. Kato R, Ogawa H. An essential gene, ESR1, is required for mitotic cell growth, DNA repair and meiotic recombination in *Saccharomyces cerevisiae. Nucleic Acids Res* 1994; 22:3104–3112.
92. Keegan KS, Holtzman DA, Plug AW, Christenson ER, Brainerd EE, Flaggs G, Bentley NJ, Taylor EM, Meyn MS, Moss SB, Carr AM, Ashley T, Hoekstra MF. The Atr and Atm protein kinases associate with different sites along meiotically pairing chromosomes. *Genes Dev* 1996; 10:2423–2437.
93. Keely PJ, Westwick JK, Whitehead IP, Der CJ, Parise LV. Cdc42 and Rac1 induce integrin-mediated cell motility and invasiveness through PI(3)K. *Nature* 1997; 390:632–636.
94. Keith CT, Schreiber SL. PIK-related kinases: DNA repair, recombination, and cell cycle checkpoints. *Science* 1995; 270:50–51.
95. Khanna KK, Lavin MF. Ionizing radiation and UV induction of p53 protein by different pathways in ataxia-telangiectasia cells. *Oncogene* 1993; 8:3307–3312.
96. Khosravi-Far R, Campbell S, Rossman KL, Der CJ. Increasing complexity of Ras signal transduction: Involvement of Rho family proteins. *Adv Cancer Res* 1998; 72:57–107.
97. Ko LJ, Prives C. p53: Puzzle and paradigm. *Genes Dev* 1996; 10:1054–1072.
98. Kostrub CF, Knudsen K, Subramani S, Enoch T. Hus1p, a conserved fission yeast checkpoint protein, interacts with Rad1p and is phosphorylated in response to DNA damage. *EMBO J* 1998; 17:2055–2066.
99. Kubbutat MH, Jones SN, Vousden KH. Regulation of p53 stability by Mdm2. *Nature* 1997; 387:299–303.
100. Kunz J, Henriquez R, Schneider U, Deuter-Reinhard M, Movva NR, Hall MN. Target of rapamycin in yeast, TOR2, is an essential phosphatidylinositol kinase homolog required for G1 progression. *Cell* 1993; 73:585–596.
101. Lane DP, Lu X, Hupp T, Hall PA. The role of the p53 protein in the apoptotic response. *Philos Trans R Soc Lond* 1994; 345:277–280.
102. Lavin MF, Davidson M. Repair of strand breaks in superhelical DNA of ataxia telangiectasia lymphoblastoid cells. *J Cell Sci* 1981; 48:383–391.
103. Lavin MF, Shiloh Y. The genetic defect in ataxia-telangiectasia. *Annu Rev Immunol* 1997; 15:177–202.
104. Lawrence JCJ, Abraham RT. PHAS/4E-BPs as regulators of mRNA translation and cell proliferation. *Trends Biochem Sci* 1997; 22:345–349.
105. Lazaris-Karatzas A, Montine KS, Sonenberg N. Malignant transformation by a eukaryotic initiation factor subunit that binds to mRNA 5′ cap. *Nature* 1990; 345:544–547.
106. Lazaris-Karatzas A, Smith MR, Frederickson RM, Jaramillo ML, Liu YL, Kung HF, Sonenberg N. Ras mediates translation initiation factor 4E-induced malignant transformation. *Genes Dev* 1992; 6:1631–1642.
107. Leber R, Wise TW, Mizuta R, Meek K. The XRCC4 gene product is a target for and interacts with the DNA-dependent protein kinase. *J Biol Chem* 1998; 273:1794–1801.
108. Lee SH, Kim DK. The role of the 34-kDa subunit of human replication protein A in simian virus 40 DNA replication in vitro. *J Biol Chem* 1995; 270:12,801–12,807.
109. Lees-Miller SP, Anderson CW. The human double-stranded DNA-activated protein kinase phosphorylates the 90-kDa heat-shock protein, hsp90 alpha at two NH2-terminal threonine residues. *J Biol Chem* 1989; 264:17,275–17,280.

110. Lees-Miller SP, Chen YR, Anderson CW. Human cells contain a DNA-activated protein kinase that phosphorylates simian virus 40 T antigen, mouse p53, and the human Ku autoantigen. *Mol Cell Biol* 1990; 10:6472–6481.

111. Lees-Miller SP, Sakaguchi K, Ullrich SJ, Appella E, Anderson CW. Human DNA-activated protein kinase phosphorylates serines 15 and 37 in the amino-terminal transactivation domain of human p53. *Mol Cell Biol* 1992; 12:5041–5049.

112. Lehman AR, Stevens S. The production and repair of double strand breaks in cells from normal humans and from patients with ataxia telangiectasia. *Biochim Biophys Acta* 1977; 474:49–60.

113. Levin NA, Brzoska P, Gupta N, Minna JD, Gray JW, Christman MF. Identification of frequent novel genetic alterations in small cell lung carcinoma. *Cancer Res* 1994; 54:5086–5091.

114. Lieber MR, Grawunder U, Wu X, Yaneva M. Tying loose ends: Roles of Ku and DNA-dependent protein kinase in the repair of double-strand breaks. *Curr Opin Genet Dev* 1997; 7:99–104.

115. Lieber MR, Hesse JE, Lewis S, Bosma GC, Rosenberg N, Mizuuchi K, Bosma MJ, Gellert M. The defect in murine severe combined immune deficiency: Joining of signal sequences but not coding segments in V(D)J recombination. *Cell* 1988; 55:7–16.

116. Lieberman HB, Hopkins KM, Nass M, Demetrick D, Davey S. A human homolog of the *Schizosaccharomyces pombe* rad9+ checkpoint control gene. *Proc Natl Acad Sci USA* 1996; 93:13,890–13,895.

117. Lin TA, Kong X, Haystead TA, Pause A, Belsham G, Sonenberg N, Lawrence JC Jr. PHAS-I as a link between mitogen-activated protein kinase and translation initiation. *Science* 1994; 266:653–656.

118. Lin TA, Kong X, Saltiel AR, Blackshear PJ, Lawrence JC Jr. Control of PHAS-I by insulin in 3T3-L1 adipocytes. Synthesis, degradation, and phosphorylation by a rapamycin-sensitive and mitogen-activated protein kinase-independent pathway. *J Biol Chem* 1995; 270:18,531–18,538.

119. Lindsay HD, Griffiths DJ, Edwards RJ, Christensen PU, Murray JM, Osman, Walworth N, Carr AM. S-phase-specific activation of Cds1 kinase defines a subpathway of the checkpoint response in *Schizosaccharomyces pombe*. *Genes Dev* 1998; 12:382–395.

120. Liu VF, Weaver DT. The ionizing radiation-induced replication protein A phosphorylation response differs between ataxia telangiectasia and normal human cells. *Mol Cell Biol* 1993; 13:7222–7231.

121. Lorenz MC, Heitman J. TOR mutations confer rapamycin resistance by preventing interaction with FKBP12-rapamycin. *J Biol Chem* 1995; 270:27,531–27,537.

122. Lu X, Lane DP. Differential induction of transcriptionally active p53 following UV or ionizing radiation: Defects in chromosome instability syndromes? *Cell* 1993; 75:765–778.

123. Lustig AJ, Petes TD. Identification of yeast mutants with altered telomere structure. *Proc Natl Acad Sci USA* 1986; 83:1398–1402.

124. Lydall D, Weinert T. Yeast checkpoint genes in DNA damage processing: Implications for repair and arrest. *Science* 1995; 270:1488–1491.

125. Mendez R, Myers MGJ, White MF, Rhoads RE. Stimulation of protein synthesis, eukaryotic translation initiation factor 4E phosphorylation, and PHAS-I phosphorylation by insulin requires insulin receptor substrate 1 and phosphatidylinositol 3-kinase. *Mol Cell Biol* 1996; 16:2857–2864.

126. Metcalfe JA, Parkhill J, Campbell L, Stacey M, Biggs P, Byrd PJ, Taylor AM. Accelerated telomere shortening in ataxia telangiectasia. *Nature Genet* 1996; 13:350–353.

127. Meyn MS. Ataxia-telangiectasia and cellular responses to DNA damage. *Cancer Res* 1995; 55:5991–6001.

128. Mimori T, Hardin JA. Mechanism of interaction between Ku protein and DNA. *J Biol Chem* 1986; 261:10,375–10,379.

129. Mimori T, Hardin JA, Steitz JA. Characterization of the DNA-binding protein antigen Ku recognized by autoantibodies from patients with rheumatic disorders. *J Biol Chem* 1986; 261:2274–2278.

130. Momand J, Zambetti GP, Olson DC, George D, Levine AJ. The mdm-2 oncogene product forms a complex with the p53 protein and inhibits p53-mediated transactivation. *Cell* 1992; 69:1237–1245.

131. Moore SP, Erdile L, Kelly T, Fishel R. The human homologous pairing protein HPP-1 is specifically stimulated by the cognate single-stranded binding protein hRP-A. *Proc Natl Acad Sci USA* 1991; 88:9067–9071.

132. Morgan SE, Kastan MB. Dissociation of radiation-induced phosphorylation of replication protein A from the S-phase checkpoint. *Cancer Res* 1997; 57:3386–3389.

133. Morgan SE, Lovly C, Pandita TK, Shiloh Y, Kastan MB. Fragments of ATM which have dominant-negative or complementing activity. *Mol Cell Biol* 1997; 17:2020–2029.

134. Morice WG, Brunn GJ, Wiederrecht G, Siekierka JJ, Abraham RT. Rapamycin-induced inhibition of p34cdc2 kinase activation is associated with G1/S-phase growth arrest in T lymphocytes. *J Biol Chem* 1993; 268:3734–3738.

135. Morice WG, Wiederrecht G, Brunn GJ, Siekierka JJ, Abraham RT. Rapamycin inhibition of interleukin-2-dependent p33cdk2 and p34cdc2 kinase activation in T lymphocytes. *J Biol Chem* 1993; 268:22,737–22,745.

136. Morrow DM, Tagle DA, Shiloh Y, Collins FS, Hieter P. TEL1, an *S. cerevisiae* homolog of the human gene mutated in ataxia telangiectasia, is functionally related to the yeast checkpoint gene MEC1. *Cell* 1995; 82:831–840.

137. Moser BA, Dennis PB, Pullen N, Pearson RB, Williamson NA, Wettenhall RE, Kozma SC, Thomas G. Dual requirement for a newly identified phosphorylation site in p70s6k. *Mol Cell Biol* 1997; 17:5648–5655.

138. Mozdarani H, Bryant PE. Kinetics of chromatid aberrations in G2 ataxia-telangiectasia cells exposed to X-rays and ara A. *Int J Radiat Biol* 1989; 55:71–84.

139. Murakami H, Okayama H. A kinase from fission yeast responsible for blocking mitosis in S phase. *Nature* 1995; 374:817–819.

140. Murata K, Wu J, Brautigan DL. B cell receptor-associated protein alpha4 displays rapamycin-sensitive binding directly to the catalytic subunit of protein phosphatase 2A. *Proc Natl Acad Sci USA* 1997; 94:10,624–10,629.

141. Nagasawa H, Latt SA, Lalande ME, Little JB. Effects of X-irradiation on cell-cycle progression, induction of chromosomal aberrations and cell killing in ataxia telangiectasia (AT) fibroblasts. *Mutat Res* 1985; 148:71–82.

142. Nagasawa H, Little JB. Comparison of kinetics of X-ray-induced cell killing in normal, ataxia telangiectasia and hereditary retinoblastoma fibroblasts. *Mutat Res* 1983; 109:297–308.

143. Nasim A, Smith BP. Genetic control of radiation sensitivity in *Schizosaccharomyces pombe. Genetics* 1975; 79:573–582.

144. Navas TA, Zhou Z, Elledge SJ. DNA polymerase epsilon links the DNA replication machinery to the S phase checkpoint. *Cell* 1995; 80:29–39.

145. Nelson WG, Kastan MB. DNA strand breaks: The DNA template alterations that trigger p53-dependent DNA damage response pathways. *Mol Cell Biol* 1994; 14:1815–1823.

146. Nourse J, Firpo E, Flanagan WM, Coats S, Polyak K, Lee MH, Massague J, Crabtree GR, Roberts JM. Interleukin-2-mediated elimination of the p27Kip1 cyclin-dependent kinase inhibitor prevented by rapamycin. *Nature* 1994; 372:570–573.

147. Oliner JD, Pietenpol JA, Thiagalingam S, Gyuris J, Kinzler KW, Vogelstein B. Oncoprotein MDM2 conceals the activation domain of tumour suppressor p53. *Nature* 1993; 362:857–860.

148. Oren M. Relationship of p53 to the control of apoptotic cell death. *Semin Cancer Biol* 1994; 5:221–227.

149. Pain VM. Initiation of protein synthesis in eukaryotic cells. *Eur J Biochem* 1996; 236:747–771.

150. Painter RB, Young BR. Radiosensitivity in ataxia-telangiectasia: A new explanation. *Proc Natl Acad Sci USA* 1980; 77:7315–7317.

151. Pan ZQ, Amin AA, Gibbs E, Niu H, Hurwitz J. Phosphorylation of the p34 subunit of human single-stranded-DNA-binding protein in cyclin A-activated G1 extracts is catalyzed by cdk-cyclin A complex and DNA-dependent protein kinase. *Proc Natl Acad Sci USA* 1994; 91:8343–8347.

152. Pan ZQ, Park CH, Amin AA, Hurwitz J, Sancar A. Phosphorylated and unphosphorylated forms of human single-stranded DNA-binding protein are equally active in simian virus 40 DNA replication and in nucleotide excision repair. *Proc Natl Acad Sci USA* 1995; 92:4636–4640.

153. Pandita TK, Hittelman WN. Initial chromosome damage but not DNA damage is greater in ataxia telangiectasia cells. *Radiat Res* 1992; 130:94–103.

154. Pandita TK, Hittelman WN. The contribution of DNA and chromosome repair deficiencies to the radiosensitivity of ataxia-telangiectasia. *Radiat Res* 1992; 131:214–223.

155. Paulovich AG, Toczyski DP, Hartwell LH. When checkpoints fail. *Cell* 1997; 88:315–321.

156. Pause A, Belsham GJ, Gingras AC, Donze O, Lin TA, Lawrence JC Jr, Sonenberg N. Insulin-dependent stimulation of protein synthesis by phosphorylation of a regulator of 5'-cap function. *Nature* 1994; 371:762–767.

157. Pearson RB, Dennis PB, Han JW, Williamson NA, Kozma SC, Wettenhall RE, Thomas G. The principal target of rapamycin-induced p70s6k inactivation is a novel phosphorylation site within a conserved hydrophobic domain. *EMBO J* 1995; 14:5279–5287.

158. Peng CY, Graves PR, Thoma RS, Wu Z, Shaw AS, Piwnica-Worms H. Mitotic and G2 checkpoint control: Regulation of 14-3-3 protein binding by phosphorylation of Cdc25C on serine-216. *Science* 1997; 277:1501–1505.

159. Peterson SR, Jesch SA, Chamberlin TN, Dvir A, Rabindran SK, Wu C, Dynan WS. Stimulation of the DNA-dependent protein kinase by RNA polymerase II transcriptional activator proteins. *J Biol Chem* 1995; 270:1449–1454.

160. Plug AW, Peters AH, Xu Y, Keegan KS, Hoekstra MF, Baltimore D, Ashley T. ATM and RPA in meiotic chromosome synapsis and recombination. *Nature Genet* 1997; 17:457–461.

161. Powis G, Bonjouklian R, Berggren MM, Gallegos A, Abraham R, Ashendel C, Zalkow L, Matter WF, Dodge J, Grindey G, et al. Wortmannin, a potent and selective inhibitor of phosphatidylinositol-3-kinase. *Cancer Res* 1994; 54:2419–2423.

162. Proud CG. p70 S6 kinase: An enigma with variations. *Trends Biochem Sci* 1996; 21:181–185.

163. Proud CG, Denton RM. Molecular mechanisms for the control of translation by insulin. *Biochem J* 1997; 328:329–341.

164. Pullen N, Thomas G. The modular phosphorylation and activation of p70s6k. *FEBS Lett* 1997; 410:78–82.

165. Rathmell WK, Kaufmann WK, Hurt JC, Byrd LL, Chu G. DNA-dependent protein kinase is not required for accumulation of p53 or cell cycle arrest after DNA damage. *Cancer Res* 1997; 57:68–74.

166. Rhind N, Furnari B, Russell P. Cdc2 tyrosine phosphorylation is required for the DNA damage checkpoint in fission yeast. *Genes Dev* 1997; 11:504–511.

167. Rosenwald IB, Kaspar R, Rousseau D, Gehrke L, Leboulch P, Chen JJ, Schmidt EV, Sonenberg N, London IM. Eukaryotic translation initiation factor 4E regulates expression of cyclin D1 at transcriptional and post-transcriptional levels. *J Biol Chem* 1995; 270:21,176–21,180.

168. Rousseau D, Kaspar R, Rosenwald I, Gehrke L, Sonenberg N. Translation initiation of ornithine decarboxylase and nucleocytoplasmic transport of cyclin D1 mRNA are increased

in cells overexpressing eukaryotic initiation factor 4E. *Proc Natl Acad Sci USA* 1996; 93:1065–1070.

169. Rudolph NS, Latt SA. Flow cytometric analysis of X-ray sensitivity in ataxia telangiectasia. *Mutat Res* 1989; 211:31–41.

170. Sabatini DM, Erdjument-Bromage H, Lui M, Tempst P, Snyder SH. RAFT1: A mammalian protein that binds to FKBP12 in a rapamycin-dependent fashion and is homologous to yeast TORs. *Cell* 1994; 78:35–43.

171. Sabers CJ, Martin MM, Brunn GJ, Williams JM, Dumont FJ, Wiederrecht G, Abraham RT. Isolation of a protein target of the FKBP12-rapamycin complex in mammalian cells. *J Biol Chem* 1995; 270:815–822.

172. Sanchez Y, Desany BA, Jones WJ, Liu Q, Wang B, Elledge SJ. Regulation of RAD53 by the ATM-like kinases MEC1 and TEL1 in yeast cell cycle checkpoint pathways. *Science* 1996; 271:357–360.

173. Sanchez Y, Wong C, Thoma RS, Richman R, Wu Z, Piwnica-Worms H, Elledge SJ. Conservation of the Chk1 checkpoint pathway in mammals: Linkage of DNA damage to Cdk regulation through Cdc25. *Science* 1997; 277:1497–1501.

174. Sarkaria JN, Tibbetts RS, Busby EC, Kennedy AP, Hill DE, Abraham RT. Inhibition of phosphoinositide 3-kinase related kinases by the radiosensitizing agent wortmannin. *Cancer Res* (in press).

175. Sasai K, Evans JW, Kovacs MS, Brown JM. Prediction of human cell radiosensitivity: Comparison of clonogenic assay with chromosome aberrations scored using premature chromosome condensation with fluorescence in situ hybridization. *Int J Radiat Oncol Biol Phys* 1994; 30:1127–1132.

176. Savitsky K, Bar-Shira A, Gilad S, Rotman G, Ziv Y, Vanagaite L, Tagle DA, Smith S, Uziel T, Sfez S, et al. A single ataxia telangiectasia gene with a product similar to PI-3 kinase. *Science* 1995; 268:1749–1753.

177. Schmidt A, Bickle M, Beck T, Hall MN. The yeast phosphatidylinositol kinase homolog TOR2 activates RHO1 and RHO2 via the exchange factor ROM2. *Cell* 1997; 88:531–542.

178. Scott PH, Brunn GJ, Kohn AD, Roth RA, Lawrence JC. Evidence of insulin-stimulated phosphorylation and activation of mammalian target of rapamycin by a protein kinase B signaling pathway. *Proc Natl Acad Sci USA* 1998; 95:7772–7777.

179. Seaton BL, Yucel J, Sunnerhagen P, Subramani S. Isolation and characterization of the *Schizosaccharomyces pombe* rad3 gene, involved in the DNA damage and DNA synthesis checkpoints. *Gene* 1991; 119:83–89.

180. Sedgwick RP, Boder E. Ataxia-telangiectasia. *Handb Clin Neurol* 1991; 16:347–423.

181. Shafman T, Khana KK, Kedar P, Spring K, Kozlov S, Yen T, Hobson K, Gatei M, Zhang N, Watters D, Egerton M, Shiloh Y, Kharbanda S, Kufe D, Lavin MF. Interaction between ATM protein and c-Abl in response to DNA damage. *Nature* 1997; 387:520–523.

182. Shieh SY, Ikeda M, Taya Y, Prives C. DNA damage-induced phosphorylation of p53 alleviates inhibition by MDM2. *Cell* 1997; 91:325–334.

183. Shiloh Y, Tabor E, Becker Y. Abnormal response of ataxia-telangiectasia cells to agents that break the deoxyribose moiety of DNA via a targeted free radical mechanism. *Carcinogenesis* 1983; 4:1317–1322.

184. Siliciano JD, Canman CE, Taya Y, Sakaguchi K, Appella E, Kastan MB. DNA damage induces phosphorylation of the amino terminus of p53. *Genes Dev* 1997; 11:3471–3481.

185. Smilenov LB, Morgan SE, Mellado W, Sawant SG, Kastan MB, Pandita TK. Influence of ATM function on telomere metabolism. *Oncogene* 1997; 15:2659–2665.

186. Smith L, Liu SJ, Goodrich L, Jacbobson D, Degnin C, Bentley N, Carr A, Flaggs G, Keegan K, Hoekstra M, Thayer MJ. Duplication of ATR inhibits MyoD, induces aneuploidy and eliminates radiation-induced G1 arrest. *Nature Genet* 1998; 19:39–46.

187. Sonenberg N, Gingras AC. The mRNA 5' CAP-binding protein eIF4E and control of cell growth. *Curr Opin Cell Biol* 1998; 10:268–275.

188. Speicher MR, Howe C, Crotty P, du MS, Costa J, Ward DC. Comparative genomic hybridization detects novel deletions and amplifications in head and neck squamous cell carcinomas. *Cancer Res* 1995; 55:1010–1013.

189. Stan R, McLaughlin MM, Cafferkey R, Johnson RK, Rosenberg M, Livi GP. Interaction between FKBP12-rapamycin and TOR involves a conserved serine residue. *J Biol Chem* 1994; 269:32,027–32,030.

190. Stilgenbauer S, Schaffner C, Litterst A, Liebisch P, Gilad S, Bar S, James MR, Lichter P, Dohner H. Biallelic mutations in the ATM gene in T-prolymphocytic leukemia. *Nature Med* 1997; 3:1155–1159.

191. Sugimoto K, Ando S, Shimomura T, Matsumoto K. Rfc5, a replication factor C component, is required for regulation of Rad53 protein kinase in the yeast checkpoint pathway. *Mol Cell Biol* 1997; 17:5905–5914.

192. Sugimoto K, Shimomura T, Hashimoto K, Araki H, Sugino A, Matsumoto K. Rfc5, a small subunit of replication factor C complex, couples DNA replication and mitosis in budding yeast. *Proc Natl Acad Sci USA* 1996; 93:7048–7052.

193. Sun Z, Fay DS, Marini F, Foiani M, Stern DF. Spk1/Rad53 is regulated by Mec1-dependent protein phosphorylation in DNA replication and damage checkpoint pathways. *Genes Dev* 1996; 10:395–406.

194. Swift M, Reitnauer PJ, Morrell D, Chase CL. Breast and other cancers in families with ataxia-telangiectasia. *N Engl J Med* 1987; 316:1289–1294.

195. Taylor AM, Metcalfe JA, Oxford JM, Harnden DG. Is chromatid-type damage in ataxia telangiectasia after irradiation at G0 a consequence of defective repair? *Nature* 1976; 260:441–443.

196. Vaziri H. Critical telomere shortening regulated by the ataxia-telangiectasia gene acts as a DNA damage signal leading to activation of p53 protein and limited life-span of human diploid fibroblasts. A review. *Biochemistry* 1997; 62:1306–1310.

197. von Manteuffel S, Gingras AC, Ming XF, Sonenberg N, Thomas G. 4E-BP1 phosphorylation is mediated by the FRAP-p70s6k pathway and is independent of mitogen-activated protein kinase. *Proc Natl Acad Sci USA* 1996; 93:4076–4080.

198. Walker AI, Hunt T, Jackson RJ, Anderson CW. Double-stranded DNA induces the phosphorylation of several proteins including the 90 000 mol. wt. heat-shock protein in animal cell extracts. *EMBO J* 1985; 4:139–145.

199. Walworth N, Davey S, Beach D. Fission yeast chk1 protein kinase links the rad checkpoint pathway to cdc2. *Nature* 1993; 363:368–371.

200. Walworth NC, Bernards R. rad-dependent response of the chk1-encoded protein kinase at the DNA damage checkpoint. *Science* 1996; 271:353–356.

201. Waskiewicz AJ, Flynn A, Proud CG, Cooper JA. Mitogen-activated protein kinases activate the serine/threonine kinases Mnk1 and Mnk2. *EMBO J* 1997; 16:1909–1920.

202. Watters D, Khanna KK, Beamish H, Birrell G, Spring K, Kedar P, Gatei M, Stenzel D, Hobson K, Kozlov S, Zhang N, Farrell A, Ramsay J, Gatti R, Lavin M. Cellular localisation of the ataxia-telangiectasia (ATM) gene product and discrimination between mutated and normal forms. *Oncogene* 1997; 14:1911–1921.

203. Weinert TA, Kiser GL, Hartwell LH. Mitotic checkpoint genes in budding yeast and the dependence of mitosis on DNA replication and repair. *Genes Dev* 1994; 8:652–665.

204. Westphal CH, Rowan S, Schmaltz C, Elson A, Fisher DE, Leder P. atm and p53 cooperate in apoptosis and suppression of tumorigenesis, but not in resistance to acute radiation toxicity. *Nature Genet* 1997; 16:397–401.

205. Wobbe CR, Weissbach L, Borowiec JA, Dean FB, Murakami Y, Bullock P, Hurwitz J. Replication of simian virus 40 origin-containing DNA in vitro with purified proteins. *Proc Natl Acad Sci USA* 1987; 84:1834–1838.

206. Wold MS. Replication protein A: A heterotrimeric, single-stranded DNA-binding protein required for eukaryotic DNA metabolism. *Annu Rev Biochem* 1997; 66:61–92.

207. Wold MS, Kelly T. Purification and characterization of replication protein A, a cellular protein required for in vitro replication of simian virus 40 DNA. *Proc Natl Acad Sci USA* 1988; 85:2523–2527.
208. Wymann MP, Bulgarelli-Leva G, Zvelebil MJ, Pirola L, Vanhaesebroeck B, Waterfield MD, Panayotou G. Wortmannin inactivates phosphoinositide 3-kinase by covalent modification of Lys-802, a residue involved in the phosphate transfer reaction. *Mol Cell Biol* 1996; 16:1722–1733.
209. Xia SJ, Shammas MA, Shmookler RR. Reduced telomere length in ataxia-telangiectasia fibroblasts. *Mutat Res* 1996; 364:1–11.
210. Xiong Y, Hannon GJ, Zhang H, Casso D, Kobayashi R, Beach D. p21 is a universal inhibitor of cyclin kinases. *Nature* 1993; 366:701–704.
211. Xu Y, Ashley T, Brainerd EE, Bronson RT, Meyn MS, Baltimore D. Targeted disruption of ATM leads to growth retardation, chromosomal fragmentation during meiosis, immune defects, and thymic lymphoma. *Genes Dev* 1996; 10:2411–2422.
212. Xu Y, Baltimore D. Dual roles of ATM in the cellular response to radiation and in cell growth control. *Genes Dev* 1996; 10:2401–2410.
213. Yaneva M, Kowalewski T, Lieber MR. Interaction of DNA-dependent protein kinase with DNA and with Ku: Biochemical and atomic-force microscopy studies. *EMBO J* 1997; 16:5098–5112.
214. Zernik-Kobak M, Vasunia K, Connelly M, Anderson CW, Dixon K. Sites of UV-induced phosphorylation of the p34 subunit of replication protein A from HeLa cells. *J Biol Chem* 1997; 272:23,896–23,904.
215. Zheng P, Fay DS, Burton J, Xiao H, Pinkham JL, Stern DF. SPK1 is an essential S-phase-specific gene of *Saccharomyces cerevisiae* that encodes a nuclear serine/threonine/tyrosine kinase. *Mol Cell Biol* 1993; 13:5829–5842.
216. Zheng XF, Florentino D, Chen J, Crabtree GR, Schreiber SL. TOR kinase domains are required for two distinct functions, only one of which is inhibited by rapamycin. *Cell* 1995; 82:121–130.

16

Integrative Signaling Through c-Abl

A Tyrosine Kinase with Nuclear and Cytoplasmic Functions

Jean Y.J. Wang

1. INTRODUCTION

The mammalian genome is estimated to encode between 100 and 200 tyrosine kinases *(1)*. Protein tyrosine kinases are found in multicellular organisms, but not in unicellular eukaryotes such as yeast *(1,2)*. Thus, tyrosine kinases are likely to be involved in regulatory processes required for the formation and the maintenance of multicellularity. Consistent with this notion, all of the known tyrosine kinases can be linked to the transduction of extracellular signals from hormones, cytokines, peptide growth factors, cell–matrix interactions, and cell–cell interactions.

Although most of these tyrosine kinases are associated with receptors at or near the plasma membrane, a few tyrosine kinases are localized to the nucleus as well *(3)*. The first tyrosine kinase shown to be in the nucleus was c-Abl *(4)*. The c-Abl tyrosine kinase was identified as the normal cellular homolog of the Gag-v-Abl oncoprotein of Abelson murine leukemia virus *(5)*. In human and mouse, c-Abl and a related tyrosine kinase, Arg, have been identified *(5)*. Abl-related tyrosine kinases have also been isolated from *Drosophila* and *Caenorhabditis elegans* *(5)*. The tyrosine kinase domain of the Abl-family members is highly conserved through evolution. The Abl family members are characterized by a large C-terminal region that is not as well conserved through evolution *(5)*. Whereas the Abl-family of tyrosine kinases contain the Src-homology domains SH3 and SH2, they are distinct from the Src family members. Both c-Abl and Arg are widely expressed in a variety of mammalian cell types *(5)*.

The murine and feline c-*abl* gene has each been transduced by a retrovirus to generate a transforming virus that causes leukemia in mice or sarcoma in cats, respectively *(5)*. The human c-*abl* gene is at the breakpoint of a chromosomal translocation, known as the Philadelphia (Ph1) chromosome, which is the cytogenetic hallmark of chronic myeloid leukemia (CML) *(6)*. The juxtaposition of another human gene *(Bcr)* and c-*abl* in the Ph1-chromosome leads to the formation of a hybrid Bcr-Abl protein with transforming activity *(6,7)*. Because the transforming proteins Bcr-Abl and Gag-v-Abl contain additional functional domains, and because c-Abl does not transform cells, the

From: Signaling Networks and Cell Cycle Control: The Molecular Basis of Cancer and Other Diseases
Edited by: J. S. Gutkind © Humana Press Inc., Totowa, NJ

transforming activity of Gag-v-Abl and Bcr-Abl may involve mechanisms unrelated to the normal physiological functions of the c-Abl tyrosine kinase.

The c-Abl protein is required for the viability of mice. The mouse c-*abl* gene was one of the first to be disrupted in embryonal stem cells (8,9). Two different germline mutations were generated in the mouse c-*abl* gene. In one mutation, the kinase function is disrupted (8); in the other, a C-terminal truncation is introduced that does not abolish kinase activity (9). Both mutations are recessive and do not exhibit any phenotype in heterozygosity with the wild-type c-*abl*. However, breeding to homozygosity caused neonatal lethality with either mutation (8,9). The cause of early death is unclear. These homozygous mutants are small and runt and exhibit a wide variety of low-penetrant phenotypes, including but not restricted to, lymphopenia (8,9). Nevertheless, these studies demonstrate that the c-Abl kinase, as well as its C-terminal functions, are essential to the proper development and the long-term survival of mice.

Although the kinase domains of Abl and Arg are virtually identical, their C-terminal regions are fairly divergent with scattered segments of conserved sequences (5,10). Homozygous mutation of the Arg tyrosine kinase does not cause lethality in mice (10a). However, mutant mice lacking both the Abl and the Arg tyrosine kinase die earlier than those deficient for Abl alone (10a). These observations suggest that Arg function can sustain the survival of Abl-deficient animals to later stages of development. These observations also suggest that Abl must have functions that Arg cannot replace. This chapter focuses on c-Abl tyrosine kinase and its biological functions.

2. THE DESIGN OF Abl PROTEIN AND IMPLICATIONS ON FUNCTION

The Abl protein is composed of several functional domains depicted in a linear map in Fig. 1. An overview of the molecular design of Abl and its functional implication are discussed below.

2.1. N-Terminal Region

The N-terminal region of Abl contains a Src-like cassette with the Src-homology domains 3 and 2 (SH3, SH2) and tyrosine kinase domain (5). Immediately C-terminal of the tyrosine kinase domain is a proline-rich region that forms several binding sites for other SH3-proteins (11,12). A number of proteins have been shown to interact with this N-terminal region of Abl, through interactions with the SH3, SH2, kinase, or proline-rich domains (summarized in Table 1). Several of the binding proteins interact with more than one domain in this N-terminal region (Table 1). Proteins that interact with this N-terminal region of Abl, in general, are either regulators or substrates of the Abl tyrosine kinase (Table 1).

2.2. C-Terminal Region

The C-terminal region of Abl contains several signals that specify the "subcellular localization" of the Abl protein. These include three distinct nuclear localization signals (NLS) (13), a nuclear export signal (NES) (14), three HMG (high mobility group)-like

c-Abl Tyrosine Kinase

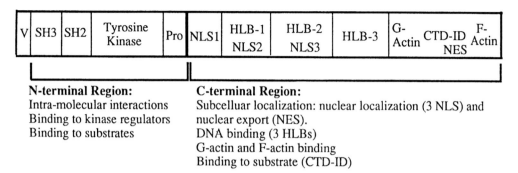

V	SH3	SH2	Tyrosine Kinase	Pro	NLS1	HLB-1 NLS2	HLB-2 NLS3	HLB-3	G-Actin	CTD-ID NES	F-Actin

N-terminal Region:
Intra-molecular interactions
Binding to kinase regulators
Binding to substrates

C-terminal Region:
Subcelluar localization: nuclear localization (3 NLS) and nuclear export (NES).
DNA binding (3 HLBs)
G-actin and F-actin binding
Binding to substrate (CTD-ID)

Fig. 1. Functional domains of the c-Abl tyrosine kinase. The N-terminal region of c-Abl contains the tyrosine kinase and kinase regulatory domains. The C-terminal region of c-Abl contains functions that specify the subcellular localization of this tyrosine kinase. V, variable 5′-exon. The murine type I (human Ia) exon encodes 26 amino acids. The murine type IV (human Ib) exon encodes 45 amino acids. SH3, Src-homology-3 domain. SH2, Src-homology-2 domain. Tyrosine kinase domain of Abl is 45 to 55% identical to the Src-family of tyrosine kinases. However, Abl and Src kinases have different substrate specificity. Pro, proline-rich region. NLS, nuclear localization signal. HLB, high-mobility group-like box. CTD-ID, CTD-interacting domain, the binding site for the C-terminal repeated domain of RNA polymerase II; NES, nuclear export signal.

boxes that bind cooperatively to A/T-rich DNA *(15)*, a G-actin binding domain *(16)*, and an F-actin binding domain with a consensus sequence found in other F-actin binding proteins *(17)* (Fig. 1). The C-terminal region also contains a substrate binding site, allowing c-Abl to interact with the C-terminal repeated domain (CTD) of RNA polymerase II *(10,18)* (Fig. 1). The presence of three NLS, binding domain for DNA, and binding site for RNA polymerase II suggests that Abl may participate in the regulation of transcription in the nucleus. The presence of G- and F-actin binding domains suggests that Abl also has a cytoplasmic function, in association with the actin cytoskeleton. Moreover, c-Abl is actively transported into and out of the nucleus through its NLS and NES *(14)*, suggesting roles in both nuclear and cytoplasmic processes.

The combination of such diverse functional domains in Abl suggests one of two possible models for the biological function of this protein. First, Abl may be partitioned to several different cytoplasmic and nuclear compartments in which it catalyzes the phosphorylation of specific substrates to regulate many independent processes. In this "partitioning" of function model, Abl would have several different biological functions that are not necessarily coordinated. With the partitioning model, the diverse functional domains of Abl may not all be relevant to the localized activity of this tyrosine kinase. This model is currently favored because it is difficult to imagine that the cytoplasmic function of Abl is dependent on its association with DNA, and its nuclear function dependent on the association with actin. The second, and entirely opposite, model proposes that the biological function of Abl is dependent on the totality of its diverse functional domains. In this "totality" of function model, Abl would have a single mission that requires all of its functional domains. The totality model is more satisfying

Table 1
Summary of Proteins Reported to Interact with c-Abl Tyrosine Kinase

Protein	Function	Binding sites in ABL	Consequences of binding
Abi-1	Adaptor	SH3 and Pro	Phosphorylated by Abl kinase
Abi-2	Related to Abi-1	SH3 and Pro	Phosphorylated by Abl kinase
APP-1	Unknown	SH3	Inhibits Abl kinase in vitro
ATM	DNA damage signaling	SH3	Activates Abl kinase
Crk	Adaptor	Pro	Phosphorylated by Abl kinase
DNA-PK	DNA repair	SH3	Activates Abl kinase
PAG	Antioxidant	SH3 and tyrosine kinase domain	Inhibits Abl autophosphorylation while phosphorylated by Abl kinase
RB	Tumor suppressor	Tyrosine kinase domain	Inhibits Abl kinase in vitro and in vivo
RNA polymerase II CTD	Transcription	SH2 and CTD-ID	Phosphorylated by Abl kinase
SHPTP1	Protein tyrosine phosphatase	SH3	Phosphorylated by Abl kinase

than the partitioning model because a single biological function provides clarity and reason for nature's design of Abl protein.

3. CURRENT KNOWLEDGE ON THE FUNCTIONAL DOMAINS OF Abl

3.1. SH3 Domain

The Abl SH3 domain exerts a negative role on Abl kinase activity. Mutation of the SH3 domain leads to an activation of Abl tyrosine kinase *(19,20)*. In a previous review on Abl, two alternative models were proposed to account for this negative regulatory role: (1) an intramolecular interaction involving the SH3 domain to keep Abl kinase is an inhibited conformation; or (2) an intermolecular interaction where the SH3 domain recruits inhibitors of the Abl kinase *(5)*. A recent study has supported the model of intramolecular interaction for the negative effect of Abl SH3 domain on kinase activity *(21)*.

The SH3-mediated intramolecular interaction was first revealed by the crystal structures of the c-Src and Hck tyrosine kinases *(22,23)*. SH3 domains are characterized by their ability to bind proline-rich peptide sequences; this was first described for the Abl SH3 domain *(24,25)*. The SH3 domain of Src or Hck can indeed bind to other proteins with proline-rich sequences, yet in the crystal structure, the SH3 domain binds to an internal proline-peptide in the linker region between the SH2 and kinase domains *(22,23)*. This intramolecular interaction affects the folding of the kinase domain to inactivate kinase activity *(22,23)*. A similar proline-peptide exists at the same linker region in Abl. Targeted mutations of this linker proline-peptide of Abl can activate tyrosine kinase *(21)*. The mutagenesis analysis strongly suggests that the Abl SH3 is involved in an intramolecular interaction similar to that observed with Src and Hck. The Nef protein of HIV has been shown to bind the SH3 domain of Hck and, by doing so, activate the Hck kinase activity *(26)*. Thus, proteins that bind to the Abl SH3 domain may exert a positive, rather than a negative, effect on the Abl tyrosine kinase.

Several Abl SH3-binding proteins have been reported and summarized in Table 1. The search for Abl SH3-binding proteins was motivated by the hypothesis that SH3 domain recruits a kinase inhibitor. As a result, the studies of Abl SH3-binding proteins have been biased toward the interpretation of negative regulation. As summarized in Table 1, two SH3-binding proteins APP-1 and PAG, have been shown to "inhibit" Abl kinase activity either in vitro or in transient co-expression assays *(27,28)*. However, PAG becomes tyrosine phosphorylated when co-expressed with Abl, an observation inconsistent with its being an "inhibitor." The "inhibitory" activity of PAG may be the result of substrate competition; that is, PAG occupies the SH3 and kinase domain to become phosphorylated and in doing so, competes for the phosphorylation of other substrates. Three other SH3-binding proteins have also been found to be phosphorylated by Abl; these include the Abl-interactor (Abi) 1 and 2 and the tyrosine phosphatase SHPTP1 *(29–31)* (Table 1). The biological significance of these phosphorylation events is unknown. In addition to the binding of substrates, the SH3 domain has also been reported to interact with ataxia telangiectasia mutated (ATM) and DNA-dependent protein kinase (DNA-PK) *(32, 33)*, which are activators of the Abl kinase *(33, 34)*.

Taken together, current data suggest that the SH3 domain of Abl can participate in intra- or intermolecular interactions. The intramolecular interaction maintains the Abl kinase in an inactive conformation, similar to the structure of the inactive Src and Hck tyrosine kinases *(21)*. The intermolecular interactions through the SH3 domain are likely to disrupt this inhibited conformation. This would explain the observations that SH3-binding proteins such as Abi-1, 2, SHPTP1, and PAG are substrates of the Abl tyrosine kinase. This might also explain the binding of two activators of Abl, ATM and DNA-PK, to the SH3-domain.

It is conceivable that some SH3-binding proteins would stabilize the intramolecular interactions to enforce the inhibition of Abl tyrosine kinase. However, such inhibitory proteins should not interact through the proline-binding pocket of the SH3 domain, as this binding pocket is engaged in the intramolecular interaction. In other words, the SH3 domain could recruit an inhibitor of Abl kinase, but such interaction must not disrupt the intramolecular interaction between the SH3 domain and the linker proline-peptide.

3.2. SH2 Domain

The Abl SH2 domain binds tyrosine-phosphorylated peptides with a preference for proline in the +2 *(35)* or +3 position *(36)*. This primary sequence preference is similar to that of the Abl kinase domain *(37)*. The convergent binding specificity of the tyrosine kinase and the SH2 domains is also true for the Src family of kinases *(36,37)*. In theory, the SH2 domain can increase the turnover rate of the phosphorylation reaction by binding to, and therefore removing, the product from the kinase domain. Indeed, the Abl SH2 domain has been shown to participate in the selection and processive phosphorylation of two substrates: the C-terminal repeated domain (CTD) of RNA polymerase II *(35)*, and the adaptor protein p130cas *(38)*. The mammalian CTD contains

52 repeats with the consensus sequence YSPTSPS, and Abl can phosphorylate the mammalian CTD to a high stoichiometry *(39)*. The Abl SH2 domain binds the tyrosine-phosphorylated CTD. Replacement of Abl SH2 with that of Src, which does not bind tyrosine-phosphorylated CTD, abolishes the high stoichiometry phosphorylation *(35)*. In vitro, Abl also phosphorylates p130cas, which contains a number of YXXP motifs, to a high stoichiometry *(38)*. Both the Abl SH2 and the Crk SH2 domains can bind to phosphorylated p130cas. With p130cas phosphorylation, both Abl SH2 and Crk SH2 can function to increase the processivity of the phosphorylation reaction *(38)*. Taken together, the current data suggest that Abl SH2 domain interacts with proteins that are tyrosine phosphorylated by the Abl kinase, and can facilitate the phosphorylation of these substrates.

3.3. Tyrosine Kinase Domain

The Abl kinase domain is ~50% identical to that of the Src kinase domain. Conservation of kinase domain is 85–95% among members of the Abl-kinase family *(5)*. The Abl kinase domain prefers tyrosine, followed by a proline in the +2 or +3 position *(37)*. The CTD of RNA polymerase II contains YSP motifs that are efficiently phosphorylated by both the Abl and the Arg tyrosine kinases, but not by Src *(10,18,35,39)*. Therefore, the Abl and Src tyrosine kinases have different substrate specificity.

The Abl tyrosine kinase can phosphorylate itself at tyrosine 412, which is equivalent to the Src autophosphorylation site at tyrosine 416. With the normal cellular c-Abl kinase, which cannot transform cells, autophosphorylation is not observed under normal physiological conditions. Autophosphorylation of c-Abl can be observed in immune complex kinase assays in vitro, or under conditions of excessive overproduction of c-Abl in transient transfection experiments *(5)*. Autophosphorylation in vivo is observed when the SH3 domain of c-Abl is mutated *(19,20)*. Thus, the SH3-mediated intramolecular interactions can suppress Abl autophosphorylation. The autokinase activity is also activated in the oncogenic derivatives of Abl: the Gag-v-Abl protein of Abelson murine leukemia virus and the Bcr-Abl protein of human CML *(5)*. The Gag-v-Abl protein lacks the Abl SH3 domain, which could account for the activation of autophosphorylation. The Bcr-Abl protein forms homo-oligomers through a coiled-coil domain in Bcr, which can activate autophosphorylation in a mechanism analogous to the ligand-mediated dimerization of receptor tyrosine kinases *(40)*. Because c-Abl is not tyrosine phosphorylated, but exhibits kinase activity, autophosphorylation is not required for substrate phosphorylation. Autophosphorylation of Abl is therefore associated with the conversion of this tyrosine kinase into a transforming agent.

A known inhibitor of the Abl kinase, which directly binds to the tyrosine kinase domain, is the retinoblastoma tumor suppressor protein, RB *(41,42)*. RB binds the N-terminal lobe of the Abl tyrosine kinase domain. Exchange of the ATP-binding lobe of Abl for that of Src generates a mutant Abl (Abl-AS2) that does not bind RB and is no longer inhibited by RB *(42)*. In RB, the binding site for Abl is mapped to the C-terminal region *(41)*. The binding of RB to the Abl kinase domain is analogous to the binding of p27Kip1 to the Cdk/cyclin complex. The three-dimensional structure of a complex containing p27Kip1, Cdk2, and cyclin A has been described *(43)*. The p27Kip1 inhibitor contacts the N-terminal ATP-binding lobe of Cdk2 *(43)*, similar to

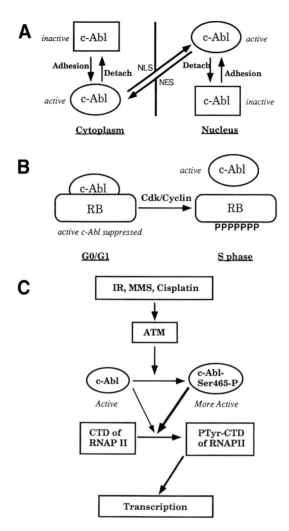

Fig. 2. Regulatory pathways of c-Abl tyrosine kinase. (**A**) Regulation of cytoplasmic and nuclear c-Abl tyrosine kinase by adhesion. In attached fibroblasts, active c-Abl tyrosine kinase is found in both the cytoplasm and the nucleus (oblong box). When fibroblasts are detached from the extracellular matrix, c-Abl kinase activity is reduced (square box). Distribution of c-Abl in the cytoplasmic and the nuclear compartments is dependent on nuclear import (mediated by three NLS in Abl) and nuclear export (mediated by an NES in Abl). Current evidence suggests that it is the active pool of c-Abl that shuttles between the nucleus and the cytoplasm. (**B**) Regulation of nuclear c-Abl tyrosine kinase during cell cycle progression. After entering nucleus, the active c-Abl is bound by RB which suppresses the Abl kinase activity. As cells progress from Go/G1 into S phase, RB becomes phosphorylated by cyclin-dependent kinases and this causes the release and the activation of nuclear c-Abl tyrosine kinase. (**C**) Regulation of nuclear c-Abl tyrosine kinase by DNA damage. When cells are exposed to DNA damaging agents such as ionizing radiation (IR), methylmethane sulfonate (MMS) or cisplatin, the nuclear c-Abl tyrosine kinase becomes more active. The stimulation of nuclear c-Abl tyrosine kinase by DNA damage requires the function of ATM and can be correlated with the phosphorylation of c-Abl at serine 465 in the tyrosine kinase domain. Increased activity of c-Abl leads to an increase in the tyrosine phosphorylation of RNA polymerase II and this may contribute to DNA damage-induced gene expression.

ECM acts through integrin receptors to activate c-Abl tyrosine kinase and the active c-Abl is then translocated into the nucleus (Fig. 2A). The precise mechanism by which integrins regulate c-Abl tyrosine kinase activity and subcellular localization is unknown.

4.2. Cell Cycle Progression

While the cytoplasmic c-Abl retains catalytic function in serum starved cells, the nuclear c-Abl is not active in quiescent cells *(42)*. In synchronized fibroblast populations, nuclear c-Abl becomes active at 12–16 h after serum stimulation, corresponding to S-phase entry and RB phosphorylation *(41,42)*. Phosphorylation of RB at two specific Serine (807, 811) leads to the inactivation of Abl binding *(56)*. Because RB inhibits Abl kinase, phosphorylation of RB should lead to kinase activation *(41)*. This conclusion is further supported by the construction of an RB-resistant Abl mutant (Abl-AS2) *(42)*. Abl-AS2 contains the ATP-binding lobe of Src. RB does not bind to Abl-AS2. When stably expressed in 3T3 cells, Abl-AS2 is found to be active in the nucleus of quiescent cells. The activity of nuclear Abl-AS2 is not further increased as cells enter S phase *(42)*. Taken together, these results support the conclusion that the nuclear c-Abl tyrosine kinase is inhibited in Go/G1 cells through an interaction with RB (Fig. 2B). The RB-inhibited c-Abl becomes active after RB is phosphorylated at G1/S transition. The phosphorylation of RB during G1/S transition is catalyzed by cyclin-dependent protein kinases *(57)*. Thus, cyclin-dependent protein kinases regulate the activity of nuclear c-Abl through RB (Fig. 2B).

Both the nuclear and the cytoplasmic c-Abl kinase activity is lost when fibroblasts are detached from the ECM *(55)* (Fig. 2A). Because RB is a nuclear protein, and the cytoplasmic c-Abl is active in quiescent cells, the inactivation of cytoplasmic c-Abl upon detachment is not mediated by RB. Detachment of cells does not cause the dephosphorylation of RB during S phase, hence, the inactivation of nuclear c-Abl after detachment is also not mediated by RB. Taken together, these results suggest two independent mechanisms for the regulation of c-Abl tyrosine kinase. The cytoplasmic pool is regulated by adhesion but not by cell cycle progression. The nuclear pool is regulated by adhesion and by cell cycle progression (Fig. 3). The cell cycle-dependent regulation of nuclear c-Abl is mediated by RB, which binds to the Abl tyrosine kinase domain to inhibit its activity. The adhesion-dependent regulatory mechanism is unknown, but it is not mediated by RB.

4.3. DNA Damage

The nuclear c-Abl kinase activity is also activated by DNA damage *(53,58)*. Of the damaging agents tested, ionizing radiation (IR), cisplatin, mitomycin C, methylmethane sulfonate (MMS), and cytosine-arabinoside can activate c-Abl, but UVC irradiation cannot activate this tyrosine kinase *(53,58)*.

The IR-induced activation of c-Abl kinase requires the function of ATM *(32,34)*. ATM is a nuclear protein kinase encoded by the gene that is mutated in the human autosomal recessive disorder ataxia tetangiectasia (AT) *(59,60)*. AT patients are characterized by pleiotropic defects including neuronal degeneration, immune dysfunction, increased cancer risk and sensitivity to killing by irradiation. In AT patient cells, c-Abl is expressed; however, its activity is not stimulated by IR *(32,34)*. The mouse ATM gene has been knocked out and these mutant mice exhibit similar phenotypes as human

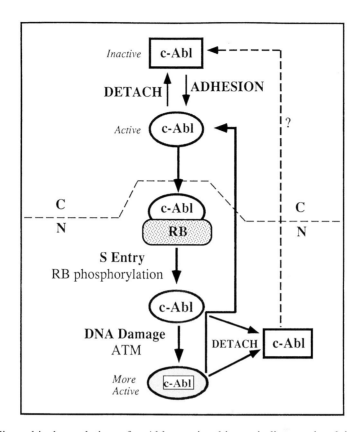

Fig. 3. Hierarchical regulation of c-Abl tyrosine kinase indicates signal integration. The current evidence suggests that c-Abl tyrosine kinase can exist in at least three functional states as determined by its CTD-kinase activity. The c-Abl without any detectable CTD-kinase activity is depicted by the square box. The c-Abl with basal CTD-kinase activity is depicted by the unfilled oblong box. The c-Abl with a stimulated CTD-kinase activity is depicted by a filled, oblong box. The CTD-kinase activity is detected with cytoplasmic and nuclear c-Abl isolated from attached fibroblasts. The CTD-kinase activity of both the cytoplasmic and the nuclear c-Abl is lost when fibroblasts are detached from the extracellular matrix (ECM). Attachment to ECM reactivates the CTD-kinase. Thus, adhesion signals regulate the conversion between the inactive and the active conformation. The mechanism for this conversion is unknown. The nuclear import of c-Abl appears to be dependent on adhesion as well. Therefore, nuclear import is depicted to occur only with c-Abl in the active conformation. Once in the nucleus, the kinase activity of c-Abl is inhibited by RB despite the active conformation. Phosphorylation of RB at G1/S transition leads to the release of c-Abl and the observed activation of nuclear c-Abl tyrosine kinase in S-phase cells. Exposure of cells to DNA damaging agents, such as ionizing radiation, can further activate the CTD-kinase activity of c-Abl. DNA damage-induced activation is mediated by the phosphorylation of c-Abl at serine 465; this is dependent on the function of ATM, encoded by the ataxia telangiectasia mutated gene. DNA damage does not activate nuclear c-Abl tyrosine kinase in G0/G1 cells or in detached cells. The cytoplasmic c-Abl originates from the nucleus because mutation of the nuclear export signal results in the exclusive nuclear localization. Adhesion to the ECM appears to regulate the nuclear import as well as the nuclear export of c-Abl. *See text* for discussion on the export of the active versus the inactive pool of c-Abl out of the nucleus during cellular attachment to the ECM. The dashed line with a question mark indicates a hypothetical export pathway that is only transiently activated at the initial stage of adhesion to allow the escape of inactive c-Abl from the nucleus.

AT patients *(61–63)*. With ATM-deficient mice, the IR-induced activation of c-Abl kinase is again defective *(34)*. Thus, the functional connection between ATM and c-Abl is conserved from mice to humans. Exposure of human or mouse cells to IR or MMS causes an increase in the tyrosine phosphorylation of RNA polymerase II *(34,53)*. This DNA damage-induced tyrosine phosphorylation of RNA polymerase II is not observed in AT patient cells or c-Abl-deficient cells *(34,53)*.

At the C-terminal end of ATM is a kinase domain that is related to PI3 kinase *(59,60)*. Co-expression of the PI3K domain of ATM with c-Abl causes a three- to fivefold increase in c-Abl kinase activity *(34)*. Serine 465 in the kinase domain of Abl is a potential phosphorylation site for PI3K. Mutation of this serine to alanine eliminates the ATM-dependent activation of c-Abl by IR. In addition, mutation of serine 465 to glutamic acid, to mimic phosphorylation, can increase the basal kinase activity (R. Baskaran and J.Y.J. Wang, unpublished observations). Co-expression of ATM PI3K domain with the S465E mutant of c-Abl did not lead to a further increase in kinase activity (R. Baskaran and J.Y.J. Wang, unpublished observations). Taken together, these results establish a DNA damage-induced signaling pathway that links ATM to the phosphorylation of c-Abl at serine 465 and then to the tyrosine phosphorylation of RNA polymerase II (Fig. 2C).

In addition to ATM, DNA-PK is also reported to activate c-Abl *(33)*. The coimmunoprecipitation of ATM and c-Abl appears to be constitutive and not affected by IR *(32)*. However, the coimmunoprecipitation of DNA-PK and c-Abl appeared to be induced by IR *(33)*. Because serine 465 is in a consensus sequence previously described for DNA-PK *(44)*, it is not surprising that DNA-PK can also activate c-Abl in vitro. The IR-induced activation of c-Abl is reduced, but not abolished, in DNA-PK-deficient cells *(44)*. DNA-PK function is necessary for V(D)J recombination that joins segments of immunoglobulin or T-cell antigen receptor genes *(64)*. Because V(D)J recombination is not defective in ATM-deficient thymocytes *(61,62)*, DNA-PK must be functional in these cells. However, c-Abl is not activated by in ATM-deficient thymocytes *(34)*. These observations can be interpreted by two models. First, ATM may recruit DNA-PK to phosphorylate c-Abl at serine 465. Second, ATM and DNA-PK can each activate c-Abl in response to IR. Because ATM and DNA-PK both bind to the SH3 domain of c-Abl and because both proteins form complex with c-Abl after IR, it is likely that ATM and DNA-PK interact with nuclear c-Abl independently of each other. Because c-Abl cannot be activated by IR in ATM-deficient cells, the formation of DNA-PK/c-Abl complex after DNA damage may in some indirect way dependent on ATM function. The second model would explain the complete abrogation of c-Abl activation by IR in ATM-deficient cells, but only a reduction in c-Abl activation by IR in DNA-PK-deficient cells.

5. INTEGRATIVE SIGNALING THROUGH C-ABL TYROSINE KINASE

Since c-Abl tyrosine kinase can be regulated by adhesion, cell cycle progression and DNA damage, it is a transducer of signals generated by the ECM, by cyclin-dependent kinases and by DNA damage. In a simplistic view, in keeping with the partitioning model, c-Abl can be considered as having three independent signaling

REFERENCES

1. Hanks S, Hunter T. The eukaryotic protein kinase superfamily: Kinase catalytic domain structure and classification. *FASEB J* 1995; 9:576–596.
2. Hunter T, Plowman G. The protein kinases of budding yeast: six score and more. *Trends Biochem* 1997; 22:18–22.
3. Wang JYJ. Nuclear protein tyrosine kinases. *Trends Biochem Sci* 1994; 19:373–376.
4. Van Etten RA, Jackson P, Baltimore D. The mouse type IV c-*abl* gene product is a nuclear protein, and activation of transforming ability is associated with cytoplasmic localization. *Cell* 1989; 58:669–678.
5. Wang JYJ. Abl tyrosine kinase in signal transduction and cell-cycle regulation. *Curr Opin Genet Dev* 1993; 3:35–43.
6. Daley GQ, Ben-Neriah Y. Implicating the *bcr/abl* gene in the pathogenesis of the Philadelphia chromososme-positive human leukemia. *Adv Cancer Res* 1991; 57:151–184.
7. Sawyers C. Signal transduction pathways involved in BCR-ABL transformation. *Baillieres Clin Haematol* 1997; 10:223–231.
8. Tybulewicz VLJ, Crawford CE, Jackson PK, Bronson RT, Mulligan RC. Neonatal lethality and lymphopenia in mice with a homozygous disruption of the c-*abl* proto-oncogene. *Cell* 1991; 65:1153–1163.
9. Schwartzberg PL, et al. Mice homozygous for the abl[m1] mutation show poor viability and depletion of selected B and T cell populations. *Cell* 1991; 65:1165–1175.
10. Baskaran R, Chiang G, Mysliwiec T, Krul G, Wang J. Tyrosine phosphorylation of RNA polymerase II carboxyl-terminal domain by Abl-related gene (Arg) encoded tyrosine kinase. *J Biol Chem* 1997; 272:18,905–18,909.
10a. Koleske AJ, Gifford AM, Scott ML, Nee M, Bronson RT, Miczek KA, Baltimore D. Essential role for the Ab and Arg tyrosine kinases in neurulation. *Neuron* 1998; 21:1259–1272.
11. Ren R, Ye Z-S, Baltimore D. Abl protein-tyrosine kinase selects the Crk adapter as a substrate using SH3-binding sites. *Genes Dev* 1994; 8:783–795.
12. Feller SM, Ren R, Hanafusa H, Baltimore D. SH2 and SH3 domains as molecular adhesives: The interactions of Crk and Abl. *Trends Biochem Sci* 1994; 19:453–458.
13. Wen S-T, Jackson PK, Van Etten RA. The cytostatic function of c-Abl is controlled by multiple nuclear localization signals and requires the *p53* and *Rb* tumor suppressor gene products. *EMBO J* 1996; 15:1583–1595.
14. Taagepera S, et al. Nuclear-cytoplasmic shuttling of c-Abl tyrosine kinase. *Proc Natl Acad Sci USA* (in press).
15. Miao Y, Wang J. Binding of A/T-rich DNA by three high mobility group like domains in c-Abl tyrosine kinase. *J Biol Chem* 1996; 271:22,823–22,830.
16. Van Etten RA, et al. The COOH terminus of the c-Abl tyrosine kinase contains distinct F- and G-actin binding domains with bundling activity. *J Cell Biol* 1994; 124:325–340.
17. McWhirter JR, Wang JYJ. An actin-binding function contributes to transformation by the Bcr-Abl oncoprotein of Philadelphia chromosome-positive human leukemias. *EMBO J* 1993; 12:1533–1546.
18. Baskaran R, Chiang GG, Wang JYJ. Identification of a binding site in c-Abl tyrosine kinase for the C-terminal repeated domain of RNA polymersase II. *Mol Cell Biol* 1996; 16:3361–3369.
19. Franz W, Berger P, Wang J. Deletion of an N-terminal regulatory domain of the c-*abl* tyrosine kinase activates its oncogenic potential. *EMBO J* 1989; 8:137–147.
20. Jackson P, Baltimore D. N-terminal mutations activate the leukemogenic potential of the myristoylated form of c-*Abl*. *EMBO J* 1989; 8:449–456.
21. Daniela B, Superti-Furga G. An intramolecular SH3-domain interaction regulates c-Abl activity. *Nature Genet* 1998; 18:280–282.

22. Sicheri F, Moarefi I, Kuriyan J. Crystal structure of the Src family tyrosine kinase Hck. *Nature* 1997; 385:602–609.

23. Xu W, Harrison S, Eck M. Three-dimensional structure of the tyrosine kinase c-Src. *Nature* 1997; 385:595–602.

24. Ren R, Mayer BJ, Cicchetti P, Baltimore D. Identification of a ten-amino acid proline-rich SH3 binding site. *Science* 1993; 259:1157–1161.

25. Cicchetti P, Mayer BJ, Thiel G, Baltimore D. Identification of a protein that binds to the SH3 region of Abl and is similar to Bcr and GAP-rho. *Science* 1992; 257:803–806.

26. Moarefi I, et al. Activation of the Src-family tyrosine kinase Hck by SH3 domain displacement. *Nature* 1997; 385:650–653.

27. Zhu J, Shore S. c-ABL tyrosine kinase activity is regulated by association with a novel SH3-domain-binding protein. *Mol Cell Biol* 1997; 16:7054–7062.

28. Wen S-T, Etten RAV. The PAG gene product, a stress-induced protein with antioxidant properties, is an Abl SH3-binding protein and a physiological inhibitor of c-bl tyrosine kinase activity. *Genes Dev* 1997; 11:2456–2467.

29. Kharbanda S, et al. The stress response to ionizing radiation involves c-Abl dependent phosphorylation of SHPTP1. *Proc Natl Acad Sci USA* 1996; 93:6898–6991.

30. Dai Z, Pendergast AM. Abi-2, a novel SH3-containing protein interacts with the c-Abl tyrosine kinase and modulates c-Abl transforming activity. *Genes Dev* 1995; 9:2569–2582.

31. Shi Y, Alin K, Goff S. Abl-interactor-1, a novel SH3-protein binding to the carboxy-terminal portion of the v-Abl protein, suppresses v-*abl* transforming activity. *Genes Dev* 1995; 9:2583–2597.

32. T. Shafman et al. Interaction between ATM protein and c-Abl in reponse to DNA damage. *Nature* 1997; 387:520–523.

33. S. Kharbanda, et al. Functional interaction between DNA-PK and c-Abl in response to DNA damage. *Nature* 1997; 386:732–735.

34. R. Baskaran, et al. Ataxia telangiectasia mutant protein activates c-Abl tyrosine kinase in response to ionizing radiation. 1997; *Nature* 387:516–519.

35. Duyster J, Baskaran R, Wang JYJ. Src homology 2 domain as a specificity determinant in the c-Abl mediated tyrosine phosphorylation of the RNA polymerase II carboxyl-terminal repeated domain. *Proc Natl Acad Sci USA* 1995; 92:1555–1559.

36. Z. Songyang, et al. SH2 domains recognize specific phosphopeptide sequences. *Cell* 1993; 72:767–778.

37. Z. Songyang, et al. Use of an oriented peptide library to determine the optimal substrates of protein kinases. *Curr Biol* 1994; 4:973–982.

38. Mayer BJ, Hirai H, Sakai R. Evidence that SH2 domains promote processive phosphorylation by protein-tyrosine kinases. *Curr Biol* 1995; 5:296–305.

39. Baskaran R, Dahmus M, Wang J. Tyrosine phosphorylation of mammalian RNA polymerase II carboxyl-terminal domain. *Proc Natl Acad Sci USA* 1993; 90:11,167–11,171.

40. McWhirter JR, Galasso DL, Wang JYJ. A coiled-coil oligomerization domain of Bcr is essential for the transforming function of Bcr-Abl oncoproteins. *Mol Cell Biol* 1993; 13:7587–7595.

41. Welch PJ, Wang YJ. A C-terminal protein-binding domain in the retinoblastoma protein regulates nuclear c-Abl tyrosine kinase in the cell cycle. *Cell* 1993; 75:779–790.

42. Welch PJ, Wang JYJ. Abrogation of retinoblastoma protein function by c-Abl through tyrosine kinase-dependent and -independent mechanisms. *Mol Cell Biol* 1995; 15:5542–5551.

43. Russo A, Jeffrey P, Patten A, Massague J, Pavletich N. Crystal structure of the p27kip1 cyclin-dependent-kinase inhibitor bound to the cyclinA-Cdk2 complex. *Nature* 1996; 382:325–331.

44. Bannister AJ, Gottlieb TM, Kouzarides T, Jackson SP. c-Jun is phosphorylated by the

DNA-dependent protein kinase in vitro–Definition of the minimal kinase recognition motif. *Nucleic Acids Res* 1993; 21:1289–1295.

45. Feller S, Knudsen B, Hanafusa H. c-Abl kinase regulates the protein binding activity of c-Crk. *EMBO J* 1994; 13:2341–2351.

46. Pawson T, Schlessinger J. SH2 and SH3 domains. *Curr Biol* 1993; 3:434–442.

47. Rosen MK, et al. Direct demonstration of an intramolecular SH2-phosphotyrosine interaction in the Crk protein. *Nature* 1995; 374:477–479.

48. Kipreos ET, Wang JYJ. Cell cycle-regulated binding of c-Abl tyrosine kinase to DNA. *Science* 1992; 256:382–385.

49. Dikstein R, Daphna H, Ben-Neriah Y, Shaul Y. c-Abl has a sequence-specific enhancer binding activity. *Cell* 1992; 69:751–757.

50. Dikstein R, Agami R, Heffetz D, Shaul Y. p140/c-Abl that binds DNA is preferentially phosphorylated at tyrosine residues. *Proc Natl Acad Sci USA* 1996; 93:2387–2391.

51. Welch P, Wang JYJ. Disruption of retinoblastoma protein function by coexpression of its C pocket fragment. *Genes Dev* 1995; 9:31–46.

52. Kipreos ET, Wang JYJ. Differential phosphorylation of c-Abl in cell cycle determined by *cdc2* kinase and phosphatase activity. *Science* 1990; 248:217–220.

53. Liu Z, et al. Three distinct signalling responses by murine fibroblasts to genotoxic stress. *Nature* 1996; 384:273–276.

54. McWhirter JR, Wang JYJ. Activation of tyrosine kinase and microfilament-binding functions of *c-abl* by bcr sequences in bcr/abl fusion proteins. *Mol Cell Biol* 1991; 11:1553–1565.

55. Lewis J, Baskaran R, Taagepera S, Schwartz M, Wang J. Integrin regulation of c-Abl tyrosine kinase activity and cytoplasmic-nuclear transport. *Proc Natl Acad Sci USA* 1996; 93:15,174–15,179.

56. Knudsen E, Wang J. Differential regulation of retinoblastoma protein function by specific cdk phosphorylation sites. *J Biol Chem* 1996; 271:8313–8320.

57. Weinberg R.A. The retinoblastoma protein and cell cycle control. *Cell* 1995; 81:323–330.

58. Kharbanda S, et al. Activation of the c-Abl tyrosine kinase in the stress response to DNA-damaging agents. *Nature* 1995; 376:785–788.

59. Savitsky K, et al. The complete sequence of the coding region of the ATM gene reveals similarity to cell cycle regulators in different species. *Hum Mol Genet* 1995; 4:2025–2032.

60. Savitsky K, et al. A single ataxia telangiectasia gene with a product similar to PI-3 kinase. *Science* 1995; 268:1749–1753.

61. Barlow C, et al. Atm-deficient mice: A paradigm of ataxia telangiectasia. *Cell* 1996; 86:159–171.

62. Xu Y, et al. Targeted disruption of ATM leads to growth redardation, chromosomal fragmentation during meiosis, immune defects and thymic lymphoma. *Genes Dev* 1996; 10:2411–2422.

63. Xu Y, Baltimore D. Dual roles of ATM in the cellular response to radiation and in cell growth control. *Genes Dev* 1996; 10:2401–2410.

64. Blunt T, et al. Defective DNA-dependent protein kinase activity is linked to V(D)J recombination and DNA repair defects associated with the murine scid mutation. *Cell* 1995; 80:813–823.

65. Walworth N, Bernards R. Rad-Dependent response of the Chkl-encoded protein kinase at the DNA damage checkpoint. *Science* 1996; 271:353–356.

66. Dahmus ME. Reversible phosphorylation of the C-terminal Domain of RNA polymerase II. *J Biol Chem* 1996; 271:19,009–19,012.

67. Dahmus ME. The role of multisite phosphorylation in the regulation of RNA polymerase II activity. *Prog Nucleic Acids Res Mol Biol* 1994; 48:143–179.

68. Dahmus ME. Phosphorylation of the C-terminal domain of RNA polymerase II. *Biochim Biophys. Acta* 1995; 1261:171–182.

69. Jones KA. Taking a new TAK on Tat transactivation. *Genes Dev* 1997; 11:2593–2599.

70. Baskaran R, Escobar SR, Wang JYJ. Nuclear c-Abl is a COOH-terminal repeated domain (CTD)-tyrosine kinase-specific for the mammalian RNA polymerase II: possible role in transcription elongation. *Cell Growth Different* 1999; 10:387–396.

71. Gong JG, Costanzo A, Yang H-Q, Melino G, Kaelin WG Jr, Levrero M, Wang JYJ. The tyrosine kinase c-Abl regulates p73 in apoptotic response to cisplatin-induced DNA damage. *Nature* 1999; 399:806–809.

72. Jose C, Marin M, Kaelin WG Jr. p73 is a human p53-related protein that can induce apoptosis. *Nature* 1997; 389:191–194.

73. Agami R, Blandino G, Oren M, Shaul Y. Interaction of c-Abl and p73 and their collaboration to induce apoptosis. *Nature* 1999; 399:809–813.

74. Yuan Z-M, Shioya H, Ishiko T, Sun X, Gu J, Huang YY, Liu H, Kharbanda S, Weichselbaum R, Kufe D. p73 is regulated by tyrosine kinase c-Abl in the apoptotic response to DNA damage. *Nature* 1999; 399:814–817.

17

Src

A Model for Regulation of Intracellular Signaling Molecules

Pamela L. Schwartzberg

1. INTRODUCTION

c-*src* was first isolated as the normal cellular homolog of v-*src*, the transforming gene of Rous sarcoma virus *(1)* and subsequently was found to be overexpressed in a number of distinct tumor types, including those affecting the colon, breast, and central nervous system (CNS) *(2,3)*. It is now known that Src is a member of a family of related tyrosine kinases, defined by a common modular structure *(4)* (Fig. 1A). This structure includes a short sequence responsible for fatty acid modification, the Src homology or SH4 domain, SH3 and SH2 protein interaction domains, a kinase domain and a regulatory tyrosine located near the C-terminus. The structures of several Src family members have recently been elucidated, providing a new understanding of how these domains help regulate these kinases.

Despite this detailed knowledge of the structure and regulation of Src, the functional role of this kinase in signaling pathways in the cell remains poorly understood. Unlike other molecules described in this book, including Ras, Raf, and MAPK, Src has not been linked into a distinct linear signaling cascade. Clues to the function of Src have resulted from (1) biochemical studies of activation, (2) studies using dominant-negative blocking mutants and antibodies, and (3) genetic studies in gene targeted mice. Together, these data suggest that Src family members are involved in signal transduction downstream from a broad range of cell surface receptors. This review will concentrate on mechanisms of Src activation and those signaling pathways in which c-Src has been directly implicated. Evidence from osteoclasts, the major cell-type affected in mice deficient in c-Src suggests that Src functions in multiple signal transduction pathways with potentially distinct functions.

2. DOMAIN STRUCTURE OF THE Src FAMILY KINASES

The nonreceptor tyrosine kinases can be divided into several groupings, including the Src, Abl, Csk, Btk, Zap70/Syk, FAK, and Jak families, based on their arrangement of protein function and lipid modification domains *(5)*. The Src family consists of at least 10 family members that share a number of these elements (Fig. 1A). Together,

From: Signaling Networks and Cell Cycle Control: The Molecular Basis of Cancer and Other Diseases
Edited by: J. S. Gutkind © Humana Press Inc., Totowa, NJ

A

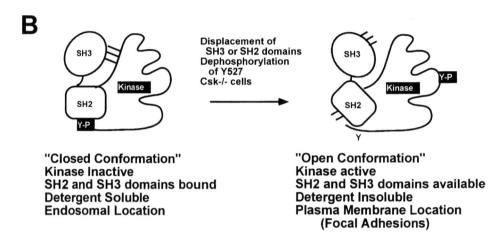

Fig. 1. (A) Domain structure of the c-Src Kinase. M, myristoylation site; U, unique domain, varies between each Src family member; SH3, Src homology 3 protein interaction domain, binds to type II proline-rich helices. Important for regulation of c-Src kinase activity by binding to a linker region of the kinase. SH2, Src homology 2 protein interaction domain, binds to phosphorylated tyrosine residues, including Y527 of Src. Kinases Tyrosine kinase catalytic domain. Contains major autophosphorylation site Y416. Y527: Negative regulatory tyrosine, binds the SH2 domain of Src via an intramolecular interaction. **(B)** Regulation of Src kinase activity. In the inactive or *closed conformation* the SH2 domain of Src binds to phosphorylated Y527 and the SH3 domain binds to the linker region of the kinase. Activation occurs by disruption of these interactions by other molecules or by dephosphorylation of Y527. The active conformation permits interaction of the SH2 and SH3 domains with other proteins and changes the subcellular localization of Src.

these domains help contribute to distinctive features and regulation of this family of kinases. However, because many of these domains are shared by other signaling molecules, knowledge about their function and regulation in Src kinases can be extended to the study of many other proteins. As one of the first described and most thoroughly dissected kinases, Src has provided important clues to the regulation of many molecules involved in signal transduction cascades.

2.1. Myristoylation Sequence

The N-termini of the Src family kinases are myristoylated, a fatty acid modification required for membrane association. Myristoylation is mediated by signals within the first seven amino acids of Src, in a region called the SH4 domain *(6)*. In addition, many of the other Src family members are palmitoylated on cysteine residues near their N-terminus. This additional fatty acid modification targets these kinases to specific glycolipid-rich regions of the plasma membrane. The importance of these fatty acid modifications was suggested by mutations in v-*src* that prevent myristoylation and prevent transformation, although the kinase activity is retained. These mutants fail to be targeted to an appropriate subcellular location and, presumably, similar mutations would interfere with the normal cellular functions of Src. Similarly, mutations that alter the palmitoylation status of Lck prevent its function in T-cell receptor (TCR) signaling *(7)*. The phenotype of such mutants underscores the importance of subcellular localization for proper function of signaling molecules.

2.2. Unique Region

A short variable region follows the N-terminus, which is unique in each Src family kinase. Functional properties of the N-terminal unique region have not been well defined, nor have crystallographic data been published for this region. This domain may be required for specific interactions between particular Src family kinases and downstream targets. Recent studies of the interaction of Src with and phosphorylation of the NMDA receptor support this view—phosphorylation of this receptor requires an intact Src unique region *(6)*. Phosphorylation of Src on specific Ser and Thr residues within the unique domain has been observed during M phase and correlates with an increase in the kinase activity of Src—mutation of these residues can lower the activation of Src during this phase of the cell cycle *(8)*. Mutation of the unique domain can also reduce transformation by v-*src,* but this requires large mutations that may also alter the SH3 domain *(9)*. Further study of this domain in the context of normal cellular functions of Src will be revealing.

2.3. SH3 Protein Interaction Domain

The next region of the protein consists of two distinct protein interaction domains, the Src homology or SH3 and 2 domains, found not only in Src family members, but also in a variety of other kinases and unrelated signaling molecules *(10)*. Important functions for these domains were suggested initially by a variety of mutants in both Src and non-Src family tyrosine kinases that exhibited host range and conditional transforming phenotypes *(9,10)*. Subsequent experiments demonstrated that these regions encode protein interaction domains that are required for normal regulation and function of the c-Src kinase. SH3 domains interact with specific proline-rich type II helices *(11,12)*. Such helices bind to SH3 domains in either orientation, suggesting that structure is more important than actual protein sequence for binding recognition *(13)*.

Evidence suggests that the SH3 domain is important for interactions with downstream effectors in Src signaling pathways. Isolation of interacting proteins through two-hybrid strategies or peptide library screens has led to a number of interesting downstream molecules, including SHC, the p85 subunit of PI3 kinase, and SIN *(14–16)*. Two other molecules that bind the Src SH3 domain are Src associated in mitosis (SAM68) and hnRNPK, both of which are found in the nucleus *(15,17,18)*. The interaction with these potential nuclear substrates may relate to the proposed role of Src in the cell cycle during M phase *(8)*. One further pathway that is regulated by SH3 interactions is the phosphorylation of the potassium channel; interactions with this channel are mediated by the Src SH3 domain *(19)*.

2.4. SH2 Protein Interaction Domain

SH2 domains bind phosphorylated tyrosine residues *(10)*. Using peptide libraries, it was determined that optimal binding involves specific amino acid sequences carboxy-terminal to the phosphorylated tyrosine residue. A consensus binding sequence for the SH2 domain of Src was found to be pYEEI *(20)*. Interestingly, specific in vivo interactions may not fit this consensus sequence—the SH2 domain of Src binds to the platelet-derived growth factor (PDGF) receptor at the sequence pYIpYV *(21)*. Binding of phosphorylated tyrosines to the SH2 domain may be a key regulatory step for activating the Src kinase by certain pathways. For example, the SH2 domain of Src family members binds to phosphorylated tyrosine residues on tyrosine kinase growth factor receptors after activation by their cognate ligands, leading to increased Src activity. Differences in binding affinities of ligands to the SH2 and SH3 domains may also contribute to regulation and activation of the Src kinase.

2.5. Kinase Domain

The next region of the protein is the catalytic or SH1 domain, responsible for the kinase activity of Src. Certain residues within this domain are strictly conserved among all kinases and are important for the binding of ATP and the phosphotransfer reaction *(22)*. Mutations of these key residues render the kinase inactive *(9,23)*. The major autophosphorylation site is located within the kinase domain in a region termed the activation loop—homologous regions contain phosphorylated tyrosine residues in the activated version of many kinases *(24)*. Phosphorylation of these tyrosines may be required for proper placement of the ATP relative to the substrate *(25,26)*, and mutation of the autophosphorylation site leads to decreased kinase activity in Src *(27,28)*. Mutation of certain other residues in the kinase domain can lead to a constitutively activated kinase *(29)*; however, the mechanism of this activation remains unclear.

Src was first defined as a tyrosine kinase and several lines of evidence strongly support a critical role for the kinase activity of Src. Mutations that inactivate the kinase prevent transformation of fibroblasts by v-*src (9,23)*. Moreover, kinase inactive mutants of Src can act as dominant-negative blocks to signal transduction in a variety of signaling pathways *(30)*. However, in some pathways kinase activity may not be strictly required for Src function, pointing to the multifaceted nature of the Src protein.

Critical downstream targets of the Src kinase remain controversial and probably depend on the particular signaling pathway that activates the kinase. Many proposed substrates of c-Src are derived from studies of proteins phosphorylated by the activated viral Src protein, including PI3 kinase, SHC, and PLC-γ *(4)*. In addition, a whole host of cytoskeletal proteins such as vinculin, paxillin, tensin, and cortactin as well as adaptor molecules such as pp130cas and c-crk are phosphorylated by v-Src and may be substrates of the endogenous Src protein *(4,31–33)*. Finally, Src was recently shown to phosphorylate and activate a number of channels and receptors influencing their activities *(19,34)*. The importance of the phosphorylation of these substrates will probably depend on the signaling pathway that activates the Src kinase.

2.6. Regulatory Carboxy-Tail

Near the C-terminus the Src family kinases have a conserved tyrosine residue that is required for the proper regulation of these molecules. This tyrosine (Y527 in Src) provides one of the critical regulatory elements for Src and, as such, is one of the defining features of the Src family kinases *(see below)* *(4)*.

3. REGULATION OF THE Src KINASE

Analyses of differences between the normal c-Src and the viral v-Src protein revealed a marked difference in the specific activities of the kinases *(4)*. The finding that either dephosphorylation or mutation of Y527 constitutively activates the c-Src kinase and enables it to transform cells, provided evidence that this residue is a key regulatory element for c-Src *(28,35,36)*. Indeed, one of the activating mutations of v-Src is loss of the C-terminus. This tyrosine is normally found phosphorylated in most cell types and is phosphorylated by members of the Csk family of kinases *(37)*. Evidence suggests that, when phosphorylated, this tyrosine interacts intramolecularly with the SH2 domain of Src, thereby inactivating the kinase *(4)*. It has been postulated that the SH2–Y527 interaction would either distort or cover the kinase domain, leading to its inactivation in this "closed conformation." As predicted, targeted deletion of Csk in mice causes constitutive activation of the Src family kinases *(38,39)*, leading to high levels of cellular phosphotyrosine. Mutations in the SH2 domain also activate c-Src, as would be predicted from disrupting this intramolecular interaction *(9)*.

Mutation of the SH3 domain also activates the Src kinase and some alleles of *v-src* contain point mutations within this domain *(9,40)*. SH3 mutants have decreased phosphorylation of Y527, suggesting that in these mutants the SH2 domain does not bind this tyrosine, leaving it accessible to cellular phosphatases *(9)*. These results suggested that the SH3 domain aided SH2 binding to phosphorylated tyrosine 527. However, until recently, the mechanism remained unclear.

New crystallographic data have provided a more detailed understanding of these regulatory interactions *(41,42)* (Fig. 1B). The crystal structures of both Src and Hck have been solved in the "closed conformation" revealing that the kinase domain remains exposed even when the SH2 domain binds phosphorylated Y527 (Fig. 1B). In fact, the SH2 and SH3 domains are found on the back side of the kinase domain, similar to their location in the active state *(26)*; thus, inactivation of the kinase cannot result from inaccessability of the kinase. However, in addition to the SH2-Y527 interaction, the SH3 domain has a separate intramolecular contact with the first portion of the kinase domain (the "linker region"). Inactivation of the kinase may, thus, be the result of torsional constraint where the dual binding of the SH2 and SH3 domains prevents free movement within the kinase domain. Mutation of either protein interaction domain would free this constraint and lead to decreased stability of the other inhibitory interactions. Interestingly, displacement of the SH3-linker interaction by an SH3 binding protein (as with Nef and the SH3 domain of Hck) leads to a more profound activation of the kinase than does displacement of the SH2 domain by a phosphorylated tyrosine peptide or displacement of the SH3 domain with a polyproline sequence *(43)*, suggesting that in vivo contacts with proteins may strongly influence binding of both domains.

Thus, both the SH2 and SH3 domains contribute to the regulation of the kinase via intramolecular interactions and disruption of these interactions, either by binding of ligands to these domains or by dephosphorylation of Y527, may be a major mechanism for activation of Src. Known SH2 ligands have higher affinities for the Src SH2 domain than that of the sequence surrounding Y527, suggesting that displacement by these ligands can readily activate Src by displacement of Y527. Furthermore, since mutations in other kinases indicate similar regulatory activity for their SH3 and SH2 domains (e.g., Fps and Abl) *(10)*, these domains may play similar roles in other molecules despite the lack of an equivalent regulatory tyrosine near the C-terminus. Not only does this mechanism of regulation allow precise regulation of kinase activity, it also regulates interactions between the SH2 and SH3 domains and other molecules, providing multiple levels of control for the Src family kinases. Indeed, regulation of the protein interaction domains may be more important for Src function than regulation of kinase activity itself. Additionally, as discussed in the next section, these regulatory interactions also help govern Src subcellular localization.

4. REGULATION OF SUBCELLULAR LOCALIZATION

Analyses of Src activation suggest that this process is associated with a change in subcellular localization. Initial studies of v-Src localization demonstrated an association with the plasma membranes at sites of cellular adhesion in a detergent insoluble fraction *(44–46)*. By contrast, later studies of the c-Src protein found it associated with endosomal membranes in a detergent soluble fraction *(47)*. Indeed, in several systems activation of Src is associated with a change in subcellular localization and detergent solubility. In platelets, Src becomes transiently activated upon activation with thrombin and cross-linking of the gpIIbIIIa integrin *(48)*. Crosslinking of this integrin is accompanied by a translocation of Src to the detergent insoluble fraction. Activation of Src by stimulation of the PDGF receptor is also associated with a translocation of Src to the plasma membrane *(49)*.

Plating of fibroblasts on fibronectin, which also activates integrins, leads to an increase in Src kinase activity accompanied by a translocation to focal adhesions and association with a detergent-insoluble fraction *(50,51)*. Interestingly, this change appears to depend on the open conformation of Src, but not on the kinase activity itself. Mutation of Y527 increased localization at focal adhesions, however, a double Y527F-kinase-inactive point mutant (Y527F-K295M) is also localized in focal adhesions, despite its lack of kinase activity. Removal of the entire kinase domain also caused a constitutive detergent-insoluble association with focal adhesions that was more pronounced than that observed in the Y527F mutant. In this truncated molecule, this subcellular localization depends on a functional SH3 domain *(50)*, arguing that the increased accessibility of this protein interaction domain causes the change in the localization of Src. Activation of Src is therefore not only associated with an increase in kinase activity, but also with increased accessibility or interactions of the protein interaction domains and a change of subcellular localization, recurrent themes in the activation of molecules in signal transduction cascades.

5. FUNCTIONAL ANALYSES OF Src IN SIGNAL TRANSDUCTION PATHWAYS

There are currently at least nine members of the Src family of kinases *(4)*. These proteins can be divided into two classes—those with wide patterns of expressions, such as Src, Fyn, and Yes, and those with more restricted patterns of expression, such as Lck, Hck, Fgr, Blk, and Lyn, in which expression is generally limited to cells in the hematopoietic or epithelial lineages. For some of these kinases, such as Lck, specific functions in defined signaling pathways have been well described (*see* Chapter 6).

For the more broadly expressed tyrosine kinases in this family, evidence suggests that there may be significant overlap in signaling function. Src is implicated in signaling pathways from a variety of cell surface receptors, including tyrosine kinase growth factor receptors, G protein-coupled receptors and integrins, cell surface adhesive receptors for the extracellular matrix. Perhaps due to the overlapping patterns of expression and potential functional redundancy of these kinases, evaluation of Src function through gene targeting in mice has produced only limited information. Although Src is expressed in most cell types, targeted disruption of Src leads to only one major phenotype— osteopetrosis or a failure to resorb bone, caused by an intrinsic defect in osteoclasts *(52,53)*. Osteoclasts express high levels of Src, and the lack of this molecule leads to dramatic defects in the ability of this cell type to resorb bone and organize its actin cytoskeleton *(54–57)*. However, the nature of the defect(s) in signal transduction in these cells remains unclear.

Understanding of the function of Src has therefore come from several sources, including biochemical examination of signaling pathways in which the Src kinase has been demonstrated to be activated, comparison of these pathways in cells derived from wild-type and $src^{-/-}$ gene-targeted mice, and overexpression of mutant Src molecules and use of blocking antibodies to manipulate Src activity in these pathways. While such studies have implicated Src in many different cascades, its contribution to downstream readouts are often poorly understood. Two of the best studied pathways are signaling downstream of growth factor and integrin adhesion receptors. The next section will focus on the function of Src in these two signaling pathways with special emphasis on the roles of the different modular domains. However, it should be emphasized that multiple signaling cascades activate c-Src, including those from G-protein-coupled receptors (GPCRs) and stress responses and that phosphorylation by Src can contribute to many signaling pathways including activation of cell surface receptors and channels (for recent reviews, see the excellent articles by Thomas and Brugge and Brown and Cooper).

6. SIGNALING FROM GROWTH FACTOR RECEPTORS

One of the first pathways shown to affect Src kinase activity was the activation of the tyrosine kinase receptors for platelet-derived growth factor (PDGF) *(58)*. Upon stimulation of fibroblasts with growth factors such as PDGF and colony-stimulating factor 1 (CSF-1), Src is found transiently associated with the receptor via its SH2 domain and there is an concommitant increase in Src kinase activity *(59,60)*. Overexpression of kinase-inactive Src has demonstrated that the kinase activity of Src family members is critical for signaling downstream of these and other growth factor receptors. Either overexpression of kinase-inactive Src or microinjection of blocking antibodies that bind Src, Fyn, and Yes will block entry into S phase of serum starved cells stimulated with PDGF, CSF, or epidermal growth factor (EGF) *(59,61,62)*. Over expression of the Fyn

SH2 domain has the same blocking effect, suggesting that the dominant-negative effects of the kinase-inactive molecules results from binding of SH2 domains to phosphorylated tyrosine residues, but failing to phosphorylate downstream targets *(62)*. Mutants affecting the SH3 domain also have a dominant-interfering phenotype in this pathway, probably by their lack of interactions with critical downstream targets *(61,63)*. Thus, both the kinase activity and the interactions of the SH3 domain of Src are essential for triggering downstream pathways leading to cell division from these receptors. It should be noted that these dominant-negative effects are observed under conditions in which these molecules are overexpressed (5- to 20-fold) and may not come under full regulation of the CSK kinase. Thus, the protein may be in an "open conformation" with the SH2 and SH3 interaction domains more accessible. In these and several other pathways, dominant-negative activities have also been demonstrated with double mutants that were not only kinase inactive, but also contained mutations of Y527, and therefore were also constitutively in an "open conformation" *(64,65)*. In these cases, the dominant-negative activities of these molecules may act more strongly because of the increased availability of the SH2 and SH3 domains.

Downstream targets in this pathway remain unclear, but a variety of proteins phosphorylated by v-Src, including PI3K, SHC, and PLC-γ, are potential substrates *(4)*. For the PDGFR-α, phosphorylation of the adaptor molecule SHC, in particular, appears to require Src activation *(66)*. For the EGFR, the receptor itself may be phosphorylated by Src, leading to increased activity *(67)*. Potential SH3 interacting molecules again include SHC, the PI3 kinase p85 subunit and SIN *(14–16)*. In the case of signaling in response to PDGF, activation of DNA synthesis occurs via a pathway that involves c-myc expression *(68)*. Overexpression of kinase-inactive Src blocks a PDGF-induced increase in c-myc expression and overexpression of c-myc can overcome the block to DNA replication, whereas overexpression of c-fos does not. However, the intermediate steps in this transcriptional activation remain unknown.

It should also be noted that multiple Src family members, particularly the widely expressed kinases, Yes and Fyn, can substitute for Src in these pathways and fibroblasts deficient in Src do not demonstrate defects in responses to the growth factors. Thus, while signaling pathways downstream from growth factor receptors clearly involve Src kinases, they provide an example where the role of Src family kinases is only observed using dominant-negative molecules. Redundancy between family members may hide functional involvement of Src in these pathways in cells from *src*[–/–] gene-targeted animals.

7. SIGNALING FROM G-PROTEIN-COUPLED RECEPTORS

The connection from G-protein-coupled receptors (GPCR) and Src is less clear; however, β-arrestin appears to be part of a complex involving c-Src and GPCR *(105)*. Nonetheless, Src family kinases are activated following stimulation of GPCRs and expression of kinase-negative versions of Src block downstream readouts from these receptors *(64,69)*. At least one effect that is blocked by such dominant-negative molecules is the activation of the EGF receptor after stimulation of the B-adrenergic receptor *(70)*. These data raise the possibility that Src family members may integrate multiple interdependent pathways (e.g., activation of receptor tyrosine kinases by GPCRs). Again, such pathways may not be evident in studies of Src deficient cells.

8. SIGNALING FROM INTEGRINS

Another major pathway in which Src has been implicated is signaling from integrin adhesion receptors. Integrins are heterodimeric receptors that bind elements of the extracellular matrix to promote cell adhesion *(71)*. Engagement of integrins is required for activation of many cellular processes, including cell division and survival. Clustering of integrins induces increased tyrosine phosphorylation and activation of a number of signaling molecules in focal adhesion complexes, the site where integrins help organize cytoskeletal and signaling proteins in response to adhesion *(71)*. After crosslinking of integrins, Src is transiently activated and found in these focal adhesions *(51)*. A very early event in this process is the activation and autophosphorylation of the focal adhesion kinase (FAK), Src and Fyn bind the autophosphorylation site of FAK via their SH2 domains *(72,73)*. FAK is itself a substrate for the Src kinase *(51,73,74)* and a variety of other proteins in the focal adhesion complex including cytoskeletal proteins, such as vinculin, paxillin, tensin, and cortactin, as well as adaptor molecules such as pp130[cas] and c-crk may also be phosphorylated by Src *(4,31–33)*.

That Src may play a critical role in signaling from integrins is indicated by the phenotypes of fibroblasts derived from *src*[-/-] mice, in which cell spreading *(51)*, phosphorylation of the adaptor molecule pp130cas *(31–33)*, and activation of MAPK are all defective in response to plating on adhesive substrates, such as fibronectin *(75)*. In contrast to the previously described signaling pathways, these integrin-mediated responses are not blocked by kinase-inactive Src. Interestingly, the defects in *src*[-/-] fibroblasts are actually partially complemented by expression of either wildtype or kinase inactive mutants of Src. For example, either a kinase-inactive point mutant of Src or a truncated molecule that removes the entire kinase domain complement the cell-spreading defect *(51)*; these molecules also increase pp 130cas phosphorylation in response to fibronectin *(75;* P. Schwartzberg, unpublished observations). A truncated Src molecule lacking the kinase domain has also been demonstrated to restore partial activation of mitogen-activated protein kinase (MAPK) in response to plating on fibronectin *(75)*. Thus, in integrin signaling, Src appears to more closely resemble an adaptor molecule that may function by recruiting or activating other tyrosine kinases. The independence from the kinase activity of Src suggests that for integrin-mediated signal transduction pathways, Src may function by a mechanism distinct from that in growth factor receptors, indicating different roles for Src in the context of different signaling systems.

9. Src FUNCTION IN THE OSTEOCLAST

Despite the nearly ubiquitous pattern of expression of c-*src* and the wide range of signaling pathways in which Src has been implicated, targeted gene disruption of the Src tyrosine kinase in mice leads to only one phenotype—osteopetrosis or a failure to break down bone *(53)*. This disease results from an intrinsic defect in osteoclasts, the cells responsible for bone resorption *(76)*. Although this appears to be a very limited phenotype, functional redundancy between Src family members may limit defects in other cells. Src is very highly expressed in osteoclasts, platelets, and neurons, yet the lack of obvious phenotypes in the other cell types suggests that expression of other Src family kinases (e.g., Fyn and Yes, which are also expressed highly in these other cells) may compensate for the lack of Src. Alternatively, there may be certain signaling pathways for which Src is specifically required in the osteoclast.

As a cell type that is dependent on Src for its normal function, the osteoclast thereore presents presents an opportunity to study Src function in a physiologic context—one that may reveal information about Src that can lead to therapeutic approaches to such diverse diseases as osteoporosis and cancer. The next section discusses potential Src functions in light of defects observed in the osteoclast.

Normal bone growth, repair, and homeostasis are regulated by a balance between two opposing cell types: the mesenchymally derived osteoblast, which lays down new bone, and the hematopoietically derived osteoclast, which resorbs bone *(77)*. Osteoclasts are tartrate-resistant acid phosphatase (TRAP)-positive multinucleated giant syncynctial cells of the monocyte–macrophage lineage, that resorb bone in response to clues from their external environment, including factors secreted by osteoblasts and other cell types and signals from the bone matrix itself *(77)*. These highly polarized cells resorb bone through a specialized region known as the ruffled border, an area of invaginated membranes adjacent to the bone matrix that secretes hydrogen ions, and enzymes, such as cathepsin K and acid phosphatase. A high concentration of vesicles containing these bone degrading enzymes and the osteoclast vacuolar H^+-ATPase secrete their contents at the ruffled border, generating the acidic environment that permits bone degradation. The ruffled border is effectively sealed off by a region called the sealing zone, where the osteoclast adheres tightly to the bone, creating a separate compartment so that the ruffled border has been described as an external lysosome. This sealing zone is responsible for the attachment of the osteoclast to the bone surface and is an area of high concentration of the αVb3 integrin, which binds to RGD-containing proteins, such as osteopontin and bone sialoprotein (BSP). The osteoclast adheres to bone via a ring of podosomes, specialized adhesion structures that are found on highly mobile cells and interestingly, cells transformed by v-*src* or v-*abl,* suggesting that high activity of these kinases may lead to the formation of these specialized adhesive structures. A cytoplasmic ring of actin is associated with these sites of attachment of the sealing zone, surrounding the areas of active resorption *(78,79)*. After a period of active resorption, this tight attachment starts to change and the osteoclast migrates to a new region of the bone to initiate a new round of resorption. Thus, proper regulation of both secretory processes and adhesive interactions are important for normal osteoclast function.

src$^{-/-}$ mice have normal or increased numbers of osteoclasts, but the cellular morphology of osteoclasts is abnormal. Microscopically, they appear flattened against the bone surface and they show little evidence of ruffled border formation *(52)*. Consistent with this lack of ruffled borders, *src*$^{-/-}$ osteoclasts are defective in bone resorption, both in vivo, as evidenced by the increased bone density of *src*$^{-/-}$ mice and in vitro as demonstrated in bone resorption assays *(76)*. Futhermore, these cells do not respond properly to physiologic stimuli that increase bone resorption; mice treated with interleukin-1 (IL-1) normally have increased numbers of osteoclasts and an increase in bone resorption that can be followed by a rise in whole blood calcium *(80)*. Osteoclasts in *src*$^{-/-}$ mice treated with IL-1 increase in number, but these cells do not resorb bone efficiently and there is no concommitant rise in whole blood calcium levels *(52)*. However, the defect in *src⁻/⁻* osteoclasts is not complete; mice deficient in both the Src and Hck kinases are more severely osteopetrotic, suggesting that there may be some degree of functional overlap between these two kinases *(55)*. The study of osteoclasts from these mice not only provides an understanding of the functions of Src family kinases within the cell but may also provide clues to the mechanisms involved in normal bone resorption by the osteoclast. In particular, since osteopetrosis is the only major finding in these mice, Src-based therapeutics have been proposed as a potential method of inhibiting osteoclast function for the treatment of osteoporosis.

The nature of defects in *src⁻/⁻* osteoclasts is unclear; several pathways have been implicated in this phenotype. Evidence suggests that the lack of ruffled border formation is associated with a defect in cellular architecture. Whereas normal osteoclasts have a distinctive actin ring formation at the site of cellular adhesion to the bone around areas of active bone resorption, *src⁻/⁻* osteoclasts have an actin organization more reminiscent of stress fibers in fibroblasts, suggesting an alteration in the mechanism or type of adhesion for this cell *(56,57)*. The demonstration that antisense to *src* leads to altered actin polymerization and adhesion-associated gelsolin-PI3 Kinase interactions, further implies that Src plays a key role in cytoskeletal architecture *(81)*. Furthermore, Src is associated with microtubule-associated vesicles and may play a key role in the polarization of this cell *(82)*. Src is highly expressed in osteoclasts, platelets and neurons *(4)*. In these other cell types, Src is also found in association with vesicles and their associated proteins and has been proposed to play a role in vesicular transport *(30)*. The association of Src with microtubular-associated vesicles in osteoclasts supports a similar possible function in the osteoclast and indeed, a recent report also suggests that expression of activated Src in osteoclasts can alter lysosomal secretion *(83)*. Whether these are the primary defects in *src⁻/⁻* osteoclasts or are secondary to altered signal transduction from other pathways remains unclear.

10. POTENTIAL DEFECTS IN *src⁻/⁻* OSTEOCLASTS

The signaling pathways in which Src has been implicated in other cell-types may provide clues to the signaling pathways defective in *src⁻/⁻* osteoclasts. For example, osteoclasts have been shown to respond to certain growth factors, including CSF-1 *(84)*, hepatocyte growth factor/scatter cell factor (HGF/SCF) *(85)*, and macrophage stimulating protein (MSP) *(86)*; such pathways may be defective in *src⁻/⁻* osteoclasts. In particular, both HGF and MSP have been reported to have modest effects on bone resorption in vitro and altered signaling from Src may lead to decreased responses to these molecules. Nonetheless, because these growth factors do not have profound effects on bone resorption by mature osteoclasts, it is unlikely that defects in responses to these signals would account for the severe phenotype observed in *src⁻/⁻* mice.

Osteoclasts are also influenced by ligands for GPCRs. For example, a major GPRC on the osteoclast is the calcitonin receptor *(77)*. However, calcitonin leads to decreased bone resorption, and thus, is an unlikely target for defective signaling leading to the phenotype of Src-deficient osteoclasts.

Integrin mediated signal transduction is also critical for proper osteoclast function. Blockage of integrins by RGD peptides or antibodies can prevent bone resorption by osteoclasts *(87)* and adhesive interactions are also required for the establishment of cell polarity, an important element of osteoclast function that may be disturbed in the $src^{-/-}$ osteoclast. Furthermore, as in $src^{-/-}$ fibroblasts, downstream effectors of integrin signaling are defective in $src^{-/-}$ osteoclasts. Thus, integrin mediated signal transduction may be a key pathway in which Src is involved in the osteoclast.

A number of the above pathways activate signal transduction molecules that themselves are required for normal osteoclast function. These include the small GTPase Rho and PI3 kinase *(88,89)*. Inhibition of these molecules by pharmocological agents can prevent bone resorption in vitro and alter osteoclast viability. Src has been implicated in activation of these molecules, both in signal transduction from growth factor receptors and from integrins. Thus Src may play a central regulatory role in signaling pathways that feed into these downstream effector molecules in the osteoclast.

11. DOWNSTREAM EFFECTORS IN THE OSTEOCLAST

To help elucidate the pathways in which Src is involved in the osteoclast, a significant effort has been made to find downstream targets for Src in the osteoclast. One such molecule is the product of the proto-oncogene *cbl*. Cbl is a widely expressed adaptor type molecule that possesses a ring-finger domain and is tyrosine phosphorylated in response to a number of signaling pathways in diverse cell types, including fibroblasts and lymphoctyes *(90–94)*. Baron and colleagues have found Cbl to be underphosphorylated and mislocalized in differentiated osteoclasts derived from $src^{-/-}$ mice *(95)*. To address whether Cbl may be a critical substrate of Src, they demonstrated that antisense oligonucleotides to *cbl* also could dramatically reduce bone resorption by osteoclast-like cells. These experiments are interesting and provocative, however, their interpretation remains unclear. In particular, in other systems, phosphorylation of Cbl is associated with downregulation of signaling pathways. It is hard to reconcile this view of Cbl with the idea of Src having an activating role in bone resorption. Secondly, it remains unclear in response to what pathway(s) Cbl may be phosphorylated in the osteoclast. In other systems, phosphorylation of Cbl has been observed in response to activation of both growth factors and integrin receptors *(96)*. It will be informative to determine whether these defects in Cbl phosphorylation are observed in response to a particular signaling pathway in osteoclasts. Alternatively, the lack of Cbl phosphorylation may point out that multiple pathways may be defective in the $src^{-/-}$ osteoclast.

A second downstream target that is of particular interest is the molecule pp130^{cas}, or Crk-associated substrate. This molecule was first described by virtue of its phosphorylated state in cells transformed by either v-*src* or v-*crk*. Subsequent cloning and studies revealed that this molecule also falls in the category of adaptor proteins, having an SH3 domain, a proline-rich region and multiple sites of potential tyrosine phosphorylation *(97)*. This molecule can be found in the focal adhesions of fibroblasts *(98)* and is phosphorylated in response to plating on fibronectin *(33)*. Interestingly, phosphorylation of pp130^{cas} in response to plating on fibronectin is reduced in fibroblasts from $src^{-/-}$ mice, but not in fibroblasts from FAK$^{-/-}$ mice *(31–33)*. Recently, it has been reported that there is increased Cas phosphorylation in osteoclasts in response to adhesion and that phosphorylation of pp130^{cas} is decreased in *src*$^{-/-}$ osteoclasts *(99)*. These results suggest that in osteoclasts, as in fibroblasts, Cas may also be an important downstream target for Src. Such results would be particularly attractive, since they would support a defect in integrin mediated signaling, consistent with those observed in *src*$^{-/-}$ fibroblasts. Futhermore, a defect in integrin-mediated signal transduction might explain the cytoskeletal defects observed in *src*$^{-/-}$ osteoclasts.

Finally, Hruska and colleagues have reported that stimulation of the αVB3 integrin with osteopontin leads to increased association of PI3 kinase with the actin-capping protein gelsolin *(81)*. This association appears to depend on Src; treatment of avian osteoclasts with antisense *src* oligos decreases this association. Together, these defects argue that integrin mediated signal transduction may be a major defective pathway in *src*$^{-/-}$ osteoclasts. Interestingly, another cell type that has shown a phenotype associated with Src deficiency is cultured cerebellar neurons from *src*$^{-/-}$ mice that have a defect in neurite outgrowth to the L1 adhesion molecule *(100)*. L1 has recently been shown to be a good ligand for the αVB3 integrin; thus, Src deficiency may lead to specific defects in responses to this integrin. If this is true, the defects in *src*$^{-/-}$ osteoclasts may result from Src-specific functions in integrin signaling.

12. GENETIC DISSECTION OF Src FUNCTION

As an alternative approach to the study of Src function in the osteoclast, we have examined the phenotypes of mice expressing mutant versions of Src. Given the differences in the ability of kinase-inactive Src mutants to affect signaling pathways, we reasoned that such mutants may provide clues to the contributions of different pathways to the phenotype of *src*$^{-/-}$ osteoclasts. As discussed above, kinase inactive molecules act as dominant-negative blocks to cell function in certain pathways, such as growth factor signaling. However, in integrin mediated pathways, defects observed in *src*$^{-/-}$ cells are at least partially complemented by kinase-inactive Src.

To address the requirement for Src kinase activity, we have generated mice expressing either wild-type or kinase-inactive versions of Src from the promoter of the gene encoding TRAP, a gene highly expressed in osteoclasts. Surprisingly, we observed that both wild-type and a kinase-inactive point mutant of Src could complement certain aspects of Src deficiency, in mice *(57)*, including tooth eruption, bone density and osteoclast response to IL-1. Although the extent of rescue is variable in the kinase-inactive background, some mice exhibit quite good degrees of complementation, suggesting that kinase-inactive Src can provide function to osteoclasts deficient in Src. The similarity of these results to that seen in the response of fibroblasts to cell adhesion suggests that a major aspect of the *src*$^{-/-}$ defect in osteoclasts may stem from a kinase-independent pathway, such as signaling from integrins. Interestingly, expression of this kinase-inactive Src molecule also restores global levels of tyrosine phosphorylation in these osteoclasts, similar to what has been observed for specific proteins such as pp130^{cas} with expression of kinase-inactive Src in *src*$^{-/-}$ fibroblasts.

Given the characteristic of kinase-inactive mutants to act as a dominant-negative molecules in various assays, it was quite remarkable that the kinase-inactive point mutant can rescue the *src*$^{-/-}$ phenotype in mice. By contrast, we have found that another kinase-deficient mutant that lacks the entire kinase domain (Src251) exhibits a dominant-negative phenotype in the osteoclast, causing variable degrees of osteopetrosis in a wild-type and heterozygous background (P. Schwartzberg, L. Xing, B. Boyce, and H.E. Varmus, manuscript in preparation). Interestingly, this mutant also exacerbates the osteopetrosis observed in the $src^{-/-}$ mice.

Histological analysis suggests that this mutant causes osteopetrosis by a novel mechanism—by increasing the rate of apoptosis of osteoclasts. The phenotype of this mutant does not appear to result from a general toxic effect of this Src mutation; the degree of apoptosis is decreased by the increased Src expression in heterozygous and wild-type mice, suggesting that wild-type Src can titrate out the apoptotic effects of this mutant. Furthermore, subsequent studies of mice expressing the kinase-inactive point mutation of Src (K295M) demonstrate that high levels of expression of this mutant also lead to increased levels of osteoclast apoptosis. The truncated Src251 mutant, by lacking the entire kinase domain, has open unregulated SH2 and SH3 interactions and in fibroblasts is constitutively found in focal adhesions, where activated Src is located. Our results suggest that this mutant (Src 251) may be a more potent dominant-negative molecule, perhaps because of the availability of its SH2 and SH3 domains. This mutant suggests that proper regulation of the protein interaction domains may be more critical for Src function in the osteoclast than kinase activity. Thus, the intertwined regulation of kinase activity, protein interactions, and subcellular localization, as evidenced by mutational and crystallogaphic analyses of Src, all may contribute to the proper function of Src.

The phenotype of these mutants also suggests that Src family kinases may have a function in signaling pathways involved in cell survival in the osteoclast. Potential signaling pathways that may be affected in the apoptotic osteoclasts include the previously discussed pathways from growth factor receptors, G-protein-coupled receptors and integrins. Blockage of all these pathways leads to decreased cell survival in other cell types. Indeed, both kinase dead and truncated Src can effectively block signaling from growth factor receptors in fibroblasts, suggesting that this pathway may be a key component of the Src-based cellular survival. The activation of PI3 kinase by Src is one potential downstream molecule that may be altered. Products of PI3 kinase activate the Akt kinase, a key regulator of cellular survival *(101)*. Whereas blocking integrin signaling also decreases cell survival *(102)*, the ability of kinase inactive Src to rescue integrin-mediated pathways in fibroblasts suggests that blockage of this pathway may not be the cause of apoptosis by the kinase-defective Src transgenes.

Finally, since $src^{-/-}$ osteoclasts do not have increased rates of apoptosis, the dominant-negative effects of these mutants may reveal Src family function in signaling pathways not affected by Src deficiency alone. Thus, this phenotype provides another example of Src family function that is only revealed by the use of dominant-negative molecules, similar to what is observed in growth factor signaling pathways in the fibroblast. Therefore, our results in the osteoclast parallel similar findings in the fibroblast where Src may be involved in multiple signal transduction pathways with distinct roles in each.

12. POTENTIAL FOR Src-BASED THERAPEUTICS

The dramatic effects on osteoclast function observed in $src^{-/-}$ mice in the absence of other obvious phenotypes suggests that blocking Src function may be of potential therapeutic value in the treatment of osteoporosis. However, the involvement of Src in signaling pathways from such diverse pathways as integrins, growth factors and GPCRs, combined with the overexpression of c-*src* in a variety of tumor types, suggests that Src based therapeutics may also be useful for treatment of certain tumors.

Based on the phenotype of *src*[-/-] mice, it could be argued that inhibition of Src function could specifically alter osteoclast function in the absence of other systemic side effects leading to an ideal treatment for osteoporosis. However, special care must be exercised in evaluating the therapeutic value of Src-based drugs. Whereas genetic alteration of Src may affect only one cell type in mice, this may result from redundancy between Src family members in other cell types. Drug intervention may interfere with more than one Src family kinase, similar to the effects observed with dominant-negative Src mutants. Thus, Src-based therapeutics may lead to unexpected effects on other cell types and organs and may therefore only be practical using highly specific molecules that interfere with the function of specified Src family members.

The type of drug intervention must also be considered. Our genetic data in mice argue that simple kinase inhibitors may not always be the drug of choice, as they may not alter certain pathways, such as integrin signaling that may be important for osteoclast function. In this regard, SH2 and SH3 inhibitors may be particularly useful. In vitro binding studies have been able to differentiate between the binding of SH3 domains of various Src members *(103,104)*. Likewise, preferred binding of certain SH2 targets may be found *(20)*. The best choice of therapeutics may ultimately depend on which target provides the best specificity of action for a given Src kinase family member in a given cell-type.

13. CONCLUSIONS

Src has provided a wealth of basic knowledge on the regulation of signal transduction molecules, yet our understanding of the function of Src remains unclear. This may result in part, from the multiplicity of pathways in which Src plays a role and the lack of clear linear activation cascades involving Src. Redundancy with other Src family members—particularly the widely expressed Yes and Fyn kinases, also complicates these studies. It is clear that, within a given cell, Src can be involved in many signaling cascades. This review has concentrated on a few well-defined pathways, including those from tyrosine kinase growth factor receptors and integrin adhesion receptors. However, Src has clearly been implicated in many different pathways, including those in response to G-protein-coupled serpentine receptors and stress, as well as those regulating receptor and channel activity. Src functions and interactions may depend on each particular pathway in which it is involved—so that for some, phosphorylation of downstream targets is required, while in others, adaptor functions may define the critical activity of Src. As a model for proteins involved in signal transduction, Src continues to provide lessons, not the least of which is that these pathways are multifaceted and may involve multiple functions for a given molecule.

REFERENCES

1. Stehelin D, Varmus HE, Bishop JM, Vogt PK. DNA related to the transforming gene(s) of avian sarcoma viruses is present in normal avian DNA. *Nature* 1976; 260:170–173.

2. Bolen JB, Veillette A, Schwartz AM, DeSeau V, Rosen N. Activation of pp60c-src protein kinase activity in human colon carcinoma. *Proc Natl Acad Sci USA* 1987; 84:2251–2255.
3. Cartwright, CA, Kamps MP, Meisler AI, Pipas JM, Eckhart W. (1989) pp60c-src activation in human colon carcinoma. *J Clin Invest* 1989; 83:2025–2033.
4. Brown, MT and Cooper JA. Regulation, substrates, and functions of Src. *Biochim Biophys Acta* 1996; 1287:121–149.
5. Neet K, Hunter T. Vertebrate non-receptor protein-tyrosine kinase families. *Genes Cells* 1996; 1:147–169.
6. Resh MD. Myristylation and palmitylation of Src family members: the fats of the matter. *Cell* 1994; 76:411–413.
7. Kabouridis PS, Magee AI, Ley SC. S-acylation of LCK protein tyrosine kinase is essential for its signalling function in T lymphocytes. *EMBO J* 1997; 16:4983–4998.
8. Shalloway D, Bagrodia S, Chackalaparampil I, Shenoy S, Lin PH, Taylor SJ. c-Src and mitosis. *Ciba Found Symp* 1992; 170:248–65; discussion 265–275.
9. Parsons JT, Weber MJ. Genetics of *src*: structural and functional organization of a protein tyrosine kinase. *Curr Top Microbiol Immunol* 1989; 147:79–127.
10. Pawson T, Gish GD. SH2 and SH3 domains: From structure to function. *Cell* 1992; 71:359–362.
11. Cicchetti P, Mayer BJ, Thiel G, Baltimore D. Identification of a protein that binds to the SH3 region of Abl and is similar to Bcr and GAP-rho. *Science* 1992; 257:803–806.
12. Ren R, Mayer BJ, Cicchetti P, Baltimore D. Identification of a ten-amino acid proline-rich SH3 binding site. *Science* 1993; 259:1157–1161.
13. Feng S, Chen JK, Yu H, Simon JA, Schreiber SL. Two binding orientations for peptides to the Src SH3 domain: Development of a general model for SH3-ligand interactions. *Science* 1994; 266:1241–1247.
14. Liu X, Marengere LE, Koch CA, Pawson T. The v-Src SH3 domain binds phosphatidylino-sitol 3±-kinase. *Mol Cell Biol* 1993; 13:5225–5232.
15. Weng Z, Thomas SM, Rickles RJ, Taylor JA, Brauer AW, Seidel-Dugan C, Michael WM, Dreyfuss G, Brugge JS. Identification of Src, Fyn, and Lyn SH3-binding proteins: implications for a function of SH3 domains. *Mol Cell Biol* 1994; 14:4509–4521.
16. Alexandropoulos K, Cheng G, Baltimore D. Proline-rich sequences that bind to Src homology 3 domains with individual specificities. *Proc Natl Acad Sci USA* 1995; 92:3110–3114.
17. Fumagalli S, Totty NF, Hsuan JJ, Courtneidge SA. A target for Src in mitosis. *Nature* 1994; 368:871–874.
18. Taylor SJ, and Shalloway D. An RNA-binding protein associated with Src through its SH2 and SH3 domains in mitosis. *Nature* 1994; 368:867–871.
19. Holmes TC, Fadool DA, Ren R, Levitan IB. Association of Src tyrosine kinase with a human potassium channel mediated by SH3 domain. *Science* 1996; 274:2089–2091.
20. Songyang Z, Shoelson SE, Chaudhuri M, Gish G, Pawson T, Haser WG, King F, Roberts T, Ratnofsky S, Lechleider RJ, et al. SH2 domains recognize specific phosphopeptide sequences. *Cell* 1993; 72:767–778.
21. Mori S, Ronnstrand L, Yokote K, Engstrom A, Courtneidge SA, Claesson-Welsh L, Heldin CH. Identification of two juxtamembrane autophosphorylation sites in the PDGF beta-receptor; involvement in the interaction with Src family tyrosine kinases. *EMBO J,* 1993; 12:2257–2264.
22. Hunter T, Cooper JA. Protein-tyrosine kinases. *Annu Rev Biochem* 1985; 54:897–930.
23. Jove R, Hanafusa H. Cell transformation by the viral *src* oncogene. *Annu Rev Cell Biol* 1987; 3:31–56.
24. Smart JE, Oppermann H, Czernilofsky AP, Purchio AF, Erikson RL, Bishop JM. Characterization of sites for tyrosine phosphorylation in the transforming protein of Rous sarcoma virus (pp60v-src) and its normal cellular homologue (pp60c-src). *Proc Natl Acad Sci USA* 1981; 78:6013–6017.

25. Russo AA, Jeffrey PD, Pavletich NP. Structural basis of cyclin-dependent kinase activation by phosphorylation. *Nature Struct Biol* 1996; 3:696–700.

26. Yamaguchi H, Hendrickson WA. Structural basis for activation of human lymphocyte kinase Lck upon tyrosine phosphorylation. *Nature* 1996; 384:484–489.

27. Piwnica-Worms H, Saundrs KB, Roberts TM, Smith AE, Cheng SH. Tyrosine phosphorylation regulates the biochemical and biological properties of pp60c-src. *Cell* 1987; 49:75–82.

28. Kmiecik TE, Shalloway D. Activation and suppresssion of pp60c-src transforming ability by mutation of its primary sites of tyrosine phosphorylation. *Cell* 1987; 49:65–73.

29. Levy JB, Iba H, Hanafusa H. Activation of the transforming potential of p60c-src by a single amino acid change. *Proc Natl Acad Sci USA* 1986; 83:4228–4232.

30. Thomas S, Brugge J. Cellular functions regulated by Src family kinases. *Annu Rev Cell Dev Biol* 1997; 13:513–609.

31. Bockholt SM, Burridge K. An examination of focal adhesion formation and tyrosine phosphorylation in fibroblasts isolated from src-, fyn-, and yes- mice. *Cell Adhes Commun* 1995 3:91–100.

32. Hamasaki K, Mimura T, Morino N, Furuya H, Nakamoto T, Aizawa S, Morimoto C, Yazaki Y, Hirai H, Nojima Y. Src kinase plays an essential role in integrin-mediated tyrosine phosphorylation of Crk-associated substrate p130Cas. *Biochem Biophys Res Commun* 1996; 222:338–343.

33. Vuori K, Hirai H, Aizawa S, Ruoslahti E. Introduction of p130cas signaling complex formation upon integrin-mediated cell adhesion: A role for Src family kinases. *Mol Cell Biol* 1996; 16:2606–2613.

34. Yu X-M, Askalan R, Keil GJ, Salter MW. NMDA channel regulation by channel-associated protein tyrosine kinase Src. *Science* 1997; 275:674–678.

35. Cartwright CA, Kaplan PL, Cooper JA, Hunter T, Eckhart W. Altered sites of tyrosine phosphorylation in pp60c-src associated with polyomavirus middle tumor antigen. *Mol Cell Biol* 1986; 6:1562–1570.

36. Courtneidge, SA. Activation of the pp60c-src kinase by middle T antigen binding or by dephosphorylation. *EMBO J* 1985; 4:1471–1477.

37. Nada S, Okada M, MacAuley A, Cooper JA, Nakagawa H. Cloning of a complementary DNA for a protein-tyrosine kinase that specifically phosphorylates a negative regulatory site of p60$^{c-src.}$ *Nature* 1991; 351:69–72.

38. Nada S, Yagi T, Takeda H, Tokunaga T, Nakagawa H, Ikawa Y, Okada M, Aizawa S. Constitutive activation of Src family kinases in mouse embryos that lack Csk. *Cell* 1993; 73:1125–1135.

39. Imamoto A, Soriano P. Disruption of the *csk* gene, encoding a negative regulator of Src family tyrosine kinases, leads to neural tube defects and embryonic lethality in mice. *Cell* 1993; 73:1117–1124.

40. Kato JY, Takeya T, Grandori C, Iba H, Levy JB, Hanafusa H. Amino acid substitutions sufficient to convert the nontransforming p60c-src protein to a transforming protein. *Mol Cell Biol* 1986; 6:4155–4160.

41. Xu W, Harrison SC, Eck MJ. Three-dimensional structure of the tyrosine kinase c-Src [see comments]. *Nature* 1997; 385:595–602.

42. Sicheri F, Moarefi I, Kuriyan J. Crystal structure of the Src family tyrosine kinase Hck [see comments]. *Nature* 1997; 385:602–609.

43. Moarefi I, LaFevre-Bernt M, Sicheri F, Huse M, Lee CH, Kuriyan J, Miller WT. Activation of the Src-family tyrosine kinase Hck by SH3 domain displacement [see comments]. *Nature* 1997; 385:650–653.

44. Rohrschneider LR. Adhesion plaques of Rous sarcoma virus-transformed cells contain the Src gene product. *Proc Natl Acad Sci USA* 1980; 77:3514–3518.

45. Krueger JG, Garber EA, Goldberg AR. Subcellular localization of pp60src in RSV-transformed cells. *Curr Top Microbiol Immunol* 1983; 107:51–124.

46. Hamaguchi M, and Hanafusa H. Association of p60src with Triton X-100-resistant cellular structure correlates with morphological transformation. *Proc Natl Acad Sci USA* 1987; 84:2312–2316.

47. Kaplan KB, Swedlow JR, Varmus HE, Morgan DO. Association of p60$^{c\text{-}src}$ with endosomal membranes in mammalian fibroblasts. *J Cell Biol* 1992; 118:321–333.

48. Clark, EA, Brugge JS. Redistribution of activated pp60c-src to integrin-dependent cytoskeletal complexes in thrombin-stimulated platelets. *Mol Cell Biol* 1993; 13:1863–1871.

49. Walker F, deBlaquiere J, Burgess AW. Translocation of pp60c-src from the plasma membrane to the cytosol after stimulation by platelet-derived growth factor. *J Biol Chem* 1993; 268:19,552–19,558.

50. Kaplan KB, Bibbins KB, Swedlow JR, Arnaud M, Morgan DO, Varmus HE. Association of the amino-terminal half of c-Src with focal adhesions alters their properties and is regulated by phosphorylation of tyrosine 527. *EMBO J* 1994; 13:4745–4756.

51. Kaplan KB, Swedlow JR, Morgan DO, Varmus HE. c-Src enhances the spreading of *src$^{-/-}$* fibroblasts on fibronectin by a kinase-independent mechanism. *Genes Dev* 1995; 9:1505–1517.

52. Boyce B, Yoneda T, Lowe C, Soriano P, Mundy G. Requirement of pp60$^{c\text{-}src}$ expression for osteoclasts to form ruffled borders and to resorb bone in mice. *J Clin Invest* 1992; 90:1622–1627.

53. Soriano P, Montgomery C, Geske R, Bradley A. Targeted disruption of the c-*src* protooncogene leads to osteopetrosis in mice. *Cell* 1991; 64:693–702.

54. Horne W, Neff L, Chatterjee D, Lomri A, Levy J, Baron R. Osteoclasts express high levels of pp60$^{c\text{-}src}$ in association with intracellular membranes. *J Cell Biol* 1992; 119:1003–1013.

55. Lowell CA, Niwa M, Soriano P, Varmus HE. Deficiency of the Hck and Src tyrosine kinases results in extreme levels of extramedullary hematopoiesis. *Blood* 1996; 87:1780–1792.

56. Neff L, Amling M, Baron R. cSrc deletion alters adhesion structures in the osteoclast: Redistribution of podosomes and formation of focal adhesions. *J Bone Miner Res* 1996; 11:S290.

57. Schwartzberg PL, Xing L, Hoffmann O, Lowell CA, Garrett L, Boyce BF, Varmus HE. Rescue of osteoclast function by transgenic expression of kinase-deficient Src in src$^{-/-}$ mutant mice. *Genes Dev* 1997; 11:2835–2844.

58. Ralston R, Bishop JM. The product of the protooncogene c-*src* is modified during the cellular response to platelet-derived growth factor. *Proc Natl Acad Sci USA* 1985; 82:7845–7849.

59. Courtneidge SA, Dhand R, Pilat D, Twamley GM, Waterfield MD, Roussel MF. Activation of Src-family kinases by colony stimulating factor-1, and their association with its receptor. *EMBO J* 1993; 12:943–950.

60. Kypta RM, Goldber Y, Ulug ET, Courtneidge SA. Association between the PDGF receptor and members of the Src-family of tyrosine kinases. *Cell* 1990; 62:481–492.

61. Broome, MA, Hunter T. Requirement for c-Src catalytic activity and the SH3 domain in platelet-derived growth factor BB and epidermal growth factor mitogenic signalling. *J Biol Chem* 1996; 271:16,798–16,806.

62. Twamley-Stein GM, Pepperkok R, Ansorge W, Courtneidge SA. The Src family tyrosine kinases are required for platelet-derived growth factor-mediated signal transduction in NIH 3T3 cells. *Proc Natl Acad Sci USA* 1993; 90:7696–7700.

63. Erpel T, Alonso G, Roche S, Courtneidge SA. The Src SH3 domain is required for DNA synthesis induced by platelet-derived growth factor and epidermal growth factor. *J Biol Chem* 1996; 271:16,807–16,812.

64. Igishi T, Gutkind JS. Tyrosine kinases of the Src family participate in signaling to MAP kinase from both Gq and Gi-coupled receptors. *Biochem Biophys Res Commun* 1998; 244:5–10.

65. Mukhopadhyay D, Tsiokas L, Zhou XM, Foster D, Brugge JS, Sukhatme VP. Hypoxic

induction of human vascular endothelial growth factor expression through c-Src activation. *Nature* 1995; 375:577–581.

66. Gelderloos JA, Rosenkranz S, Bazenet C, Kazlauskas A. A role for Src in signal relay by the platelet-derived growth factor alpha receptor. *J Biol Chem* 1998; 273:5908–5915.

67. Wilson LK, Parsons SJ. Enhanced EGF mitogenic response is associated with enhanced tyrosine phosphorylation of specific cellular proteins in fibroblasts overexpressing c-*src*. *Oncogene* 1990; 5:1471–1480.

68. Barone MV, and Courtneidge SA. Myc but not Fos rescue of PDGF signalling block caused by kinase-inactive Src. *Nature* 1995; 378:509–512.

69. Luttrell LM, BE H, T v.B, DK; L, TJ; L, and RJ L. Role of c-Src tyrosine kinase in G protein-coupled receptor- and Gbetagamma subunit-mediated activation of mitogen-activated protein kinases. *J Biol Chem* 1996; 271:19,443–19,450.

70. Della Rocca GJ, van Biesen T, Daaka Y, Luttrell DK, Luttrell LM, Lefkowitz R.J. Ras-dependent mitogen-activated protein kinase activation by G protein-coupled receptors. Convergence of Gi- and Gq-mediated pathways on calcium/calmodulin, Pyk2, and Src kinase. *J Biol Chem* 1997; 272:19,125–19,132.

71. Clark EA, Brugge JS. (1995) Integrins and signal transduction pathways: The road taken. *Science* 1995; 268:233–239.

72. Richardson A, Parsons J. Signal transduction through integrins: A central role for focal adhesion kinase? *BioEssays* 1995; 229–236.

73. Schaller MD, Hildebrand JD, Shannon JD, Fox JW, Vines RR, Parsons JT. Autophosphorylation of the focal adhesion kinase, pp125FAK, directs SH2-dependent binding of pp60src. *Mol Cell Biol* 1994; 14:1680–1688.

74. Schlaepfer DD, Hanks SK, Hunter T, van der Geer P. Integrin-mediated signal transduction linked to Ras pathway by GRB2 binding to focal adhesion kinase. *Nature* 1994; 372:786–791.

75. Schlaepfer DD, Broome MA, Hunter T. Fibronectin-stimulated signaling from a focal adhesion kinase-c-Src complex: Involvement of the GRB2, p130[cas] and Nck adaptor proteins. *Mol Cell Biol* 1997; 17:1702–1713.

76. Lowe C, Yoneda T, Boyce BF, Chen H, Mundy GR, Soriano P. Osteopetrosis in Src-deficient mice is due to an autonomous defect of osteoclasts. *Proc Natl Acad Sci USA* 1993; 90:4485–4489.

77. Baron R, Revesloot J-H, Neff L, Chakraborty M, Chatterjee D, Lomri A, Horne W. Cellular and molecular biology of the osteoclast, in *Cellular and Molecular Biology of bone,* Academic Press, San Diego, 1993, pp 445–495.

78. Lakkakorpi P, Vaananen HK. Kinetics of osteoclast cytoskeleton during the resorption cycle in vitro. *J Bone Miner Res* 1991; 6:817—825.

79. Teti A, Marchisio PC, Zamonin Zallone A. Clear zone in osteoclast function: Role of podosomes in regulation of bone-resorbing activity. *Am J Physiol* 1991; 261:C1–7.

80. Boyce BF, Aufdemorte TB, Garrett IR, Yates AJP, Mundy GR. Effects of interleukin-1 on bone turnover in normal mice. *Endocrinology* 1989; 125:1142–1150.

81. Chellaiah M, Hruska K. Osteopontin stimulates gelsolin-associated phosphoinositide levels and phosphatidylinositol triphosphate-hydroxyl kinase. *Mol Biol Cell* 1996; 7:743–753.

82. Abu-Amer Y, Ross FP, Schlesinger P, Tondravi MM, Teitelbaum SL. Substrate recognition by osteoclast precursors induces c-Src/microtubule association. *J Cell Biol* 1997; 137:247–258.

83. Brubaker KD, Gay CV. Evidence for plasma membrane estrogen receptors and rapid signaling events in osteolasts. *J Bone Miner Res* 1997; 12:S134.

84. Insogna KL, Sahni M, Grey AB, Tanaka S, Horne WC, Neff L, Mitnick M, Levy JB, Baron R. Colony-stimulating factor-1 induces cytoskeletal reorganization and c-src-dependent tyrosine phosphorylation of selected cellular proteins in rodent osteoclasts. *J Clin Invest* 1997; 100:2476–2485.

85. Grano M, Galimi F, Zambonin G, Colucci S, Cottone E, Zallone AZ, Comoglio PM. Hepatocyte growth factor is a coupling factor for osteoclasts and osteoblasts in vitro. *Proc Natl Acad Sci USA* 1996; 93:7644–7648.

86. Kurihara N, Iwama A, Tatsumi J, Ikeda K, Suda T. Macrophage-stimulating protein activates STK receptor tyrosine kinase on osteoclasts and facilitates bone resorption by osteoclast-like cells. *Blood* 1996; 87:3704–3710.

87. Horton MA, Taylor ML, Arnett TR, Helfrich MH. Arg-Gly-Asp (RGD) peptides and the anti-vitronectin receptor antibody 23C6 inhibit dentine resorption and cell spreading by osteoclasts. *Exp Cell Res* 1991; 195:386–375.

88. Lakkakorpi PT, Wesolowski G, Zimolo Z, Rodan GA, Rodan SB. Phosphatidylinositol 3-kinase association with the osteoclast cytoskeleton, and its involvement in osteoclast attachment and spreading. *Exp Cell Res* 1997; 237:296–306.

89. Zhang D, Udagawa N, Nakamura I, Murakami H, Saito S, Yamasaki K, Shibasaki Y, Morii N, Narumiya S, Takahashi N, et al. The small GTP-binding protein, rho p21, is involved in bone resorption by regulating cytoskeletal organization in osteoclasts. *J Cell Sci* 1995; 108:2285–2292.

90. Bowtell DD, Langdon WY. The protein product of the c-cbl oncogene rapidly complexes with the EGF receptor and is tyrosine phosphorylated following EGF stimulation. *Oncogene* 1995; 11:1561–1567.

91. Fusaki N, Iwamatsu A, Iwashima M, Fujisawa J. Interaction between Sam68 and Src family tyrosine kinases, Fyn and Lck, in T cell receptor signaling. *J Biol Chem* 1997; 272:6214–6219.

92. Husson H, Mograbi B, Schmid-Antomarchi H, Fischer S, Rossi B. CSF-1 stimulation induces the formation of a multiprotein complex including CSF-1 receptor, c-Cbl, PI 3-kinase, Crk-II and Grb2. *Oncogene* 1997; 14:2331–2338.

93. Panchamoorthy G, Fukazawa T, Miyake S, Soltoff S, Reedquist K, Druker B, Shoelson S, Cantley L, Band H. p120cbl is a major substrate of tyrosine phosphorylation upon B cell antigen receptor stimulation and interacts in vivo with Fyn and Syk tyrosine kinases, Grb2 and Shc adaptors, and the p85 subunit of phosphatidylinositol 3-kinase. *J Biol Chem* 1996; 271:3187–3194.

94. Soltoff SP, Cantley LC. p120cbl is a cytosolic adapter protein that associates with phospho-inositide 3-kinase in response to epidermal growth factor in PC12 and other cells. *J Biol Chem* 1996; 271:563–567.

95. Tanaka S, Amling M, Neff L, Peyman A, Uhlmann E, Levy JB, Baron R. c-Cbl is downstream of c-Src in a signalling pathway necessary for bone resorption. *Nature* 1996; 383:528–531.

96. Ojaniemi M, Martin SS, Dolfi F, Olefsky JM, Vuori K. The proto-oncogene product p120(cbl) links c-Src and phosphatidylinositol 3′-kinase to the integrin signaling pathway. *J Biol Chem* 1997; 272:3780–3787.

97. Sakai R, Iwamatsu A, Hirano N, Ogawa S, Tanaka T, Mano H, Yazaki Y, Hirai H. A novel signaling molecule, p130, forms stable complexes in vivo with v-Crk and v-Src in a tyrosine phosphorylation-dependent manner. *EMBO J* 1994; 13:3748–3756.

98. Nakamoto T, Sakai R, Honda H, Ogawa S, Ueno H, Suzuki T, Aizawa S, Yazaki Y, Hirai H. Requirements for localization of p130cas to focal adhesions. *Mol Cell Biol* 1997; 17:3884–3897.

99. Nakamura I, Jimi E, Duong LT, Sasaki T, Takahashi N, Rodan GA, Suda T. Tyrosine phosphorylation of p130Cas is involved in actin organization in osteoclasts. *J Biol Chem* 1998: 273:11,144–11,149.

100. Ignelzi MA, Miller DR, Soriano P, Maness PF. Impaired neurite outgrowth of Src-minus neurons on the cell adhesion molecule L1. *Neuron* 1994; 12:873–884.

101. Marte BM, Downward J. PKB/Akt: Connecting phosphoinositide 3-kinase to cell survival and beyond. *Trends Biochem Sci* 1997; 22:355–358.

102. Frisch SM, Ruoslahti E. Integrins and anoikis. *Curr Opin Cell Biol* 1997; 9:701–706.
103. Cheng G, Ye ZS, Baltimore D. Binding of Bruton's tyrosine kinase to Fyn, Lyn, or Hck through a Src homology 3 domain-mediated interaction. *Proc Natl Acad Sci USA* 1994; 91:8152–8155.
104. Rickles RJ, Botfield MC, Zhou XM, Henry PA, Brugge JS, Zoller MJ. Phage display selection of ligand residues important for Src homology 3 domain binding specificity. *Proc Natl Acad Sci USA* 1995: 92:10909–10913.
105. Luttrell LM, Ferguson SS, Daaka Y, Miller WE, Mandsley S, Della Rocca GJ, Lin F, Kauakatsu H, Owada K, Luttrell DK, Caron MG, Lefkowitz RJ. Beta-Arrestin-dependent formation of beta 2 adrenergic receptor-Src protein kinase complexes. *Science* 1999; 283:655–661.

18

Inhibitors of Protein Kinase C and Related Receptors for the Lipophilic Second-Messenger sn-1,2-Diacylglycerol

Peter M. Blumberg, Peter Acs, Dipak K. Bhattacharyya, and Patricia S. Lorenzo

1. INTRODUCTION

Toxic natural products, selected by evolution both for activity against crucial biological targets and for potency, have made major contributions in highlighting such targets and in defining their functions. The phorbol esters, initially isolated on the basis of their activity as tumor promoters and as acute irritants, were found to have dramatic biological effects in virtually every system in which they were examined *(1)*. We now appreciate that the phorbol esters function as ultrapotent analogs of the lipophilic second messenger sn-1,2-diacylglycerol (DAG) and that phorbol ester receptors identify high-affinity targets in DAG signaling *(2)*, of which protein kinase C (PKC) has been most thoroughly studied *(3–7)*.

DAG is the common second messenger generated by a wide array of receptors which are coupled either through G-protein or tyrosine phosphorylation mechanisms to activation of phospholipase C activity specific for phosphatidylinositol 4,5-bisphosphate *(8)*. The other product of this hydrolysis is inositol 4,5-bisphosphate, which causes elevation of intracellular Ca^{2+} arising from release from intracellular stores. DAG can also be produced in a two-step process via production of phosphatidic acid by phospholipase D *(9)*. Unlike the phospholipase C pathway, this latter route is not associated with elevated intracellular Ca^{2+}. Other lipophilic second-messenger/co-messengers include free fatty acids and lysophospholipids. An important concept, emphasized by Nishizuka *(3)* is that coordinate control by DAG in the context of these other co-messengers may differentially mediate DAG sensitive effectors.

2. PKC IS ONLY ONE OF FOUR EFFECTORS OF DAG SIGNALING

The high affinity interaction of phorbol ester/DAG with its targets is mediated through a so-called C1 domain *(2)*. Currently, this C1 domain has been identified in four families of proteins, three of which are positioned to play prominent roles in cellular signaling. These four families are PKC, the chimerins, RasGRP, and Unc-13 (Fig. 1).

From: Signaling Networks and Cell Cycle Control: The Molecular Basis of Cancer and Other Diseases
Edited by: J. S. Gutkind © Humana Press Inc., Totowa, NJ

Cys motif $= H X_{12} C X_2 C X_{13/14} C X_2 C X_4 H X_2 C X_7 C$
C= cysteine; H: histidine; X= any other amino acid

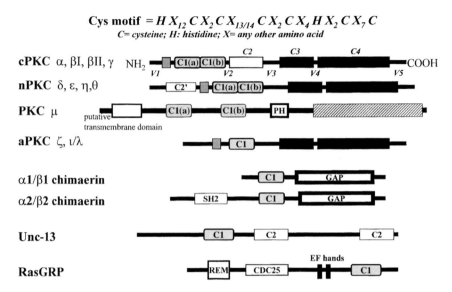

Fig. 1. Differences in structure between PKC isozymes, α/β chimaerins, Unc-13 and RasGRP. C1, cysteine-rich motif; PH, putative pleckstrin domain; GAP, GTPase-activating protein; RasGRP, Ras guanyl-releasing protein; REM, Ras exchange motif; CDC25, prototype Ras activator from *Saccharomyces cerevisiae*.

The PKC family consists of 11 members, dividing into four subfamilies *(3,4,6,7)*. The classical PKCs α, βI, βII, and γ possess a regulatory domain with tandem C1 domains and a C2 domain involved in Ca^{2+} responsiveness and phospholipid binding; the C-terminal catalytic domain is a serine/threonine-specific protein kinase. The novel PKCs δ, ε, η, and ξ differ from the classical PKCs in lacking the C2 domain; however, the function of this domain appears to be replaced by a Ca^{2+} unresponsive homolog N-terminal to the C1 domains *(10)*. The atypical PKCs ζ and iota/λ lack the C2 domain and possess only a single C1-like domain; this latter domain, however, contains several sequence changes that render it inactive for phorbol ester/DAG binding *(11,12)*. Finally, PKC μ shows multiple structural differences compared to the other three subfamilies. The tandem C1 domains are more widely separated; the pseudosubstrate region found in the other PKCs is missing; there is a putative transmembrane region; and the kinase domain shows lower homology with those of the other PKCs and is more closely related to that of the Ca^{2+}/calmodulin-dependent protein kinase type II *(13)*.

In the chimerins, a single C1 domain is linked to a distinct effector region, homologous to that in the Bcr protein, with p21Rac GAP activity *(14,15)*. The four family members are generated from two genes by alternate splicing *(16–18)*. The β splice variants possess an SH2 domain.

Unc-13 family numbers contain a single C1 domain as well as two or three C2 domains, similar to the classical PKCs *(19)*. Although the nature of the effector region has not been identified, the protein is found associated with synaptic vesicles and may be involved in neurotransmitter release *(20)*. RasGRP possesses a single C1 domain, a pair of structures resembling modified EF-hands—a Ca^{2+} binding motif distinct from that in the C2 domains—and a catalytic domain with Ras guanyl releasing activity *(21)*.

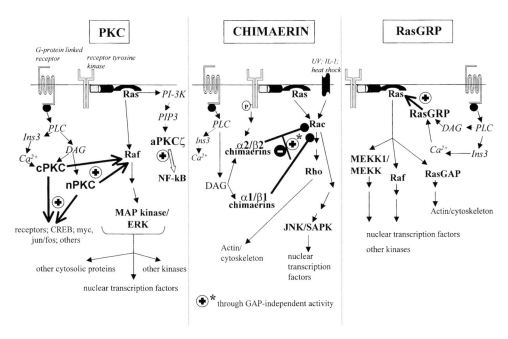

Fig. 2. Schematic pathways for PKC, chimerin, and RasGRP proteins.

3. DAG SIGNALING PATHWAYS

The role of PKC in cellular signaling has been studied in considerable detail. The other classes of phorbol ester/DAG transducers have been explored experimentally in much less depth, although they are positioned in controlling positions in major signaling pathways. Both for the chimerins and for RasGRP, a central difference compared with PKC is their more restricted tissue distribution. The chimaerins are found predominantly in brain and testis, but with lower-level expression of β2 chimerin in heart and pancreas and detectable expression in other tissues *(17,18)*. Interestingly, the level of β2 chimerin expression is reduced in malignant glial tumors relative to low-grade astrocytomas or normal brain *(22)*. RasGRP is expressed in brain and T-lymphocytes *(21,21a)*. The schematic pathways for these different phorbol ester/DAG receptors are illustrated in Fig. 2. The chimerins are positioned as inhibitors of the sapk/jnk pathway and of rearrangements in the actin cytoskeleton mediated by Rac. RasGRP stimulates the Ras pathway, a pathway into which PKC acts as well.

4. IMPLICATIONS OF MULTIDOMAIN RECEPTORS ON INHIBITOR DESIGN

The multidomain structure of the phorbol ester/DAG effectors provides multiple opportunities for inhibitor design. Because these domains may also be expressed in other families of proteins, the choice of domain to which the inhibitor is targeted will carry with it the profile for potential crossreactivity or lack of activity. PKC aptly illustrates this issue. For ligands targeted to the C1 domain, the above four families of receptors pose the challenge for effecting selectivity. For inhibitors of the catalytic domain, selectivity becomes an issue of distinguishing between kinase catalytic domains. Here, the chimerin, RasGRP, and Unc-13 classes are irrelevant. By contrast, the akt1/PKB family, which possesses a regulatory domain distinct from PKC, is homologous in its kinase domain to the classical and novel PKCs *(23,24),* whereas PKC mu falls outside the family. In addition, for inhibitors targeted to the kinase domain the very large number of protein kinases in the cell, estimated at perhaps 1000, poses a substantial problem; a clear implication is that screening against a modest set of kinases, as is often done, cannot be extrapolated to more general conclusions about selectivity. Finally, inhibitors that are selective for membrane enzymes will appear to be selective for PKC if screened against typical kinases, but will be recognized to be unselective if screened against other membrane proteins. As described below, all these problems have arisen in practice.

An additional conceptual issue for inhibitor design is that proteins are often multifunctional. Inhibition of one function may thus not be equivalent to abrogation of all functions of the protein. In the case of PKC, its primary effector function is as a serine-threonine kinase. However, a number of reports suggest that PKC can stimulate phospholipase D activity in a kinase-independent fashion, perhaps mediated via its C2 domain *(25).* Finally, proper functioning of PKC, like many other kinases, is affected by specific protein–protein interactions. Overexpression of catalytically inactive enzyme or of regulatory domain fragments has been shown to lead to dominant negative activity, presumably by competition with active PKC at these required sites of interaction *(26,27).* Similar behavior of PKC upon inhibition of its catalytic activity may contribute to the effects of an exogenous inhibitor.

5. MECHANISMS OF PKC REGULATION

PKC activity is regulated by its state of folding, by its localization, and by downregulation. Each of these processes thus affords opportunities for inhibitor design. The state of PKC folding and the associated level of intrinsic PKC activity has received the greatest attention. A central concept is that multiple factors contribute to the energetics of folding, and it is their combined effects that determine outcome. Within the regulatory domain of PKC is a so-called pseudosubstrate region, which embodies the substrate requirements for PKC, but with an alanine residue in lieu of a serine/threonine residue at which phosphorylation could take place *(28).* The inhibition of catalytic activity by the regulatory domain is thought to reflect the intramolecular binding of this pseudosubstrate region to the catalytic site of the enzyme. PKC is activated by association with anionic lipids, notably phosphatidylserine, interacting with the C1 and C2 domains, by binding of ligands to the C1 domains, and, for the classical PKC isoforms, by Ca^{2+} enhancing the membrane interaction of the C2 domain *(4,29).* All these factors stabilize an open form of the enzyme in which the pseudosubstrate is displaced from the catalytic site. Protein–protein interactions can provide further stabilization, as exemplified by the RACK (receptor for activated C kinase) proteins *(30).* Because these various interactions contribute to the global energetics of unfolding, the effect of a specific activating factor will depend on the magnitude of the contributions of the other coactivators present.

5.1. Regulation Through the C1 Domain

Phorbol ester/diacylglycerol functions by binding to the twin C1 domains of PKC. The solution structure of the C1 domain has been determined by nuclear magnetic resonance (NMR), and the crystal structure has been determined in both the absence and presence of ligand *(31)*. Further insights have been provided by molecular modeling, using the NMR and crystal structures as a starting point *(32)*. The C1 domains are highly conserved zinc finger structures. The top half is hydrophobic except for a hydrophilic cleft formed from the separated strands of a β sheet. The phorbol ester inserts into this hydrophilic cleft, providing a hydrophobic cap. It thereby functions as a hydrophobic switch to facilitate association of the C1 domain with the bilayer. At least two factors contribute to this hydrophobic cap. The first is the phorbol ester moiety itself, which fits into the cleft; the second is the nature of the side chains on the phorbol ester or diacylglycerol. The side chains extend beyond the cleft but can contribute, depending on their size, orientation, and specific structure, to the hydrophobic interactions with the lipid bilayer. This latter effect is particularly difficult to model, because it depends on the ternary complex of PKC–ligand–phospholipid. By contrast, the analysis of the patterns of biological response to structural variants of the phorbol esters have unambiguously demonstrated the importance of the side chains. Unsaturation in the side chains generates compounds that are inflammatory but either not tumor promoting or only weakly tumor promoting *(33);* mezerein exemplifies this behavior *(34,35)*. Even more striking, both 12-deoxyphorbol 13-acetate and its long-chain substituted homolog 12-deoxyphorbol 13-tetradecanoate fully activate PKC in vitro. However, whereas the long-chain substituted homolog is a potent tumor promoter, 12–deoxyphorbol 13-acetate is only weakly inflammatory, fails to induce either acute or chronic skin hyperplasia, and dramatically inhibits phorbol ester induced tumor promotion *(36,37)*. The model of phorbol ester action that emerges is thus that of a hydrophobic cap and tassel, functioning as a hydrophobic switch.

Although the classical and novel PKCs contain two C1 domains, the significance of tandem domains remains uncertain. To address this issue, we introduced mutations into either the first (C1a), the second (C1b), or both domains to reduce phorbol ester binding affinity, but not to destroy the integrity of the C1 domain or abolish phorbol ester interaction with it. The mutated PKCs were reintroduced into NIH 3T3 cells and ligand interaction was measured by its ability to induce translocation. We found that the dependence on the C1 domains for translocation depended both on the ligand and on the specific isoform, PKC α or δ, examined *(38,39,39a)*. Three patterns were observed: (1) the C1a and C1b domains were not equivalent, and the C1b domain played the more prominent role in translocation; (2) the C1a and C1b domains were equivalent, with the C1a/C1b double mutant showing further loss of affinity; and (3) the C1a/C1b domains were equivalent, but the C1a/C1b double mutant did not show further loss of affinity. The conclusion that different ligands show different dependence on the C1a and C1b domains is supported by several other experimental approaches, although specific details differ *(40,41)*. In contrast to the agreement, using intact PKC, that both C1 domains can function for phorbol ester binding, some studies with isolated C1 domains have suggested a lack of activity for the C1a domains of some isoforms

(42). A possible reconciliation of the conflict is that the isolated domains may be unstable under the conditions of assay.

For intact PKC, DAG/phorbol ester binding depends not only on the C1 domains themselves, but also on other factors that influence the energetics of PKC unfolding/ activation. Both potency and structure–activity relations are influenced by other domains in PKC. For example, the structure–activity relationships between the PKC δ C1b domain and the intact enzyme differed by up to 30-fold *(43,44)*. Likewise, in NIH 3T3 cells, PMA was 29-fold more potent for inducing translocation of the chimera formed from the PKC α regulatory domain and the PKC ε catalytic domain than it was for inducing translocation of PKC α itself *(45)*. Structure–activity relations are also influenced markedly by the cellular context in which PKC is found. Thus, PMA was highly selective for PKC δ compared with PKC α in mouse keratinocytes, whereas it was much less selective in NIH 3T3 cells; bryostatin 1 showed appreciably less difference in selectivity between the two cell lines *(46,47)*. Similarly, the selectivity of 12-deoxyphorbol 13-acetate for PKC δ compared with PKC α in mouse keratinocytes differed dramatically from that determined with the purified isoforms assayed in vitro. In contrast to fivefold selectivity for PKC α in the in vitro binding assay, 12-deoxyphorbol 13-phenylacetate was 70-fold selective for translocation of PKC δ in the mouse keratinocytes—an overall difference of 350-fold *(43,48)*. These findings have three important implications for drug discovery efforts targeted at the C1 domains. First, modeling of the C1 domain by itself will not be sufficient to predict the influence of these context-dependent factors. Second, assay of cloned isoforms in vitro is insufficient for establishing isotype selectivity in the intact cell. Third, the large contribution of varying cellular context to selectivity complements the intrinsic differences between PKC isoforms to generate abundant opportunities for drug design.

5.2. Role of Phosphorylation in Regulating PKC

The activity of PKC, as well as its conformation, is dependent on its state of phosphorylation *(4,49)*. As characterized for PKC β, there are three sites of serine/ threonine phosphorylation: Thr-500, Thr-641, and Ser-660. The latter two sites are sites of autophosphorylation; Thr-500 is phosphorylated by a distinct kinase. Phosphorylation at Thr-500 is required for conversion of PKC to a state capable of activation. As such, the kinase which carries out this phosphorylation represents an interesting potential target for inhibition of PKC. The two autophosphorylation sites stabilize the activatable conformation, with the site at Ser-660 also enhancing the affinity of the enzyme for Ca^{2+}.

Emerging evidence also suggests a role for tyrosine phosphorylation in PKC regulation *(50–53)*. Two types of behavior have been observed. First, PKC δ, but not other PKCs, is phosphorylated at multiple sites on tyrosine in response to receptor activation or phorbol ester treatment *(50–53)*. The specific sites of phosphorylation depend on the stimulus. For stimulation through the FcεRI receptor in RBL-2H3 cells, PKC δ is phosphorylated on Tyr52 *(51)*. In the same cells, stimulation with phorbol 12-myristate 13-acetate (PMA) causes tyrosine phosphorylation at additional sites. Using chimeras, the sites of tyrosine phosphorylation are localized to the regulatory domain of PKC δ expressed in either NIH 3T3 cells *(54)* or in C6 glioma cells *(54a)*. The functional effect of tyrosine phosphorylation appears to be to change the substrate selectivity of the enzyme, either stimulating or inhibiting the enzyme depending on the substrate examined *(55)*. In both the NIH 3T3 and C6 cell systems, mutation of the sites of tyrosine phosphorylation leads to a dominant negative phenotype.

Oxidative stress induces a different pattern of tyrosine phosphorylation *(56)*. In this case, phosphorylation is in the catalytic domain and is associated with enzymatic activation. Inhibition of protein tyrosine kinase activity thus appears to be a potential strategy for interfering with aspects of the PKC signaling pathway.

5.3. Regulation of PKC Through Protein–Protein Interactions

One of the emerging themes of protein regulation is the control of substrate selectivity through protein protein interactions. Mochly-Rosen has characterized in detail the existence of receptors for activated C kinase (RACKs) that bind to PKC, drive its localization, and maintain PKC in an active conformation *(30,57)*. A factor contributing to the energetics of maintaining PKC in a closed conformation is the intramolecular interaction between sequences in PKC corresponding to a RACK binding site and a complementary peptide. Peptides corresponding to the RACK binding sites on PKC, when introduced into the intact cell, prevent its proper localization and can thereby function as inhibitors *(57)*. Conversely, specific PKC isoforms can be activated through the use of peptides which interact with the RACK binding site on PKC and displace the complementary sequence in the PKC itself. Because these sequences are not conserved between isoforms, this approach represents an exciting strategy for isoform selective activation or inhibition. Outside of experimental situations, however, the problematic pharmacology of peptides suggests the need for peptidomimetic analogs.

Isoform specific interactions of PKC have also been identified with actin *(58–60)* and with scaffolding proteins, such as caveolin *(61)* and AKAP79 *(62,63)*.

5.3. Downregulation of PKC

For PKC, downregulation associated with chronic activation represents a major mechanism of control. The susceptibility to downregulation, like many other properties, depends on the cellular context. Thus, PKC ε is down regulated by either PMA or bryostatin 1 in NIH 3T3 cells *(46)*.In mouse keratinocytes it is fully downregulated by 12-deoxyphorbol 13-phenylacetate but only partially by PMA and bryostatin 1 *(47,48)*. Downregulation of PKC has been used as one approach for implication of PKC in various biochemical pathways. Likewise, downregulation represents one strategy for inhibition of PKC activity.

Breakdown of PKC has been described to proceed through at least three mechanisms: calpain, caspase, and the proteosome pathway *(64–66)*. Susceptibility depends both on the isoform and on the state of phosphorylation, presumably coupled to the state of folding. At least through the calpain pathway, the initial intermediates in the breakdown are the regulatory and the catalytic domains. On the one hand, the liberation of the catalytic domain generates a constitutively active enzyme *(64)*. On the other hand, the localization of the enzyme is shifted to the cytosol from the membrane, leading to a difference in substrate accessibility. It is also more labile, although appreciable accumulation is observed in some systems. Experimentally, the catalytic domain has been shown to retain some but not other biological activities *(67,68)*. Although accumulation of the regulatory domain has received less attention, current evidence suggests that this should have dominant-negative activity *(27,69)*.

In addition to cleavage between the catalytic and regulatory domains of PKC, other patterns of susceptibility to proteolysis have been observed, and these depend on the specific patterns of phosphorylation *(70)*.

6. FUNCTIONAL SPECIFICITY OF PKC ISOZYMES

Because of the ubiquitous presence of PKC in cells, a severe initial concern with PKC as a therapeutic target was that of specificity. Factors that have proved to largely mitigate this concern are the existence of the multiple PKC isoforms, different functional roles for different PKC isoforms, and the role of cellular context in generating yet further diversity in the PKC pathway. Numerous studies demonstrate functional specificity. For example, we have shown that, in RBL-2H3 cells stimulated with antigen, PKC β and δ preferentially support secretion *(71)*, PKC α and ε inhibit phospholipase C *(72)*, PKC β and ε stimulate fos/jun expression *(73)*, and PKC δ phosphorylates the γ chain of the FcεRI receptor *(74)*. In 32D mouse promyelocytic cells, PKC α and δ stimulate myeloid differentiation *(75)*. In NIH 3T3 cells, cell growth is stimulated by PKC ε; conversely, NIH 3T3 cell growth is inhibited by PKC α and δ *(54,76)*. Such cellular approaches are complemented by emerging studies with knockout mice. For example, PKC γ knockout mice fail to show hypersensitivity to pain in response to inflammatory injury, suggesting this isoform as a selective therapeutic target in the treatment of allodynia *(77)*. PKC β knockout mice show defects in B-cell functioning *(78)*.

For strategies of therapeutic intervention, a crucial concept emerging from the analysis of the specific functions of individual PKC isoforms is that isoforms may be functionally antagonistic. In NIH 3T3 cells, for example, PKC ε stimulates cell growth, whereas PKC δ and α inhibit it. In the RBL-2H3 cells, PKC γ antagonized the effect of the other isoforms *(79)*. Physiological control through the balance of antagonistic receptor pathways, physiological tone, is a classical concept in pharmacology. It appears to apply to aspects of control by PKC. An alternative to intervention using inhibitors targeted to a specific isoform, thus, is through agonists selective for a functionally antagonistic isoform.

7. INHIBITORS AND ACTIVATORS AS PROBES OF PKC INVOLVEMENT IN BIOLOGICAL RESPONSES

7.1. Activators of PKC Function

The easiest approach for implicating PKC in a biological response is by treatment with a potent phorbol ester. The typical ligand employed is PMA, phorbol 12-myristate 13-acetate, also referred to as 12-O-tetradecanoylphorbol 13-acetate (TPA). Standard negative controls are 4-α-PMA or phorbol. Phorbol 12, 13-dibutyrate (PDBu) is the ligand normally used for quantitating phorbol ester binding to PKC, since it has reduced nonspecific binding compared with PMA *(80)*. For greater comparability with binding analysis, PDBu may also be used as a PKC activator. PKC activators do not distinguish PKC from the more recently identified classes of phorbol ester/DAG responsive targets *(44,81,82)*. In addition, phorbol esters may be subject to degradation by esterases, distorting response particularly under conditions of chronic treatment. Finally, because of its substantially greater potency than DAG, the phorbol esters may be able to drive responses through PKC that DAG is unable to achieve.

Although DAG is the endogenous ligand for PKC, its rapid metabolism and lipophilicity, which prevent it from transferring from medium into cells, make it problematic. One approach has been to treat cells with bacterial phospholipase C to generate DAG *in situ*, avoiding the problem of transfer. Alternatively, more hydrophilic DAG analogs can be used for exogenous addition. *sn*-1,2-Dioctanoylglycerol is most widely used; *sn*-1-oleoyl-2-acetylglycerol is also suitable. Because of the lower potency and rapid metabolism, a concern with interpretation is that effects may reflect membrane perturbation by the relatively hydrophilic DAG and its metabolites.

7.2. PKC Activators That Paradoxically Function as PKC Inhibitors in Intact Cells

Two classes of natural products have been identified that, although they act as complete agonists for PKC in vitro, function as partial antagonists of phorbol ester-mediated responses in cellular systems. Bryostatin 1, currently in phase 2 clinical trials for myeloma, lymphoma, melanoma, renal cell carcinoma, and glioma, is a macrocyclic lactone isolated from the marine organism *Bugulaneritina (83)*. In intact cells, bryostatin 1 induces only some of the responses induced by the phorbol esters *(84)*. For all those responses that can be induced by the phorbol esters, but not by the bryostatins, bryostatin 1 blocks the response to the phorbol ester upon coapplication. Although bryostatin 1 in general appears to cause PKC translocation and downregulation consistent with its being an ultrapotent ligand for PKC, it shows a unique pattern of downregulation of PKC δ *(46,47)*. Whereas low doses of bryostatin 1 lead to PKC δ downregulation, higher doses fail to down regulate PKC δ and, consistent with the biology, protect PKC δ from downregulation by phorbol ester. Inhibition of a number of phorbol ester responses occurs at similar potencies to those for protection from downregulation. By the use of chimeras between the regulatory and catalytic domains of PKCs α and δ, the catalytic domain of PKC δ was shown to be essential for protection from downregulation, but the potency of byrostatin 1 for protection (as well as for downregulation) depended on the regulatory domain *(85)*. These results demonstrate that (1) the protection is a direct effect of interaction of bryostatin 1 with PKC δ, and (2) that PKC δ can bind bryostatin 1 with two distinct affinities.

Two mechanisms can thus be visualized for the antagonism by bryostatin 1. On the one hand, translocation of PKC δ to a distinct membrane compartment might block that subset of responses requiring activated PKC δ at the plasma membrane. Alternatively, by protecting PKC δ from down regulation while concomitantly causing downregulation of PKC isoforms (e.g., PKC ε), with opposite effects it could shift the balance toward a PKC δ driven pattern of response. Different mechanisms may apply for different endpoints. In the case of inhibition of glutamine synthetase expression in C6 glioma cells, protection of PKC δ accounts for the observed effects *(54a)*. For the inhibition of arachidonic acid release in C3H10T1/2 cells by bryostatin 1 *(86)*, the former mechanism seems more probable.

Prostratin (12-deoxyphorbol 13-acetate) and 12-deoxyphorbol 13-phenylacetate also activate PKC but block some responses in intact cells. The range of antagonism is more limited than in the case of bryostatin 1 but is nonetheless of great interest. In mouse skin, pretreatment with these compounds dramatically suppresses acute and chronic hyperplasia induced by a typical phorbol ester (PMA) and substantially (approx 70%) inhibits PMA-induced acute inflammation *(36,87)*. Consistent with its effects on hyperplasia, 12-deoxyphorbol 13-phenylacetate blocks tumor promotion by PMA by up to 97% *(37)*. A very important conclusion is that PKC activation is not inherently linked to tumor promotion.

A possible mechanism for 12-deoxyphorbol 13-phenylacetate is through selective downregulation. In mouse keratinocytes, 12-deoxyphorbol 13-phenylacetate but neither bryostatin 1 nor PMA causes complete downregulation of PKC ε *(47,48)*. Like bryostatin 1, 12-deoxyphorbol 13-phenylacetate thus shifts the balance between PKC δ and ε, although it uses the opposite strategy: depletion of PKC ε rather than protection of PKC δ. In a number of other systems (e.g., NIH 3T3 or RBL-2H3 cells), 12-deoxyphorbol does not show such antagonistic activity. Likewise, in these systems, it does not show differential downregulation.

Bryostatin 1 and the 12-deoxyphorbol 13-monoesters validate the strategy that ligands targeted to the regulatory domain of PKC can function as antagonists. Although the mechanisms may be more complicated than in the case of inhibitors targeted to the catalytic site, the inherent greater specificity makes this an interesting alternative approach.

7.3. Nonspecific Inhibitors Targeted to the Regulatory Domain

Sphingosine and calphostin C were initially suggested to be specific PKC inhibitors *(88–91)*. It is now recognized that they are more generally active. Sphingosine is positively charged, whereas PKC requires an anionic membrane surface under usual activation conditions *(92,93)*. Many other membrane proteins, likewise, are sensitive to the surface charge. In addition, sphingosine metabolites are involved as signaling molecules in their own right. Calphostin C requires photoactivation, a source of confusion in early studies. Upon photoactivation, calphostin C causes free radical reactions with lipids and inhibits multiple lipid-associated membrane proteins *(94–96)*. The initial conclusion that calphostin C was a specific inhibitor of PKC arose from comparisons in which only soluble kinases were compared with PKC. Like calphostin C, chelerythrine leads to free radical generation and inhibits many proteins *(97,98)*.

7.4. Catalytic Site-Directed Inhibitors of PKC

A number of extensive reviews of catalytic site directed inhibitors of PKC have been published *(99–101)*. The initially described inhibitors showed only modest specificity. H7 is selective relative to myosin light chain kinase; however, its affinity for the cyclic adenosine monophosphate (cAMP)-dependent protein kinase, for example, is similar to that for PKC *(102)*. Staurosporine attracted attention as a highly potent PKC inhibitor with nM affinity *(103)*. By contrast, it has very low specificity, even inhibiting tyrosine kinases with similar affinity to PKC. Its main impact has been as a lead structure for the development of potent, more selective inhibitors. Those currently used as research tools include GF109203X (or bisindolylmaleimide I) *(104)*, Gö9678, Ro31-8330, and Ro31-8425. These all appear to have improved specificity, although it must be emphasized that the specificity is not absolute *(105)*. Because of the imperfect selectivity, such inhibitors provide corroborative evidence for the involvement of PKC in a response but are insufficient by themselves.

Along with enhanced selectivity for PKC relative to other kinases, inhibitors have been developed which demonstrate PKC isoform selectivity. Of particular interest is LY333531, which displays 50-fold selectivity for PKC β relative to the other isoforms examined *(106)*. PKC β has been implicated in vascular proliferation in diabetes, and LY333531 is currently being clinically evaluated for that indication *(107)*. Balanol derivatives selective for PKC β, δ, ε, and η have also been described *(108,109)*. At least in vitro, Gö9678 is selective for the classical PKCs relative to the novel isoforms *(110)*. The initial success in obtaining isotype selective inhibitors, together with the development of knockout mice to define the physiological roles of individual isoforms at the whole animal level, should provide strong impetus for further developments in this area.

7.5. Other Strategies for Obtaining Isoform Selective Inhibitors

As research tools, antisense constructs provide a powerful approach for implicating specific PKC isoforms in pathways of biological response, complementing the use of constructs for overexpression *(111)*. A significant obstacle remains the necessity to optimize conditions carefully for uptake. The species specificity of antisense constructs has both advantages and disadvantages. For example, in mice bearing human xenotransplanted tumors, antisense to human PKC α can be shown to inhibit tumor growth without interfering toxicity because of inhibition of the PKC α of the murine host *(112)*. By contrast, that same specificity makes the system unsuitable for evaluating potential toxicity in a clinical setting in which PKC α would be affected not only in the tumor but also in the normal tissues of the patient. As for other applications of antisense in therapy, the pharmacological problems of delivery and uptake will be of major importance.

Peptides interfering with RACK interactions have been used to specifically inhibit the activity of PKC β and ε *(57)*. The reciprocal peptides leading to PKC activation have been described for PKC β. Peptides based on the pseudosubstrate regions of the PKC isoforms inhibit PKC activity with modest selectivity relative to other kinases *(28,113)*. On the other hand, the substrate requirements of the different isoforms show marked overlap *(43,114)*.

8. FUTURE PROSPECTS

The central role of PKC in cellular signaling makes it an attractive target for drug development. The multiplicity of functionally distinct isoforms of PKC and the depth of modification of their properties in a cell context-specific fashion provide abundant opportunities for generating therapeutic specificity. The emerging elucidation of the complexities of regulation of PKC folding and localization affords novel strategies for intervention, complementing the promising efforts directed at the design of selective catalytic site inhibitors. Although PKC initially attracted the attention of cancer researchers through its identification as the receptor for the phorbol ester tumor promoters, its general role in signal transduction affords a much broader field of opportunity. The evaluation of LY333531 for treatment of the vascular complications of diabetes exemplifies this more mature understanding.

REFERENCES

1. Blumberg PM. In vitro studies on the mode of action of the phorbol esters, potent tumor promoters. *Crit Rev Toxicol* 1980; 8:153–234.
2. Hurley JH, Newton AC, Parker PJ, Blumberg PM, Nishizuka Y. Taxonomy and function of C1 protein kinase C homology domains. *Protein Sci* 1997; 6:477–480.
3. Nishizuka Y. Intracellular signaling by hydrolysis of phospholipids and activation of protein kinase C. *Science* 1992; 258:607–614.
4. Newton AC. Protein kinase C: Structure, function, and regulation. *J Biol Chem* 1995; 270:28495–28498.
5. Asaoka Y, Nakamura S, Yoshida K, Nishizuka, Y. Protein kinase C, calcium and phospholipid degradation. *Trends Biochem Sci* 1992; 17:414–417.
6. Nishizuka Y. Protein kinase C and lipid signaling for sustained cellular responses. *FASEB J*, 1995; 9:484–496.
7. Newton AC. Cofactor regulation of protein kinase C, in *Protein Kinase C* (Dekker LV, Parker PJ, eds), RG Landes, Austin, TX, 1997, 25–44.
8. Rhee SG, Bae YS. Regulation of phosphoinositide-specific phospholipase C isozymes. *J Biol Chem* 1997; 272:15,045–15,048.
9. Exton JH. Phospholipase D: Enzymology, mechanisms of regulation, and function. *Physiol Rev* 1997; 77:303–320.
10. Sossin WS, Schwartz JH. Ca^{2+}-independent protein kinase Cs contain an amino-terminal domain similar to the C2 consensus sequence. *Trends Biochem Sci* 1993; 18:207,208.
11. Nishizuka Y. Protein kinase C and lipid signalling for sustained cellular responses. *Curr Opin Struct Biol* 1995; 5:396–402.
12. Kazanietz MG, Bustelo XR, Barbacid M, Kolch W, Mischak H, Wong G, Bruns JD, Blumberg PM. Zinc finger domains and the phorbol ester pharmacophore: Analysis of binding to a mutated form of PKC ζ, and the vav and c-raf protooncogene products. *J Biol Chem* 1994; 269:11,590–11,594.
13. Dekker LV, Palmer RH, Parker PJ. The protein kinase C and protein kinase C related gene families. *Curr Opin Struct Biol* 1995; 5:396–402.
14. Lim L. N-chimaerin and neuronal signal transduction mechanisms. *Biochem Soc Trans* 1992; 20:611–614.
15. Hall C, Monfries C, Smith P, Lim HH, Kozma R, Ahmed S, Vanniasingham V, Leung T, Lim L. Novel human-brain cDNA-encoding a 34,000 Mr protein n-chimaerin, related to both the regulatory domain of protein kinase C and BCR, the product of the breakpoint cluster region gene. *J Mol Biol* 1990; 211:11–16.
16. Hall C, Sin WC, Teo M, Michael GJ, Smith P, Dong JM, Lim HH, Manser E, Spurr NK, Jones TA, Lim L. α2-chimaerin, a SH2-containing GTPase-activating protein for the Ras-related protein p21RAC derived by alternate splicing of the human n-chimaerin gene, is selectively expressed in brain-regions and testes. *Mol Cell Biol* 1993; 13:4986–4998.
17. Leung T, How BE, Manser E, Lim L. Germ cell β-chimaerin, a new GTPase-activating protein for p21*rac,* is specifically expressed during the acrosomal assembly stage in rat testis. *J Biol Chem* 1993; 268:3813–3816.
18. Leung T, How BE, Manser E, Lim L. Cerebellar β-chimaerin, a GTPase-activating protein for the p21RAS-related Rac, is specifically expressed in granule cells and has a unique N-terminal SH2 domain. *J Biol Chem* 1994; 269:12,888–12,892.
19. Ahmed S, Maruyana IN, Kozma R, Lee J, Brenner S, Lim L. The Caenorhabditis elegans Unc-13 gene-product is a phospholipid-dependent high affinity phorbol ester receptor. *Biochem J* 1992; 287:995–999.
20. Betz A, Telemanakis I, Hofmann K, Broze N. Mammalian Unc-13 homologues as possible regulators of neurotransmitter release. *Biochem Soc Trans* 1996; 24:661–666.

21. Ebinu JO, Bottorff DA, Chan EYW, Stang SL, Dunn RJ, Stone JC. RasGRP, a Ras Guanyl nucleotide-releasing protein with calcium- and diacylglycerol-binding motifs. *Science* 1998; 280:1082–1086.

21a. Tognon CE, Kirk HE, Passmore LA, Whitehead IP, Der CJ, Kay RJ. Regulation of RasGRP via a phorbol ester-responsive C1 domain. *Mol Cell Biol* 1998; 18:6995–7008.

22. Yuan S, Miller DW, Barnett GH, Hahn JF, Williams BR. Identification and characterization of human beta 2-chimaerin: Association with malignant transformation in astrocytoma. *Cancer Res* 1995; 55:3456–3461.

23. Franke TF, Yang SI, Chan TO, Datta K, Kazlauskas A, Morrison DK, Kaplan DR, Tsichlis PN. The protein kinase encoded by the Akt proto-oncogene is a target of the PDGF-activated phosphatidylinositol 3-kinase. *Cell* 1995; 81:727–736.

24. Burgering BMT, Coffer PJ. Protein kinase B (c-Akt) in phosphatidylinositol-3-OH kinase signal transduction. *Nature* 1995; 376:599–602.

25. Singer WD, Brown HA, Jiang X, and Sternweis PC. Regulation of phospholipase D by protein kinase C is synergistic with ADP-ribosylation factor and independent of protein kinase activity. *J Biol Chem* 1996; 271:4504–4510.

26. Li W, Yu JC, Shin DY, Pierce JH. Characterization of a protein kinase C-δ (PKC-δ) ATP binding mutant. An inactive enzyme that competitively inhibits wild type PKC-δ enzymatic activity. *J Biol Chem* 1995; 270:8311–8318.

27. Liao L, Hyatt SL, Chapline C, Jaken S. Protein kinase C domains involved in interactions with other proteins. *Biochemistry* 1994; 33:1229–1233.

28. House C, Kemp BE. Protein kinase C contains a pseudosubstrate prototope in its regulatory domain. *Science* 1987; 238:1729–1728.

29. Quest AFG. Regulation of protein kinase C: A tale of lipids and proteins. *Enzyme Protein* 1996; 49:231–261.

30. Mochly-Rosen D, Khaner H, Lopez J. Identification of intracellular receptor proteins for activated protein kinase C. *Proc Natl Acad Sci USA* 1991; 88:3987–4000.

31. Zhang G, Kazanietz MG, Blumberg PM, Hurley JH. Crystal structure of the cys2 activator-binding domain of protein kinase Cδ in complex with phorbol ester. *Cell* 1995; 81:917–924.

32. Wang S, Kazanietz MG, Blumberg PM, Marquez VE, Milne WA. Molecular modeling and site-directed mutagenesis studies of a phorbol ester-binding site in protein kinase C. *J Med Chem* 1996; 39:2541–2553.

33. Zayed S, Sorg B, Hecker E. Structure activity relations of polyfunctional diterpenes of the tigliane type, VI. Irritant and tumor promoting activities of semi-synthetic mono and diesters of 12-deoxyphorbol. *Planta Med* 1984; 1:65–69.

34. Slaga T, Fisher SM, Nelson K, Gleason GL. Studies on the mechanism of skin tumor promotion: Evidence for several stages in promotion. *Proc Natl Acad Sci USA* 1980; 77:3659–3663.

35. Argyris TS. Nature of the epidermal hyperplasia produced by mezerein, a weak tumor promoter, in initiated skin of mice. *Cancer Res* 1983; 43:1768–1773.

36. Szallasi Z, Blumberg PM. Prostratin, a non-promoting phorbol ester, inhibits induction of phorbol 12-myristate 13-acetate of ornithine decarboxylase, edema, and hyperplasia in CD-1 mouse skin. *Cancer Res* 1991; 51:5355–5360.

37. Szallasi Z, Krsmanovich L, Blumberg PM. Non-promoting 12-deoxyphorbol 13-esters inhibit phorbol 12-myristate 13-acetate induced tumor promotion in CD-1 mouse skin. *Cancer Res* 1993; 53:2507–2512.

38. Szallasi Z, Bogi K, Gohari S, Biro T, Acs P, Blumberg PM. Non-equivalent roles for the first and second zinc fingers of protein kinase Cδ. Effect of their mutation on phorbol ester-induced translocation in NIH 3T3 cells. *J Biol Chem* 1996; 271:18,299–18,301.

39. Bogi K, Lorenzo PS, Szallasi Z, Acs P, Wagner GS, Blumberg PM. Differential selectivity of ligands for the C1a and C1b phorbol ester binding domains of protein kinase Cδ: Possible correlation with tumor-promoting activity. *Cancer Res* 1998; 58:1423–1428.

39a. Bogi K, Lorenzo PS, Acs P, Szallasi Z, Wagner GS, Blumberg PM. Comparison of the roles of the C1a and C1b domains of protein kinase C alpha in ligand induced translocation in NIH3T3 cells. *FEBS Lett* 1999; 456:27–30.

40. Shieh HL, Hansen H, Zhu J, Riedel H. Differential protein kinase C ligand regulation detected in vivo by a phenotypic yeast assay. *Mol Carcinog* 1995; 12:166–176.

41. Slater SJ, Ho C, Kelly, MB, Larkin JD, Taddeo FJ, Yeager MD, Stubbs CD. Protein kinase C α contains two activator binding sites that bind phorbol esters and diacylglycerol with opposite affinities. *J Biol Chem* 1996; 271:4627–4631.

42. Hunn M, Quest AF. Cysteine-rich regions of protein kinase Cδ are functionally non-equivalent. Differences between cysteine-rich regions of non-calcium dependent protein kinase Cδ and calcium-dependent protein kinase Cγ. *FEBS Lett* 1997; 400:226–232.

43. Kazanietz MG, Areces LB, Bahador A, Mischak H, Goodnight J, Mushinski JF, Blumberg PM. Characterization of ligand and substrate specificity for the calcium-dependent and calcium-independent PKC isozymes. *Mol Pharmacol* 1993; 44:298–307.

44. Kazanietz MG, Lewin NE, Bruns JD, Blumberg PM. Characterization of the cysteine-rich region of the *Caenorhabditis elegans* protein Unc-13 as a high affinity phorbol ester receptor: analysis of ligand-binding interactions, lipid cofactor requirements, and inhibitor-sensitivity. *J Biol Chem* 1995; 270:10,777–10,783.

45. Acs P, Bogi K, Lorenzo PS, Marquez VE, Biro T, Szallasi Z, Blumberg PM. The catalytic domain of protein kinase C chimeras modulates the affinity and targeting of phorbol ester-induced translocation. *J Biol Chem* 1997; 272:22,148–22,153.

46. Szallasi Z, Smith CB, Pettit, GR, Blumberg PM. Differential regulation of protein kinase C isozymes by bryostatin 1 and phorbol 12-myristate 13-acetate in NIH 3T3 fibroblasts. *J Biol Chem* 1994; 269:2118–2124.

47. Szallasi Z, Denning MF, Smith, CB, Dlugosz AA, Yuspa SH, Pettit GR, Blumberg PM. Bryostatin 1 protects PKC δ from down-regulation in mouse keratinocytes in parallel with its inhibition of phorbol ester induced differentiation. *Mol Pharmacol* 1994; 46:840–850.

48. Szallasi Z, Kosa K, Smith CB, Dlugosz AA, Williams EK, Yuspa SH, Blumberg PM. Differential regulation by the anti-promoting 12-deoxyphorbol 13-phenylacetate reveals distinct roles of the classical and novel protein kinase C isozymes in biological responses of primary mouse keratinocytes. *Mol Pharmacol* 1995; 47:258–265.

49. Tsutakawa SE, Medzihradszky KF, Flint AJ, Burlingame AL, Koshland DE. Determination of in vitro phosphorylation sites in protein kinase C. *J Biol Chem* 1995; 45: 26,807–26,812.

50. Li W, Yu, J, Michieli P, Beeler JF, Ellmore N, Heidaran MA, Pierce JH. Stimulation of the platelet-derived growth factor beta receptor signaling pathway activates protein kinase C-δ. *Mol Cell Biol* 1994; 14:6727–6735.

51. Szallasi Z, Denning MF, Chang E-Y, Rivera J, Yuspa SH, Lehel C, Olah Z, Anderson WB, Blumberg PM. Development of a rapid approach to identification of tyrosine phosphorylation sites: application to PKCδ phosphorylated upon activation of the high affinity receptor for IgE in rat basophilic leukemia cells. *Biochem Biophys Res Commun* 1995; 214:888–894.

52. Denning MF, Dlugosz AA, Threadgill DW, Magnuson T, Yuspa SH. Activation of the epidermal growth factor receptor signal transduction pathway stimulates tyrosine phosphorylation of protein kinase C-δ. *J Biol Chem* 1996; 271:5325–5331.

53. Li W, Chen X-H, Kelley CA, Alimandi M, Zhang J, Chen Q, Bottaro DP, Pierce JH. Identification of tyrosine 187 as a protein kinase C-δ phosphorylation site. *J Biol Chem* 1996; 271:26,404–26,409.

54. Acs P, Wang QJ, Bogi K, Marquez VE, Lorenzo PS, Biro T, Szallasi Z, Mushinski JF, Blumberg PM. Both the catalytic and the regulatory domains of protein kinase C chimeras modulate the proliferation properties of NIH 3T3 cells. *J Biol Chem* 1997; 272:28,793–28,799.

54a. Brodie C, Bogi K, Acs P, Lorenzo PS, Baskin L, Blumberg PM. Protein kinase Cδ (PKCδ) inhibits the expression of glutamine synthetase in glial cells via the PKCδ regulatory domain and its tyrosine phosphorylation. *J Biol Chem* 1998; 273:30,713–30,718.

55. Haleem-Smith H, Chang E-Y, Szallasi Z, Blumberg PM, Rivera J. Tyrosine phosphorylation of protein kinase C-δ in response to the activation of the high affinity receptor for immunoglobulin E modifies its substrate recognition. *Proc Natl Acad Sci USA* 1995; 92:9112–9116.

56. Konishi H, Tanaka M, Takemura Y, Matsuzaki H, Ono Y, Kikkawa U, Nishizuka Y. Activation of protein kinase C by tyrosine phosphorylation in response to H_2O_2. *Proc Natl Acad Sci USA* 1997; 94:11,233–11,237.

57. Mochly-Rosen D, Gordon AS. Anchoring proteins for protein kinase C: A means for isozyme selectivity. *FASEB J* 1998; 12:35–42.

58. Keenan C, and Kelleher D. Protein kinase C and the cytoskeleton. *Cell Signal* 1993; 10:225–232.

59. Gomez J, Martinez de Aragon A, Bonay P, Pitton C, Garcia A, Silvia A, Fresno M, Alvarez F, Rebollo A. Physical association and functional relationship between protein kinase C ζ and the actin cytoskeleton. *Eur J Immunol* 1995; 25:2673–2678.

60. Hu YL, Chien S. Effects of shear stress on protein kinase C distribution in endothelial cells. *J Histochem Cytochem* 1997; 45:237–249.

61. Oka, N, Yamamoto, M, Schwencke, C, Kwabe, J, Ebina, T, Ohno, S, Couet, S, Lisanti, M.P., Ishikawa, Y. Caveolin interaction with protein kinase C: Isoenzyme-dependent regulation of kinase activity by the caveolin scaffolding domain peptide. *J Biol Chem* 1997; 272:33,416–33,421.

62. Faux MC, Scott JD. Molecular glue: Kinase anchoring and scaffold proteins. *Cell* 1996; 85:9–12.

63. Klauck TM, Faux MC, Labudda K, Langeberg LK, Jaken S, Scott JD. Coordination of three signaling enzymes by AKAP79, a mammalian scaffold protein. *Science* 1996; 271:1589–1592.

64. Susuki K, Saido TC, Hirai S. Modulation of cellular signals by calpain. *Ann NY Acad Sci* 1992; 31:218–227.

65. Ghayur T, Hugunin M, Talanian RV, Ratnofky S, Quinlan C, Emoto Y, Pandey P, Datta R, Huang Y, Kharbanda S, Allen H, Kamen R, Wong W, Kufe D. Proteolytic activation of protein kinase C δ by an ICE/CED 2-like protease induces characteristics of apoptosis. *J Exp Med* 1996; 184:2399–2404.

66. Lee H-W, Smith L, Pettit GR, Vinitsky A, Smith JB. Ubiquitination of protein kinase C-α and degradation by the proteasome. *J Biol Chem* 1996; 271:20,973–20,976.

67. Nakakuma H, Willingham MC, Blumberg PM. Effect of microinjected catalytic fragment of protein kinase C on morphological change in Swiss 3T3 cells. *Cancer Comm* 1989; 1:127–132.

68. Muramatsu M, Kaibuchi K, Irai K. A protein kinase C cDNA without the regulatory domain is active after transfection in vivo in the absence of phorbol ester. *Mol Cell Biol* 1989; 9:831–836.

69. Parissenti AM, Kirwan AF, Colantonio CM, Schimmer BP. Molecular strategies for the dominant negative inhibition of protein kinase C. *Endocr Res* 1996; 22:621–630.

70. Edwards AS, Newton AC. Phosphorylation at conserved carboxyl-terminal hydrophobic motif regulates the catalytic and regulatory domains of protein kinase C. *J Biol Chem* 1997; 272:18,382–18,390.

71. Ozawa K, Szallasi Z, Kazanietz MG, Blumberg PM, Mischak H, Mushinski JF, Beaven MA. Ca^{++}-dependent and Ca^{++}-independent isozymes of protein kinase C mediate exocytosis in antigen-stimulated rat basophilic RBL-2H3 cells: Reconstitution of secretory responses with Ca^{++} and purified isozymes in washed permeabilized cells. *J Biol Chem* 1993; 268:1749–1756.

72. Ozawa K, Yamada K, Kazanietz MG, Blumberg PM, Beaven MA. Different isozymes of

protein kinase C mediate feedback inhibition of phospholipase C and stimulatory signals for exocytosis in rat RBL-2H3 cells. *J Biol Chem* 1993; 268:2280–2283.

73. Razin E, Szallasi Z, Kazanietz MG, Blumberg PM, Rivera J. Protein kinase C-β and ε link the mast cell high affinity receptor for IgE to the expression of c-fos and c-jun. *Proc Natl Acad Sci USA* 1994; 91:7722–7726.

74. Germano P, Gomez J, Kazanietz MG, Blumberg PM, and Rivera J. Phosphorylation of the γ chain of the high affinity receptor for immunoglobulin E by receptor-associated protein kinase C-δ. *J Biol Chem* 1994; 269:23,102–23,107.

75. Mischak H, Pierce JH, Goodnight J, Kazanietz MG, Blumberg PM, and Mushinski JF. Phorbol ester-induced myeloid differentiation is mediated by protein kinase C-α and -δ and not by protein kinase C-βII, -ε, -ζ, and -η. *J Biol Chem* 1993; 268:20,110–20,115.

76. Mischak H, Goodnight J, Kolch W, Martiny-Baron G, Schaechtele C, Kazanietz MG, Blumberg PM, Pierce JH, Mushinski JF. Overexpression of protein kinase C-δ and -ε in NIH 3T3 cells induces opposite effects on growth, morphology, anchorage dependence, and tumorigenicity. *J Biol Chem* 1993; 268:6090–6096.

77. Malmberg AB, Chen C, Tonegawa S, Basbaum AI. Preserved acute pain and reduced neuropathic pain in mice lacking PKC-γ. *Science* 1997; 278:279–283.

78. Leitges M, Schmedt C, Guinamard R, Davoust J, Schaal S, Stabel S, and Tarakhovsky A. Immunodeficiency in protein kinase C-β-deficient mice. *Science* 1996; 273:788–791.

79. Baumgartner RA, Ozawa K, Cunha-Melo JR, Yamada K, Gusovsky F, Beaven MA. Studies with transfected and permeabilized RBL-2H3 cells reveal unique inhibitory properties of protein kinase C-γ. *Mol Biol Cell* 1994; 5:475–484.

80. Driedger PE, Blumberg PM. Specific binding of phorbol ester tumor promoters. *Proc Natl Acad Sci USA* 1980; 77:567–571.

81. Areces LB, Kazanietz MG, Blumberg PM. Close similarity of baculovirus expressed n-chimaerin and protein kinase C α as phorbol ester receptors. *J Biol Chem* 1994; 269:19,553–19,558.

82. Caloca MJ, Fernandez MN, Lewin NE, Ching D, Modali R, Blumberg PM, Kazanietz MG. β2-Chimaerin is a high affinity receptor for the phorbol ester tumor promoters. Analysis of phorbol ester binding and subcellular distribution after phorbol ester treatment. *J Biol Chem* 1997; 227:26,488–26,496.

83. Pettit GR, Herald CL, Doubek DL, Herald DL, Arnold E, Clardy J. Isolation and structure of bryostatin 1. *J Am Chem Soc* 1982; 104:6846–6848.

84. Blumberg PM, Pettit GR. The bryostatins, a family of protein kinase C activators with therapeutic potential, in *New Leads and Targets in Drug Research, Alfred Benzon Symposium 33* (Krogsgaard-Larsen P, Christensen SB, Kofod H, eds), Munksgaard International, Copenhagen, Denmark, 1992; pp 273–285.

85. Lorenzo PS, Bogi K, Acs P, Pettit GR, Blumberg PM. The catalytic domain of protein kinase Cδ confers protection from down-regulation induced by bryostatin 1. *J Biol Chem* 1997; 272:33,338–33,343.

86. Dell'Aquila ML, Herald CL, Kamano Y, Petit GR, Blumberg PM. Differential effects of bryostatins and phorbol esters in arachidonic acid metabolite release and epidermal growth factor binding in C3H10T1/2 cells. *Cancer Res* 1988; 48:3702–3708.

87. Szallasi Z, Krausz K, Blumberg PM. Non-promoting 12-deoxyphorbol 13-esters as potent inhibitors of phorbol 12-myristate 13-acetate induced acute and chronic biological responses in CD-1 mouse skin. *Carcinogenesis* 1992; 13:2161–2167.

88. Gordge PC, Ryves WJ. Inhibition of protein kinase C. *Cell Signal* 1994; 6:871–872.

89. Hannun YA, Merrill AH Jr, Bell RM. Use of sphingosine as an inhibitor of protein kinase C. *Methods Enzymol* 1991; 201:316–328.

90. Kobayashi E, Nakano H, Morimoto M, Tamaoki T. Calphostin C (UCN-1028C), a novel microbial compound, is a highly potent and specific inhibitor of protein kinase C. *Biochem Biophys Res Commun* 1989; 159:548–553.

91. Tamaoki T, Takahashi I, Kobayashi E, Nakano H, Akinaga S, Suzuki K. Calphostin (UCN1028) and calphostin related compounds, a new class of specific and potent inhibitor of protein kinase C. *Adv Second Messenger Phosphoprotein Res* 1990; 24:497–501.

92. Bottega R, Epand RM, Ball EH. Inhibition of protein kinase C by sphingosine correlates with the presence of positive charge. *Biochem Biophys Res Commun* 1989; 164:102–107.

93. Bazzi MD, Nelsestuen GL. Mechanism of protein kinase C inhibition by sphingosine. *Biochem Biophys Res Commun* 1987; 146:203–207.

94. Gamou S, Shimizu N. Light-dependent induction of early-response gene expression by calphostin-C. *Cell Struct Funct* 1994; 19:195–200.

95. Gopalakrishna R, Chen ZH, Gundimeda U. Irreversible oxidative inactivation of protein kinase C by photosensitive inhibitor calphostin C. *FEBS Lett* 1992; 314:149–154.

96. Rotenberg SA, Huang MH, Zhu J, Su L, Riedel H. Deletion analysis of protein kinase C inactivation by calphostin C. *Mol Carcinog* 1995; 12:42–49.

97. Herbert JM, Augereau JM, Gleye J, Maffrand JP. Chelerythrine is a potent and specific inhibitor of protein kinase C. *Biochem Biophys Res Commun* 1990; 172:993–999.

98. Drsata J, Ulrichova J, Walterova D. Sanguinarine and chelerythrine as inhibitors of aromatic amino acid decarboxylase. *J Enzyme Inhib* 1996; 10:231–237.

99. Hofmann J. The potential for isoenzyme-selective modulation of protein kinase C. *FASEB J* 1997; 11:649–669.

100. Bradshaw D, Hill CH, Nixon JS, Wilkinson SE. Therapeutic potential of protein kinase C inhibitors. *Agents Actions* 1993; 38:135–147.

101. Hu H. Recent discovery and development of selective protein kinase C inhibitors. *Drug Discov Today* 1996; 1:438–447.

102. Hidaka H, Inagaki M, Kawamoto S, Sasaki Y. Isoquinolinesulfonamides, novel and potent inhibitors of cyclic nucleotide dependent protein kinase and protein kinase C. *Biochemistry* 1984; 23:5036–5041.

103. Tamaoki T, Nomoto H, Takahashi I, Kato Y, Morimoto M, Tomita F. Staurosporine, a potent inhibitor of phospholipid/Ca^{++} dependent protein kinase. *Biochem Biophys Res Commun* 1986; 135:397–402.

104. Toullec D, Pianetti P, Coste H, Bellevergue P, Grand-Perret T, Ajakane M, Baudet V, Boissin P, Boursier E, Loriolle F. The bisindolylmaleimide GF 109203X is a potent and selective inhibitor of protein kinase C. *J Biol Chem* 1991; 266:15,771–15,781.

105. Alessi DR. The protein kinase C inhibitors Ro 318220 and GF 109203X are equally potent inhibitors of MAPKAP kinase-1β (RSK-2) and p70 S6 kinase. *FEBS Lett* 1997; 402:121–123.

106. Ishii H, Jirousek MR, Koya D, Takagi C, Xia P, Clermont A, Bursell SE, Kern TS, Ballas LM, Heath WF, Stramm LE, Feener EP, King GL. Amelioration of vascular dysfunctions in diabetic rats by an oral PKC-β inhibitor. *Science* 1996; 277:728–731.

107. Ishii H, Koya D, King GL. Protein kinase C activation and its role in the development of vascular complications in diabetes mellitus. *J Mol Med* 1998; 76:21–31.

108. Lai YS, Mendoza JS, Jagdmann GE Jr, Menaldino DS, Biggers CK, Heerding JM, Wilson JW, Hall SE, Jiang JB, Janzen WP, Ballas LM. Synthesis and protein kinase C inhibitory activities of balanol analogs with replacement of the perhydroazepine moiety. *J Med Chem* 1997; 40:226–235.

109. Defauw JM, Murphy MM, Jagdmann GE Jr, Hu H, Lampe JW, Hollinshead SP, Mitchell TJ, Crane HM, Heerding JM, Mendoza JS, Davis JE, Darges JW, Hubbard FR, Hall SE. Synthesis and protein kinase C inhibitory activities of acyclic balanol analogs that are highly selective for protein kinase C over protein kinase A. *J Med Chem* 1996; 39:5215–5227.

110. Martiny-Baron G, Kazanietz MG, Mischak H, Blumberg PM, Kochs G, Hug H, Marme D, Schaechtele C. Selective inhibition of protein kinase C isozymes by the indolocarbazole Gö6976. *J Biol Chem* 1993; 268:9194–9197.

111. McGraw K, McKay R, Miraglia L, Boggs RT, Pribble JP, Muller M, Geiger T, Fabbro

D, Dean NM. Antisense oligonucleotide inhibitors of isozymes of protein kinase C: In vitro and in vivo activity and clinical development as anti-cancer therapeutics. *Anticancer Drug Design* 1997; 12:315–326.

112. Dean N, McKay R, Miraglia L, Howard R, Cooper S, Giddings J, Nicklin P, Meister L, Ziel R, Geiger T, Muller M, Fabbro D. Inhibition of growth of human tumor cell lines in nude mice by an antisense oligonucleotide inhibitor of protein kinase C-α expression. *Cancer Res* 1996; 56:3499–3507.

113. Soderling TR. Protein kinases. Regulation by autoinhibitory domains. *J Biol Chem* 1990; 265:1823–1826.

114. Nishikawa K, Toker A, Johannes FJ, Songyang Z, Cantley LC. Determination of the specific substrate sequence motifs of protein kinase C isozymes. *J Biol Chem* 1997; 272:952–956.

Although the establishment of a physiological role for ROS in cell signaling is an important first step, there are still large gaps in our understanding of how ROS act. This is particularly true with respect to defining the role of ROS in the already extraordinarily complex area of proliferative signaling. For example, there is emerging, although sometimes conflicting, evidence for ROS in apoptotic pathways as well *(81)*. There is no doubt that identifying the salient participants in redox signaling pathways (i.e., sources and molecular targets of ROS) will go a long way toward resolving many of the conflicts that exist today. In addition to providing fresh insight into a host of biological questions, it is reasonable to hope that these studies might also provide new direction and therapeutic approach to a wide assortment of human disease in which ROS are implicated.

Note Added in Proof

A recent manuscript (Su YA, Arnold RS, Lassegue B, Shi J, Xu XX, Sorescu D, Chung AB, Griendling KK, Lambeth JD. Cell transformation by the superoxide-generating oxidase Mox1. *Nature* 1999; 401:79–82) describes the isolation of a new gene product, mox1, that is expressed in non-phagocytic cells but that shows extensive homology to the phagocytic protein gp91^{phox}. Expression of mox1 in NIH373 cells increases superoxide production and leads to cellular transformation.

REFERENCES

1. Finkel T. Oxygen radicals and signaling. *Curr Opin Cell Biol* 1998; 10:243–253.
2. Rosner JL, Storz G. Regulation of bacterial responses to oxidative stress. *Curr Top Cell Regul* 1997; 35:163–177.
3. Demple B. Study of redox-regulated transcription factors in prokaryotes. *Methods* 1997; 11:267–278.
4. Storz G, Tartaglia LA, Ames BN. Transcriptional regulator of oxidative stress-inducible genes: Direct activation by oxidation. *Science* 1990; 248:189–194.
5. Hennet T, Richter C, and Peterhans E. Tumour necrosis factor-alpha induces superoxide anion generation in mitochondria of L929 cells. *Biochem J* 1993; 289:587–592.
6. Matsubara T, Ziff M. Superoxide anion release by human endothelial cells: Synergism between a phorbol ester and a calcium ionophore. *J Cell Physiol* 1986; 127:207–210.
7. Rosen GM, Freeman BA. Detection of superoxide generated by endothelial cells. *Proc Natl Acad Sci USA* 1984; 81:7269–7273.
8. Griendling KK, Minieri CA, Ollerenshaw JD, and Alexander RW. Angiotensin II stimulates NADH and NADPH oxidase activity in cultured vascular smooth muscle cells. *Circ Res* 1994; 74:1141–1148.
9. Lo YY, Cruz TF. Involvement of reactive oxygen species in cytokine and growth factor induction of c-fos expression in chondrocytes. *J Biol Chem* 1995; 270:11,727–11,730.
10. Cui XL, Douglas JG. Arachidonic acid activates c-jun N-terminal kinase through NADPH oxidase in rabbit proximal tubular epithelial cells. *Proc Natl Acad Sci USA* 1997; 94:3771–3776.
11. Jones SA, Wood JD, Coffey MJ, Jones OT. The functional expression of p47-phox and p67-phox may contribute to the generation of superoxide by an NADPH oxidase-like system in human fibroblasts. *FEBS Lett* 1994; 355:178–182.
12. Ushio-Fukai M, Zafari AM, Fukui T, Ishizaka N, Griendling KK. p22^{phox} is a critical component of the superoxide-generating NADH/NADPH oxidase system and regulates

angiotensin II-induced hypertrophy in vascular smooth muscle cells. *J Biol Chem* 1996; 271:23317–23321.

13. Segal AW, Abo A. The biochemical basis of the NADPH oxidase of phagocytes. *Trends Biochem Sci* 1993; 18:43–47.

14. Bokoch GM. Regulation of the human neutrophil NADPH oxidase by the Rac GTP-binding proteins. *Curr Opin Cell Biol* 1994; 6:212–218.

15. Sundaresan M, Yu ZX, Ferrans VJ, Sulciner DJ, Gutkind JS, Irani K, Goldschmidt-Clermont PJ, Finkel T. Regulation of reactive-oxygen-species generation in fibroblasts by Rac1. *Biochem J* 1996; 318:379–382.

16. Abate C, Patel L, Rauscher F, Curran T. Redox regulation of fos and jun DNA-binding activity in vitro. *Science* 1990; 249:1157–1161.

17. Xanthoudakis S, Curran T. Identification and characterization of Ref-1, a nuclear protein that facilitates AP-1 DNA-binding activity. *EMBO J* 1992; 11:653–665.

18. Xanthoudakis S, Miao G, Wang F, Pan YC, Curran T. Redox activation of Fos-Jun DNA binding activity is mediated by a DNA repair enzyme. *EMBO J* 1992; 11:3323–3335.

19. Schenk H, Klein M, Erdbrugger W, Droge W, Schulze OK. Distinct effects of thioredoxin and antioxidants on the activation of transcription factors NF-kappa B and AP-1. *Proc Natl Acad Sci USA* 1994; 91:1672–1676.

20. Hirota K, Matsui M, Iwata S, Nishiyama A, Mori K, Yodoi J. AP-1 transcriptional activity is regulated by a direct association between thioredoxin and Ref-1. *Proc Natl Acad Sci USA* 1997; 94:3633–3638.

21. Doan TN, Gentry DL, Taylor AA, Elliott SJ. Hydrogen peroxide activates agonist-sensitive Ca^{2+}-flux pathways in canine venous endothelial cells. *Biochem J* 1994; 297:209–215.

22. Dreher D, Jornot L, Junod AF. Effects of hypoxanthine-xanthine oxidase on Ca^{2+} stores and protein synthesis in human endothelial cells. *Circ Res* 1995; 76:388–395.

23. Rooney TA, Renard DC, Sass EJ, Thomas AP. Oscillatory cytosolic calcium waves independent of stimulated inositol 1,4,5-trisphosphate formation in hepatocytes. *J Biol Chem* 1991; 266:12,272–12,282.

24. Roveri A, Coassin M, Maiorino M, Zamburlini A, van AF, Ratti E, Ursini F. Effect of hydrogen peroxide on calcium homeostasis in smooth muscle cells. *Arch Biochem Biophys* 1992; 297:265–270.

25. Sweetman LL, Zhang NY, Peterson H, Gopalakrishna R, Sevanian A. Effect of linoleic acid hydroperoxide on endothelial cell calcium homeostasis and phospholipid hydrolysis. *Arch Biochem Biophys* 1995; 323:97–107.

26. Grover AK, Samson SE, Fomin VP. Peroxide inactivates calcium pumps in pig coronary artery. *Am J Physiol* 1992; 263:H537–H543.

27. Suzuki YJ, Ford GD. Inhibition of Ca^{2+}-ATPase of vascular smooth muscle sarcoplasmic reticulum by reactive oxygen intermediates. *Am J Physiol* 1991; 261:H568–H574.

28. Henschke PN, Elliott SJ. Oxidized glutathione decreases luminal Ca^{2+} content of the endothelial cell ins(1,4,5)P$_3$-sensitive Ca^{2+} store. *Biochem J* 1995; 312:485–489.

29. Missiaen L, Taylor CW, Berridge MJ. Spontaneous calcium release from inositol trisphosphate-sensitive calcium stores. *Nature* 1991; 352:241–244.

30. Renard DC, Seitz MB, Thomas AP. Oxidized glutathione causes sensitization of calcium release to inositol 1,4,5-trisphosphate in permeabilized hepatocytes. *Biochem J* 1992; 284:507–512.

31. Koshio O, Akanuma Y, Kasuga M. Hydrogen peroxide stimulates tyrosine phosphorylation of the insulin receptor and its tyrosine kinase activity in intact cells. *Biochem J* 1988; 250:95–101.

32. Hayes GR, Lockwood DH. Role of insulin receptor phosphorylation in the insulinomimetic effects of hydrogen peroxide. *Proc Natl Acad Sci USA* 1987; 84:8115–8119.

33. Nakamura K, Hori T, Sato N, Sugie K, Kawakami T, Yodoi J. Redox regulation of a src family protein tyrosine kinase p56[lck] in T cells. *Oncogene* 1993; 8:3133–3139.

34. Schieven GL, Kirihara JM, Burg DL, Geahlen RL, Ledbetter JA. p72^{syk} tyrosine kinase is activated by oxidizing conditions that induce lymphocyte tyrosine phosphorylation and Ca^{2+} signals. *J Biol Chem* 1993; 268:16,688–16,692.

35. Larsson R, Cerutti P. Translocation and enhancement of phosphotransferase activity of protein kinase C following exposure in mouse epidermal cells to oxidants. *Cancer Res* 1989; 49:5627–5632.

36. Gopalakrishna R, Anderson WB. Ca^{2+}- and phospholipid-independent activation of protein kinase C by selective oxidative modification of the regulatory domain. *Proc Natl Acad Sci USA* 1989; 86:6758–6762.

37. Sundaresan M, Yu ZX, Ferrans VJ, Irani K, Finkel T. Requirement for generation of H$_2$O$_2$ for platelet-derived growth factor signal transduction. *Science* 1995; 270:296–299.

38. Stevenson MA, Pollock SS, Coleman CN, Calderwood SK. X-irradiation, phorbol esters, and H$_2$O$_2$ stimulate mitogen-activated protein kinase activity in NIH-3T3 cells through the formation of reactive oxygen intermediates. *Cancer Res* 1994; 54:12–15.

39. Guyton KZ, Liu Y, Gorospe M, Xu Q, Holbrook NJ. Activation of mitogen-activated protein kinase by H$_2$O$_2$. Role in cell survival following oxidant injury. *J Biol Chem* 1996; 271:4138–4142.

40. Kamata H, Tanaka C, Yagisawa H, Matsuda S, Gotoh Y, Nishida E, Hirata H. Suppression of nerve growth factor-induced neuronal differentiation of PC12 cells. N-Acetylcysteine uncouples the signal transduction from ras to the mitogen-activated protein kinase cascade. *J Biol Chem* 1996; 271: 33,018–33,025.

41. Wilhelm D, Bender K, Knebel A, Angel P. The level of intracellular glutathione is a key regulator for the induction of stress-activated signal transduction pathways including Jun N-terminal protein kinases and p38 kinase by alkylating agents. *Mol Cell Biol* 1997; 17:4792–4800.

42. Fischer EH, Charbonneau H, Tonks NK. Protein tyrosine phosphatases: A diverse family of intracellular and transmembrane enzymes. *Science* 1991; 253:401–406.

43. Hecht D, Zick Y. Selective inhibition of protein tyrosine phosphatase activities by H$_2$O$_2$ and vanadate in vitro. *Biochem Biophys Res Commun* 1992; 188:773–779.

44. Knebel A, Rahmsdorf HJ, Ullrich A, Herrlich P. Dephosphorylation of receptor tyrosine kinases as target of regulation by radiation, oxidants or alkylating agents. *EMBO J* 1996; 15:5314–5325.

45. Schreck R, Rieber P, Baeuerle PA. Reactive oxygen intermediates as apparently widely used messengers in the activation of the NF-kappa B transcription factor and HIV-1. *EMBO J* 1991; 10:2247–2258.

46. Schmidt KN, Amstad P, Cerutti P, Baeuerle PA. Identification of hydrogen peroxide as the relevant messenger in the activation pathway of transcription factor NF-kappaB. *Adv Exp Med Biol* 1996; 387:63–68.

47. Sulciner DJ, Irani K, Yu ZX, Ferrans VJ, Goldschmidt CP, Finkel T. rac1 regulates a cytokine-stimulated, redox-dependent pathway necessary for NF-kappaB activation. *Mol Cell Biol* 1996; 16:7115–7121.

48. Perona R, Montaner S, Saniger L, Sanchez-Perez I, Bravo R, Lacal JC. Activation of the nuclear factor-kappaB by Rho, CDC42, and Rac-1 proteins. *Genes Dev* 1997; 11:463–475.

49. Wang GL, Jiang BH, Rue EA, and Semenza GL. Hypoxia-inducible factor 1 is a basic-helix-loop-helix-PAS heterodimer regulated by cellular O$_2$ tension. *Proc Natl Acad Sci USA* 1995; 92:5510–5514.

50. Wang GL, Jiang BH, Semenza GL. Effect of altered redox states on expression and DNA-binding activity of hypoxia-inducible factor 1. *Biochem Biophys Res Commun* 1995; 212:550–556.

51. Huang LE, Arany Z, Livingston DM, Bunn HF. Activation of hypoxia-inducible transcription factor depends primarily upon redox-sensitive stabilization of its alpha subunit. *J Biol Chem* 1996; 271:32,253–32,259.

52. Shang F, Gong X, Taylor A. Activity of ubiquitin-dependent pathway in response to oxidative stress. Ubiquitin-activating enzyme is transiently up-regulated. *J Biol Chem* 1997; 272: 23,086–23,093.

53. Salceda S, Caro J. Hypoxia-inducible factor 1alpha (HIF-1alpha) protein is rapidly degraded by the ubiquitin-proteasome system under normoxic conditions. Its stabilization by hypoxia depends on redox-induced changes. *J Biol Chem* 1997; 272:22,642–22,647.

54. Karin M, Liu ZG, Zandi E. AP-1 function and regulation. *Curr Opin Cell Biol* 1997; 9:240–246.

55. Murrell GA, Francis MJ, Bromley L. Modulation of fibroblast proliferation by oxygen free radicals. *Biochem J* 1990; 265:659–665.

56. Stirpe F, Higgins T, Tazzari PL, Rozengurt E. Stimulation by xanthine oxidase of 3T3 Swiss fibroblasts and human lymphocytes. *Exp Cell Res* 1991; 192:635–638.

57. Burdon RH, Gill VM, Rice-Evans C. Oxidative stress and heat shock protein induction in human cells. *Free Radic Res Commun* 1987; 3:129–139.

58. Shibanuma M, Kuroki T, Nose K. Stimulation by hydrogen peroxide of DNA synthesis, competence family gene expression and phosphorylation of a specific protein in quiescent Balb/3T3 cells. *Oncogene* 1990; 5:1025–1032.

59. Craven PA, Pfanstiel J, DeRubertis FR. Role of reactive oxygen in bile salt stimulation of colonic epithelial proliferation. *J Clin Invest* 1986; 77:850–859.

60. Nose K, Shibanuma M, Kikuchi K, Kageyama H, Sakiyama S, Kuroki T. Transcriptional activation of early-response genes by hydrogen peroxide in a mouse osteoblastic cell line. *Eur J Biochem* 1991; 201:99–106.

61. Rao GN, Berk BC. Active oxygen species stimulate vascular smooth muscle cell growth and proto-oncogene expression. *Circ Res* 1992; 70:593–599.

62. Burdon RH, Gill V. Cellularly generated active oxygen species and HeLa cell proliferation. *Free Radic Res Commun* 1993; 19:203–213.

63. Church SL, Grant JW, Ridnour LA, Oberley LW, Swanson PE, Meltzer PS, Trent JM. Increased manganese superoxide dismutase expression suppresses the malignant phenotype of human melanoma cells. *Proc Natl Acad Sci USA* 1993; 90:3113–3117.

64. Irani K, Xia Y, Zweier JL, Sollott SJ, Der CJ, Fearon ER, Sundaresan M, Finkel T, Goldschmidt CP. Mitogenic signaling mediated by oxidants in Ras-transformed fibroblasts. *Science* 1997; 275: 1649–1652.

65. Ohba M, Shibanuma M, Kuroki T, Nose K. Production of hydrogen peroxide by transforming growth factor-beta 1 and its involvement in induction of egr-1 in mouse osteoblastic cells. *J Cell Biol* 1994; 126:1079–1088.

66. Lo YYC, Wong JMS, Cruz TF. Reactive oxygen species mediate cytokine activation of c-Jun NH_2-terminal kinases. *J Biol Chem* 1996; 271:15,703–15,707.

67. Frenkel K. Carcinogen-mediated oxidant formation and oxidative DNA damage. *Pharmacol Ther* 1992; 53:127–166.

68. Santos L, Tipping PG. Attenuation of adjuvant arthritis in rats by treatment with oxygen radical scavengers. *Immunol Cell Biol* 1994; 72:406–414.

69. Stefanovic RM, Stadler J, Evans CH. Nitric oxide and arthritis. *Arthritis Rheum* 1993; 36:1036–1044.

70. Szatrowski TP, Nathan CF. Production of large amounts of hydrogen peroxide by human tumor cells. *Cancer Res* 1991; 51:794–798.

71. Williams LT. Signal transduction by the platelet-derived growth factor receptor. *Science* 1989; 243:1564–1570.

72. Bae YS, Kang SW, Seo MS, Baines IC, Tekle E, Chock PB, Rhee SG. Epidermal growth factor (EGF)-induced generation of hydrogen peroxide. Role in EGF receptor-mediated tyrosine phosphorylation. *J Biol Chem* 1997; 272:217–221.

73. Diaz MN, Frei B, Vita JA, Keaney JF. Jr. Antioxidants and atherosclerotic heart disease. *N Engl J Med* 1997; 337:408–416.

74. Harrison DG, Ohara Y. Physiologic consequences of increased vascular oxidant stresses in hypercholesterolemia and atherosclerosis: Implications for impaired vasomotion. *Am J Cardiol* 1995; 75:75B–81B.

75. Li YS, Shyy JY, Li S, Lee J, Su B, Karin M, Chien S. The Ras-JNK pathway is involved in shear-induced gene expression. *Mol Cell Biol* 1996; 16:5947–5954.

76. Jo H, Sipos K, Go YM, Law R, Rong J, McDonald JM. Differential effect of shear stress on extracellular signal-regulated kinase and N-terminal Jun kinase in endothelial cells. G_{i2-} and G beta/gamma-dependent signaling pathways. *J Biol Chem* 1997; 272:1395–1401.

77. Topper JN, Cai J, Falb D, Gimbrone MA Jr. Identification of vascular endothelial genes differentially responsive to fluid mechanical stimuli: Cyclooxygenase-2, manganese superoxide dismutase, and endothelial cell nitric oxide synthase are selectively up-regulated by steady laminar shear stress. *Proc Natl Acad Sci USA* 1996; 93:10,417–10, 422.

78. Inoue N, Ramasamy S, Fukai T, Nerem RM, Harrison DG. Shear stress modulates expression of Cu/Zn superoxide dismutase in human aortic endothelial cells. *Circ Res* 1996; 79:32–37.

79. Rajagopalan S, Kurz S, Munzel T, Tarpey M, Freeman BA, Griendling KK, Harrison DG. Angiotensin II-mediated hypertension in the rat increases vascular superoxide production via membrane NADH/NADPH oxidase activation. Contribution to alterations of vasomotor tone. *J Clin Invest* 1996; 97:1916–1923.

80. Fukui T, Ishizaka N, Rajagopalan S, Laursen JB, Capers Q/T, Taylor WR, Harrison DG, de LH, Wilcox JN, Griendling KK. p22phox mRNA expression and NADPH oxidase activity are increased in aortas from hypertensive rats. *Circ Res* 1997; 80:45–51.

81. Jacobson MD. Reactive oxygen species and programmed cell death. *Trends Biochem Sci* 1996; 21:83–86.

20

Sphingolipid Metabolites in Signal Transduction

Sarah Spiegel, PhD and Sheldon Milstien, PhD

1. INTRODUCTION

The importance of intracellular signaling molecules derived from sphingolipids, a major class of membrane lipids, has only recently begun to be appreciated. Sphingolipids contain a long-chain sphingoid base backbone, of which sphingosine is the most common; an amide-linked fatty acid; and a polar head group (hydroxyl for ceramide, phosphorylcholine for sphingomyelin, and carbohydrate residues of varying complexity for glycosphingolipids). Biological activity is exhibited not only by the more complex species of sphingolipids, but also by their metabolic products, with such metabolites as ceramide, sphingosine, and sphingosine 1-phosphate (SPP) emerging as a distinct class of lipid second messengers *(1–5)*.

Branching pathways of sphingolipid metabolism mediate growth arrest, stress responses, or proliferation of cells, depending on cell type and the nature of the stimulus. Ceramide is an important regulator of stress responses as well as of apoptosis, or programmed cell death, induced by tumor necrosis factor-α (TNF-α) or FAS ligand, both members of the TNF superfamily of proteins *(3,6–8)*. By contrast, we have implicated a further metabolite of ceramide, SPP, as a second messenger in cellular proliferation and survival induced by platelet-derived growth factor (PDGF), nerve growth factor (NGF), or serum *(9–11)*. This chapter reviews the current knowledge of the role of sphingolipid metabolites in the actions of growth factors and cytokines, with emphasis on the second messenger roles of ceramide and SPP in the regulation of cellular processes.

2. CERAMIDE AND APOPTOSIS

Within the last several years, our understanding of the mechanism by which events at the cell surface can trigger apoptosis has increased greatly *(12–15)* (Fig. 1). Protein–protein interactions link intracellular regions, known as death domains, of cell surface receptors for TNF-α (TNFR1) or FAS ligand (known as CD95, FAS, or APO1) to a cascade of proteases that are homologous to interleukin-1β-converting enzyme (ICE) and *Caenorhabditis elegans* CED-3. This family of more than 10 aspartate-specific cysteine proteases (caspases) can be phylogenetically classified into three subfamilies: (1) the CED-3 subfamily, consisting of caspase-3 (also known as CPP32, Yama, and

From: Signaling Networks and Cell Cycle Control: The Molecular Basis of Cancer and Other Diseases
Edited by: J. S. Gutkind © Humana Press Inc., Totowa, NJ

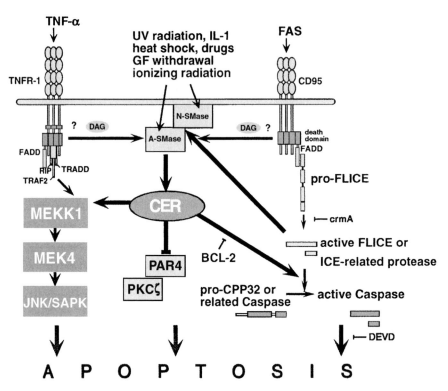

Fig. 1. Sphingolipid metabolites and apoptotic signals. Various stress stimuli, including FAS ligand, tumor necrosis factor-α (TNF-α), interleukin-1 (IL-1), growth factor (GF) withdrawal, anticancer drugs, ionizing or ultraviolet (UV) radiation, and heat shock, activate A-SMase or N-SMase, resulting in a marked and sustained increase in the cellular concentration of ceramide, an activator of JNK (SAPK) signaling. In stress, stimuli can also stimulate an ICE-like protease (possibly related to caspase-8, or FLICE), activating a SMase in a *CrmA*-dependent manner. Ceramide, in turn, can activate CPP32 (caspase-3) or a related caspase, resulting in amplification of the caspase cascade that leads to apoptosis. Higher concentrations of ceramide also induce conformational changes in PKCζ that increase its interaction with PAR4, resulting in its enzymatic inactivation and promotion of apoptosis. PARP, poly(ADP-ribose) polymerase.

apopain) *(16,17)*, caspase-6 (MCH2), caspase-7 (MCH3, ICE-LAP3, CMH1), caspase-8 (FLICE, MACH, MCH5), caspase-9 (ICE-LAP6, MCH6), caspase-10 (MCH4), and caspase 10/b (FLICE2); (2) the ICE subfamily, which includes caspase-1, caspase-4 (TX, ICH2, ICE rel-II), caspase-5 (TY, ICE rel-III), and caspase-11 (ICH3); and (3) the NEDD2 subfamily, which is represented by caspase-2 (ICH1, NEDD2). Binding of the adapter protein FADD, which also contains a death domain, either to CD95 directly or to TNFR1 through the death domain-containing protein TRADD *(12)* results in the recruitment of caspase-8 to the plasma membrane and thereby triggers autocatalytic activation of various proapoptotic proteases and consequent apoptosis *(15)*. TRADD also serves as a platform for recruitment of two additional proteins, RIP and TRAF2. Whereas FADD mediates activation of the apoptotic machinery, RIP and TRAF2 trigger activation of the protein kinase JNK and the transcription factor NF-κB *(14)*.

A variety of stress stimuli, including FAS ligand, TNF-α, growth factor withdrawal, oxidative stress, heat shock, ionizing radiation, ultraviolet (UV) light, and anticancer drugs such as arabinosylcytosine, daunorubicin, and vincristine, activate sphingomyelinase (SMase), which catalyzes the hydrolysis of sphingomyelin to produce ceramide. Moreover, cell-permeable analogs of ceramide mimic the effects of these stimuli in inducing the hallmarks of apoptosis—cell growth arrest and DNA fragmentation—whereas closely related compounds are ineffective, suggesting that ceramide may act as a common mediator of downstream events leading to apoptosis *(3)*. Both ceramide production and apoptosis induced by REAPER, a protein that plays an important role in apoptosis during embryogenesis in *Drosophila melanogaster,* are suppressed by an inhibitor of ICE-like proteases, z-VAD-fmk *(18)*. Similarly, CRMA, a poxvirus serpin that inhibits ICE-like proteases but does not affect caspase-3, blocks ceramide formation in response to TNF-α. Overexpression of the *CrmA* gene blocks TNF-α-induced apoptosis but does not affect the response to exogenous ceramide. Thus, ceramide appears to act downstream of an ICE-like protease and upstream of caspase-3 (or a related caspase).

The mechanisms by which cellular insults are coupled to activation of SMase are not well defined, but several hypotheses have been proposed. Ligation of several members of the TNF receptor family results in activation of neutral SMase (N-SMase) and acidic SMase (A-SMase). The death domains of TNFR1 and CD95 have been implicated in activation of A-SMase, possibly through activation of phosphatidylcholine-specific phospholipase C *(19)*. Moreover, A-SMase plays an essential role in radiation-induced apoptosis *(8)*. Lymphocytes from patients with Niemann-Pick disease, who have an inherited deficiency of A-SMase, do not generate ceramide or undergo apoptosis in response to ionizing radiation or CD95 ligation. These deficits are reversible by restoration of A-SMase activity *(8)*. Similar observations have been made with A-SMase knockout mice *(8),* further substantiating the obligatory role for ceramide generation in these apoptotic responses. TNF-α-induced activation of A-SMase was recently shown to be mediated through TRADD and FADD and activation of a protease distinct from caspase-8 *(20)*. Although A-SMase was originally localized predominantly to the acidic endosome compartment, more recently it has been shown to be associated with caveolae of the plasma membrane that are enriched in sphingomyelin.

Another potentially important signaling pathway initiated by TNF-α and FAS ligand involves the activation of membrane-bound N-SMase as a result of the binding of a WD-repeat protein, FAN (factor associated with N-SMase activation), to the corresponding receptor. FAN binds to TNFR1 at a distinct membrane-proximal sequence of 11 amino acids directly adjacent to the death domain *(21)*. In addition, depletion of glutathione also may contribute to activation of N-SMase. Given that glutathione depletion occurs in a variety of cells during the response to cellular injury and apoptosis, it may serve as a link between oxidative stress and signaling through the products of sphingomyelin hydrolysis *(22)*. N-SMase also may play a role in mitogenic and proinflammatory cellular responses to TNF-α *(21),* because it can couple TNFR1 to the growth-stimulatory mitogen-activated protein (MAP) kinase cascade through the activation of a ceramide-activated protein kinase (CAPK). This latter enzyme is a member of the family of proline-directed serine-threonine protein kinases that activate RAF1 *(23)* and was recently identified as a kinase suppressor of RAS (KSR) *(24)*. However, the recent cloning of N-SMase revealed no indication that this enzyme plays an important role in apoptosis or inflammation (25). A different cytosolic form of N-SMase that is magnesium independent is also activated in response to TNF-α, vitamin D_3, or NGF and acts on a specific pool of sphingomyelin located in the inner leaflet of the membrane bilayer (3). Indeed, whether TNF-α exerts a proliferative or apoptotic effect on two myeloid leukemia cell lines has been shown to correlate with the transverse distribution of sphingomyelin in the plasma membrane.

Although the stimulus-induced increase in the cellular concentration of ceramide occurs rapidly in some cell types, in others it is delayed and persistent (3,18). Biphasic ceramide responses similar to the biphasic increases in the cellular concentration of the second messenger diacylglycerol have also been observed. The existence of several different forms of SMase that might be differentially activated by stress stimuli may be responsible for these different ceramide responses. Both the extent and persistence of ceramide accumulation may determine the cellular response. Furthermore, ceramide formed in distinct cellular compartments might be linked to specific signaling pathways.

An important issue is whether activation of SMase and generation of ceramide are the cause of apoptosis or merely a consequence of activation of the death program. Several lines of evidence support the former scenario. First, exogenous ceramide mimics many of the physiological effects of apoptotic stimuli in a highly specific manner. Furthermore, in an in vitro reconstitution system in which extracts prepared from cells treated with antibodies to CD95 or exposed to UV radiation induce typical apoptotic morphological changes and internucleosomal DNA cleavage in added nuclei, the addition of ceramide alone to untreated cell extracts also induced similar nuclear changes. By contrast, dihydroceramide, which lacks apoptotic signaling activity in intact cells, had no effect in the in vitro system (26). Second, overexpression of the proto-oncogene BCL2, a homolog of the C. elegans antiapoptotic gene ced-9, did not interfere with ceramide formation induced by various stimuli yet did protect against apoptosis (3). Moreover, BCL2, as well as other members of the BCL2 family, such as BCL-x_L and A1, inhibits ceramide-mediated death in lymphoid and endothelial cells. These results also suggest that ceramide acts upstream of the caspases that are targets of BCL2 action. In addition, DEVD, a relatively selective inhibitor of caspase-3, prevents ceramide-induced apoptosis. Variant Jurkat T cells with a defect in caspase-3 activation are also resistant to apoptosis induced by antibodies to FAS or by ceramide, indicating that ceramide functions upstream of caspase-3. Finally, activation of protein kinase C (PKC) by diacylglycerol or pharmacological activators antagonizes apoptosis induced by TNF-α, FAS, or ionizing radiation, as well as that mediated by ceramide, suggesting that an increase in the cellular concentration of ceramide alone is not necessarily sufficient to initiate the death process.

3. SPP AND CELL GROWTH

SPP was initially described as an intermediate in the degradation of long-chain sphingoid bases (27). However, our recent observations provide new insight into a possible physiological function of this metabolite. The concentration of SPP in cells is low and is determined by the balance between its formation, catalyzed by sphingosine kinase (28), and its degradation, catalyzed by a pyridoxal phosphate-dependent lyase in the endoplasmic reticulum and a phosphatase (29,30). Because it can be rapidly

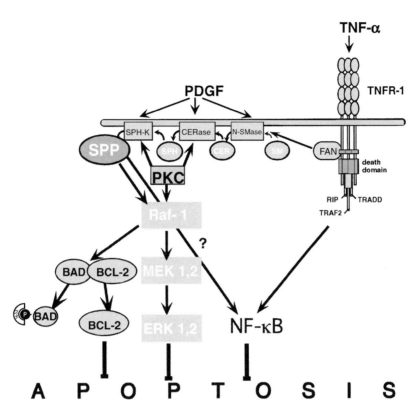

Fig. 2. Sphingolipid metabolites and cell survival signals. The scheme illustrates the effects of tumor necrosis factor α (TNF-α) and growth factors such as platelet-derived growth factor (PDGF) on sphingolipid metabolism, which result in the activation of ERK and NF-κB and in cell survival. Both TNF-α and PDGF induce small and transient increases in ceramide (CER), as a result of activation of N-SMase. Subsequent activation of ceramidase (CERase) and sphingosine kinase (SPH-K) results in accumulation of SPP. SPP not only stimulates ERKs, but it also prevents SAPK/JNK activation by ceramide and consequent apoptosis. In addition to its role at the plasma membrane as an activator of the ERK signaling pathway, RAF1 can also translocate to mitochondria, where it phosphorylates BAD and thereby releases Bcl2 to perform its antiapoptotic function. SPP also activates NF-κB, which has been implicated as an antiapoptotic signal.

produced and degraded, we hypothesized that SPP may function as an intracellular second messenger *(4)*. Indeed, SPP triggers a distinct pathway of calcium mobilization *(31)*, as well as activation of phospholipase D (PLD) *(32)* and the RAF-MEK-ERK signaling cascade *(33)* (Fig. 2). The latter MAP kinase pathway results in activation of the transcription factor AP1, thus linking signal transduction by sphingolipid metabolites to gene expression *(34)*.

We demonstrated that the SPP concentration is low in quiescent cultures of Swiss 3T3 fibroblasts, and that it increases rapidly on exposure of the cells to PDGF or serum *(10)*, but not to other mitogens, such as epidermal growth factor (EGF). Both PDGF and serum, but not EGF, also transiently increased sphingosine kinase activity *(10)*. Both D,L-*threo*-dihydrosphingosine and *N,N*-dimethylsphingosine, competitive inhibitors of sphingosine kinase, prevented formation of SPP and blocked cellular proliferation induced by PDGF or serum, but not proliferation induced by EGF *(10)*, further supporting a role for SPP in cellular proliferation. PDGF was subsequently shown to increase the concentration of SPP in both arterial *(35)* and airway *(36)* smooth muscle cells. Furthermore, PDGF, but not endothelin-1, induces proliferation of glomerular mesangial cells through ceramidase-regulated generation of sphingosine and, subsequently, SPP *(37)*.

In addition to PDGF, other mitogens, including PKC activators, the β subunit of cholera toxin, and NGF, stimulate sphingosine kinase activity, with a concomitant increase in SPP concentration, in diverse cell types *(4,9,11,38,39)*. Collectively, these results provide insight into the biological function of SPP, and they demonstrate that the importance of sphingosine kinase is not restricted to the simple catabolism of sphingolipids as originally proposed *(40)*. The properties, structure, and mechanism of regulation of sphingosine kinase remain largely unknown. We recently purified the enzyme from rat kidney by a factor of $6 \times 10_5$ to apparent homogeneity. The apparent molecular mass of the purified protein was approx 49 kDa, as determined by sodium dodecyl sulfate-polyacrylamide gel electrophoresis SDS-PAGE under denaturing conditions. Because a similar molecular size was obtained by gel-filtration analysis, the active form of sphingosine kinase is likely a monomer. With sphingosine as substrate, the enzyme showed a broad pH optimum of 6.6–7.5 and exhibited Michaelis-Menten kinetics, with K_m values of 5 and 93 μM for sphingosine and ATP, respectively *(41)*.

4. SIGNALING DOWNSTREAM OF SPP

Although the mechanism by which SPP modulates cell growth is not completely understood, several studies have recently begun to unravel the signaling pathways involved. One important downstream effect of SPP is calcium mobilization *(31,42–45)*. In most cell lines studied, SPP-mediated calcium mobilization occurs via an inositol trisphosphate (IP_3)-independent pathway *(31,42)* from stores within the endoplasmic reticulum that also contain sphingosine kinase *(42)*. Calcium mobilization in response to engagement of FcεR1 receptors for immunoglobulin E requires activation of sphingosine kinase and the generation of SPP *(43)*; inhibitors of sphingosine kinase, such as D,L-*threo*-dihydrosphingosine, block-FcεR1-mediated calcium mobilization as well as partially inhibit histamine release *(43)*. The effect of SPP on calcium mobilization resembles that of IP_3, which is mediated by direct activation of a specific calcium channel. However, the SPP-targeted calcium channel remains to be identified.

Evidence suggests that SPP may mediate mitogenesis, in part, by regulation of kinase cascades *(9,33–36,46–48)*. In Swiss 3T3 fibroblasts, D,L-*threo*-dihydrosphingosine blocked the PDGF-induced (but not EGF-induced) activation of two cyclin-dependent kinases (p34^{cdc2} and CDK2) and that of the MAP kinase ERK2, tyrosine phosphorylation of the adapter protein CRK, and increase in the DNA binding activity of AP1, without an effect on PDGF receptor autophosphorylation, SHC phosphorylation, or phosphatidylinositol 3-kinase activation *(46)*. Inhibition of PDGF-stimulated CDK activation and DNA synthesis *(10)* was reversed by SPP, demonstrating that the effects of D,L-*threo*-dihydrosphingosine were due to inhibition of sphingosine kinase *(46)*. SPP induced tyrosine phosphorylation of CRK, which links growth factor receptors to RAS activation, in NIH 3T3 cells, and CRK overexpression also enhanced SPP-induced mitogenesis *(48)*.

SPP also induces rapid reorganization of the actin cytoskeleton *(35,47)*, resulting in stress fiber formation and concomitant assembly of focal adhesions as well as tyrosine phosphorylation of both focal adhesion kinase (FAK) and paxillin in Swiss 3T3 fibroblasts *(47)*. The exoenzyme C3 transferase, which inactivates the small GTP-binding protein RHO by ADP-ribosylation, inhibited both SPP-induced protein tyrosine phosphorylation and stress fiber formation, indicating the existence of a RHO-mediated signaling pathway that is modulated by SPP *(47)*.

SPP induces the proliferation of Swiss 3T3 fibroblasts, in part, by activating PLD, which results in an increase in the concentration of the second messenger phosphatidic acid (PA) *(32)*. Activation of PLD by SPP occurs independent of PKC or G_i or G_o protein-linked receptor pathways *(49)*. In many cell types, SPP increases the PA concentration, whereas ceramide inhibits PLD *(50,51)*. Thus, increased concentrations of ceramide may induce growth arrest by blocking the PLD signaling pathway that mediates the mitogenic effects of SPP. The effects of sphingolipid metabolites on PA concentration suggest that the sphingolipid cycle might regulate the glycerophospholipid cycle.

In addition to inducing calcium mobilization and PA accumulation, SPP also regulates the intracellular concentration of another second messenger, cyclic adenosine monophosphate (cAMP)*(5)*. In most cell types, SPP induces inactivation of adenylate cyclase and a consequent decrease in cAMP concentration *(52–54)*. However, the relevance of changes in cAMP concentration to the mitogenic effects of SPP remains unclear.

5. THE CERAMIDE-SPP RHEOSTAT

Activation of PKC prevents ceramide-mediated apoptosis *(6,9,55,56)*. Although the mechanism of this antiapoptotic action of PKC is unknown, we observed that activation of PKC in many cell types results in increased sphingosine kinase activity and the consequent conversion of sphingosine to SPP. In turn, SPP suppresses ceramide-mediated apoptosis *(9)*. Furthermore, inhibition of either PKC or sphingosine kinase induces apoptosis, an effect that can be prevented by the addition of SPP *(9,11)*. Activation of PKC also blocks the TNF-α-induced increase in ceramide concentration. Conversely, TNF-α reduces sphingosine kinase activity and markedly decreases the concentration of SPP. Thus, growth factors and TNF-α exert opposing actions on the intracellular concentrations of ceramide and SPP; substantially affecting the ratio of the concentrations of these metabolites *(9)*. Dissociation of cytokine-induced apoptosis from growth factor-induced mitogenesis may thus be determined by distinct sphingolipid-derived second messengers *(9,11,37,57)*. Stress stimuli activate SMase, but not ceramidase, leading to an accumulation of ceramide, whereas growth signals stimulate both ceramidase and sphingosine kinase, resulting in increased concentrations of sphingosine and SPP. We propose that the balance between the cellular concentration of ceramide, which promotes cell death, and that of SPP, which inhibits death, is a critical determinant of cell fate.

How do sphingolipid metabolites regulate life and death? Three MAP kinases that participate in distinct, but related, signaling pathways, play crucial roles in cell survival and death. The importance of the extracellular signal-regulated kinases ERK1 and ERK2 in the RAS-RAF-MEK-ERK signaling cascade triggered by growth factors has been well established *(58)*. By contrast, stress-activated protein kinases (SAPKs), also known as c-JUN N-terminal kinases (JNKs), and p38 are activated by various environmental stresses and cytokines. Cell survival and death are most likely determined by the dynamic balance between ERK signaling and that mediated by JNKs and p38 *(59)*. Ceramide and SPP have opposing effects on these pathways. In many cell types, ceramide-induced apoptosis has been correlated with stimulation of JNKs, and overexpression of dominant-negative mutant forms of components of the JNK pathway inhibits ceramide-mediated apoptosis *(7)*. Conversely, SPP not only stimulates ERKs *(33)*, but also prevents JNK activation by ceramide and consequent apoptosis *(9)*. The duration of JNK activation also appears to be important in determining the outcome of signaling. Transient JNK activation results in cellular proliferation, whereas sustained activation results in apoptosis *(60)*. In a similar manner, transient ERK activation stimulates cell growth, whereas prolonged activation leads to differentiation *(58)*. Therefore, a single kinase signaling pathway may have distinct functions that depend on the induction pattern within the context of other signaling pathways.

In addition to its role in the signaling cascade leading to ERK activation, RAF is translocated in a BCL2-dependent manner to mitochondria resulting in phosphorylation of the proapoptotic BCL2 family member BAD. Phosphorylated BAD preferentially binds to protein 14-3-3 and translocates to the cytosol, thereby precluding its interaction with BCL2 and BCL-x_L and allowing these latter proteins to carry out their antiapoptotic functions. The ability of SPP to activate RAF1 may be important for its antiapoptotic effects (Fig. 2). In this regard, the sphingosine kinase inhibitor *N,N,*-dimethylsphingosine induces phosphorylation of protein 14-3-3, which might interfere with either the function of RAF or the sequestration of BAD.

Recent attention has focused on the potential roles for ceramide in the caspase cascade of apoptosis *(61)*. Ceramide appears to act downstream of an ICE-like protease and upstream of caspase-3 or a related caspase *(62,63)*. Ceramide formed in response to stress stimuli may act in a positive-feedback manner to amplify the action of the death proteases. In support of this proposal, ceramide links cellular stress responses induced by γ-irradiation or anticancer drugs to the CD95 pathway of apoptosis by upregulating CD95 expression *(64)*. In contrast to activation of the caspase cascade by ceramide, we showed that SPP suppresses the apoptotic pathway downstream of caspase-8 but upstream of caspases-3, -6, and -7 *(65)*. Although the relations between the caspase cascade and the JNK cascade have not yet been clarified, ceramide and SPP have opposing effects on both of these apoptotic signaling pathways. Thus, we have proposed that control of the ceramide-SPP rheostat and consequent differential regulation of various MAP kinases and caspases are important determinants of whether cells survive or die *(9)*. Although the ceramide-SPP rheostat may be an inherent characteristic of each cell type, external stimuli can reset this ratio.

The ceramide-SPP rheostat appears to be an evolutionarily conserved stress regulatory mechanism. Ceramide induces arrest in the G_1 phase of the cell cycle and cell death in *Saccharomyces cerevisiae (66)*. Moreover, heat stress in this yeast results in the accumulation of phytosphingosine, dihydrosphingosine, and ceramide *(67,68)*, and activates transcription from the global stress response element *(68)*. We have identified two genes in *S. cerevisiae* that regulate the cellular concentrations of phosphorylated sphingoid bases and ceramide: *LBP1* and its homolog *LBP2* encode hydrophobic proteins that function as specific long-chain sphingoid base phosphate phosphatases. Deletion of *LBP1* and *LBP2* results in reduced concentrations of ceramide and increased concentrations of long-chain base phosphates, as well as in markedly increased cell survival after exposure to severe heat shock *(69)*.

6. DUAL ACTIONS OF SPP

Although many studies indicate an intracellular site of action for SPP, some of the biological effects of this metabolite, when added exogenously, such as inhibition of motility and changes in cell shape, may be mediated extracellularly by cell surface receptors. SPP is stored in high concentrations in human platelets, from which it is released on cell activation by physiological stimuli, possibly to play a role in platelet aggregation *(70)*. We have shown that pertussis toxin-sensitive G proteins participate in some of the signaling pathways triggered by SPP, suggesting that SPP might activate a receptor coupled to a G_i or G_o protein *(33, 53)*. Consistent with this hypothesis, low concentrations of SPP activate G_i protein-coupled inward-rectifying potassium channels only when applied at the extracellular face of atrial myocytes *(52)*. Moreover, nanomolar concentrations of SPP rapidly induce RHO-dependent neurite retraction and cell rounding in mouse N1E-115 neuronal cells *(71)*, and SPP markedly inhibits melanoma cell motility by binding to an extracellular receptor *(72)*.

The structure of SPP is highly similar to that of lysophosphatidic acid, another lysophospholipid present in serum that acts through a specific G protein-coupled receptor to regulate multiple cellular responses *(73)*. The product of *ventricular zone gene-1*, also known as *EDG2*, was recently shown to act as a functional receptor for lysophosphatidic acid *(74,75)*, and to share 37% sequence identity with the G_i-linked orphan receptor EDG1 and 30–32% sequence identity with the cannabinoid and melanocortin receptors. *EDG1* was cloned as an immediate-early gene induced by phorbol ester treatment of human umbilical vein endothelial cells *(76)* and is thought to be important in endothelial cell differentiation. However, the endogenous ligand for EDG1 has not been identified. Recently, we have shown that SPP acts as a specific ligand for EDG1, with a dissociation constant of 8 n*M (77,78)*. Other phospholipids and sphingolipids, including lysophosphatidic acid, *N,N*-dimethylsphingosine, sphingosine, and sphingosinephosphorylcholine, did not compete with SPP for binding to EDG1. Binding of SPP to HEK 293 cells stably expressing recombinant EDG1-induced inhibition of cAMP accumulation, activation of ERK, RHO-dependent cell aggregation, expression of cadherins, and formation of well-developed adherens junctions *(77,78)*. By contrast, two well-characterized biological responses to SPP, mitogenesis and prevention of apoptosis, were unrelated to the interaction of SPP with EDG1, but instead correlated with intracellular uptake *(78)*. SPP-induced calcium mobilization, activation of PLD, and tyrosine phosphorylation of FAK were also independent of EDG1 expression. Moreover, DNA synthesis in Swiss 3T3 fibroblasts was substantially and specifically increased by microinjection of SPP. Finally, SPP suppresses apoptosis in HL60 and PC12 cells, which do not exhibit specific SPP binding or contain *EDG1* mRNA. Conversely, sphinganine 1-phosphate, which differs structurally from SPP by only a single double bond and binds to and signals via EDG1, does not exert a significant cytoprotective effect. Hence, SPP may be the prototype for a new class of lipid mediators that act both extracellularly as ligands for cell surface receptors and intracellularly as second messengers.

ACKNOWLEDGMENTS

We thank the many members of the Spiegel laboratory for their contributions to the studies that were quoted in this review, especially Drs. Ana Olivera, Olivier Cuvillier, Takafumi Kohama, and James R. Van Brocklyn. This work was supported by research grants RO1 CA61774 and R01CA61774 from the National Institutes of Health and BE-275 from The American Cancer Society.

REFERENCES

1. Kolesnick R, Golde DW. The sphingomyelin pathway in tumor necrosis factor and interleukin-1 signaling. *Cell* 1994; 77:325–328.
2. Hannun YA. The sphingomyelin cycle and the second messenger function of ceramide. *J Biol Chem* 1994; 269:3125–3128.
3. Hannun Y. Functions of ceramide in coordinating cellular responses to stress. *Science* 1996; 274:1855–1859.
4. Spiegel S, Milstien S. Sphingolipid metabolites: Members of a new class of lipid second messengers. *J Membr Biol* 1995; 146:225–237.
5. Spiegel S, Foster D, Kolesnick R. (1996) Signal transduction through lipid second messengers. *Curr Opin Cell Biol* 1996; 8:159–167.
6. Obeid LM, Lindaric CM, Karolak LA, Hannun YA. Programmed cell death induced by ceramide. *Science* 1993; 259:1769–1771.
7. Verheij M, Bose R, Lin XH, Yao B, Jarvis WD, Grant S, Birrer MJ, Szabo E, Zon LI, Kyriakis JM, Haimovitz-Friedman A, Fuks Z, Kolesnick RN. Requirement for ceramide-initiated SAPK/JNK signalling in stress-induced apoptosis. *Nature* 1996; 380:75–79.
8. Santana P, Peña LA, Haimovitz-Friedman A, Martin S, Green D, McLoughlin M, Cordon-Cardo C, Schuchman EH, Fuks Z, Kolesnick R. Acid sphingomyelinase-deficient human lymphoblasts and mice are defective in radiation-induced apoptosis. *Cell* 1996; 86:189–199.
9. Cuvillier O, Pirianov G, Kleuser B, Vanek PG, Coso OA, Gutkind S, Spiegel S. Suppression of ceramide-mediated programmed cell death by sphingosine-1-phosphate. *Nature* 1996; 381:800–803.
10. Olivera A, Spiegel S. Sphingosine-1-phosphate as a second messenger in cell proliferation induced by PDGF and FCS mitogens. *Nature* 1993; 365:557–560.
11. Edsall LC, Pirianov GG, Spiegel S. Involvement of sphingosine 1-phosphate in nerve growth factor-mediated neuronal survival and differentiation. *J Neurosci* 1997; 17:6952–6960.
12. Hsu H, Shu HB, Pan MG, Goeddel DV. TRADD-TRAF2 and TRADD-FADD interactions define two distinct TNF receptor 1 signal transduction pathways. *Cell* 1996; 84:299–308.
13. Chinnaiyan AM, Orth K, O'Rourke K, Duan H, Poirier GG, Dixit VM. Molecular ordering of the cell death pathway. Bcl-2 and Bcl-xL function upstream of the CED-3-like apoptotic proteases. *J Biol Chem* 1996; 271:4573–4576.
14. Liu Z-G, Hsu H, Goeddel DV, Karin M. Dissection of the TNF receptor 1 effector functions: JNK activation is not linked to apoptosis while NF-κB activation prevents cell death. *Cell* 1996; 87:565–576.
15. Muzio M, Chinnaiyan AM, Kischkel FC, O'Rourke K, Shevchenko A, Ni J, Scaffidi C, Bretz JD, Zhang M, Gentz R, Mann M, Krammer PH, Peter ME, Dixit VM. FLICE, a novel FADD-homologous ICE/CED-3-like protease, is recruited to the CD95 (Fas/APO-1) death-inducing signaling complex. *Cell* 1996; 85:817–827.

16. Fernandes-Alnemri T, Litwak G, and Alnemri ES. (1994) CPP32, a novel human apoptotic protein with homology to *Caenorhabditis elegans* cell death protein Ced-3 and mammalian interleukin-1β-converting enzyme. *J Biol Chem* 1994; 269:30,761–30,764.

17. Nicholson DW, Thornberry NA. Caspases: Killer proteases. *Trends Biochem Sci* 1997; 22:299–306.

18. Pronk GJ, Ramer K, Amiri P, Williams LT. Requirement of an ICE-like protease for induction of apoptosis and ceramide generation by REAPER. *Science* 1996; 271:808–810.

19. Wiegmann K, Schutze S, Machleidt T, Witte D, Kronke M. Functional dichotomy of neutral and acidic sphingomyelinases in tumor necrosis factor signaling. *Cell* 1994; 78:1005–1015.

20. Schwandner R, Wiegmann K, Bernardo K, Kreder D, Kronke M. TNF receptor death domain-associated proteins TRADD and FADD signal activation of acid sphingomyelinase. *J Biol Chem* 1998; 273:5916–5922.

21. Adam-Klages S, Adam D, Wiegmann K, Struve S, Kolanus W, Schneider-Mergener J, Kronke M. FAN, a novel WD-repeat protein, couples the p55 TNF-receptor to neutral sphingomyelinase. *Cell* 1996; 86:937–947.

22. Liu B, Hannun, YA. Inhibition of the neutral magnesium-dependent sphingomyelinase by glutathione. *J Biol Chem* 1997; 272:16,281–16,287.

23. Yao B, Zhang Y, Dellkat S, Mathias S, Basu S, Kolesnick R. Phosphorylation of raf by ceramide-activated protein kinase. *Nature* 1995; 378:307–310.

24. Zhang Y, Yao B, Delikat S, Bayoumy S, McGinley M, Chan-Hui P-Y, Lichenstein H, Kolesnick R. Kinase suppressor of ras is ceramide-activated protein kinase. *Cell* 1997;89:63–72.

25. Tomiuk S, Hofmann K, Nix M, Zumbansen M, Stoffel W. Cloned mammalian neutral sphingomyelinase: functions in sphingolipid signaling? *Proc Natl Acad Sci USA* 1998; 95:3638–3643.

26. Martin SJ., Newmeyer DD, Mathias S, Farschon DM, Wang HG, Reed J. C, Kolesnick RN, Green DR. Cell-free reconstitution of Fas-, UV radiation-and ceramide-induced apoptosis. *EMBO J* 1995; 14:5191–5200.

27. Stoffel W, Assmann G. Enzymatic degradation of 4t-sphingenine 1-phosphate (sphingosine-1-phosphate) to 2t-hexadecen-1-al and ethanolamine phosphate. *Hoppe-Seylers Z Physiol Chem* 351:1041–1049.

28. Olivera A, Rosenthal J, Spiegel S. Effect of acidic phospholipids on sphingosine kinase. *J Cell Biochem* 1996; 60:529–537.

29. Van Veldhoven PP, Mannaerts GP. Subcellular localization and membrane topology of sphingosine-1-phosphate lyase in rat liver. *J Biol Chem* 1991; 266:12,502–12,507.

30. Van Veldhoven PP, Mannaerts GP. Sphinganine 1-phosphate metabolism in cultured skin fibroblasts: Evidence for the existence of a sphingosine phosphatase. *Biochem J* 1994; 299:597–601.

31. Mattie M, Brooker G, Spiegel S. Sphingosine-1-phosphate, a putative second messenger, mobilizes calcium from internal stores via an inositol trisphosphate-independent pathway. *J Biol Chem* 1994; 269:3181–3188.

32. Desai NN, Zhang H, Olivera A, Seki T, Brooker G, Spiegel S. Sphingosine-1-phosphate, a metabolite of sphingosine, increases phosphatidic acid levels by phospholipase D activation. *J Biol Chem* 1992; 267:23,122–23,128.

33. Wu J, Spiegel S, Sturgill TW. Sphingosine 1-phosphate rapidly activates the mitogen-activated protein kinase pathway by a G protein-dependent mechanism. *J Biol Chem* 1995; 270:11,484–11,488.

34. Su Y, Rosenthal D, Smulson M, Spiegel S. Sphingosine 1-phosphate, a novel signaling molecule, stimulates DNA binding activity of AP-1 in quiescent Swiss 3T3 fibroblasts. *J Biol Chem* 1994; 269:16,512–16,517.

35. Bornfeldt KE, Graves LM, Raines EW, Igarashi Y, Wayman G, Yumamura S, Yatomi Y,

Sidhu JS, Krebs EG, Hakomori S, Ross R. Sphingosine-1-phosphate inhibits PDGF-induced chemotaxis of human arterial smooth muscle cells: Spatial and temporal modulation of PDGF chemotactic signal transduction. *J Cell Biol* 1995; 130:193–206.

36. Pyne S, Chapman J, Steele L, Pyne NJ. Sphingomyelin-derived lipids differentially regulate the extracellular signal-regulated kinase 2 (ERK-2) and c-Jun N-terminal kinase (JNK) signal cascades in airway smooth muscle cells. *Eur J Biochem* 1996; 237:819–826.

37. Coroneos E, Martinez M, McKenna S, Kester M. Differential regulation of sphingomyelinase and ceramidase activities by growth factors and cytokines. *J Biol Chem* 1995; 270:23,305–23,309.

38. Wang F, Buckley NE, Olivera A, Goodemote KA, Su Y, Spiegel S. Involvement of sphingolipid metabolites in cellular proliferation modulated by ganglioside GM1. *Glycoconjugate J* 1996; 13:937–945.

39. Mazurek N, Megidish T, Hakomori S-I, Igarashi Y. Regulatory effect of phorbol esters on sphingosine kinase in BALB/C 3T3 fibroblasts (variant A31): Demonstration of cell type-specific response. *Biochem Biophys Res Commun* 198:1–9.

40. Stoffel W, Hellenbroich B, Heimann G. Properties and specificities of sphingosine kinase from blood platelets. *Hoppe-Seylers Z Physiol Chem* 1973; 354:1311–1316.

41. Olivera A, Kohama T, Tu Z, Milstien S, Spiegel S. Purification and characterization of rat kidney sphingosine kinase. *J Biol Chem* 1998; 273:12,576–12,583.

42. Ghosh TK, Bian J, Gill DL. Sphingosine 1-phosphate generated in the endoplasmic reticulum membrane activates release of stored calcium. *J Biol Chem* 1994; 269:22,628–22,635.

43. Choi OH, Kim J-H, Kinet, J-P. Calcium mobilization via sphingosine kinase in signalling by the FcεRI antigen receptor. *Nature* 1996; 380:634–636.

44. Fatatis A, Miller RJ. Platelet-derived growth factor (PDGF)-induced Ca^{2+} signaling in the CG4 oligodendroglial cell line and in transformed oligodendrocytes expressing the β-PDGF receptor. *J Biol Chem* 1997; 272:4351–4358.

45. Fatatis A, Miller RJ. Sphingosine and sphingosine 1-phosphate differentially modulate platelet-derived growth factor-BB-induced Ca^{2+} signaling in transformed oligodendrocytes. *J Biol Chem* 1996; 271:295–301.

46. Rani CS, Berger A, Wu, J, Sturgill TW, Beitner-Johnson D, LeRoith D, Varticovski L, Spiegel S. Divergence in signal transduction pathways of PDGF and EGF receptors: Involvement of sphingosine-1-phosphate in PDGF but not EGF signaling. *J Biol Chem* 1997; 272:10,777–10,783.

47. Wang F, Nobes CD, Hall A, Spiegel S. Sphingosine 1-phosphate stimulates Rho-mediated tyrosine phosphorylation of focal adhesion kinase and paxillin in Swiss 3T3 fibroblasts. *Biochem J* 1997; 324:481–488.

48. Blakesly VA, Beitner-Johnson D, Van Brocklyn JR, Rani S, Shen-Orr Z, Stannard BS, Spiegel S, LeRoith D. Sphingosine 1-phosphate stimulates tyrosine phosphorylation of Crk. *J Biol Chem* 1997; 272:16,211–16,215.

49. Spiegel S, Milstien S. Sphingoid bases and phospholipase D activation. *Chem Phys Lipids* 1996; 80:27–36.

50. Venable ME, Blobe GC, Obeid, LM. Identification of a defect in the phospholipase D/diacylglycerol pathway in cellular senescence. *J Biol Chem* 1994; 269:26,040–26,044.

51. Gomez-Munoz A, Martin A, O'Brien L, Brindley DN. Cell-permeable ceramides inhibit the stimulation of DNA synthesis and phospholipase D activity by phosphatidate and lysophosphatidate in rat fibroblasts. *J Biol Chem* 1994; 269:8937–8943.

52. van Koppen CJ, Meyer zu Heringdorf D, Laser KT, Zhang C, Jakobs KH, Bünnemann M, Pott L. Activation of a high affinity G_i protein-coupled plasma membrane receptor by sphingosine-1-phosphate. *J Biol Chem* 1996; 271:2082–2087.

53. Goodemote KA, Mattie ME, Berger A, Spiegel S. Involvement of a pertussis toxin sensitive G protein in the mitogenic signaling pathways of sphingosine 1-phosphate. *J Biol Chem* 1995; 270:10,272–10,277.

54. Okajima F, Tomura H, Sho K, Kimura T, Sato K, Im DS, Akbar M, Kondo Y. Sphingosine 1-phosphate stimulates hydrogen peroxide generation through activation of phospholipase C-Ca^{2+} system in FRTL-5 thyroid cells: Possible involvement of guanosine triphosphate-binding proteins in the lipid signaling. *Endocrinology* 1997;138:220–229.

55. Jarvis WD, Fornari FA, Jr, Browning JL, Gewirtz DA, Kolesnick RN, Grant S. Attenuation of ceramide-induced apoptosis by diglyceride in human myeloid leukemia cells. *J Biol Chem* 1994; 269:31,685–31,692.

56. Tepper CG, Jayadev S, Liu B, Bielawska A, Wolff R, Yonehara S, Hannun YA, Seldin MF. Role for ceramide as an endogenous mediator of Fas-induced cytotoxicity. *Proc Natl Acad Sci USA* 1995; 92:8443–8447.

57. Nikolova-Karakashian M, Morgan ET, Alexander C, Liotta DC, Merrill AH Jr. Bimodal regulation of ceramidase by interleukin-1beta. Implications for the regulation of cytochrome p450 2C11. *J Biol Chem* 1997; 272:18,718–18,724.

58. Marshall CJ. Specificity of receptor tyrosine kinase signaling: Transient versus sustained extracellular signal-regulated kinase activation. *Cell* 1995; 80:179–185.

59. Xia Z, Dickens M, Raingeaud J, Davis RJ, Greenberg ME. Opposing effects of ERK and JNK-p38 MAP kinases on apoptosis. *Science* 1995; 270:1326–1331.

60. Chen Y-R, Meyer CF, Tan T-Y. Persistent activation of c-jun N-terminal kinase 1 (JNK1) in γ radiation-induced apoptosis. *J Biol Chem* 1996; 271:631–634.

61. Chinnaiyan AM, O'Rourke K, Lane BR, Dixit VM. Interaction of CED-4 with CED-3 and CED-9: A molecular framework for cell death. *Science* 1997; 275:1122–1126.

62. Smyth MJ, Perry DK, Zhang J, Poirier GG, Hannun YA, Obeid LM. prICE: A downstream target for ceramide-induced apoptosis and for the inhibitory action of Bcl-2. *Biochem J* 1996; 316:25–28.

63. Dbaibo GS, Perry DK, Gamard CJ, Platt R, Poirier GG, Obeid LM, Hennun YA. Cytokine response modifier A (CrmA) inhibits ceramide formation in response to tumor necrosis factor (TNF)-α: CrmA and Bcl-2 target distinct components in the apoptotic pathway. *J Exp Med* 1997; 185:481–490.

64. Herr I, Wilhelm D, Bohler T, Angel P, Debatin KM. Activation of CD95 (APO-1/Fas) signaling by ceramide mediates cancer therapy-induced apoptosis. *EMBO J* 1997; 16:6200–6208.

65. Cuvillier O, Rosenthal DS, Smulson ME, Spiegel S. Sphingosine-1-phosphate inhibits activation of caspases that cleave poly(ADP-ribose) polymerase and lamins during Fas- and ceramide-mediated apoptosis in Jurkat T lymphocytes. *J Biol Chem* 1998; 273:2910–2916.

66. Nickels JT, Broach JR. A ceramide-activated protein phosphatase mediates ceramide-induced G$_1$ arrest of *Sacharromyces cerevisiae*. *Genes Dev* 1996; 10:382–394.

67. Jenkins GM, Richards A, Wahl T, Mao C, Obeid L, Hannun Y. Involvement of yeast sphingolipids in the heat stress response of saccharomyces cerevisiae. *J Biol Chem* 1997; 272:32,566–32,572.

68. Dickson RC, Nagiec EE, Skrzypek M, Tillman P, Wells GB, Lester RL. Sphingolipids are potential heat stress signals in *Saccharomyces*. *J Biol Chem* 1997; 272:30,196–30,200.

69. Mandala S, Thornton R, Tu Z, Kurtz M, Nickels J, Broach J, Menzeleev R, Spiegel S. Sphingoid base 1-phosphate phosphatase, a key regulator of sphingolipid metabolism and stress response. *Proc Natl Acad Sci USA* 1997; 95:150–155.

70. Yatomi Y, Ruan F, Hakomori S, Igarashi Y. Sphingosine-1-phosphate: A platelet-activating sphingolipid released from agonist-stimulated human platelets. *Blood* 1995; 86:193–202.

71. Postma FR, Jalink K, Hengeveld T, Moolenaar WH. Sphingosine-1-phosphate rapidly induces rho-dependent neurite retraction: Action through a specific cell surface receptor. *EMBO J* 1996; 15:2388–2392.

72. Yamamura S, Yatomi Y, Ruan F, Sweeney EA, Hakomori S, Igarashi Y. Sphingosine 1-phosphate regulates melanoma cell motility through a receptor-coupled extracellular action and in a pertussis toxin-insensitive manner. *Biochemistry* 1997; 36:10,751–10,759.

73. Moolenaar WH, Kranenburg O, Postma FR, Zondag GCM. Lysophosphatidic acid: G-protein signalling and cellular responses. *Curr Opin Cell Biol* 1997; 9:168–173.
74. Hecht JH, Weiner JA, Post SR, Chun J. Ventricular zone gene-1 (vzg-1) encodes a lysophosphatidic acid receptor expressed in neurogenic regions of the developing cerebral cortex. *J Cell Biol* 1996; 135:1071–1083.
75. An S, Dickens MA, Bleu T, Hallmark OG, Goetzel EJ. Molecular cloning of the human Edg2 protein and its identification as a functional cellular receptor for lysophophatidic acid. *Biochem Biophys Res Commun* 1997; 231:619–622.
76. Hla T, Maciag T. An abundant transcript induced in differentiating human endothelial cells encodes a polypeptide with structural similarities to G-protein coupled receptors. *J Biol Chem* 1990; 265:9308–9313.
77. Lee M-J, Van Brocklyn JR, Thangada S, Liu CH, Hand AR, Menzeleev R, Spiegel S, Hla T. Sphingosine-1-phosphate as a ligand for the G protein-coupled receptor Edg-1. *Science* 1998; 279:1552–1555.
78. Van Brocklyn JR, Lee MJ, Menzeleev R, Olivera A, Edsall L, Cuvillier O, Dianne MT, Coopman PJP, Thangada S, Hla T, Spiegel S. Dual actions of sphingosine-1-phosphate: Extracellular through the G_i-coupled orphan receptor edg-1 and intracellular to regulate proliferation and survival. *J Cell Biol* 1998; 142:229–240.

21

The Jak/Stat Signaling Cascade

Its Role in the Biological Effects of Interferons

Andrew C. Larner, MD, PhD and Andrew Keightley, PhD

1. INTRODUCTION

Transmission of information from the environment into cells by polypeptide growth factors and cytokines is accomplished by a variety of mechanisms that share numerous common features. Initiation of signals requires binding of the polypeptide to specific cell surface receptors and clustering of the engaged receptors, which then results in the activation of receptor-intrinsic or cytoplasmic protein kinase(s). Subsequent to stimulation of thes kinase(s), rapid increases occur in the rates of transcription of cellular genes whose protein products mediate the biological actions of cytokines and growth factors. It has become recently apparent that a given cytokine or growth factor does not activate a unique protein kinase, which then functions in a linear signaling pathway to produce a distinct biological effect. Rather, two or more signaling cascades can be activated simultaneously, allowing for combinatorial effects that permit more refined regulation of a given biological end point or several distinct endpoints.

A widely employed signaling cascade, whose function is important for the actions of polypeptide growth regulators, and for cytokines that mediate cell differentiation or organogenesis, has been elaborated over the past several years. It contains at least two common components: (1) signal transducers and activators of transcription (Stats), which are Src homology 2 (SH2) domain-containing transcription factors required for the activation of immediate early response genes by interferons, as well as numerous other cytokines and growth factors; and (2) the Janus tyrosine kinases (Jaks), whose activity is required for ligand-induced tyrosine phosphorylation of Stats. This chapter provides a broad outline of the Jak/Stat signaling cascade and reviews the evidence suggesting that this pathway regulates and is regulated by other well-defined signaling cascades. As many of the details concerning the Jak and Stat proteins were defined within the context of understanding the mechanism by which interferons stimulate the expression of immediate early genes, the control of the Jak/Stat pathway by interferons is used as a paradigm for much of the information communicated in this review. However, other cytokines that activate the Jak/Stat pathway use mechanisms similar to those employed by interferons.

From: Signaling Networks and Cell Cycle Control: The Molecular Basis of Cancer and Other Diseases
Edited by: J. S. Gutkind © Humana Press Inc., Totowa, NJ

2. INTERFERON ACTION

The antiviral, antigrowth, and immunomodulatory activities of interferons appear to be controlled in part by sets of cellular genes that are rapidly induced upon interferon-α/β (IFN-α/β) or IFN-γ binding to specific cell surface receptors. Incubation of cells with interferons induces the synthesis of several proteins, which can be prevented by the RNA synthesis inhibitor actinomycin D *(1–6)*. Isolation of IFN-induced RNAs confirmed that unique, although partially overlapping, sets of cellular genes were transcriptionally activated by treatment of cells with either IFN-α/β (type I) or IFN-γ (type II) *(7–9)*. Analysis of the promoters of IFN-α/β-stimulated genes led to the identification of an enhancer termed the interferon-stimulated response element (ISRE), which proved necessary and sufficient for activation of these genes by IFN-α/β *(10)*. Likewise, a distinct consensus element was mapped in the promoters of genes that are activated by IFN-γ. This element has been given a variety of acronyms, including γ-response region (GRR) or IFN-γ activation sequence (GAS) *(11,12)*. IFN-α/β can also activate GRR-regulated genes such as IRF-1 *(13)*. Interferon-stimulated gene factors (ISGFs), later termed Stats, bind to the enhancers in the promoters of IFN-α/β- and IFN-γ-induced genes to mediate transcription *(10,14)*. Stats are required for the activation of early response genes by interferons and are posttranslationally modified through tyrosine phosphorylation. Subsequently, they translocate to the nucleus where they interact with enhancers. The Jak family of tyrosine kinases (Jak1, Jak2 Jak3, and Tyk2) are also an integral component in these signaling cascades *(15)*. A model that reflects our knowledge of this process as it relates to IFN-α/β signaling is shown in Fig. 1.

The receptor that binds type 1 interferons consists of two subunits termed IFNAR1 and IFNAR2. IFNAR2 is expressed in three isoforms (IFNAR2a, IFNAR2b, and IFN-AR2c) that contain cytoplasmic domains of different lengths *(16,17)*. Only IFNAR2c allows for IFN-α/β activation of the Jak/Stat pathway. Both subunits appear to bind type 1 interferons. Tyk2 is constitutively associated with IFNAR1, whereas Jak1, Stat1, and Stat2 bind IFNAR2. Upon binding of ligand, IFNAR1 and IFNAR2 heterodimerize, followed by Tyk2 and Jak1 activation, presumably as a consequence of transphosphorylation. Activated Jak1 and Tyk2 can then phosphorylate both subunits of the receptor. Tyrosine phosphorylated receptors provide docking sites for the SH2 domains of Stat proteins. Although this appears to be a common mechanism to recruit Stats to activated cytokine receptors, it is clear that, in many cases, including Stat activation by IFN-α/β, it is unnecessary for the receptor to undergo tyrosine phosphorylation in order for the cascade to function *(18,19)*. Under such circumstances, another signaling component may recruit Stats into the complex. For example, it has been reported that tyrosine phosphorylated Jak2 can serve as a docking site for Stat5 in cells triggered with IL-6 *(20)*. The fact that Stat1 and Stat2 interact with IFNAR2 in the absence of ligand implies that other domains in addition to the SH2 domains of these Stats can interact with the receptor *(21)*.

In addition to the Jaks and Stats, several other kinases and phosphatases associate with the type 1 IFN receptor, as well as with other cytokine receptors. The SH2 domain-containing tyrosine phosphatases SHP-1 and SHP-2 interact with IFNAR1 and appear to function as negative and positive regulators of IFN-α/β signaling, respectively *(22,23)*. Raf-1 (unpublished results), Erk2 *(24)*, arginine methyltransferase *(25)*, PKA *(26)* and

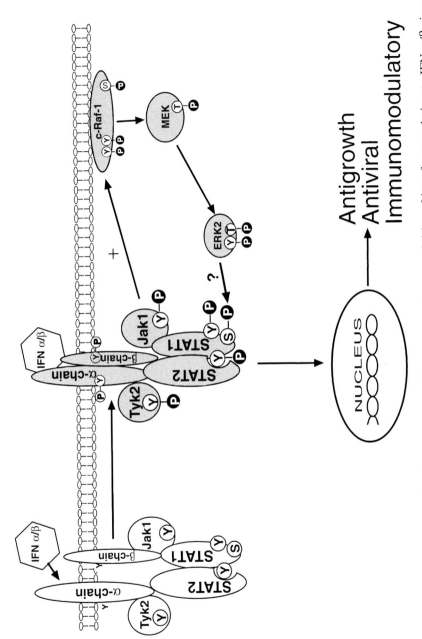

Fig. 1. Model of the antiviral, antigrowth and immunomodulatory activities of interferons relating to IFN-α/β signaling.

phosphatidylinositol 3-kinase *(27)* are also components of this signaling complex. The tyrosine phosphatase CD45, and the tyrosine kinases Lck and ZAP-70 associate with IFNAR1 in a ligand-dependent manner in primary lymphocytes and Jurkat cells *(28)*. The function of these proteins with respect to the biological actions of IFN-α/β is addressed later in this chapter.

In summary, evidence indicates that IFN-α/β and other cytokine receptors exist in preformed complexes before ligand binding. The role of some of these proteins in the biological actions of this cytokine have been elucidated, whereas the function of others remains unknown. Subsequent reactions that occur as a result of ligand binding are more appropriately viewed as events that are not diffusion controlled, but rather regulated by solid-state chemistry.

3. IFN ACTIVATION OF THE Stat-PROTEINS

Stat1 and Stat2 were purified and cloned as the regulatory component of the ISRE binding complex ISGF3 *(29,30)*. Whereas Stat1 is the primary Stat protein that undergoes tyrosine phosphorylation in response to IFN-γ, both Stat1 and Stat2 become tyrosine phosphorylated in response to IFN-α/β *(31–37)*. In certain cells IFN stimulation can also result in the tyrosine phosphorylation of Stat3, Stat4 and Stat5 *(38–40)*. Phosphopeptide mapping showed that IFN-γ and IFN-α/β-induced phosphorylation of Stat1 on tyrosine 701 and that a tyrosine in Stat2 (Y-690) adjacent to a relatively similar sequence becomes phosphorylated by IFN-α/β treatment *(41,42)*. Stat3, Stat4, Stat5a, Stat5b, and Stat6 also contain a conserved tyrosine in their C-terminus which is phosphorylated upon incubation of cells with the appropriate cytokine. After Stats are tyrosine phosphorylated they form homo- or heterodimers via their SH2 domains, which allows them to bind DNA *(43)*. A domain required for Stat1 and Stat3 to bind DNA has been located between residues 400 and 500 *(44)*. Under circumstances in which adjacent DNA binding sites are present in a promoter, Stats can also form multimers *(45)*. Recently the crystal structure of tyrosine-phosphorylated Stat1-bound to DNA has been elucidated *(126)*. The Stat1 dimer forms a c-shaped clamp around DNA that is stabilized by interactions between the SH2 domain of one monomer and the phosphorylated tyrosine of the other monomer *(126)*.

Although it has been appreciated for several years that Stat proteins require tyrosine phosphorylation for dimerization and DNA binding, recent evidence suggests that unphosphorylated Stat1 can also control the expression of certain genes *(46)*. Stat1-deficient cells are insensitive to TNF-α-induced apoptosis and express certain caspase family members (ICE, Cpp32, and Ich-1) at 10- to 15-fold lower levels than cells reconstituted with wild-type Stat1 or with Stat1 (Y701F) *(46)*. A functional Stat1 is also required for IFN and oncostatin M to activate the serine kinase Raf-1 *(47)*, since Stat1 (Y701F) is unable to reconstitute cytokine activation of Raf-1. The mechanisms by which constitutive expression of Stat1 and possibly other Stats functions to regulate gene expression and/or activation of other signaling cascades is unclear.

The mechanisms by which tyrosine phosphorylated Stat proteins when bound to DNA stimulate the transcription of cellular genes is also not well defined. Both Stat1 and Stat2 bind to the general transcriptional coactivators p300 and CBP *(48–50)*. These proteins appear to open chromatin near transcriptional start sites and link enhancer binding factors to the basal transcriptional machinery. Several other transcriptional activators synergize with Stat proteins. Examples include the apparent function of the glucocorticoid receptor as a transcriptional coactivator of Stat5 *(51)*. SP1, which has a binding site adjacent to a GAS element in the ICAM promoter interacts with tyrosine phosphorylated Stat1 *(52)*. Stat3 reportedly enhances the transcriptional effects of c-jun *(53)*, and Stat 6 forms a direct association with NFκB, resulting in synergistic transcriptional activation of an interleukin-4 inducible reporter gene *(54)*.

Two other experimental approaches have provided further information regarding the components required for IFN activation of Stat proteins. The selection of cell lines defective in either IFN-α/β or IFN-γ signaling allowed for the reconstitution of IFN signaling in these lines with cDNAs encoding the defective proteins (for review, see 55). The first mutant (U1) defective in IFNα signaling was rescued by complementation with the protein tyrosine kinase Tyk2 *(56)*. This observation not only provided evidence for a functional role for Tyk2, but also suggested that other tyrosine kinases structurally related to Tyk2 (Jak1, Jak2, and Jak3) may function in a similar manner. Subsequently, several other mutants have been rescued by cDNAs encoding Jak1, Jak2, or other components that comprise ISGF3 *(57,58)*.

The other approach was the development of a cell-free system in which IFN-α/β-stimulated Stat binding to the ISRE or GAS was reenacted in either cell homogenates or partially purified plasma membranes *(32,34,59,60)*. The development of a system that permitted formation of ISGF3 in homogenized cells not only provided another indication for the role of tyrosine kinases in activation of this transcription complex, but also shed light on several other essential features of the activation process *(59,60)*. Treatment of a plasma membrane fraction with IFN-α/β activates the DNA binding of Stat1 and Stat2. This result indicated that the preassociated signaling cascade is localized to the plasma membrane. The role of tyrosine phosphatases both in the initiation and in the downregulation of IFN-stimulated Stat1 and Stat2 tyrosine phosphorylation was also inferred from the use of the cell free system *(32,60)*. The two SH2-domain-containing PTPases SHP-1 and SHP-2 are at least in part responsible for initiating and downregulating IFN-α/β activation of the Jak/Stat pathway *(22,23)*. In addition to SHP-1, three other mechanisms have been delineated that suppress cytokine activation of the Jak/Stat pathway. A nuclear tyrosine phosphatase that acts on tyrosine-phosphorylated Stats inactivates Stat-dependent gene expression *(61)*. In addition, there are reports indicating that a ubiquitin-proteosome pathway mediates degradation of IFNγ activated Stat1 and IL-2 activated Stat5 *(62,63)*. A family of seven cytokine-inducible proteins (CIS), all of which contain SH2 domains, act as negative regulators of cytokine action by inactivating the Jak/Stat pathway *(64–67)*. These RNAs, which encode CIS protein, are induced as a result of treatment of cells with a variety of cytokines. CIS proteins bind to either tyrosine phosphorylated receptors, activated Jak kinases, or tyrosine phosphorylated Stats, inactivating each of these essential signaling components *(68)*.

4. MULTIPLE CYTOKINES AND GROWTH FACTORS ACTIVATE THE Jak/Stat PATHWAY

Electrophoretic mobility shift assays with the GRR and related enhancers and Stat1 immunoprecipitations have shown that numerous growth factor receptors with or without intrinsic tyrosine kinase activity can stimulate tyrosine phosphorylation and DNA-binding of Stat1 *(10,69–76).* Table 1 lists the cytokines that use Stat and Jak proteins in their signaling cascades. Cytokine-stimulated formation of complexes that bind to GRR related enhancers occurs very rapidly, followed by their translocation from the cytoplasm to the nucleus *(77–79).* Many genes activated by Stat proteins in response to cytokines such as IFN, interleukin-6 (IL-1), or prolactin are well characterized *(80,81).* However, in other instances, the cellular genes that are presumably regulated by Stat proteins have not been defined. Characterization of such genes is of clear interest in terms of understanding the specificity of cytokine signaling and in obtaining more information about how such proteins mediate their biological actions.

In most cases in which Stat1 is activated by a given mitogen there has also been shown to be Jak kinase involvement in the signaling cascade. The exceptions to this observation include epidermal growth factor (EGF) and platelet-derived growth factor (PDGF), both of which stimulate tyrosine phosphorylation of Stats and Jak1. However, these growth factors are still capable of stimulating tyrosine phosphorylation of Stats in Jak1-deficient cells *(82–84).* It has also been reported that expression of v-src, v-abl, or BCR-Abl and various other oncoproteins and tumor viruses such as HTLV-2 results in constitutive activation of Stat1, Stat3, Stat5, and Stat6 *(85–89).* Expression of some, if not all, of these oncoproteins activates one or several of the Jak kinases, so it remains uncertain whether these oncoproteins phosphorylate Stats directly or do so by activating a Jak. However, a recent report suggests that the two pathways can, in fact, be separated *(90).*

5. PHYSIOLOGIC ROLES FOR THE Jak KINASES AND Stat TRANSCRIPTION FACTORS

In addition to cell lines lacking individual Jak kinases or Stat proteins, mice with targeted deletions of Stat1, 4, 5a, 5b, and 6 have been described *(91–103).* Table 2 summarizes the phenotypes of these mice. Most of the defects reflect the biological activities of the primary cytokines that activate the given Jak or Stat. For example, some of the most potent activators of Stat1 are IFN-γ and IFN-α. Consequently Stat1-null mice are very sensitive to viral infections and resistant towards the antiviral actions of IFNs *(91,92).* HT1080 human fibrosarcoma cells which do not express Stat1 are also insensitive to the antiviral and antigrowth effects of interferons *(104,105).* However, Stat1 is activated by many other cytokines in cell culture, yet Stat1-null mice raised in a pathogen-free environment appear to be normal. Therefore, it is surprising that it has no obligatory role in mouse development. Like Stat1 knockout mice, targeted deletions in Stat4, Stat5a, Stat5b, and Stat6 lead to well-defined defects consistent with the function of the cytokines which are regulate their activation. Stat3-null mice display embryonic lethality and die before gastrulation *(106).* It is interesting to note that it has been reported that Stat3 can function as an oncogene, and is required for cell transformation by oncogenic src, ros, and insulin-like growth factor-1 *(127–130).* Drosophila appear to express a single Stat protein (Stat92). Expression of this protein occurs in embryonic development a targeted deletion of Stat92 *(marelle)* also results in an embryonic lethal phenotype *(107,108).* A Stat-like protein has also been decribed in *Dictyostelium discoideum,* where it is required for prestalk cell differentiation *(109).*

Table 1
JAK STAT Components Implicated in the Signaling Response Induced by the Indicated Cytokines and Growth Factors

Ligands	JAKs				STATs					
	JAK1	TYK2	JAK2	JAK3	1α/β	2	3	4	5α/β	6
IFN family										
IFN-α/β	+	+	−	−	+	+	+	+	+	−
IFNγ	+	−	+	−	+	−	−	−	+	−
IL-10	+	+	−	−	+	−	+	−	+	−
gp130 family										
LIF	+	+	+	−	+	−	+	−	−	−
IL-6	+	+	+	−	+	−	+	−	−	−
IL-11	+	−	−	−	+	−	+	−	−	−
IL12	−	+	+	−	−	−	+	+	−	−
CNTF	+	+	+	−	+	−	+	−	−	−
OSM	+	+	+	−	+	−	+	−	−	−
CT-1	+	+	+	−	−	−	+	−	−	−
Leptin	−	−	+	+	+	−	+	−	−	−
γ-C family										
IL-1	+	−	−	+	+	−	+	−	+	−
IKL-4	+	−	+	+	−	−	−	−	−	+
IL-7	+	−	−	+	−	−	−	−	+	−
IL-9	+	−	−	+	−	−	−	−	+	−
IL-13	+	+	+	−	+	−	+	−	+	+
IL-15	+	−	−	+	−	−	−	−	+	−
β-chain family										
IL-3	−	−	+	−	−	−	−	−	+	−
IL-5	−	−	+	−	−	−	−	−	+	−
GM-CSF	−	−	+	−	+	−	+	−	+	+
Homodimer receptors										
EPO	−	−	+	−	−	−	−	−	+	−
G-CSF	+	+	+	−	+	−	−	−	+	−
GH	+	−	+	−	+	−	+	−	+	−
PRL	+	+	+	−	+	−	−	−	+	−
TPO	+	+	+	−	+	−	+	−	+	−
Receptor tyrosine kinases (RTKs)										
EGF	+	−	+	−	+	−	+	−	−	−
Eyk	+	−	−	−	+	−	+	−	−	−
FGF	−	−	−	−	+	−	+	−	−	−
PDGF	+	+	+	−	+	−	+	−	+	+
CSF-1	+	−	+	−	+	−	+	−	−	−
c-kit	−	−	+	−	+	−	−	−	−	−
vSis (via PDGFR activation)					−	−	+	−	−	−
Other receptors										
TNF	+	+	+	−	+	−	+	−	+	+
HTLV1	+	−	−	+	+	−	+	−	+	−
AngII	−	+	+	−	+	−	+	−	+	+
lipopolysaccharide and IL-1 (and IL-6)					uncharacterized "LIL STAT" activation					
Nonreceptor tyrosine kinases										
Abl	+	−	+	−	−	−	−	−	+	−
v-Src	−	−	−	−	−	−	+	−	+	−
c-Fes (v-Fps)	−	−	−	−	−	−	+	−	−	−
Bmx	−	−	−	−	+	−	+	−	+	−
Lck	+	−	+	−	−	−	+	−	+	−
polyomavirus middle T-antigen (activites Src family kinases)					−	+	−	−	−	

Table 2
Phenotypes Expressed in Organisms with Targeted Disruptions of Jaks and Stats

Disrupted gene	Species	Phenotype
Stat	Drosophila	Abnormal expression of pair rule genes, such as *even-skipped*
Stat	Dictyostelium discoideum	Disruptions in prestalk cell differentiation
Stat1	Mouse	Highly sensitive to microbial and bacterial infections; no developmental abnormalities
Stat3	Mouse	Early embryonic lethal
Stat4	Mouse	Disrupted T_H1 cell function
Stat5a	Mouse	Disrupted mammary gland development and lactogenesis
Stat5b	Mouse	Disrupted mammary gland development and lactogenesis
Stat6	Mouse	Disrupted T_H2 cell function
Jak	Mouse	Disrupted embryonic patterning, cell proliferation (hematopoietic)
Jak1	Mouse	Perinatal lethal, failure to nurse
Jak2	Mouse	Embryonic lethal, absence of definitive erythropoiesis
Jak3	Mouse	Defects in B lymphocyte maturation
Jak3	Human	X-linked severe combined immunodeficiency-like syndrome with defects in B-cell signaling.

Jak1$^{-/-}$, Jak2$^{-/-}$, and Jak3$^{-/-}$ mice have also been generated *(98,100–103)*. Jak3-null mice display a severe block in B-cell development at the pre-B stage. Although these animals have small thymuses, their T-cell development is relatively normal. Mutations in Jak3 in humans leads to a phenotype similar to X-linked severe combined immunedeficiency with impaired B-cell signaling *(99)*. Disruption of the Jak2 gene causes embryonic lethality as a result of defects in erythropoiesis *(102,103)*. Although primative myeloid progenitors are found in liver, evidence suggests that these cells can not respond to IL-3, granulocyte/macrophage colony-stimulating factor (CSF) or IFN-γ. It is interesting to note that the Jak homologue in drosophila *(hopscotch)* is involved in both embryonic patterning and cell proliferation. A gain-of-function mutation in *hopscotch* leads both to the formation of melanotic tumors and to hypertrophy of larval lymph glands that represent the *Drosophila* hematopoietic organs *(110,111)*. Jak1-deficient mice are runted at birth, fail to nurse, and die perinatally. Cells from these mice do not respond to receptors that use the γ_c subunit or gp130 subunits for signaling.

6. ROLE OF OTHER SIGNALING CASCADES IN REGULATION OF IFN-STIMULATED EARLY RESPONSE GENES

Several reports indicate that IFN-α can activate signaling cascades that are distinct from the Jak/Stat pathway. Treatment of cells with IFN-α activates the cytosolic form of phospholipase A_2 *(112)*, certain isoforms of protein kinase C (PKC) *(113)*, induces an association of the p85 subunit of PI3-kinase with IRS-1 *(114)* and increase intracellular concentrations of inositol trisphosphate *(115)*. The GTP exchange protein Vav, and the adaptor proteins IRS1, Cbl, and CrkL are also tyrosine phosphorylated in response to treatment of certain cells with IFN-α *(116–118)*. The aforementioned studies indicate that IFN treatment modifies a number of signaling proteins known to function in cascades that are distinct from the Jak/Stat pathway. However, the role of IFN-α stimulation of these enzymes and subsequent phosphorylation of downstream substrates in the biological actions of this cytokine is unclear. Several reports provide convincing evidence that IFN activation of the Jak/Stat pathway is not sufficient by itself to account for the biological actions of either IFN-γ and IFN-α. Results from Kerr's laboratory indicate that whereas a kinase inactive mutant of Jak1 can sustain IFN-γ-inducible Stat activation and Stat-regulated gene expression, it does not allow for the antiviral activity of this cytokine *(119)*. It has also been demonstrated that certain deletions of the IFNAR2 receptor that do not effect IFN-β activation of the Jak/Stat pathway result in the loss of the antiviral activity of IFN-β *(120)*. Interestingly, in these lines where the antiviral activity of IFNβ is lost, the antiviral activity of IFN-α is maintained suggesting that the antiviral actions of IFN-α and IFN-β can also be distiguished even though both ligands bind the same receptor. Petricoin and colleagues reported that, in primary T cells, IFN-α induces the rapid association of components involved in T-cell receptor signaling such as the tyrosine kinases Lck and ZAP-70 and the tyrosine phosphatase CD45 with the alpha chain of the IFN-α receptor (IFNAR1). Although the absence of ZAP-70, Lck, or CD45 did not effect IFN-α stimulation of the Jak/Stat pathway and its antiviral activity, the antiproliferative effects of IFN-α were completely abrogated in cell lines missing one of these enzymes. Reconstitution of CD45, Lck or ZAP-70 activity in cells deficient in expression of these signaling components restored the antiproliferative actions of IFN-α. Although the downstream substrates modified by CD45, Lck, and ZAP-70 have not been defined, these studies provide evidence for an IFN-α activated signaling cascade in T cells that requires components of the T-cell receptor for this cytokine to exert its antiproliferative actions T cells. They also support the hypothesis that IFN-α/β activation of the Jak/Stat pathway is not sufficient by itself for the biological activities of this cytokine.

Another well-characterized "alternative" signaling cascade regulated by IFNs is the p42MAP kinase pathway. Although it was initially thought that cytokine activation of the Jak/Stat and Raf/MEK/MAPK signaling cascades were independent events, several reports have clearly shown that these two pathways are intimately linked *(24,121–124)*. Stat1β lacking the 39-amino acids at its C-terminus failed to support the expression of IFN-γ stimulated genes *(125)*. A serine residue located at position 727 in Stat1 α was shown to be phosphorylated in response to IFNs. Mutation of S727 decreased activation of several Stat-regulated genes by IFN-γ *(123)* and also abrogated its antiviral and antiproliferative effects *(104,105)*. Serine 727 of Stat1 α is conserved in Stat3 and Stat4, and is a consensus site for proline-directed serine kinases such as MAP kinases. Studies from this lab have demonstrated that IFNs rapidly stimulate p42 MAP kinase activity and its association with both the IFNAR1 receptor and Stat1 α *(24)*. In addition, expression of dominant-negative forms of p42 MAPK inhibits stimulation of luciferase reporter constructs that contain either GAS or ISRE enhancers by IFN-α/β and IFN-γ *(24)*. IFN-α/β or IFN-γ activates Raf-1 as well as B-Raf, two serine kinases ultimately responsible for the activation of p42MAPK *(124)*. Activation of Raf-1 by IFNs requires both Jak1 and Stat1 *(47,124)*. It appears that activation of MAP kinase is an essential modulator of Stat-mediated gene expression in response to IFNs, and probably to other cytokines as well. Embryonic stem cells derived from mice embryos with targeted deletions of B-Raf indicate that the expression of B-Raf but not Raf-1 is an integral component of the antigrowth and antiviral actions of IFN-α (A.C. Larner, unpublished data). Interestingly, IFN-α stimulation of B-Raf$^{+/+}$ or B-Raf$^{-/-}$ cells results in equivalent stimulation of the Jak/Stat pathway, providing yet another example for additional signaling cascades in the biological actions of this cytokine.

7. CONCLUSIONS

The purification and cloning of Stat proteins, and the discovery that they are tyrosine phosphorylated in a Jak kinase-dependent manner in reponse to numerous cytokines and growth factors has defined a new signaling cascade whose biological functions are still being fully delineated. The development of both cell lines and mice with deletions in components of the Jak/Stat pathway have provided an outline for many of the biological effects that are regulated either directly or indirectly by this cascade. However, many questions still need to be addressed, to understand how this signaling cascade modulates the biological effects of such a diverse group of growth regulators. Areas that still need investigation include (1) the mechanism by which certain cytokines activate different Stats in a cell or tissue-specific manner; (2) the mechanisms by which unphosphorylated Stat1 can regulate the expression of proteins that control apoptosis, and whether other "inactive" Stats also regulate gene expressions; (3) the complex interrelationships between activation of the Jak/Stat signaling cascade and several other cascades that are coordinately regulated by the same growth factors; and (4) the mechanism(s) that controls the subcellular distribution of Stat proteins. The merger of the Jak/Stat pathway with many other established signaling cascades that play pivotal roles in the biological actions of many growth factors and cytokines creates exciting opportunities for new discoveries.

REFERENCES

1. Knight E Jr, Korant BD. Fibroblast interferon includes synthesis of four proteins in human fibroblast cells. *Proc Natl Acad Sci USA* 1979; 76:1824–1827.
2. Gupta SL, Rubin BY, Holmes SL. Interferon action: Inductioon of specific proteins in mouse and human cells by homologous interferons. *Proc Natl Acad USA* 1979; 76:4817–4821.
3. Farrell PJ, Broeze RJ, Lengyel P. Accumulation of an mRNA and protein in interferon-treated Ehrlich ascites tumour cells. *Nature* 1979; 279:523–525.
4. Weil J, Epstein J, Epstein LB, Sedmak JJ, Sabran JL, Grossberg SE. A unique set of polypeptides is induced by γ interferon in addition to those induced in common with α and β interferons. *Nature* 1983; 301:437–439.
5. Hovanessian AG, Meurs E, Aujean O, Vaquero C, Stefanos S, Falcoff E. Antiviral response and induction of specific proteins in cells treated with immune t (type II) interferon analogous to that from viral interferon (type I)-treated cells. *Virology* 1980; 104:195–204.
6. Rubin BY, Gupta SL. Interferon-induced proteins in human fibroblasts and development of the antiviral state. *J Virol* 1980; 34:446–454.
7. Ladoux A, Abita J-P, Geny B. Retinoic-acid-induced differentiation of HL-60 cells is associated with biphasic activation of the Na$^+$-K$^+$ pump. *Differentiation* 1986; 33:142–147.

8. Larner AC, Jonak G, Cheng Y-SE, Korant B, Knight E, Darnell JE. Transcriptional induction of two genes in human cells by β interferon. *Proc Natl Acad Sci USA* 1984; 81:6733–6737.

9. Friedman RL, Manley SP, McMahon M, Kerr IM, Stark GR. Transcriptional and posttranscriptional regulation of interferon-induced gene expression in human cells. *Cell* 1984; 38:745–755.

10. Larner AC, Finbloom DS. Protein tyrosine phosphorylation as a mechanism which regulates cytokine activation of early response genes. *Biochim Biophys Acta* 1995; 1266:278–287.

11. Lew DJ, Decker T, Strehlow I, Darnell JE. Overlapping elements in the guanylate-binding protein gene promoter mediate transcriptional induction by alpha and gamma interferons. *Mol Cell Biol* 1991; 11:182–191.

12. Pearse RN, Feinman R, Ravetch JV. Characterization of the promoter of the human gene encoding the high-affinity IgG receptor: Transcriptional induction by γ interferon is mediated through common DNA response elements. *Proc Natl Acad Sci USA* 1991; 88:11,305–11,309.

13. Haque SJ, Williams BRG. Identification and Characterization of an interferon (IFN)-stimulated response element-IFN-stimulated gene factor 3-independent signaling pathway for IFN-α. *J Biol Chem* 1994; 269:19,523–19,529.

14. Darnell JE, Kerr IM, Stark GR. Jak-STAT pathways and transcriptional activation in response to IFNs and other extracellular signaling proteins. *Science* 1994; 264:1415–1421.

15. Ihle JN, Witthuhn BA, Quelle FW, Yamamoto K, Thierfelder WE, Kreider B, Silvennoinen O. Signaling by the cytokine receptor superfamily: JAKS and STATS. *Trends Biochem* 1994; 19:222–227.

16. Novick D, Cohen B, Rubinstein M. The human interferon α/β receptor: Characterization and molecular cloning. *Cell* 1994; 77:391–400.

17. Domanski P, Witte M, Kellum M, Rubinstein M, Hackett R, Pitha P, Colamonici OR. Cloning and expression of a long form of the β-subunit of the interferon α/β receptor that is required for signaling. *J Biol Chem* 1995; 270:21,606–21,611.

18. Wang Y-D, Wong K, Wood WI. Intracellular tyrosine residues of the growth hormone receptor are not required for the signaling of proliferation of Jak-STAT activation. *J Biol Chem* 1995; 270:7021–7024.

19. Hackett RH, Wang Y-D, Larner AC. Mapping of the cytoplasmic domain of the human growth hormone receptor required for the activation fo Jak2 and Stat proteins. *J Biol Chem* 1995; 270:21,326–21,330.

20. Fujitani Y, Hibi M, Fukada T, Takahashi-Tezuka M, Yoshida H, Yamaguchi T, Sugiyama K, Yamanaka Y, Nakajima K, Hirano T. An alternative pathway for STAT activation that is mediated by the direct inteaction between JAK and STAT. *Oncogene* 1997; 14:751–761.

21. Li X, Leung S, Ker IM, Stark GR. Functional subdomains of STAT2 required for preassociation with the alpha interferon receptor and for signaling. *Mol Cell Biol* 1997; 17:2048–2056.

22. David M, Zhou G, Pine R, Dixon JE, Larner AC. The SH2-domain containing tyrosine phosphatase PTP1D is required for IFNα/β-induced gene expression. *J Biol Chem* 1996; 271:15,862–15,865.

23. David M, Chen HE, Goelz S, Larner AC, Neel BG. Differential regulation of the IFNα/β-stimulated Jak/Stat pathway by the SH2-domain containing tyrosine phosphatase SHPTP1. *Mol Cell Biol* 1995; 15:7050–7058.

24. David M, Petricoin EF, III, Benjamin C, Pine R, Weber MJ, Larner AC. Requirement for MAP kinase (ERK2) activity in interferonα/β-stimulated gene expression through Stat proteins. *Science* 1995; 269:1721–1723.

25. Abramovich C, Yakobson B, Chebath J, Revel M. A protein-arginine methyltransferase binds to the intracytoplasmic domain of the IFNaR1 chain in the type 1 interferon receptor. *EMBO J* 1997; 16:260–266.

26. David M, Petricoin E, Larner AC. Activation of protein kinase A inhibits IFN induction of the Jak/Stat/Pathway in U266 cells. *J Biol Chem* 1996; 271:4585–4588.

27. Pfeffer LM, Mullersman JE, Pfeffer SR, Murti A, Shi W, Yang CH. STAT3 as an adapter to couple phosphatidylinositol 3-kinase to the IFNAR1 chain of the type1 interferon receptor. *Science* 1997; 276:1418–1420.

28. Petricoin EF, 111, Ito S, Williams BL, Audet S, Stancato LF, Gamero A, Clouse K, Grimley P, Weiss A, Beeler J, Finbloom DS, Shores EW, Abraham R, Larner AC. Antiproliferative action of interferon-α requires components of T-cell receptor signalling. *Nature* 1997; 390:629–632.

29. Fu X-Y, Schindler C, Improta T, Aebersold R, Darnell JEJ. The proteins of ISGF-3, the interferon α-induced transcriptional activator, define a gene family involved in signal transduction. *Proc Natl Acad Sci USA* 1992; 89:7840–7843.

30. Schindler C, Fu X-Y, Improta T, Aebersold R, Darnell JE Jr. Proteins of transcription factor ISGF-3: One gene encodes the 91- and 84-kDa ISGF-3 proteins that are activated by interferon α. *Proc Natl Acad Sci USA* 1992; 89:7836–7839.

31. Schindler C, Shuai K, Prezioso VR, Darnell JE Jr. Interferon-dependent tyrosine phosphorylation of a latent transcription factor. *Science* 1992; 257:809–813.

32. Igarashi K, David M, Finbloom DS, Larner AC. In vitro activation of the transcription factor gamma interferon activation factor by gamma interferon: Evidence for a tyrosine phosphatase/kinase signaling cascade. *Mol Cell Biol* 1993; 13:1634–1640.

33. Shuai K, Schindler C, Prezioso VR, Darnell JE Jr. Activation of transcription by IFN-γ: Tyrosine phosphorylation of a 91-kD DNA binding protein. *Science* 1992; 258:1808–1812.

34. Igarashi K, David M, Larner AC, Finbloom DS. In vitro activation of a transcription factor by IFNγ requires a membrane associated tyrosine kinase and is mimicked by vanadate. *Mol Cell Biol* 1993; 13:3984–3989.

35. Shuai K, Stark GR, Kerr IM, Darnell JE Jr. A single phosphotyrosine residue of Stat91 required for gene activation by interferonγ. *Science* 1993; 261:1744–1746.

36. McKendry R, John J, Flavell D, Muller M, Kerr IM, Stark GR. High-frequency mutagensis of human cells and characterization of a mutant unresponsive to both α and γ interferons. *Proc Natl Acad Sci USA* 1991; 88:11,455–11,459.

37. Improta T, Schindler C, Horvath CM, Kerr IM, Stark GR, Darnell JE Jr. Transcription factor ISGF-3 formation requires phosphorylated Stat91 protein, but Stat113 protein is phosphorylated independently of Stat91 protein. *Proc Natl Acad Sci USA* 1994; 91:4776–4780.

38. Raz R, Durbin JE, Levy DE. Acute phase response factor and additional members of the interferon-stimulated gene factor 3 family integrate diverse signals from cytokines, interferons, and growth factors. *J Biol Chem* 1994; 269:24,391–24,395.

39. Cho SS, Bacon CM, Sudarshan C, Rees RC, Finbloom D, Pine R, O'Shea JJ. Activation of STAT4 by IL-12 and IFN-α. *J Immunol* 1996; 157:4781–4789.

40. Meinke A, Barahmand-Pour F, Wohrl S, Stoiber D, Decker T. Activation of different Stat5 isoforms contributes to cell-type-restricted signaling in response to interferons. *Mol Cell Biol* 1996; 16:6937–6944.

41. Pellegrini S, John J, Shearer M, Kerr IM, Stark GR. Use of a selectable marker regulated by alpha interferon to obtain mutations in the signaling pathway. *Mol Cell Biol* 1989; 9:4605–4612.

42. John J, McKendry R, Pellegrini S, Flavell D, Kerr IM, Stark GR. Isolation and characterization of a new mutant cell line unresponsive to alpha and beta interferons. *Mol Cell Biol* 1991; 11:4189–4195.

43. Shuai K, Horvath CM, Tsai Huang LH, Qureshi SA, Cowburn D, Darnell JE Jr. Interferon activation of the transcription factor Stat91 involves dimerization through SH2-phosphotyrosyl peptide interactions. *Cell* 1994; 76:821–828.

44. Horvath CM, Wen Z, Darnell JE Jr. A STAT protein domain that determines DNA sequence recognition suggests a novel DNA-binding domain. *Genes Dev* 1995; 9:984–994.

45. Xu X, Sun Y-L, Hoey T. Cooperative DNA binding and sequence—selective recognition conferred by the STAT amino-terminal domain. *Science* 1996; 273:794–797.

46. Kumar A, Commane M, Flickinger TW, Horvath CM, Stark GR. Defective TNF-α-induced apoptosis in STAT1-null cells due to low constitutive levels of caspases. *Science* 1997; 278:1630–1632.

47. Stancato LF, Yu C-R, Petricoin EF III, Larner AC. Activation of Raf-1 by interferon gamma and oncostatin M requires expression of the Stat1 transcription factor. *J Biol Chem* 1998; 273:18,701–18,704.

48. Bhattacharya S, Eckner R, Grossman S, Oldread E, Arany Z, D'Andrea A, Livingston DM. Cooperation of Stat2 and p300/CBP in signalling induced by interferon-α. *Nature* 1996; 383:344–347.

49. Horvai AE, Xu L, Korzus E, Brard G, Kalafus D, Mullen T-M, Rose DW, Rosenfeld MG, KGC. Nuclear integration of JAK/STAT and Ras/AP-1 signaling by CBP and p300. *Proc Natl Acad Sci USA* 1997; 94:1074–1079.

50. Zhang JJ, Vinkemeier U, Gu W, Chakravarti D, Horvath CM, Darnell JE Jr. Two contact regions between Stat1 and CBP/p300 in interferon γ signaling. *Proc Natl Acad Sci USA* 1996; 93:15092–15096.

51. Stocklin E, Wissler M, Gouilleux F, Gronner B. Functional interactions betwen Stat5 and the glucocorticoid receptor. *Nature* 1996; 383:726–728.

52. Look DC, Pelletier MR, Tidwell RM, Roswit RM, Holtzman MJ. Stat1 depends on transcriptional synergy with Sp1. *J Biol Chem* 1995; 270:30,264–30,267.

53. Schaefer TS, Sanders LK, Nathans D. Cooperative transcriptional activity of Jun and Stat3β, a short form of Stat3. *Proc Natl Acad Sci USA* 1995; 92:9097–9101.

54. Shen CH, Stavnezer J. Interaction of STAT6 and NF-κB: Direct association and synergistic activation of IL-4-induced transcription. *Mol Cell Biol* 1998; 18:3395–3404.

55. Leaman DW, Leung S, Li X, Stark GR. Regulation of STAT-dependent pathways by growth factors and cytokines. *FASEB J* 1996; 10:1578–1588.

56. Velazquez L, Fellous M, Stark GR, Pellegrini S. A protein tyrosine Kinase in the interferon α/β signaling pathway. *Cell* 1992; 70:313–322.

57. Watling D, Guschin D, Muller M, Silvennoinen O, Witthuhn BA, Quelle FW, Rogers NC, Schindler C, Ihle JN, Stark GR, Kerr IM. Complementation by the protein tyrosine kinase JAK2 of a mutant cell line defective in the interferon-γ signal transduction pathway. *Nature* 1993; 366:166–170.

58. Muller M, Briscoe J, Laxton C, Guschin D, Ziemiecki A, Silvennoinen O, Harpur AG, Barbieri G, Withuhn BA, Schindler C, Pellegrini S, Wilks AF, Ihle JN, Stark GR, Kerr IM. The protein tyrosine kinase JAK1 complements defects in the interferon-α/β and -γ signal transduction. *Nature* 1993; 366:129–135.

59. David M, Larner AC. Activation of transcription factors by interferon alpha in a cell free system. *Science* 1992; 257:813–815.

60. David M, Romero G, Zhang ZY, Dixon JE, Larner AC. In vitro activation of the transcription factor ISGF3 by IFNα involves a membrane associated tyrosine phosphatase and kinase. *J Biol Chem* 1993; 268:6593–6599.

61. David M, Grimley PM, Finbloom DS, Larner AC. A nuclear tyrosine phosphatase downregulates interferon-induced gene expression. *Mol Cell Biol* 1993; 13:7515–7521.

62. Yu CL, Burakoff SJ. Involvement of proteasomes in regulating Jak/STAT pathways upon interleukin-2 stimulation. *J Biol Chem* 1997; 272:14,017–14,020.

63. Kim TK, Maniatis T. Regulation of interferon-γ-activated STAT1 by the ubiquitin-proteosome pathway. *Science* 1996; 273:1717–1719.

64. Yoshimura A, Ohkubo T, Kiguchi T, Jenkins NA, Gilbert DJ, Copelaand NG, Hara T, Miyajima A. A novel cytokine-inducible gene CIS encodes an SH2-containing protein

that binds tyrosine-phosphorylated interleukin 3 and erythropoietin receptors. *EMBO J* 1995; 14:2816–2826.

65. Starr R, Willson TA, Viney EM, Murray LJL, Rayner JR, Jenkins BJ, Gonda TJ, Alexander WS, Metcalf D, Nicola NA, Hilton DJ. A family of cytokine-inducible inhibitors of signalling. *Nature* 1997; 387:917–921.

66. Endo TA, Masuhara M, Yokouchi M, Suzuki R, Sakamoto H, Mitsui K, Matsumoto A, Tanimura S, Ohtsubo M, Misawa H, Miyazaki T, Leonor N, Taniguchi T, Fujita T, Kanakura Y, Komiya S, Yoshimura A. A new protein containing an SH2 domain that inhibits JAK kinases. *Nature* 1997; 387:921–924.

67. Naka T, Narazaki M, Hirata M, Matsumoto T, Minamoto S, Aono A, Nishimoto N, Kajita T, Taga T, Yoshizaki K, Akira S, Kishimoto T. Structure and function of a new STAT-induced STAT inhibitor. *Nature* 1997; 387:924–929.

68. Javad Aman M, Leonard WJ. Cytokine signaling: cytokine-inducible signaling inhibitors. *Curr Biol* 1997; 7:784–788.

69. Larner AC, David M, Feldman GM, Igarashi K, Hackett RH, Webb DAS, Sweitzer SM, Petricoin EF III, Finbloom DS. Tyrosine phosphorylation of DNA binding proteins by multiple cytokines. *Science* 1993; 261:1730–1733.

70. Fu X-Y, Zhang J-J. Transcription factor p91 interacts with the epidermal growth factor receptor and mediates activation of the c-*fos* gene promoter. *Cell* 1993; 74:1135–1145.

71. Finbloom DS, Petricoin EFI, Hackett RH, David M, Feldman GM, Igarashi K, Fibach E, Weber MJ, Thorner MO, Silva CM, Larner AC. Growth hormone and erythropoietin activate DNA-binding proteins by tyrosine phosphorylation. *Mol Cell Biol* 1994; 14:1477–1486.

72. Silvennoinen O, Schindler C, Schlessinger J, Levy DE. Ras-independent growth factor singaling by transcription factor tyrosine phosphorylation. *Science* 1993; 261:1736–1739.

73. Ruff-Jamison S, Chen K, Cohen S. Induction by EGF and interferon γ of tyrosine phosphory-lated DNA binding protein in mouse liver nuclei. *Science* 1993; 261:1733–1736.

74. Sadowski HB, Shuai K, Darnell JE Jr, Gilman MZ. A common nuclear signal transduction pathway activated by growth factor and cytokine receptors. *Science* 1993; 261:1739–1744.

75. Gilmour KC, Reich NC. Receptor to nucleus signaling by prolactin and interleukin 2 via activation of latent DNA-biinding factors. *Proc Natl Acad Sci USA* 1994; 91:6850–6854.

76. Bonni A, Frank DA, Schindler C, Greenberg ME. Characterization of a pathway for ciliary neurotrophic factor signaling to the nucleus. *Science* 1993; 262:1575–1579.

77. Decker T, Lew DJ, Mirkovitch J, Darnell JE Jr. Cytoplasmic activation of GAF, an IFN-γ-regulated DNA-binding factor. *EMBO J* 1991; 10:927–932.

78. Schindler C, Kashleva H, Pernis A, Pine R, Rothman P. STF-IL4: A novel IL-4-induced signal transducing factor. *EMBO J* 1994; 13:1350–1356.

79. David M, Petricoin EF III, Igarashi K, Feldman GM, Finbloom DS, Larner AC. Prolactin activates the interferon-regulated p91 transcription factor and the Jak2 kinase by tyrosine phosphorylation. *Proc Natl Acad Sci USA* 1994; 91:7174–7178.

80. Wegenka UM, Lutticken C, Buschmann J, Yuan J, Lottspeich F, Muller-Esterl W, Schindler C, Roeb E, Heinrich PC, Horn F. The interleukin-6-activated acute phase response factor is antigenically and functionally related to members of the signal transducer and activator of transcription (STAT) family. *Mol Cell Biol* 1994; 14:3186–3196.

81. Wakao H, Gouilleux F, Groner B. Mammary gland factor (MGF) is a novel member of the cytokine regulated transcription factor gene family and confers prolactin response. *EMBO J* 1994; 13:2182–2191.

82. Leaman DW, Pisharody S, Flickinger TW, Commane MA, Schlessinger J, M KI, Levy DE, Stark GR. Roles of JAKS in activation of STATa and stimulation of c-fos gene expression by epidermal growth factor. *Mol Cell Biol* 1996; 16:369–375.

83. Vignais M-L, Sadowski HB, Watling D, Rogers NC, Gilman M. Platelet-derived growth

factor induces phosphorylation of multiple JAK kinases and STAT proteins. *Mol Cell Biol* 1996; 16:1759–1769.

84. David M, Wong L, Flavell R, Thompson S, Larner AC, Johnson G. STAT activation by EGF and amphiregulin: Requirement for the EGF receptor kinase, but not for tyrosine phosphorylation sites or JAK1. *J Biol Chem* 1996; 271:9185–9188.

85. Yu C-L, Meyer DJ, Campbell GS, Larner AC, Carter-Su C, Schwartz J, Jove R. Enhanced DNA-binding of a Stat3-related protein in cells transformed by the Src oncoprotein. *Science* 1995; 269:81–83.

86. Migone TS, Lin JX, Cereseto A, Mullot JC, O'Shea JJ, Franchini G, Leonard WJ. Constitutively activated Jak/STAT pathway in T cells transformed with HTLV-1. *Science* 1995; 269:79–81.

87. Lund TC, Garcia R, Medveczky M, Jove R, Medveczky PG. Activation of STAT transcription factors by herpes saimiri Tip-484 requires p56^{lck}. *J Virol* 1997; 71:6677–6682.

88. Garcia R, Yu C-L, Hudnall A, Catlett R, Nelson KL, Smithgall T, Fujita DJ, Ethier SP, Jove R. Consitutive activation of Stat3 in fibroblasts transformed by diverse oncoproteins and in breast carcinoma cells. *Cell Growth Diff* 1997; 8:1267–1276.

89. Danial NN, Pernis A, Rothman PB. Jak-STAT signaling induced by the v-*abl* oncogene. *Science* 1995; 269:1875–1877.

90. Chaturvedi P, Ramana Reddy MV, Premkumar Reddy E. Src kinases and not JAKs activate STATs during IL-3 induced myeloid cell proliferation. *Oncogene* 1998; 16:1749–1758.

91. Meraz MA, White JM, Sheehan KCF, Bach EA, Rodig SJ, Dighe AS, Kaplan DH, Riley JK, Greenlund AC, Campbell D, Carver-Moore K, DuBois RN, Clark R, Aguet M, Schreiber RD. Targeted disruption of the *Stat1* gene in mice reveals unexpected physiologic specificity in the JAK-STAT signaling pathway. *Cell* 1996; 84:431–442.

92. Durbin JE, Hackenmiller R, Simon MC, Levy DE. Targeted Disruption of the mouse *Stat1* gene results in compromised innate immunity to viral disease. *Cell* 1996; 84:443–450.

93. Takeda K, Tanaka T, Shi W, Matsumoto M, Minami M, Kashiwamura S, Nakanishi K, Yoshida N, Kishimoto T, Akira S. Essential role of Stat6 in IL-4 signalling. *Nature* 1996; 380:627–630.

94. Thierfelder WE, van Deursen JM, Yamamoto K, Tripp RA, Sarawar SR, Carson RT, Sangster MY, Vignali DAA, Doherty PC, Grosveld GC, Ihle JN. Requirement for Stat4 in interleukin-12-mediated responses of natural killer cells and T cells. *Nature* 1996; 382:171–174.

95. Kaplan MH, Sun Y-L, Hoey T, Grusby MJ. Impaired IL-12 responses and enhanced development of Th2 cells in Stat4-deficient mice. *Nature* 1996; 32:174–177.

96. Liu X, Robinson GW, Wagner K-U, Wynshaw-Boris A, Henninghausen L. Stat5a is mandatory for adult mammary gland development and lactogenesis. *Genes Dev* 1997; 11:179–186.

97. Udy GB, Towers RP, Snell RG, Wilkens RJ, Park S-H, Ram PA, Waxman DJ, Davey HW. Requirement of Stat5b for sexual dimorphism of body growth rates and liver gene expression. *Proc Natl Acad Sci USA* 1997; 94:7239–7244.

98. Nosaka T, A vDJM, Tripp RA, Thierfelder WE, Witthun BA, McMickle AP, Doherty PC, Grosveld GC, Ihle JN. Defective lymphoid development in mice lacking Jak3. *Science* 1995; 270:800–802.

99. Russell SM, Tayebi N, Nakajima H, Riedy MC, Roberts JL, Aman MJ, Migone T-S, Noguchi M, Markert ML, Buckley RH, O'Shea JJ, Leonard WJ. Mutation of Jak3 in a patient with SCID: Essential role of Jak3 in lymphoid development. *Science* 1995; 270:797–800.

100. Thomis DC, Gurniak CB, Tivol E, Sharpe AH, Berg LJ. Defects in B lymphocyte maturation and T lymphocyte activation in mice lacking Jak3. *Science* 1995; 270:794–797.

101. Rodig SJ, Meraz MA, White JM, Lampe PA, Riley JK, Arthur CD, King KL, Sheehan KCF, Yin L, Pennica D, Johnson EM Jr, Schreiber RD. Disruption of the Jak1 gene

demonstrates obligatory and nonredundant roles of the Jaks in cytokine-induced biological responses. *Cell* 1998; 93:373–383.

102. Parganas E, Wang D, Stravopodis D, Topham DJ, ChristopheMarine J, Teglund S, Vanin EF, Bodner S, Colamonici OR, van Deursen JM, Grosveld G, Ihle JN. Jak2 is essential for signaling through a variety of cytokine receptors. *Cell* 1998; 93:385–395.

103. Neubauer H, Cumano A, Muller M, Wu H, Huffstadt U, Pfeffer K. Jak2 deficiency defines an essential developmental checkpoint in definitive hematopoiesis. *Cell* 1998; 93:397–409.

104. Horvath CM, Darnell JE Jr. The antiviral state induced by alpha interferon and gamma interferon requires transcriptionally active Stat1 protein. *J Virol* 1996; 70:647–650.

105. Bromberg JF, Horvath CM, Wen Z, Schreiber RD, Darnell JE Jr. Transcriptionally active Stat1 is required for the antiproliferative effects of both interferon α and interferon γ. *Proc Natl Acad Sci USA* 1996; 93:7673–7678.

106. Tekeda K, Noguchi K, Shi W, Tanaka T, Matsumoto M, Yoshida N, Kishimoto T, Akira S. Targeted disruption of the mouse *Stat3* gene leads to early embryonic lethality. *Proc Natl Acad Sci USA* 1997; 94:3801–3804.

107. Hou XS, Meinick MB, Perrimon N. *marelle* Acts downstream of the *Drosophila* HOP/JAK kinase and encodes a protein similar to the mammalian STATs. *Cell* 1996; 84:411–419.

108. Yan R, Small S, Desplan C, Dearolf CR, Darnell JE Jr. Identification of a Stat gene that functions in *Drosophila* development. *Cell* 1996; 84:421–430.

109. Kawata T, Shevchenko A, Fukuzawa M, Jermyn KA, Totty NF, Zhukovskaya NV, Sterling AE, Mann M, Williams JG. SH2 Signaling in a lower eukaryote: A STAT protein that regulates stalk cell differentiation in *Dictyostelium*. *Cell* 1997; 89:909–916.

110. Binari R, Perrimon N. Stripe-specific regulation of pair rule genes by hopscotch, a putative Jak family tyrosine kinase in *Drosophila*. *Genes Dev* 1994; 8:300–312.

111. Luo H, Hanratty WP, Dearolf CR. An amino acid substitution in the *Drosophila* hop^{Tum-1} Jak kinase causes leukemia-like hematopoietic defects. *EMBO J* 1995; 14:1412–1420.

112. Flati V, Haque SJ, Williams BRG. Interferon-α-induced phosphorylation and activation of cytosolic phospholipase A$_2$ is required for the formation of interferon-stimulated gene factor three. *EMBO J* 1996; 15:1566–1571.

113. Pfeffer LM, Strulovici B, Saltiel AR. Interferon-α selectively activates the β isoform of protein kinase C through phosphatidylcholine hydrolysis. *Proc Natl Acad Sci USA* 1990; 87:6537–6541.

114. Uddin S, Yenush L, Sun X-J, Sweet ME, White MF, Platanias LC. Interferon-α engages the insulin receptor substrate-1 to associate with the phosphatidylinositol 3′-kinase. *J Biol Chem* 1995; 270:15,938–15,941.

115. Yap WH, Teo TS, Tan YH. An early event in the interferon-induced transmembrane signaling process. *Science* 1986; 234:355–358.

116. Platanias LC, Sweet ME. Interferon α induces rapid tyrosine phosphorylation of the *vav* proto-oncogene product in hematopoietic cells. *J Biol Chem* 1994; 269:3143–3146.

117. Platanias LC, Uddin S, Yetter A, Sun XJ, White MF. The type I interferon receptor mediates tyrosine phosphorylation of insulin receptor substrate 2. *J Biol Chem* 1996; 271:278–282.

118. Uddin S, Gardziola C, Dangat A, Yi T, Platanias LC. Interaction of the c-cbl proto-oncogene product with the Tyk-2 protein tyrosine kinase. *Biochem Biophys Res Commun* 1996; 225:833–838.

119. Briscoe J, Rogers NC, Witthuhn BA, Watling D, Harpur AG, Wilks AF, Stark GR, Ihle JN, Kerr IM. Kinase-negative mutants of JAK1 can sustain interferon-γ-inducible gene expression but not an antiviral state. *EMBO J* 1996; 15:799–809.

120. Domanski P, Nadeau OW, Platanias LC, Fish E, Kellum M, Pitha P, Colamonici OR. Differential use of the β$_L$ subunit of the type I interferon (IFN) receptor determines signaling specificity for IFNα2 and IFNβ. *J Biol Chem* 1998; 273:3144–3147.

121. Winston LA, Hunter T. JAK2, Ras, and Raf are required for activation of extracellular

the prevention of cancer development. The generation of *p53*-deficient mice not only supported a role for *p53* as a tumor suppressor, but also demonstrated that p53 function is not essential for normal growth and development, although some subtle abnormalities in the development of the *p53*-deficient mice have since been noted *(28,29)*. Interestingly, generation of mice with p53-inducible reporter gene expression has revealed striking p53-dependent gene expression in some tissues during development, although the contribution of this activity to embryonic development is unclear *(30–32)*. These studies also showed striking age and tissue dependent differences in the DNA damage induced p53 response. In normal cycling cells the very short half-life of p53 keeps the protein levels very low and essentially no p53 function is detected in these cells. It seems that p53 function becomes important when the protein is activated in response to various stress signals and, as such, p53 is thought to act to monitor for potentially oncogenic changes in cells and prevent the growth of abnormal or damaged cells. Clearly, loss of such function might lead to increased tumor incidence because of an inability to eliminate or repair cells in danger of becoming malignant.

One of the most extensively studied activators of the p53 response is DNA damage, and exposure of cells to radiation or DNA damaging drugs leads to a very rapid elevation of p53 and manifestation of p53 function *(26)*. Analysis of both cells in culture and *p53* deficient animals has shown that loss of *p53* results in the accumulation of genetic abnormalities which might arise from the continued replication of cells with damaged DNA, the loss of a direct p53 function in the DNA repair process, or abnormal mitotic divisions resulting from an inability to regulate centromere duplication *(33–36)*.

The ability of p53 to monitor for and prevent the replication of damaged cells could clearly contribute to protection against the acquisition of oncogenic genetic lesions and defend against tumor development. However, it has recently become clear that p53 functions at other stages in carcinogenic progression, and activation by other signals may be of equal importance in tumor progression. In addition to DNA damage, p53 is activated by a broad range of signals that lead to abnormal proliferation, particularly signals mediated by the activation of oncogenes or loss of the function of other tumor suppressor proteins such as pRB *(37–40)*. The molecular basis for this link is discussed later, but such an activity for p53 might eliminate cells that have already begun the process of tumorigenic conversion. Finally, activation of p53 by hypoxia may play a role during later stages of tumor development, as the size of the tumor increases *(41)*. Indeed, p53 itself appears to contribute to the generation of hypoxic conditions within the tumor by negatively regulating angiogenesis, and as such may also prevent the spread of metastases *(42)*.

It is of interest to note that loss of p53 function is not necessarily an initiation event during tumorigenesis, but often occurs at later stages in response to the accumulation of other oncogenic mutations, such as activation of Ras or Myc *(43,44)*. It is therefore likely that loss of p53 contributes to tumor development at a number of steps; in the accumulation of genetic damage, the tolerance of abnormal proliferation and by allowing survival under hypoxic conditions. It is clear that mutation of other components of these pathways could substitute for loss of p53 at some stages of tumor progression, but the ability of p53 to function protectively at several stages during the tumorigenic process may well explain why loss of function of the p53 protein itself is so strongly selected for in such a broad range of cancers.

4. MECHANISMS OF P53 FUNCTION

By far the best understood function of p53 is as a transcription factor, an activity that contributes to both cell cycle arrest and apoptotic functions *(45,46)*. A large number of cellular genes that are potentially transcriptionally regulated by p53 have now been described, although many of these have not yet been verified as bona fide mediators of the p53 response. Furthermore, it is clear that the function of p53 cannot depend on the activation of a single target gene, and the response to p53 is dependent on the coordinate expression of several p53-responsive gene products *(6)*.

Activation of p53 in cycling cells leads to an arrest at both G1 and G2 phases of the cell cycle which is mediated primarily through the transcriptional activation of $p21^{Waf1/Cip1}$, an inhibitor of the cyclin-dependent kinases, which are essential for cell cycle progression *(47)*. Deletion of the $p21^{Waf1/Cip1}$ gene in either mice or a human cell line dramatically impedes the cell cycle arrest response to p53 activation, although the retention of some growth arrest in the mouse cells indicates that other p53-dependent functions can also contribute to this response *(48–50)*. Nevertheless, expression of $p21^{Waf1/Cip1}$ itself results in G1 and G2 arrests indistinguishable from those seen in response to p53. Several other p53-inducible genes may also contribute to the activation of both G1 or G2 arrests, including IGF-BP3, a secreted protein that binds and blocks the activity of the mitogen IGF *(51)*, the 14-3-3 protein which induces a G2 arrest by interfering with the normal activity of CDC25 phosphotase *(52)* and Siah, the human homolog of the *Drosophila* seven in absentia gene *(53)*. In addition to genes directly activated by p53, recent studies have shown that p53 can also participate indirectly in the transcriptional activation of other genes that could participate in mediating a cell cycle arrest. p53-dependent activation of GADD45, a protein which interacts with PCNA and potentially plays a role in signaling cell cycle arrest and DNA repair, is mediated both through direct p53/DNA interactions and through interaction of p53 with WT1, the product of the Wilm's tumor gene *(54)*. WT1 binds sequences in the GADD45 promoter and the WT1/p53 complex stimulates transcription. This added layer of complexity suggests that a number of p53 responsive genes which lack p53 binding sites in their promoters may remain to be identified.

Identification of components of p53's apoptotic response has proved more difficult. In contrast to the role of p21[Waf1/Cip1] in mediating the p53-induced cell cycle arrest, it is clear that expression of this cdk inhibitor does not generally result in cell death and there is some evidence that p21[Waf1/Cip1] may even exhibit an antiapoptotic effect *(55,56)*. One p53 inducible gene with a clear potential contribution to apoptosis is *bax*, encoding a pro apoptotic member of the Bcl2 family *(57)*. Although cells from *bax*-deficient mice are still able to undergo p53-dependent apoptosis *(58)*, illustrating that Bax cannot be the only mediator of this function, a role for Bax is supported by the observation that these cells did show some reduction in apoptotic rate *(59–61)*. Other potential apoptotic targets of p53 include IGF-BP3 *(51)*, which would be expected to inhibit the function of IGF as a survival factor and another novel proapoptotic gene, *PAG608* *(62)*. p53 has also been shown to activate expression of the death receptors Fas/Apo1 and DR5, which would result in sensitization of the cell to extracellular death promoting signals. *(63)*. A less specific mechanism for p53-induced apoptosis has also been suggested by the observation that several genes that are activated in a p53-dependent manner are involved in generating or responding to oxidative stress, and it is possible that p53 induces apoptosis by generating reactive oxygen species within the cell *(64)*.

Despite the clear contribution of transcriptional activation of apoptotic targets to p53-induced apoptosis, several observations suggest that p53 may contribute to an apoptotic signal by mechanisms distinct from its function as a transcription factor. One activity of p53 that has been suggested to play a role in mediating the apoptotic signal is the ability to function as a transcriptional repressor *(65,66)*. Although many promoters have been shown to be repressed by p53, interpretation of these data is complicated by the observation that the apoptotic response to p53 may in itself lead to down-regulation of expression from these promoters *(67)*. Nevertheless, it is clear that p53 can repress expression of some cellular genes, although the contribution of this activity to mediating a p53 response remains to be determined. p53 also shows apoptotic activities that are entirely transcriptionally independent and are likely to reflect direct interaction of p53 with other proteins *(68,69)*. The proline rich domain towards the N-terminus of p53 may mediate interactions with SH3 domain-containing proteins and deletion of this region impairs the growth suppressive activity of p53, although whether this reflects loss of cell cycle arrest or apoptotic activity is not yet clear *(70,71)*. Numerous proteins have been shown to interact with p53, including SH3 domain containing proteins such as Abl *(72)* and p53-BP2 *(73)*, although the consequences of these interactions remain unclear.

Sequences in the extreme C-terminus of p53 have also been shown to contribute to the apoptotic response. Several components of the transcription-repair complex TFIIH have been shown to bind to this region of p53 with evidence that this interaction can contribute to cell death *(74,75)*. Overall, however, there is no clear consensus on how transcriptionally independent activities of p53 contribute to cell death, or even what the relative contribution of such activities are to the overall function of p53 as a tumor suppressor.

5. CHOICE OF RESPONSE: GROWTH ARREST OR APOPTOSIS

The identification of distinct groups of cell cycle arrest and apoptotic target genes for p53 indicated that these are independent functions of p53 and that apoptosis is not simply the consequence of cell cycle arrest. Several p53 mutants that retain the ability to induce cell cycle arrest, but that fail to activate apoptosis, have now been described *(67,76)*. These mutants show interesting promoter selectivity in that they remain capable of activating expression of $p21^{Waf1/Cip1}$ (a cell cycle arrest target for p53) but show varying degrees of loss of the ability to activate expression of *bax* and *IGF-BP3* (both potential apoptotic targets of *p53*) *(67,77,78)*. The observation that several tumor-associated p53 mutants retain the ability to induce cell cycle arrest but lose apoptotic function suggests that it is the apoptotic activity of p53 that is of primary importance in tumor suppression.

Not all cells respond to p53 by undergoing both cell cycle arrest and apoptosis, and it is clear that cell type, extent of DNA damage, the accumulation of other oncogenic abnormalities and cell environment can all contribute to the choice of response. It seems likely that the first response to p53 is a cell cycle arrest, because the $p21^{Waf1/Cip1}$ promoter shows a very high affinity for p53, and expression of $p21^{Waf1/Cip1}$ is activated by very low levels of p53. Higher levels of p53, mediated perhaps by sustained or more extensive stress or damage, would further activate apoptotic targets leading to cell death *(79)*. The presence of survival factors can also influence the response to *p53*, and protection from apoptotic death after treatment with survival factors reveals the underlying cell cycle arrest *(80–82)*. In some cells, survival factor-mediated rescue from p53-induced death has been shown to be mediated through Jak kinase-dependent pathways *(83)*. Perhaps of greatest interest in terms of using p53 in tumor therapy is the observation that cells that have undergone additional oncogenic changes, such as loss of the pRB tumor suppressor protein, show enhanced apoptosis in response to p53 activation *(39,84,85)*. This raises the appealing possibility that activation of p53 would kill tumor cells but induce only a reversible cell cycle arrest in normal cells.

6. REGULATION OF p53 ABUNDANCE AND ACTIVITY

6.1. p53 Stability

Activation of a p53 response by DNA damage, proliferative abnormalities, or hypoxia is accompanied by a rapid increase in the intracellular levels of p53, as a result of both increased protein half-life and enhanced translation *(86)*. p53 is normally very rapidly degraded through ubiquitin-dependent proteolysis and recent studies have shown that the Mdm2 protein is a key component of this pathway *(87,88)*. Mdm2 is the product of a p53-inducible gene, which, unlike the other p53 targets, plays no clear role in mediating downstream effects of p53 *(89)*. The importance of Mdm2 is in the regulation of p53 activity itself, and Mdm2 inhibits both p53 transcriptional activity directly by binding to the N-terminal transactivation domain of p53, as well as targeting p53 for degradation through the proteasome *(87,88,90)*. The importance of Mdm2 in this negative feedback loop of p53 function is illustrated by mice deleted of the *Mdm2* gene, which show an extremely early embryonic lethality unless simultaneously deleted for *p53 (91,92)*. The complete rescue of this lethality by loss of p53 suggests that the principal role of Mdm2 during development is to control p53 activity. The intimate relationship between p53 and Mdm2 expression has also provided an explanation for the observation that p53 mutant proteins seen in tumor cells are almost always expressed to very high levels. These mutant proteins fail to activate transcription of targets such as $p21^{Waf1/Cip1}$ and *bax* and therefore cannot inhibit tumor cell growth. However, these *p53* mutants also fail to activate expression of Mdm2 and then fail to promote the expression of the cell protein necessary to target their own degradation *(86)*. When expressed with wild-type p53 that can activate Mdm2, or in the presence of exogenously expressed Mdm2, tumor-derived p53 mutants are degraded like the wild-type protein and maintained in such cells at low levels *(93)*.

The precise contribution of Mdm2 to p53 degradation has not been elucidated, although it is clear that regions of both Mdm2 and p53, which are independent of the binding domains, are necessary for degradation. The Mdm2 protein has been shown to contain sequences that permit nuclear export and this activity of Mdm2 is important for p53 degradation *(94)*, suggesting that Mdm2 carries p53 out of the nucleus for degradation in the cytoplasm. Another study has suggested that Mdm2 can function as a ubiquitin ligase, and thus functions directly to target p53 to the proteasome *(95)*.

Mdm2 appears to be the principal regulator of p53 stability in cells, and activation of the p53 response is very likely to involve signals that inhibit the degradative function of Mdm2. One of the most straightforward mechanisms to achieve this would be to prevent interaction between the two proteins, as binding to Mdm2 is essential for degradation of p53 to occur. Several kinases have been shown to phosphorylate p53 close to the Mdm2 binding domain; phosphorylation of p53 by DNA-PK was shown to reduce the interaction between p53 and Mdm2 *(96)*. Another study showed a similar effect after phosphorylation of Mdm2 by DNA-PK *(97)*. DNA-PK is an attractive candidate for the mediator of a DNA damage response, as it is activated by double-stranded DNA breaks, and the sites identified as targets for DNA-PK in p53 are clearly phosphorylated in vivo following DNA damage *(98)*. However, analysis of cells from mice that are defective for DNA-PK has not revealed a clear defect in their ability to stabilize p53 in response to DNA damage *(99)*. The ATM protein, a kinase in the same family as DNA-PK, is another potential participant in this pathway, although phosphorylation of p53 by ATM has yet to be demonstrated. Nevertheless, cells defective for ATM function show a substantial delay in elevation of p53 levels in response to IR, although the UV-induced response was found to be normal *(100)*. Such results present a model in which some forms of DNA damage activate a kinase, which, by phosphorylating p53 or Mdm2, prevent interaction between the two proteins and thereby lead to the stabilization of p53. However, p53 proteins mutated at all the known phosphorylation sites can be stabilized in response to DNA damage (M. Ashcroft, unpublished observations), indicating that phosphorylation-independent mechanisms can also regulate p53 stability.

The independence of binding and degradation functions on both p53 and Mdm2 *(87,101)* indicates that p53 could be stabilized by mechanisms that do not prevent Mdm2 binding, and under some circumstances elevation in p53 protein is seen without a clear loss of the ability to interact with Mdm2 (S. Bates, unpublished observations). Recently p14[ARF] has been identified as an Mdm2 binding protein that inhibits the ability of Mdm2 to degrade p53 without disrupting the Mdm2/p53 interaction *(102–104)*. p14[ARF] (the mouse homolog of this protein is called p19[ARF]) is encoded by the *CDKN2A* locus, which also encodes the cyclin-dependent kinase inhibitor p16[INK4A] *(105)*. The amino acid sequences of these two proteins are completely unrelated, as they are produced using separate first exons and translation of the common second exon in different reading frames *(106)*. This locus is a frequent site for mutation in tumors, however, and both p16[INK4A] and p14[ARF] are likely to function as tumor suppressor proteins. Although p14[ARF] activates p53 very efficiently by preventing degradation by Mdm2, it does not appear to play a role in the DNA damage response, since p14[ARF] levels are not elevated by DNA damage and cells deficient in p14[ARF] retain the ability to induce p53 in response to DNA damage *(105)*. The importance of p14[ARF] has been demonstrated by recent studies showing that deregulated expression of E2F1, a transcription factor intimately associated with cell proliferation, activates expression of p14[ARF] *(107)* (Fig. 2). This finding suggests that any signal that can induce abnormal or uncontrolled proliferation might result in deregulated E2F1 activity, leading to

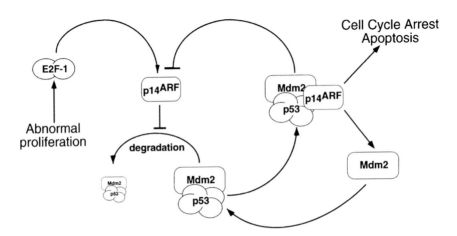

Fig. 2. The link between abnormal proliferative signals and activation of p53 is, at least in part, through activation of p14[ARF]. The transcription factor E2F-1, which is normally tightly regulated through the cell cycle by interaction with pRB, is activated by proliferative signals such as oncogene activation. E2F-1 directly activates expression of p14[ARF], which interacts with Mdm2 and prevents the degradation of p53. The p53 protein is therefore stabilized and activates cell cycle arrest and apoptotic responses.

increased levels of p14[ARF], and then to activation of a p53 response, showing how the cell can be protected from potentially oncogenic changes through activation of p14[ARF]. This model not only highlights the importance of p14[ARF], but also indicates that E2F1, a protein inherently activated by cell cycle progression, is part of a failsafe mechanism to protect against aberrant cell growth. This is entirely consistent with the initially puzzling observation that E2F1, a protein known to have growth-promoting functions, can also function as a tumor suppressor *(108,109)*. As yet there is no direct information on how p53 stability is regulated in response to hypoxic signals, although the hypoxia inducible factor HIF1-α has been shown to bind and stabilize p53, and is therefore an excellent candidate for another protein that somehow interferes with Mdm2-mediated degradation of p53 *(41)*. Interestingly, HIF-1α has recently been shown to be required for the development of certain tumors suggesting that hypoxic induction of HIF-1α results in both tumor promoting and tumor suppressive signals *(110)*.

Another mechanism by which p53 stability might be regulated is at the level of transcriptional activation of Mdm2 by p53. The transcriptional co-activator p300 has been shown to bind the N-terminus of p53 and enhance the ability of *p53* to function as a transcription factor *(111–113)*. p300 binding to p53 appears to be more important in the activation of some p53 responsive genes than others and may be essential for activation of Mdm2, but not mediators of the p53 response such as p21[Waf1/Cip1] or Bax *(114)*. Oncogenic changes that deplete the cell of p300 activity, such as expression of the adenoviral oncoprotein E1A, would therefore result in the downregulation of Mdm2 expression and consequently stabilization of p53.

Taken together, these recent observations suggest that the different signals that activate p53 may use different pathways which ultimately converge to perturb the same point of p53 regulation; degradation of p53 by Mdm2 (Fig. 3).

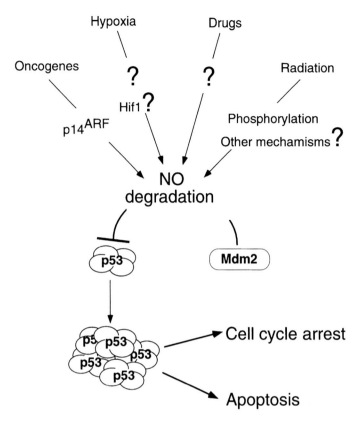

Fig. 3. A model showing how multiple signals can activate a p53 response by allowing stabilization of p53. This is likely to be through the shared ability to interfere with the ability of Mdm2 to target *p53* for degradation, either by preventing the p53/Mdm2 interaction (e.g., phosphorylation of the N-terminus of p53 in response to radiation) or more indirectly by binding to the p53/Mdm2 complex (p14^{ARF}). The pathways mediating the response to other signals such as hypoxia and DNA damaging drugs have not yet been described.

6.2. Activation of p53 DNA Binding

Despite the obvious importance of regulation of protein stability to activation of p53 function there is considerable evidence from in vitro studies that regulation of the conformation of the p53 protein, allowing a switch from a latent to an active form, is also an important regulatory step *(11,115–117)*. Activation of the latent non-DNA binding form of *p53* can be achieved by several mechanisms, many of which involve modification of the extreme C-terminus of the protein. Phosphorylation *(118)*, glycosylation *(119)*, acetylation *(120)*, binding to short single strands of DNA *(12)*, or a C-terminal antibody (PAb 421) *(11)*, or deletion of this region leads to the activation of the sequence specific DNA binding activity of p53 in vitro *(11)*, and it has been proposed that the C-terminal regulatory domain of p53 can block the activity of the central DNA binding domain by an allosteric mechanism that is relieved in response to an activating signal. The mechanism regulating this switch in vivo remains unclear, although a role for an ATM-dependent dephosphorylation the C-terminus of p53, allowing interaction with 14-3-3 (also the product of a p53-responsive gene), has been suggested *(121)*.

Changes in the cellular redox state can also shift p53 from the latent to active form
(122); proteins that contribute to the modification of chromatin structure may also play
a role, either directly or indirectly. The p300 transcriptional coactivator that binds to
the N-terminus of p53 shows both histone acetylase activity and the ability to acetylate
the C-terminus of p53, thereby activating DNA binding function *(120)*. By contrast,
the high-mobility group protein-1 (HMG-1), a chromatin-associated protein that bends
DNA to allow access for transcription factors, can enhance p53/DNA binding without
clearly changing the conformation of the p53 protein itself *(123)*.

Although it is clear that p53 can adopt latent and active forms, the contribution of
regulation of p53 conformation to controlling p53 activity in cells is less obvious. In
several studies, the dissociation between p53 activity and accumulation of p53 protein
has been attributed to the activation of low levels of latent p53 by conformational
switch without stabilization of the protein *(118,124,125)*. Stabilization of the p53 protein
without activation of function has also been described, and the very high levels of
wild-type p53 in teratocarcinoma cells is likely to be maintained in a latent form *(126)*.
In addition to conformational shift, cytoplasmic sequestration can regulate the activity
of wild-type p53, which needs to be in the nucleus to function. Inactive wild-type p53
that fails to localize to the nucleus is seen in some tumors *(127,128)* and in ES cells *(129)*.

Stabilization of p53 without activation of function may also play an important role
in determining the carcinogenic potential of DNA binding chemicals. Strongly potent
carcinogens such as the polycyclic aromatic hydrocarbon BgChDE can stabilize p53
very efficiently, but the p53 protein that accumulates in response to the carcinogens
is not transcriptionally active and fails to enhance expression of p53 target genes such
as p21$^{Waf1/Cip1}$ *(130,131)*. This ability of carcinogens to evade activation of a normal
p53 response could contribute to their high carcinogenic potential, because cells exposed
to these agents continue DNA synthesis in the presence of DNA damage and subsequently accumulate potentially oncogenic genetic alterations. The defect in the p53
protein produced in response to carcinogens is unknown, although it is possible that
the inactivity reflects a failure to switch from latent to active conformation or a failure
to localize to the nucleus.

7. PERSPECTIVES

The two findings that *p53* is the most frequently mutated gene in human cancer and
that reactivation of p53 function is likely to cause programmed cell death specifically
in tumor cells have led to intense interest as to the use of p53 as a therapeutic agent.
Although direct mutation within the p53 gene itself is a very common mechanism by
which p53 function is lost, it is becoming clear that cancers that retain wild-type p53
have frequently lost p53 function by an alternative mechanisms, affecting either the
regulators upstream of p53 or the downstream mediators of p53 function *(132–135)*.
These alternative mechanisms for loss of p53 activity offer additional targets for therapeutic intervention, which are discussed in much greater detail in the subsequent
chapters. It is now 20 years since p53 was first described as a cellular protein expressed
in tumor cells and associated with viral transforming proteins, and our understanding
of how this protein functions to protect from tumor development has increased enor-
mously. We are now at a stage where the advances made during the past two decades

can be applied to the development of new strategies for the treatment of human disease, and it seems likely that the future will hold great scientific and clinical rewards.

ACKNOWLEDGMENTS

We are grateful to Margaret Ashcroft and Stewart Bates for advice and sharing unpublished results. This work was sponsored by the National Cancer Institute, DHHS, under contract with A.B.L.

REFERENCES

1. Hollstein M, Rice K, Greenblatt MS, Soussi T, Fuchs R, Sørlie T, Hovig E, Smith-Sørensen B, Montesano R, Harris CC. Database of *p53* gene somatic mutations in human tumors and cell lines. *Nucleic Acids Res* 1994; 22:3551–3555.
2. Donehower LA, Harvey M, Slagle BL, McArthur MJ, Montgomery CA Jr, Butel JS, Bradley A. Mice deficient for *p53* are developmentally normal but susceptible to spontaneous tumors. *Nature* 1992; 356:215–221.
3. Levine AJ. *p53*, the cellular gatekeeper for growth and division. *Cell* 1997; 88:323–331.
4. Haffner R, Oren M. Biochemical properties and biological effects of *p53*. *Curr Opin Genet Dev* 1995; 5:84–90.
5. Field S, Jang SJ. Presence of a potent transcription activating sequence in the *p53* protein. *Science* 1990; 249:1046–1049.
6. Hansen R, Oren M. *p53*; from inductive signal to cellular effect. *Curr Opin Genet Dev* 1997; 7:46–51.
7. Bates S, Vousden KH *p53* in signalling checkpoint arrest or apoptosis. *Curr Opin Genet Dev* 1996; 6:1–7.
8. Walker KK, Levine AJ. Identification of a novel *p53* functional domain that is necessary for efficient growth suppression. *Proc Natl Acad Sci USA* 1996; 93:15,335–15,340.
9. Shaulsky, G, Goldfinger N, Tosky MS, Levine A, Rotter V. Nuclear localization is essential for the activity of *p53* protein. *Oncogene* 1991: 6:2055–2065.
10. Wang P, Reed M, Wang Y, Mayr G, Stenger J, Anderson M, Schwedes JF, Tegtmeyer P. *p53* domains: Structure, oligomerization, and transformation. *Mol Cell Biol* 1994; 14:5182–5191.
11. Hupp TR, Meek DW, Midgley CA, Lane DP. Regulation of the specific DNA binding function of *p53*. *Cell* 1992; 71:875–886.
12. Jayaraman L, Prives C. Activation of *p53* sequence-specific DNA binding by short single strands of DNA requires the *p53* C-terminus. *Cell* 1995; 81:1021–1029.
13. Soussi T, Caron de Fromentel C, May P. Structural aspects of the *p53* protein in relation to gene evolution. *Oncogene* 1990; 5:945–952.
14. Finlay CA, Hinds PW, Tan T-H, Eliyahu D, Oren M, Levine AJ. Activating mutations for transformation by *p53* produce a gene product that forms an hsc70-*p53* complex with an altered half life. *Mol Cell Biol* 1988; 8:531–539.
15. Iggo R, Gatter K, Bartek J, Lane D, Harris AL. Increased expression of mutant forms of *p53* oncogene in primary lung cancer. *Lancet* 1990; 335:675–679.
16. Kern SE, Kinzler KW, Baker SJ, Nigro JM, Rotter V, Levine AJ, Friedman P, Prives C, Vogelstein B. Mutant *p53* proteins bind DNA abnormally in vitro. *Oncogene* 1991; 6:131–136.
17. Milner J, Medcalf EA. Co-translation of activated mutant *p53* with wild type drives the wild type *p53* protein into the mutant conformation. *Cell* 1991; 65:765–774.
18. Milner J, Medcalf EA, Cook AC. Tumor suppressor *p53*: Analysis of wild-type and mutant *p53* complexes. *Mol Cell Biol* 1991; 11:12–19.

19. Dittmer D, Pati S, Zambetti G, Chu S, Teresky AK, Moore M, Finlay C, Levine AJ. Gain of function mutations in *p53*. Nature Genet 4:42–46.

20. Lin J, Teresky AK, Levine AJ. Two critical hydrophobic amino acids in the N-terminal domain of the *p53* protein are required for the gain of function phenotypes of human *p53* mutants. *Oncogene* 1995; 10:2387–2390.

21. Li R, Sutphin PD, Schwartz D, Matas D, Almog N, Wolkowicz R, Goldfinger N, Pei H, Prokocimer M, Rotter V. Mutant *p53* protein expression interferes with *p53*-independent apoptotic pathways. *Oncogene* 1998; 16:3269–3277.

22. Kaghad M, Bonnet H, Yang A, Creancier L, Biscan J-C, Valent A, Minty A, Chalon P, Lelias J-M, Dumont X, Ferrara P, McKeon F, Caput D. Monoallelically expressed gene related to *p53* at 1p36, a region frequently deleted in neuroblastoma and other human cancers. *Cell* 1997; 90:809–819.

23. Bian J, and Sun Y. *p53*CP, a putative *p53* competing protein that specifically binds to the consensus *p53* DNA binding sites: A third member of the *p53* family? *Proc Nat Acad Sci USA* 1997; 94:14,753–14,758.

24. Schmale H, Bamberger C. A novel protein with strong homology to the tumor suppressor *p53*. *Oncogene* 1997; 15:1363–1367.

25. Jost CA, Marin MC, Kaelin WG Jr p73 is a human *p53*-related protein that can induce apoptosis. *Nature* 1997; 389:191–194.

26. Kuerbitz SJ, Plunkett BS, Walsh WV, Kastan MB. Wild-type *p53* is a cell cycle checkpoint determinant following irradiation. *Proc Natl Acad Sci USA* 1992; 89:7491–7495.

27. Yonish-Rouach E, Resnitzky D, Lotem J, Sachs L, Kimchi A, Oren M. Wild-type *p53* induces apoptosis of myeloid leukaemic cells that is inhibited by interleukin-6. *Nature* 1991; 353:345–347.

28. Sah VP, Attardi LD, Mulligan GJ, Williams BO, Bronson RT, Jacks T. A subset of *p53*-deficient embyos exhibit exencephaly. *Nature Genet* 1995; 10:175–180.

29. Armstrong JF, Kaufman MH, Harrison DJ, Clarke AR. High-frequency developmental abnormalities in *p53*-deficient mice. *Curr Biol* 1995; 5:931–936.

30. MacCullum DE, Hupp TR, Midgley CA, Stuart D, Campbell SJ, Harper A, Walsh FS, Wright EG, Balmain A, Lane DP, Hall PA. The *p53* response to ionising radiation in adult and developing murine tissues. *Oncogene* 1996; 13:2575–2587.

31. Gottlieb E, Haffner R, King A, Asher G, Gruss P, Lonai P, Oren M. Transgenic mouse model for studying the transcriptional activity of the *p53* protein: Age- and tissue-dependent changes in radiation-induced activation during embryogenesis. *EMBO J* 1997; 16:1381–1390.

32. Komarova EA, Chernov MV, Franks R, Wang K, Armin G, Zelnick CR, Chin DM, Bacus SS, Stark GR, Gudkov AV. Transgenic mice with *p53*-responsive *lacZ: p53* activity varies dramatically during normal development and determines radiation and drug sensitiivy in vivo. *EMBO J* 1997; 16:1391–1400.

33. Livingstone LR, White A, Sprouse J, Livanos E, Jacks T, Tlsty TD. Altered cell cycle arrest and gene amplification potential accompany loss of wild-type *p53*. *Cell* 1992; 70:923–935.

34. Fukasawa K, Choi T, Kuriyama R, Rulong S, Vande Woude GF. Abnormal centrosome amplification in the absence of *p53*. *Science* 1996; 271:1744–1747.

35. Smith ML, Chen I-T, Zhan Q, O'Conner PM, Fornace AJ. Involvement of *p53* tumor suppressor in repair of u.v.-type DNA damage. *Oncogene* 1995; 10:1053–1059.

36. Yin Y, Tainsky MA, Bischoff FZ, Strong LC, Wahl GM. Wild-type *p53* restores cell cycle control and inhibits gene amplification in cells with mutant *p53* alleles. *Cell* 1992; 70:937–948.

37. Hicks GG, Egan SE, Greenberg AH, Mowat M. Mutant *p53* tumor suppressor alleles release *ras*-induced cell cycle growth arrest. *Mol Cell Biol* 1991; 11:1344–1352.

38. Hiebert SW, Packham G, Strom DK, Haffner R, Oren M, Zambetti G, Cleveland JL. E2F-1:DP-1 induces *p53* and overrides survival factors to trigger apoptosis. *Mol Cell Biol* 1995; 15:6864–6874.

39. Morgenbesser SD, Williams BO, Jacks T, DePinho RA. *p53*-dependent apoptosis produced by *Rb*-deficiency in the developing mouse lens. *Nature* 1994; 371:72–74.

40. Serrano M, Lin AW, McCurrach ME, Beach D, Lowe SW. Oncogenic *ras* provokes premature cell senescence associated with accumulation of *p53* and p16[INK4a]. *Cell* 1997; 88:593–602.

41. An WG, Kanekal M, Simon MC, Maltepe E, Blagosklonny MV, Neckers LM. Stabilization of wild-type by hypoxia-inducible factor 1alpha. *Nature* 1998; 392:405–408.

42. Dameron KM, Volpert OV, Tainsky MA, Bouck N. Control of angiogenesis in fibroblasts by *p53* regulation of thrombospondin-1. *Science* 1994; 265:1582–1584.

43. Fearon ER, Vogelstein B. A genetic model for colorectal tumorigenesis. *Cell* 1990; 61:759–767.

44. Kemp CJ, Burns PA, Brown K, Nagase H, Balmain A. Transgenic approaches to the analysis of and *p53* function in multistage carcinogenesis. *Cold Spring Harb Symp Quant Biol* 1994; 59:427–434.

45. Pietenpol JA, Tokino T, Thiagaligam S, El-Deiry W, Kinzler KW, Vogelstein B. Sequence-specific transcriptional activation is essential for growth suppression by *p53*. *Proc. Natl. Acad. Sci. USA* 1994; 91:1998–2002.

46. Attardi LD, Lowe SW, Brugarolas J, Jacks T. Transcriptional activation by *p53*, but not induction of the p21 gene, is essential for oncogene-mediated apoptosis. *EMBO J* 1996; 15:3639–3701.

47. El-Deiry W, Tokino T, Velculescu VE, Levy DB, Parson VE, Trent JM, Lin D, Mercer WE, Kinzler KW, Vogelstein B. WAF1, a potential mediator of *p53* tumour suppression. *Cell* 1993; 75:817–825.

48. Waldman T, Kinzler KW, Vogelstein B. p21 in necessary for the *p53*-mediated G1 arrest in human cancer cells. *Cancer Res* 1995; 55:5187–5190.

49. Deng C, Zhang P, Harper JW, Elledge SJ, Leder P. Mice lacking p21[CIP1/WAF1] undergo normal development, but are defective in G1 checkpoint control. *Cell* 1995; 82:675–684.

50. Brugarolas J, Chandrasekaran C, Gordon JI, Beach D, Jacks T, Hannon GJ. Radiation-induced cell cycle arrest compromised by p21 deficiency. *Nature* 1995; 377:552–556.

51. Buckbinder L, Talbott R, Velasco-Miguel S, Takenaka I, Faha B, Seizinger BR, Kley N. Induction of the growth inhibitor IGF-binding protein 3 by *p53*. Nature 1995; 377:646–649.

52. Hermeking H, Lengauer C, Polyak K, He T-C, Zhang L, Thiagalingam S, Kinzler KW, Vogelstein B. *14-3-3σ* is a *p53*-regulated inhibitor of G2/M progression. *Mol Cell* 1997; 1:3–11.

53. Amson RB, Nemani M, Roperch J-P, Israeli D, Bougueleret L, LeGall I, Medhioub M, Linares-Cruz G, Lethrosne F, Pasturaud P, Piouffre L, Prieur S, Susini L, Alvaro V, Millasseau P, Guidicelli C, Bui H, Massart C, Cazes L, Dufour F, Bruzzoni-Giovanelli H, Owadi H, Hennion C, Charpak G, Dausset J, Calvo F, Oren M, Cohen D, Telerman A. Isolation of 10 differentially expressed cDNAs in *p53*-induced apoptosis: Activation of the vertebrate homologue of the *Drosophila* seven in absentia gene. *Proc Natl Acad Sci USA* 1996; 93:3953–3957.

54. Zhan Q, Chen IT, Antimore MJ, Fornace AJ. Tumor suppressor *p53* can participate in transcriptional induction of the GADD45 promoter in the absence of direct DNA binding. *Mol Cell Biol* 1998; 18:2768–2778.

55. Polyak K, Waldman T, He T-C, Kinzler KW, Vogelstein B. Genetic determinants of *p53*-induced apoptosis and growth arrest. *Genes Dev* 1996; 10:1945–1952.

56. Gorospe M, Cirielli C, Wamg X, Seth P, Capogrossi MC, Holbrook NJ. p21[Waf1/Cip1] protects against *p53*-mediated apoptosis of human melanoma cells. *Oncogene* 1997; 14:929–935.

57. Miyashita T, Reed JC. Tumor suppressor *p53* is a direct transcriptional activator of the human bax gene. *Cell* 1995; 80:293–299.

58. Knudson MC, Tung KSK, Tourtellotte WG, Brown GAJ, Korsmeyer SJ. Bax-deficient mice with lymphoid hyperplasia and male germ cell death. *Science* 1995; 270:96–98.

59. McCurrach ME, Connor TMF, Knudson MC, Korsmeyer SJ, Lowe SW. *bax*-deficiency promotes drug resistance and oncogenic transformation by attenuating *p53*-dependent apoptosis. *Proc Natl Acad Sci USA* 1997; 94:2345–2349.

60. Yin C, Knudson CM, Korsmeyer SJ, Van Dyke T. Bax suppresses tumorigenesis and stimulates apoptosis in vivo. *Nature* 1997; 385:637–640.

61. Wu G, Burns TF, McDonald ER, Jiang W, Meng R, Krantz ID, Kao G, Gan DD, Zhou JY, Muschel R, Hamilton SR, Spinner NB, Markowitz S, Wu G, El-Deiry WS. KILLER/DR5 is a DNA damage-inducible *p53*-regulated death receptor gene. *Nature Genet* 1997; 17:141–143.

62. Israeli D, Tessler E, Haupt Y, Elkeles A, Wilder S, Amson R, Telerman A, Oren M. A novel *p53*-inducible gene, *PAG608,* encodes a nuclear zinc finger protein whose expression promotes apoptosis. *EMBO J* 1997; 16:4384–4392.

63. Owen-Schaub LB, Zhang W, Cusack JC, Angelo LS, Santee SM, Fujiwara T, Roth JA, Deisseroth AB, Zhang W-W, Kruzel E, Radinsky R. Wild-type human *p53* and a temperature sensitive mutant induce Fas/APO-1 expression. *Mol Cell Biol* 1995; 15:3032–3040.

64. Polyak K, Xia Y, Zweier JL, Kinzler KW, Vogelstein B. A model for *p53*-induced apoptosis. *Nature* 1997; 389:300–305.

65. Sabbatini P, Chiou S-K, Rao L, White E. Modulation of *p53*-mediated transcriptional repression and apoptosis by the adenovirus E1B 19K protein. *Mol Cell Biol* 1995; 15:1060–1070.

66. Shen YQ, Shenk T. Relief of *p53*-mediated transcriptional repression by the adenovirus E1B 19-kDa protein or the cellular bcl-2 protein. *Proc Natl Acad Sci USA* 1994; 91:8940–8944.

67. Ryan KM, Vousden KH. Characterization of structural *p53* mutants which show selective defects in apoptosis, but not cell cycle arrest. *Mol Cell Biol* 1998; 18:3692–3698.

68. Haupt Y, Rowan S, Shaulian E, Vousden KH, Oren M. Induction of apoptosis in HeLa cells by trans-activation deficient *p53*. Genes Dev 1995; 9:2170–2183.

69. Caelles C, Helmberg A, Karin M. *p53*-dependent apoptosis in the absence of transcriptional activation of *p53*-target genes. *Nature* 1994; 370:220–223.

70. Sakamuro D, Sabbatini P, White E, Prendergast GC. The polyproline region of *p53* is required to activate apoptosis but not growth arrest. *Oncogene* 1997; 15:887–898.

71. Ruaro EM, Collavin L, Del Sal G, Haffner R, Oren M, Levine AJ, Schneider C. A proline-rich motif in *p53* is required for transactivation-independent growth arrest as induced by Gas 1. *Proc Natl Acad Sci USA* 1997; 94:4675–4680.

72. Goga A, Liu X, Hambuch TM, Senechal K, Major E, Berk AJ, Witte ON, Sawyers CL. *p53* dependent growth suppression by the c-Abl nuclear tyrosine kinase. *Oncogene* 1995; 11:791–799.

73. Iwabuchi K, Bartel PL, Li B, Marraccino R, Fields S. Two cellular proteins that bind to wild-type but not mutant *p53*. Proc Natl Acad Sci USA 1994; 91:6098–6102.

74. Wang XW, Yeh H, Schaeffer L, Roy R, Moncollin V, Egly J-M, Wang Z, Friedberg EC, Evans MK, Taffe BG, Bohr VA, Weeda G, Hoeijmakers JHJ, Forrester K, Harris CC. *p53* modulation of TFIIH-associated nucleotide excision repair activity. *Nature Genet* 1995; 10:188–195.

75. Wang XW, Vermeulen W, Coursen JD, Gibson M, Lupold SE, Forrester K, Xu G, Elmore L, Yeh H, Hoeijmakers JH, Harris CC. The XPB and XPD DNA helicases are components of the *p53*-mediated apoptosis pathway. *Genes Dev* 1996; 10:1219–1232.

76. Rowan S, Ludwig RL, Haupt Y, Bates S, Lu X, Oren M, Vousden KH. Specific loss of apoptotic but not cell cycle arrest funtion in a human tumour derived *p53* mutant. *EMBO J* 1996; 15:827–838.

77. Ludwig RL, Bates S, Vousden KH. Differential transcriptional activation of target cellular promoters by *p53* mutants with impaired apoptotic function. *Mol Cell Biol* 1996; 16:4952–4960.

78. Friedlander P, Haupt Y, Prives C, Oren M. A mutant *p53* that discriminated between *p53* responsive genes cannot induce apoptosis. *Mol Cell Biol* 1996; 16:4961–4971.

79. Chen X, Ko LJ, Jayaraman L, Prives C. *p53* levels, functional domains, and DNA damage determine the extent of the apoptotic response of tumor cells. *Genes Dev* 1996; 10:2438–2451.

80. Gottlieb E, Haffner R, von Ruden T, Wagner EF, Oren M. Down-regulation of wild-type *p53* activity interferes with apoptosis of IL-3 dependent hematopoietic cells following IL-3 withdrawal. *EMBO J* 1994; 13:1368–1374.

81. Lin Y, Benchimol S. Cytokines inhibit *p53*-mediated apoptosis but not *p53*-mediated G1 arrest. *Mol Cell Biol* 1995; 15:6045–6054.

82. Guillouf C, Grana X, Selvakumaran M, De Luca A, Giordano A, Hoffman B, Liebermann DA. Dissection of the genetic programs of *p53*-mediated G1 growth arrest and apoptosis: Blocking *p53*-induced apoptosis unmasks G1 arrest. *Blood* 1995; 85:2691–2698.

83. Quelle FW, Wang J, Feng J, Wang D, Cleveland JL, Ihle JN, Zambetti GP. Cytokine rescue of *p53*-dependent apoptosis and cycle arrest is mediated by distinct Jak kinase signaling pathways. *Genes Dev* 1998; 12:1099–1107.

84. Qin X-Q, Livingston DM, Kaelin WG, Adams PD. Deregulated transcription factor E2F-1 expression leads to S-phase entry and *p53*-mediated apoptosis. *Proc Natl Acad Sci USA* 1994; 91:10,918–10,922.

85. Hickman ES, Bates S, Vousden KH. Perturbation of the *p53* response by human papillomavirus type 16 E7. *J Virol* 1997; 71:3710–3718.

86. Kubbutat MHG, Vousden KH. Keeping an old friend under control: regulation of *p53* stability. *Mol Med Today* 1998; 4:250–256.

87. Kubbutat MHG, Jones SN, Vousden KH. Regulation of *p53* stability by Mdm2. *Nature* 1997; 387:299–303.

88. Haupt Y, Maya R, Kazaz A, Oren M. Mdm2 promotes the rapid degradation of *p53*. *Nature* 1997; 387:296–299.

89. Marston NJ, Crook T, Vousden KH. Interaction of *p53* with MDM2 is independent of E6 and does not mediate wild type transformation suppressor function. *Oncogene* 1994; 9:2707–2716.

90. Momand J, Zambetti GP, George DL, Levine AJ. The mdm-2 oncogene product forms a complex with the *p53* protein and inhibits *p53*-mediated transactivation. *Cell* 1992; 69:1237–1245.

91. Jones SN, Roe AE, Donehower LA, Bradley A. Rescue of embyonic lethality in Mdm2-deficient mice by absence of *p53*. *Nature* 1995; 378:206–208.

92. Montes de Oca Luna R, Wagner DS, Lozano G. Rescue of early embryonic lethality in *mdm2*-deficient mice by deletion of *p53*. Nature 1995; 378:203–206.

93. Midgley CA, Lane DP. *p53* protein stability in tumour cells is not determined by mutation but is dependent on Mdm2 binding. *Oncogene* 1997; 15:1179–1189.

94. Roth J, Dobbelstein M, Freedman DA, Shenk T, Levine AJ. Nucleo-cytoplasmic shuttling of the hdm2 oncoprotein regulates the levels of the *p53* protein via a pathway used by the human immunodeficiency virus rev protein. *EMBO J* 1998; 17:554–564.

95. Honda R, Tanaka H, Yasuda H. Oncoprotein MDM2 is a ubiquitin ligase E3 for tumor suppressor *p53*. *FEBS Lett* 1997; 420:25–27.

96. Shieh S-Y, Ikeda M, Taya Y, Prives C. DNA damage-induced phosphorylation of *p53* alleviates inhibition by MDM2. *Cell* 1997; 91:325–334.

97. Mayo LD, Turchi JJ, Berberich SJ. Mdm-2 phosphorylation by DBA-dependent protein kinase prevents interaction with *p53*. *Cancer Res* 1997; 57:5013–5016.

98. Siliciano JD, Canman CE, Taya Y, Sakaguchi K, Appella E, Kastan MB. DNA damage induces phosphorylation of the amino terminus of *p53*. *Genes Dev* 1997; 11:3471–3481.

99. Fried LM, Koumenis C, Peterson SR, Green SL, van Zijl P, Allalunis-Turner J, Chen DJ,

Fishel R, Giaccia AJ, Brown JM, Kirchgessner CU. The DNA damage response in DNA-dependent protein kinase-deficient SCID mouse cells: Replication protein A hyperphosphorylation and *p53* induction. *Proc Natl Acad Sci USA* 1996; 93:13,825–13,830.

100. Kastan MB, Zhan Q, El Deiry W-S, Carrier F, Jacks T, Walsh WV, Plunkett BS, Vogelstein B, Fornace A-J Jr. A mammalian cell cycle checkpoint pathway utilizing *p53* and GADD45 is defective in ataxia-telangiectasia. *Cell* 71:587–597.

101. Kubbutat MHG, Ludwig RL, Ashcroft M, Vousden KH. Regulation of Mdm2 directed degradation by the C-terminus of *p53*. *Mol Cell Biol* 1993; 18:5690–5698.

102. Stott F, Bates SA, James M, McConnell BB, Starborg M, Brookes S, Palmero I, Hara E, Ryan KM, Vousden KH, Peters G. The alternative product from the human CDKN2A locus, p14^ARF, participates in a regulatory feedback loop with *p53* and MDM2. *EMBO J* 1998; 17:5001–5014.

103. Zhang Y, Xiong Y, Yarbrough WG. ARF promotes MDM2 degradation and stabilizes *p53*: *ARF-INK4a* locus deletion impairs both the Rb and *p53* tumor suppression pathways. *Cell* 1998; 92:725–734.

104. Pomerantz J, Schreiber-Agus N, Liégeois NJ, Silverman A, Alland L, Chin L, Potes J, Chen K, Orlow I, Lee H-W, Cordon-Cardo C, DePinho RA. The *Ink4a* tumor suppressor gene product, p19^Arf, interacts with MDM2 and neutralizes MDM2's inhibition of *p53*. *Cell* 1998; 92:713–723.

105. Kamijo T, Zindy F, Roussel MF, Quelle DE, Downing JR, Ashmun RA, Grosveld G, Sherr CJ. Tumor suppression at the mouse *INK4a* locus mediated by the alternative reading frame product p19^ARF. *Cell* 1997; 91:649–659.

106. Quelle DE, Zindy F, Ashmun RA, Sherr CJ. Alternative reading frames of the INK4a tumor suppressor gene encode two unrelated proteins capable of inducing cell cycle arrest. *Cell* 1995; 83:993–1000.

107. Bates S, Phillips AC, Stott F, Ludwig RL, Peters G, Vousden KH. E2F-1 regulation of p14^ARF links pRB and *p53* tumor suppressor functions. *Nature* 1998; 395:124, 125.

108. Yamasaki L, Jacks T, Bronson R, Goillot E, Harlow E, Dyson N. Tumor induction and tissue atrophy in mice lacking E2F-1. *Cell* 1996; 85:537–548.

109. Field SJ, Tsai F-Y, Kuo F, Zubiaga AM, Kaelin WG, Livingston DM, Orkin SH, Greenberg ME. E2F-1 functions in mice to promote apoptosis and suppress proliferation. *Cell* 1996; 85:549–561.

110. Ryan HE, Lo J, Johnson RS. HIF-1α is required for solid tumor formation and embyonic vascularization. *EMBO J* 1998; 17:3005–3015.

111. Avantaggiati ML, Ogryzko V, Gardner K, Giordano A, Levine AS, Kelly K. Recruitment of p300/CBP in *p53*-dependent signal pathways. *Cell* 1997; 89:1175–1184.

112. Gu W, Shi X-L, Roeder RG. Synergistic activation of transcription by CBP and *p53*. *Nature* 1997; 387:819–823.

113. Lill NL, Grossman SR, Ginsberg D, DeCaprio J, Livingston DM. Binding and modulation of *p53* by p300/CBP coactivators. *Nature* 1997; 387:823–827.

114. Thomas A, White E. Suppression of the p300-dependent *mdm2* negative-feedback loop induced the *p53* apoptotic function. *Genes Dev* 1998; 12:1975–1985.

115. Hupp TR, Sparks A, Lane DP. Small peptides activate the latent sequence-specific DNA binding function of *p53*. *Cell* 1995; 83:237–245.

116. Hupp TR, Lane DP. Regulation of the cryptic sequence-specific DSA-binding function of *p53* by protein kinases. *CSH Symp Quant Biol* 1994; 59:195–206.

117. Halazonetis TD, Kandil AN. Conformational shifts propagate from the oligomerization domain of *p53* to its tetrameric DNA binding domain and restore DNA binding to select *p53* mutants. *EMBO J* 1993; 12:5057–5064.

118. Hupp TR, Lane DP. Two distinct signaling pathways activate the latent DNA binding

function of *p53* in a casein kinase II-independent manner. *J Biol Chem* 1995; 270:18,165–18,174.

119. Shaw P, Freeman J, Bovey R, Iggo R. Regulation of specific DNA binding by *p53*: Evidence for a role of O-glycosylation and charged residues at the carboxy-terminus. *Oncogene* 1996; 12:921–930.

120. Gu W, Roeder RG. Activation of *p53* sequence-specific DNA binding by acetylation of the C-terminal domain. *Cell* 1997; 90:595–606.

121. Waterman MJ, Stavridi ES, Waterman JL, Halazonetis TD. ATM-dependent activation of *p53* involves dephosphorylation and association with 14-3-3 proteins. *Nature Genet* 1998; 19:175–178.

122. Jayaraman L, Murthy KGK, Zhu C, Curran T, Xanthoudakis S, Prives C. Identification of redox/repair protein Ref-1 as a potent activator of *p53*. *Genes Dev* 1997; 11:558–570.

123. Jayaraman L, Moorthy NC, Murthy KG, Manley JL, Bustin M, Prives C. High mobility group protein-1 (HMG-1) is a unique activator of *p53*. *Genes Dev* 1998; 12:462–472.

124. Lu X, Burbridge SA, Griffin S, Smith HM. Discordance between accumulated *p53* protein levels and its transcriptional activity in response to U.V. radiation. *Oncogene* 1997; 13:413–418.

125. Sun Y, Bian J, Wang Y, Jacobs C. Activation of *p53* transcriptional activity by 1,10-phenanthroline, a metal chelator and redox sensitive compound. *Oncogene* 1997; 14:385–393.

126. Lutzker SG, Levine AJ. A functionally inactive *p53* protein in teratocarcinoma cells is activated by either DNA damge or cellular differentiation. *Nature Med* 1996; 2:804–810.

127. Moll UM, Riou G, Levine AJ. Two distinct mechanisms alter *p53* in breast cancer: Mutation and nuclear exclusion. *Proc Natl Acad Sci USA* 1992; 89:7262–7266.

128. Takahashi K, Suzuki K. DNA synthesis-associated nuclear exclusion of *p53* in normal human breast epithelial cells in culture. *Oncogene* 1994; 9:183–188.

129. Alagjem MI, Spike BT, Rodewald LW, Hope TJ, Klemm M, Jaenisch R, Wahl GM. ES cells do not activate *p53*-dependent stress responses and undergo *p53*-independent apoptosis in response to DNA damage. *Curr Biol* 1998; 8:145–155.

130. Khan QA, Vousden KH, Dipple A. Cellular response to DNA damage from a potent carcinogen involves stabilization of *p53* without induction of p21$^{wafl/cip1}$. *Carcinogenesis* 1997; 18:2313–1218.

131. Khan Q, Agarwal R, Seidel A, Frank H, Vousden KH, Dipple A. Effects of optical isomers of benzo(g)chryses antidihydrodiol epoxide in passage of MCF-7 cells through the cell cycle. *Mol Carcinog* 1998; 23:115–120.

132. Oliner JD, Kinzler KW, Meltzer PS, George DL, Vogelstein B. Amplification of a gene encoding a *p53*-associated protein in human sarcomas. *Nature* 1992; 358:80–83.

133. Leach FS, Tokino T, Meltzer P, Burrell M, Oliner JD, Smith S, Hill DE, Sidransky D, Kinzler KW, Vogelstein B. *p53* mutation and MDM2 amplification in human soft tissue sarcomas.*Cancer Res* 1993; 53:2231–2234.

134. Reifenberger G, Liu L, Ichimura K, Schmidt EE, Collins VP. Amplification and overexpression of the MDM2 gene in a subset of human malignant gliomas without *p53* mutations. *Cancer Res* 1993; 53:2736–2739.

135. Rampino N, Yamamoto H, Ionov Y, Li Y, Sawai H, Reed JC, Perucho M. Somatic frameshift mutations in the BAX gene in colon cancers of the microsatellite mutator phenotype. *Science* 1997; 275:967–969.

23

Regulation of NF-κB Function
Novel Molecular Targets for Pharmacological Intervention

Frank Mercurio, PhD and Anthony M. Manning, PhD

1. INTRODUCTION

Malignant tumor cells have usually accumulated mutations that affect a variety of cellular processes, including those that sustain cell growth, that block growth inhibition and apoptosis, that affect DNA repair, and that allow the tumor to escape immune surveillance. The Rel/NF-κB transcription factor family participates in the induction of a variety of cellular and viral genes involved in these processes. Although NF-κB was originally identified as a transcription factor required for B-cell-specific gene expression, subsequent studies demonstrated that it is ubiquitously expressed and serves as a critical regulator of the inducible expression of many genes. For this reason, the pharmaceutical industry has focused significant attention on this pathway for the identification of novel therapeutic agents. However, much remains to be understood as to how NF-κB is regulated and the specific role played by this transcription factor in the spectrum of tumors in man. This chapter briefly summarizes recent findings on the mechanisms of NF-κB regulation in cells and on the potential role of NF-κB in cancer. This information suggests that NF-κB inhibitors will represent agents with broad potential for the treatment of cancer.

2. NF-κB AND IκB PROTEINS

NF-κB exists in the cytoplasm of most cell types as homo- or heterodimers of a family of structurally related proteins (1,2). Each member of this family contains a conserved N-terminal region called the Rel-homology domain (RHD), within which lie the DNA-binding and dimerization domains and the nuclear localization signal (NLS). To date, five proteins belonging to the NF-κB family have been identified in mammalian cells: RelA (also known as p65), c-Rel, RelB, NF-κB1 (p50/105), and NF-κB2 (p52/100). The first three of these are produced as transcriptionaly active proteins, the latter are synthesized as longer precursor molecules of 105 and 100 kDa, respectively, which are further processed to smaller, transcriptionally active forms. The classical NF-κB dimer contains RelA and NF-κB1, but a variety of other Rel-containing dimers are also known to exist (3–5).

From: Signaling Networks and Cell Cycle Control: The Molecular Basis of Cancer and Other Diseases
Edited by: J. S. Gutkind © Humana Press Inc., Totowa, NJ

NF-κB exisits in the cytoplasm in an inactive form associated with inhibitory proteins termed IκB's, of which the most important may be IκBα, IκBβ, and IκBε *(3,6)*. The IκB family members, which share common ankyrin-like repeat domains, regulate the DNA binding and subcellular localization of Rel/NF-κB proteins by masking a nuclear localization signal (NLS) located near the C-terminus of the Rel homology domain *(7)*.

3. NF-κB ACTIVATION PATHWAY

NF-κB can be activated in cells by a wide variety of stimuli associated with stress, injury and inflammation. Potent inducers of NF-κB include cytokines, such as interleukin-1β (IL-1β) and tumor necrosis factor-α (TNF-α); bacterial and viral products, such as lipopolysaccharide (LPS), sphingomyelinase, double-stranded RNA, and the Tax protein from human T-cell leukemia virus 1 (HTLV-1); and proapoptotic and necrotic stimuli, such as oxygen free radicals, ultraviolet (UV) light, and γ-irradiation *(8)*. This diversity of inducers highlights an intriguing aspect of NF-κB regulation, namely the ability of many different signal transduction pathways emanating from a wide variety of induction mechanisms to converge on a single target: the cytosolic NF-κB–IκB complex. The recent discovery of several key enzyme components of the NF-κB activation pathway suggests a molecular basis for signal integration in this pathway.

NF-κB activation is achieved through the signal-induced proteolytic degradation of IκB in the cytoplasm (Fig. 1). Extracellular stimuli initiate a signaling cascade leading to activation of two IκB kinases—IKK-1 (IKKα) and IKK-2 (IKKβ)—which phosphorylate IκB at specific N-terminal serine residues (S32 and S36 for IκBα, S19 and S23 for IκBβ) *(9–13, reviewed in refs. 14–16)*. Phosphorylated IκB is then selectively ubiquitinated, presumably by an E3 ubiquitin ligase, the terminal member of a cascade of ubiquitin-conjugating enzymes *(17,18)*. In the last step of this signaling cascade, phosphorylated and ubiquitinated IκB, which is still associated with NF-κB in the cytoplasm, is selectively degraded by the 26S proteasome *(19)*. This process exposes the NLS, freeing NF-κB to interact with the nuclear import machinery and translocate to the nucleus *(7)*, where it binds its target genes to initiate transcription.

The IκB kinases IKK-1 (IKKα) and IKK-2 (IKKβ) are related members of a new family of intracellular signal transduction enzymes, containing an N-terminal kinase domain and a C-terminal region with two protein interaction motifs: a leucine zipper and a helix-loop-helix motif (Fig. 2). These motifs mediate the heterodimerization of IKK-1 and IKK-2, although it is unknown whether heterodimerization is essential for function. There is strong evidence that IKK-1 and IKK-2 are themselves phosphorylated and activated by one or more upstream activating kinases, which are likely to be members of the MAP kinase kinase kinase (MAPKKK) family of enzymes *(9–13,20)*. One such upstream kinase, NF-κB inducing kinase (NIK), was identified by its ability to bind directly to TRAF2, an adapter protein thought to couple both TNF-α and IL-1 receptors to NF-κB activation *(21)*. A second MAPKKK, MEKK-1, was shown to be present in the IKK signalsome complex *(12)*. Coexpression of either NIK or MEKK enhances the ability of the IKKs to phosphorylate IκB and activate NF-κB *(9,10,12,13)*. The likely sites of activating phosphorylation on the IKKs have been identified as two serine residues within the kinase activation loop that lie within a short region of

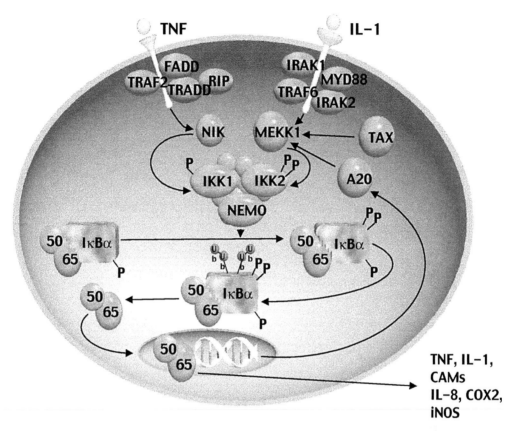

Fig. 1. Schematic representation of components of the NF-κB signal transduction pathway leading from the tumor necrosis factor (TNF) and interleukin-1 (IL-1) receptors. A number of signal transduction proteins have been identified as associated with these recpetors, including TNF-receptor associated factors 2 and 6 (TRAF2 and 6), death domain-containing proteins (TRADD and FADD), kinases associated with the IL-1 recpetor (IRAK1 and 2, and MYD88). Other proteins, such as ring-finger interacting protein (RIP), have been identified based on their ability to interact with several of these proteins. Signals emanating from the TNF and IL-1 receptors activate members of the MEKK-related family, including NIK and MAKK1. These proteins are involved in activation of IKK1 and IKK2, the IkB kinase components of the IKK signalsome. These kinase phosphorylate members of the IkB family at specific serines within their N-termini, leading to site-specific ubiquitination and degradation by the 26S proteosome. Several NF-kB-induced genes act to autoregulate this pathway, including IκBα and A20. Tax, a protein encoded by the HTLV-1 virus, acts to transactivate NF-κB through activation of MEKK-1 and the NF-κB cascade.

homology to the MEK (MAP kinase kinase) family of proteins *(12)*. Phosphorylation of these two serine residues in the MEKs is required for their activation. In IKK-2, mutation of the two corresponding serine residues to alanine yields an inactive dominant-negative protein capable of blocking the activation of endogenous NF-κB *(12)*. In both IKK-1 and IKK-2, mutation of these residues to glutamate yields a constitutively active kinase, presumably because the glutamate residues mimic to some degree the phosphoserines obtained after phosphorylation by the upstream activating kinase *(12)*.

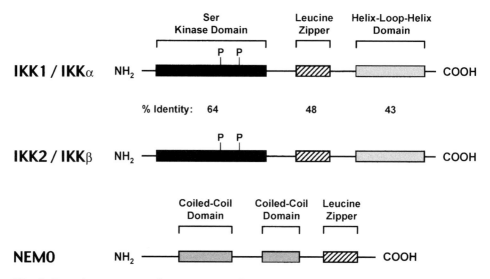

Fig. 2. Domain structures of components of the IKK signalsome. IKK1 and 2 (also known as IKKα and β) represent the IκB kinases. The overall identity of these kinases at the amino acid level is noted. NEMO was identified as a non-kinase component of this complex, and specifically binds IKK2.

The precise role of NIK and MEKK-1 in IKK activation has been the subject of several recent reports. NIK preferentially phosphorylates IKK1 on ser 176 in the activation loop between subdomain VII and VIII, leading to the activation of IKK1 kinase activity *(22)*. Overexpression of NIK in cells leads to activation of both IKK1 and IKK2, suggesting that IKK1 activation soemhow leads to activation of IKK2. Of note, MEKK-1 specifically phosphorylates the corresponding serines in the activation loop of IKK2, leading to activation of IKK2 kinase activity, but not IKK1 activity *(22,23)*. Because NIK and MEKK-1 are activated by discrete stimuli, they appear to provide a mechanism for the differential activation of members of the IKK complex. Extracellular stimuli that selectively activate IKK1 or IKK2 have not been identified, and the physiologic consequences of selective IKK activation remain unknown. It is intriguing to speculate that this mechanism may somehow play a role in the selective activation of different complexes of Rel family members within the cytoplasm. Clearly, additional characterization of the biochemical components of the IKK signalsome complex and the mechanism of recruitment and phosphorylation of different IκB-containing complexes is essential to further understanding the role of selective IKK activation. Recently, a non-kinase component of the IKK signalsome was identified through genetic complementation of a flat cellular variant of HTLV-1 Tax-transformed rat fibroblasts, known as 5R, which is unresponsive to all tested NF-κB activating stimuli *(24)*. This protein, named NEMO [NF-κB-essential modulator], represents a 48-kDa protein, which contains a putative leucine zipper (Fig. 2). In vitro NEMO can homodimerize and directly interact with IKK2. The protein is absent from 5R cells, and another NF-κB-unresponsive cell line, 1.3E2, is present in the IKK signalsome complex and is essential for its formation. The NEMO protein was able to complement both cell lines, and restore NF-κB activation induced by lipopolysaccharide (LPS), phorbol myristate acetate (PMA), and IL-1. Using biochemical techniques, we recently identified the presence of two distinct IKK-containing complexes in cells: one a hetero-dimer containing IKK1 and IKK2, the other a homodimer containing IKK2 *(25)*. Both complexes contained NEMO, presumably through its interaction with IKK2. The assembly of distinct IKK-containing complexes that can be differentially activated by upstream activators such as NIK or MEKK provides an additional mechanism for selective activation of NF-κB complexes in cells.

κB phosphorylation serves as a molecular tag leading to rapid ubiquitination and degra-dation of IκB by components of the ubiquitin-proteasome system. The sites of ubiquitin conjugation are two adjacent lysine residues (Lys-20 and Lys-21 in IκBα) located just N-terminal to the two serines that are targets for phosphorylation by the IKKs *(26)*. Using peptides as substrate mimics, it was established that IκBα phosphorylation generates a binding site for the specific ubiquitin ligase(s) responsible for conjugation of ubiquitin to IκBα, and that microinjection of these phosphopeptides into cells could interfere with NF-κB activation *(27)*. These results emphasize the importance of the ubiquitin ligase system in IκB degradation. The IκB-specific E3 ligase awaits molecular identification.

The IκB kinases IKK1 and IKK2, their upstream activating kinases MEKK and NIK, and their downstream effector, the putative E3 ligase, all represent attractive targets for the discovery of drugs that selectively regulate NF-κB function. These proteins may all be part of a large 600- to 800-kDa protein complex, the IKK signalsome *(12)*. Particularly interesting is the crosstalk between the NF-κB and AP-1 activation pathways, exemplified by the homology between IKKs and MEKs, the presence of MEKK in the IKK signalsome complex, and the fact that the upstream kinases of the IKKs are members of the MAPKKK family.

Posttranslational modification of the NF-κB complex, occurring subsequent to IκB degradation have been reported to enhance transcriptional activation of NF-κB-depen-dent genes. The transcriptional activity of NF-κB is stimulated upon phosphorylation of its p65 subunit on serine 276 by protein kinase A (PKA) *(28)*. The transcriptional coactivator CBP/p300 was found to associate with NF-κB RelA through two sites: an N-terminal domain that interacts with the C-terminal region of unphosphorylated RelA, and a second domain that interacts with RelA phosphorylated on serine 276 *(29)*. Accessibility to both sites is blocked in unphosphorylated RelA through an intramolecu-lar masking of the N-terminus by the C-terminal region of RelA. Phosphorylation by PKA both weakens the interaction between the N- and C-terminal regions of RelA and creates an additional site for interaction with CBP/p300 *(30)*. Because PKA phosphory-lates a range of substrates in vivo, it is unlikely that PKA inhibitors could achieve selective modulation of NF-κB-dependent gene transcription. Of note, RelA is phosphor-ylated by IKK1 and IKK2 in vitro on several other residues in addition to Ser 276 *(12,25)*. The precise residues phosphorylated by these enzymes, as well as their effects on NF-κB-dependent transcription in-vivo, have yet to be reported.

4. NF-κB AND CANCER

Cancer is a group of diseases characterized by uncontrolled cell growth and spread of abnormal cells. Cancer is the second leading cause of death in the United States, with 500,000 deaths and an estimated 1.3 million new cases in 1996. The American Cancer Society estimates that in 1997 the approximate economic cost of cancer in the United States alone amounted to $104 billion.

Malignant tumor cells have usually accumulated mutations that affect a variety of processes, including those that sustain cell growth, that block growth inhibition and apoptosis, that affect DNA repair, and that allow the tumor to escape immune surveillance. Several lines of evidence suggest that NF-κB family members are involved in tumor growth and metastasis. The genes for c-rel, NFKB1 (p105), NFKB2 (p52), RelA, and Bcl-3 are located at sites of recurrent tranlsocation and genomic rearrangements in cancer *(31–33)*. Several Hodgkin's lymphoma cell lines contain constitutively nuclear NF-κB complexes, and inhibition of NF-κB activation by overexpression of a nondegradable IκBα molecule inhibits proliferation and tumorigenicity of these cells *(34)*. Many breast cancer cells also contain high levels of nuclear NF-κB DNA-binding activity, which is essential for the survival of these cells in culture *(35)*. Of note, chemically induced breast cancers in rats and many primary human breast cancer samples have high levels of nuclear NF-κB. High levels of activated NF-κB are also associated with the progression of breast cancer cells to estrogen-independent growth *(36)*. High levels of NF-κB activity have been reported in diverse solid tumor-derived cell lines *(37)*. Human thyroid carcinoma cells require nuclear NF-κB activity for proliferation and malignant transformation in vitro *(38)*. The Tax protein from the leukemogenic virus HTLV-1 is a potent activator of NF-κB *(39)*. Oncogenic forms of *ras,* the most common defect in human tumors, can activate NF-κB, and NF-κB inhibition can block *ras*-mediated cellular transformation *(40)*. Insights into the molecular mechanims by which NF-κB promotes these effects are being elucidated. Many cancer therapies function to kill transformed cells through apoptotic mechanisms. Resistance to apoptosis provides protection against cell killing by these therapies and may represent a major mechanism of tumor drug resistance *(41)*. The activation of NF-κB by TNF-α, ionizing radiation, and chemotherapeutic agents was found to protect tumor cells from cell killing *(42–44)*. Inhibition of NF-κB activation in this setting enhanced apoptotic killing by these reagents, but not by apoptotic stimuli that do not activate NF-κB. NF-κB can induce the expression of antiapoptotic genes such as IAP proteins (cellular inhibitor of apoptosis-1 *(45,46)*, superoxide dismutase (SOD), and A20, or genes that contribute to proliferation, such as c-*myc* and Bcl-2 (Fig. 3). Recently, NF-κB activation was shown to result in transcriptional activation of the genes encoding a novel factor IEX-1L *(77)* and TRAF1 and 2, and result in supression of caspase 8 activation *(78)*. In this way, persistent activation of NF-κB represents a unique mechanism by which these cells express genes that protect against apoptotic stimuli. NF-κB also regulates the expression cell adhesion molecules that facilitate cell adhesion and migration *(50,51)*. Inhibition of NF-κB activation, using either antisense oligonucleotides or transcription factor decoys, results in loss of adhesion in tumor cells in culture *(79)* and reduction in tumor formation in nude mice *(80)*. Inhibition of NF-κB represents a novel approach to cancer drug development, and when used as combination therapy with established therapeutics, these agents could provide a more effective treatment of drug-resistant forms of cancer.

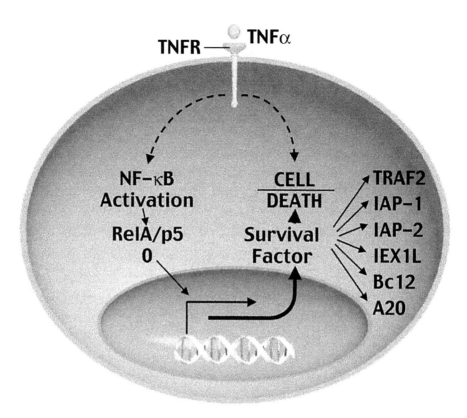

Fig. 3. Mechanism by which NF-κB protects cells from tumor necrosis factor (TNF)-induced apoptosis. NF-κB activation results in the transcriptional activation of a range of anti-apoptosis proteins, including TRAF2, IAP-1 and -2, IEX-1L, Bcl2, and A20. 30.

5. CONCLUDING REMARKS

During the 10 years since the identification of NF-κB, this transcription factor has been revealed as an important regulator of a broad range of genes implicated in human disease. Recent studies using human tissues and animal models of human disease have substantiated a key role for NF-κB in cancer. The elucidation of enzyme components of the NF-κB signal transduction pathway are providing molecular targets for the development of potent and selective small molecular inhibitors of NF-κB activation. The availability of these inhibitors will permit complete evaluation of the potential of NF-κB as a novel target for anticancer therapies.

REFERENCES

1. Baldwin AS. The NF-κB and IκB proteins: New discoveries and insights. *Annu Rev Immunol* 1996; 14:649–681.
2. Kopp E, Ghosh S. NF-κB and Rel proteins in innate immunity. *Adv Immunol* 1995; 58:1–27.
3. Baeuerle PA, Baltimore D. NF-κB: Ten years after. *Cell* 1996; 87:13–20.
4. Baeuerle PA, Henkel T. Function and activation of NF-κB in the immune system. *Annu Rev Immunol* 1994; 12:141–179.

5. May MJ, Ghosh S. Signal transduction through NF-κB. *Immunol Today* 1998; 19:80–88.
6. Whiteside ST, Epinat JC, Rice NR, Israel A. IκB epsilon, a novel member of the IκB family, controls RelA and cRel NF-κB activity. *EMBO J* 1997; 16:1413–1426.
7. Henkel T, Zabel U, Van Zee K, Muller JM, Fanning E, Baeuerle P. Intramolecular masking of the nuclear location signal and dimerization domain in the precursor for the p50 NF-κB subunit. *Cell* 1992; 68:1121–1133.
8. Bauerle PA, Baichwal VR. NF-κB as a frequent target for immunosuppressive and anti-inflammatory molecules. *Adv Immunol* 1997; 65:111–136.
9. Regnier CH, Song H, Gao H, Goeddel DV, Cao Z, Rothe M. Identification and characterization of an IκB Kinase. *Cell* 1997; 90:373–383.
10. DiDonato JA, Hayakawa M, Rothwarf DM, Zandi E, Karin M. A cytokine-responsive IκB kinase that activates the transcription factor NF-κB. *Nature* 1997; 388:853–862.
11. Zandi E, Rothwarf DM, Delhasse M, Hayakawa M, Karin M. The IκB kinase complex (IKK) contains two kinase subunits, IKKα and IKKβ, necessary for IκB phosphorylation and NF-κB activation. *Cell* 1997; 91:243–252.
12. Mercurio F, Zhu H, Murray BW, Shevchenko A, Bennett BL, Li J, Young D, Barbosa M, Mann M, Manning AM, Rao A. IKK-1 and IKK-2: Cytokine-activated IκB kinases essential for NF-κB activation. *Science* 1997; 278:860–866.
13. Woronicz JD, Gao X, Cao Z, Rothe M, Goeddel DV. IκB kinase-β: NF-κB activation and complex formation with IκB kinase-α and NIK. *Science* 1997; 278:866–869.
14. Stancovski I, Baltimore D. NF-κB activation: The IκB kinase revealed? *Cell* 1997; 91:299–302.
15. Maniatis T. Catalysis by a multiprotein IκB kinase complex. *Science* 1997; 278:818–819.
16. Verma IM, Stevenson J. IκB kinase: Beginning, not end. *Proc Nat Acad Sci USA* 1997; 94:11758–11760.
17. Alkalay I, Yaron A, Hatzubai A, Orian A, Ciechanover A, Ben-Neriah Y. Stimulation-dependent IκBα phosphorylation marks the NF-κB inhibitor for degradation via the ubiquitin-proteasome pathway. *Proc Natl Acad Sci USA* 1995; 92:10,599–10,603.
18. Yaron A, Gonen H, Alkalay I, Hatzubai A, et al. Inhibition of NF-κB cellular function via specific targeting of the IκB ubiquitin ligase. *EMBO J* 1997; 16:6486–6494.
19. Chen Z, Hagler J, Palombella VJ, Melandri F, Scherer D, Ballard D, Maniatis T. Signal-induced site-specific phosphorylation targets IκB α to the ubiquitin-proteasome pathway. *Genes Dev* 1995; 9:1586–1597.
20. Lee FS, Hagler J, Chen ZJ, Maniatis T. Acitvation of the IκBα complex by MEKK1, a kinase of the JNK pathway. *Cell* 1997; 88:213–222.
21. Malinin NL, Boldin MP, Kovalenko AV, Wallach D. MAP3K-related kinase involved in NF-κB induction by TNF, CD95 and IL-1. *Nature* 1997; 385:540–544.
22. Nakano H, Shindo M, Sakon S, Nishinaka S, Mihara M, Yagita H, Okumura K. Differential regulation of IκB kinase α and κ by two upstream kinases, NF-κB-inducing kinase and mitogen-activated protein kinase/ERK kinase kinase-1. *Proc Natl Acad Sci USA* 1998; 95:3537–3542.
23. Yin M-J, Christerson LB, Yamamoto Y, Kwak Y-T, Xu S, Mercurio F, Barbosa M, Cobb MH, Gaynor RB. HTLV-I Tax protein binds to MEKK1 to stimulate IκB kinase activity and NF-κB activation. *Cell* 1998; 93:875–884.
24. Yamaoka S, Courtois G, Bessia C, Whiteside ST, Weil R, Agou F, Kirk H, Kay RJ, Israël A. Complementation cloning of NEMO, a component of the IκB kinase complex essential for NF-κB activation. *Cell* 1998; 93:1231–1240.
25. Mercurio F, Murray B, Bennett BL, Pascaul G, Shevchenko A, Zhu H, Young D, Li J, Mann M, Manning A. IKKAP-1, a novel regulator of NF-κB activation, reveals heterogeneity in IκB complexes. *Mol Cell Biol* 1999; 19:1526–1538.
26. Orian A, Whiteside S, Israel A, Stancovski I, Schwartz AL, Ciechanover A. Ubiquitin-mediated processing of NF-κB transcriptional activator precursor p105. Reconstitution of

a cell-free system and identification of the ubiquitin-carrier protein, E2, and a novel ubiquitin-protein ligase, E3, involved in conjugation. *J Biol Chem* 1995; 270:21,707–21,714.

27. Yaron A, Alkalay I, Hatzubai A, Jung S, Beyth S, Mercurio F, Manning AM, Gonen H, Ciechanover A, Ben-Neriah Y. Inhibition of NF-κB cellular function via specific targeting of the IκB ubiquitin ligase. *EMBO J* 1997; 16:101–107

28. Zhong H, Yang HS, Erdjument-Bromage H, Tempst P, Ghosh S. The transcriptional activity of NF-κB is regulated by the IκB-associated PKAc subunit through a cyclic AMP-independent mechanism. *Cell* 1997; 89:413–424.

29. Perkins ND, Felzien LK, Betts JC, Leung K, Beach DH, Nabel GJ. Regulation of NF-κB by cyclin-dependent kinases associated with the p300 coactivator. *Science* 1997; 275:523–527.

30. Zhong H, Voll RE, Ghosh S. Phosphorylation of NF-κB p65 by PKA stimulates transcriptional activity by promoting a novel bivalent interaction with the coactivatorCBP/p300. *Mol Cell* 1998; 1:661–671.

31. Matthew S, Murty VV, Dalla-Favera R, Chaganti R.S. Chromosomal localization of genes encoding the transcription factors c-Rel, NF-κB p50, NF-κB p65 and lyt10 by fluoresence in situ hybridization. *Oncogene* 1993; 8:191–193.

32. Gilmore TD, Morin PJ. The IκB proteins: Members of a multifunctional family. *Trends Genet.* 1993; 9:427–433.

33. Bargou RC, Emmerich F, Krappmann D, Bommert K, Mapara MY, Arnold W, Royer HD, Grinstein E, Greiner A, Scheidereit C, Dorken B. Constitutive NF-κB RelA activation is required for proliferation and survival of Hodgkin's disease tumor cells. *J Clin Invest* 1997; 100:2961–2969.

34. Sovak MA, Bellas RE, Kim DW, Zanieski GJ, Rogers AE, Traish AM, Sonenshein GE. Aberrant NF-κB expression and the pathogenesis of breast cancer. *J Clin Invest* 1997; 100:2952–2960.

35. Nakshatri H, Bhat-Nakshatri P, Martin D, Goulet R, Sledge G. Constitutive activation of NF-κB during progression of breast cancer to hormone-independent growth. *Mol Cell Biol* 1997; 17:3629–3639.

36. Bours V, Dejardin E, Goujon-Letawe F, Merville MP, Castronovo V. The NF-κB transcription factor and cancer: High expression of NF-κB and IκB-related proteins in tumor cell lines. *Biochem Pharmacol* 1994; 47:145–149.

37. Visconti R, Cerutti J, Battista S, Fedele M, Trapasso F, Zeki K, Miano MP, de Nigris F, Casalino L, Curcio F, Santoro M, Fusco A. Expression of the neoplastic phenotype by human thyroid carcinoma cell lines requires NF-κB p65 protein expression. *Oncogene* 1997; 15:1987–1994.

38. Hammarskjold ML, Simurda MC. Epstein Barr virus latent membrane protein transactivates the human immunodeficiency virus type 1 long terminal repeat through induction of NF-κB activity. *J Virol* 1992; 66:6496–6501.

39. Finco TS, Westwick JK, Norris JL, Beg AA, Der CJ, Baldwin AS. Oncogenic Ha-Ras-induced signalling activates NF-κB transcriptional activity, which is required for cellular transformation. *J Biol Chem* 1997; 272:24,113–24,116.

40. Fisher DE. Apoptosis in cancer therapy: Crossing the threshold. *Cell* 1994; 78:539–542.

41. Wang C, Mayo M, Baldwin AS. TNF- and cancer therapy-induced apoptosis: potentiation by inhibition of NF-κB. *Science* 1996 274:784–787.

42. Van Antwerp DJ, Martin SJ, Kafri T, Green DR, Verma IM. Suppression of TNFα-induced apoptosis by NF-κB. *Science* 1996; 274:787–789.

43. Beg AA, Baltimore D. An essential role for NF-κB in preventing TNFα-induced cell death. *Science* 1996; 274:782–784.

44. Chu ZL, McKinsey TA, Liu L, Gentry JJ, Malim MH, Ballard DW. Suppression of TNF-induced cell death by inhibitor of apoptosis c-IAP2 is under NF-κB control. *Proc Natl Acad Sci USA* 1997, 94:10,057–10,062.

45. You M, Ku PT, Hrdlickova R, Bose HR. ch-IAP1, a member of the inhibitor of apoptosis

family, is a mediator of the anti-apoptotic activity of the v-Rel oncoprotein. *Mol Cell Biol* 1997; 17:7328–7341.

46. Wu MX, Ao Z, Prasad KV, Wu R, Schlossman SF. IEX-1L, an apoptosis inhibitor involved in NF-κB-mediated cell survival. *Science* 1998; 281:998–1001.

47. Wang C-Y, Mayo MW, Korneluk RG, Goeddell DV, Baldwin AS. NF-κB antiapoptosis: Induction of TRAF1 and TRAF2 and c-IAP1 and c-IAP2 to supress caspase 8 activation. *Science* 1998; 281:1680–1683.

48. Sokoloski JA, Sartorelli AC, Rosen CA, Narayanan R. Antisense oligonucleotides to the p65 subunit of NF-κB block CD11b expression and adhesion properties of differentiated HL-60 granulocytes. *Blood* 1993; 82:625–632.

49. Higgins KA, Perez JR, Coleman TA, Dorshkind K, McComas WA, Sarmiento UM, Rosen CA, Narayanan R. Antisense inhibition of the p65 subunit of NF-κB blocks tumorigenicity and causes tumor regression. *Proc Natl Acad Sci USA* 1993; 90:9901–9905.

24

Using Protein–Interaction Domains to Manipulate Signaling Pathways

Bruce J. Mayer

1. INTRODUCTION

The signal transduction machinery of eukaryotes is driven by changes in protein–protein associations. We have traditionally thought of signal transmission as being mediated by the altered activities of enzymes such as kinases and GTPases; in most cases, however, such changes in enzymatic activity are the result of changes in protein–protein binding. Furthermore, the activation of enzymes involved in signaling often leads in turn to further changes in their binding interactions or those of their substrates. The central importance of protein–protein binding is reinforced by the realization that most enzymes involved in signaling pathways consist of multiple protein-interaction domains (and, in some cases, lipid interaction domains) in addition to the catalytic domain itself. This modular design allows the activity of the enzyme and its local concentration relative to potential activators and substrates to be regulated by interactions with other proteins.

A number of protein-interaction modules have been identified, including Src Homology 2 (SH2) and SH3, PTB, WW, and PDZ domains *(1–3)*. These share the characteristics of being found in a wide variety of protein contexts, being able to fold independently and confer binding activity that is relatively insensitive to the protein context, and binding to linear peptide determinants as opposed to large protein surfaces. For each of these domains, it has been possible to establish consensus binding sites for specific domains (e.g., the SH2 domain of Src vs. that of Grb2) and numerous high-resolution crystal and nuclear magnetic resonance (NMR) structures exist that reveal the underlying basis of specificity at the atomic level. These characteristics make such domains attractive targets for experimental disruption, not only as a means to understand the logic of specific signaling networks but also as potential targets for therapeutic drugs. This brief chapter explores some experimental approaches to inhibition of protein-protein interactions in signaling with an emphasis on SH2- and SH3-mediated interactions.

2. SH2 AND SH3 DOMAINS

The specifics of the structures and binding specificity of SH2 and SH3 domains have been extensively reviewed *(1–4)*. Briefly, SH2 domains bind with high affinity

From: Signaling Networks and Cell Cycle Control: The Molecular Basis of Cancer and Other Diseases
Edited by: J. S. Gutkind © Humana Press Inc., Totowa, NJ

to tyrosine-phosphorylated peptides; because they have negligible affinity for unphosphorylated sites, they therefore serve as *switches* to regulate binding in response to changes in tyrosine phosphorylation. Individual SH2 domains exhibit specificity for different tyrosine-phosphorylated sites, with most of the specificity conferred by the three residues C-terminal to the phosphorylated tyrosine. SH3 domains bind to proline-rich sites that adopt the left-handed proline-II helix conformation. There is also specificity among SH3 domains for different binding sites, but the determinants of specificity are less clear-cut than in the case of the SH2 domains and there is often considerable overlap in the spectrum of sites that bind different SH3 domains. In addition many proteins contain multiple SH3 domains and many target proteins contain multiple binding sites, resulting in increased affinity caused by multidentate interactions.

The specificity of these interactions is a critical parameter if we are to ultimately understand how a particular signaling network operates and how it might be disrupted experimentally. Specificity is conferred not only by the intrinsic dissociation constants of the domain–peptide interactions (for high-affinity peptide ligands, measured dissociation constants are within the range of 10^{-7} M for SH2-phosphopeptide binding, and 10^{-6}–10^{-5} M for SH3–peptide interactions) but is also necessarily influenced by the local concentration of potential binding partners. One can imagine an SH3 domain might have a very different spectrum of binding partners at equilibrium in the cytosol compared to the same domain in the same cell if were localized on the plasma membrane, where the local concentration of potential partners will be quite different. Such local concentration effects might explain some instances where proteins bound to a specific SH3 domain appear to change upon signal-induced relocalization *(5,6)*. We are severely hampered by our inability to accurately measure the effective local concentration of proteins and their potential ligands in various compartments of the cell. These parameters will be crucial to understanding the dynamic aspects of signaling, especially those that govern spatially organized phenomena such as motility and the cytoskeleton.

The issue of specificity is also critical if we wish to interpret the results of experiments designed to disrupt particular interactions. As discussed below we might introduce dominant negative mutants of a signaling protein, or peptides that mimic a specific binding site, and measure the ability of such reagents to block a particular signal. One must constantly be aware that such approaches often rely on quite high concentrations of the inhibitors, and at such concentrations they are likely to bind to a broad spectrum of endogenous proteins, not only those for which they were designed. Even if the disruption strategy does not involve high concentrations of inhibitors, the overlapping specificities of many SH2 and SH3 domains at physiological concentrations must be kept in mind. While these considerations might make it impossible to definitively assign a role for a specific interaction in a specific signal output, such approaches are still useful. In some ways they probably reflect the realities of intracellular signaling, which are likely to depend on complex equilibria of many different competing interactions, more accurately than more linear approaches that assume a single interaction is uniquely important to signal output.

To illustrate this point, one might consider the response of cells to an extracellular stimulus such as the peptide mitogen, platelet-derived growth factor (PDGF). The PDGF receptor has intrinsic tyrosine kinase activity, and upon ligand binding rapidly autophosphorylates on a number of sites on its intracellular catalytic domain. The first signal that is interpreted by the interior of the cell, therefore, is the presence of a new constellation of tyrosine phosphorylated sites that can serve as binding sites for cytosolic proteins containing SH2 or PTB domains. In the case of the PDGF receptor, these include PLCγ, Ras-GAP, Pl-3 kinase, the protein-tyrosine phosphatase SHP-2, and Src-family nonreceptor tyrosine kinases, in addition to adaptor proteins which do not contain catalytic domains such as Shc, Grb2, and Nck *(7)*. Some of these proteins can themselves be phosphorylated by the receptor, thereby creating additional binding sites for other cytosolic proteins. Although phosphorylation can to some extent directly regulate the enzymatic activity of some of these proteins, it is likely that their relocalization to the membrane (in proximity to their substrates) is far more important to the ultimate signal output.

One way to define the "signaling state" of a cell is the array of tyrosine-phosphorylated sites, each with a different spectrum of potential ligands, which serves as a sort of bar-code representation of the extracellular environment. Indeed, one can consider the cytosolic SH2- and PTB-containing proteins as a sensing apparatus for detecting changes in the concentration and/or localization of such sites. Because there are several different phosphorylation sites even on a single receptor, each of which can interact with a spectrum of proteins with varying affinities, intracellular responses cannot be thought of in linear terms; a more accurate representation would be changes in the binding equilibria of complex populations of proteins. Indeed, experiments in which single PDGF receptor phosphorylation sites have been mutated, or added back to a receptor in which all major sites had been eliminated by mutation, have yielded somewhat enigmatic results *(8,9)*. Add to this the realization that the population of phosphorylated sites on a receptor can change over time following stimulation *(10)*, and the fact that most cells exist in an environment in which multiple tyrosine kinase-mediated pathways are constantly stimulated at least at basal levels, and it is apparent that attempts to ascribe a signal output to a specific single protein or interaction might be unrealistic. The approaches outlined, however, allow us to perturb entire classes of interactions, thereby complementing techniques such as genetic knock-outs that are designed to address the role of a single gene product.

3. "PROTEIN GENETICS"

The use of dominant negative mutants has become a popular approach to inhibiting the function of a protein of interest. To act as a dominant negative, a mutant protein must retain the ability to interact with normal endogenous binding partners, but be impaired in some other function so that the endogenous binding partners are sequestered in inactive complexes. Proteins containing protein-interaction modules such as SH2 or SH3 domains are ideal candidates for such an approach. For example, if the biological activity of an enzyme is dependent on SH2-mediated relocalization to membranes, overexpression of a mutant in which the SH2 is intact but the catalytic domain is nonfunctional would be predicted to prevent activation of the endogenous enzyme by blocking its access to the tyrosine phosphorylated sites on the membrane. SH2/SH3 adaptors, such as Grb2, also lend themselves to this approach. These adaptors consist entirely of SH2 and SH3 domains, and function as inducible crosslinkers during signaling. In this case SH2 mutants inhibit by sequestering SH3-binding proteins in cytosolic complexes, whereas SH3 mutants block access of endogenous proteins to their tyrosine phosphorylated SH2-binding sites (Fig. 1).

Several caveats must be considered when using any dominant negative approach. The most important of these is that such mutants are very different from genetic nulls: A phenotype engendered by a dominant negative mutant does not imply that the endogenous protein is involved in the phenotype, but that proteins that bind to the protein are involved. This potential disadvantage can be turned to advantage however. If one considers a case in which there might be multiple family members with similar binding activities (the closely related adaptors Crk and Crkl, for example), a dominant negative mutant of either would inhibit the function of both, whereas a genetic null (generated by targeted gene disruption or antisense approaches) would have no phenotype if the multiple family members function redundantly. Because dominant approaches are relatively rapid and likely to give phenotypic effects, they can be very informative provided the results are interpreted thoughtfully.

One can think of such an approach, especially in the case of proteins with clearly defined domains with well-understood functions, as a type of "protein genetics." If one obtains a phenotype of interest by overexpression of a mutant, the effects must be attributable to the sequestration or mislocalization of proteins that bind to the unmutated domains. For example, if a Grb2 SH2 mutant blocks mitogenesis, then its effects must be via proteins that bind its SH3 domains. Such information is useful because the domain now provides a biochemical handle to identify the culprits; the SH3 domains can be used to screen for binding proteins by a variety of methods. While it might require several additional steps to then prove that any particular SH3-binding protein or set of proteins is responsible for the phenotype, an important logical link is forged between a biological effect and a class of proteins with specific binding properties.

4. DOMINANT NEGATIVE APPROACHES

A wide variety of experiments designed to dominantly inhibit signaling pathways by interfering with SH2- or SH3-mediated interactions have been undertaken, and a few examples (by no means an exhaustive or even representative list) are outlined below. Such approaches involve introduction of mutant protein or the DNA or RNA encoding it, and can involve expression of isolated SH2 or SH3 domains or full-length enzymes in which the catalytic activity has been ablated. Finally, as discussed at the end of this chapter, it is also possible to introduce peptide or peptidomimetic ligands to block SH3- or SH2-mediated interactions in vivo.

4.1. Microinjection of Purified Protein

Perhaps the simplest experiments conceptually are those involving microinjection of purified, bacterially-produced SH2 or SH3 domains into tissue culture cells. The microinjected domains inhibit signaling by binding to endogenous proteins and thereby preventing their association with their normal partners. Because proteins are injected directly into the cytosol, the phenotypic effects are expected to be quite rapid (essentially only limited by diffusion of the injected protein and the rate of dissociation of pre-existing endogenous complexes). The signal outputs that can be analyzed, however, are limited to those that can be assayed at the single-cell level, usually by microscopy.

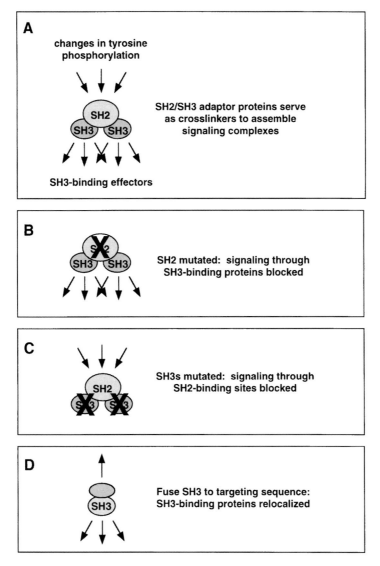

Fig. 1. Inhibition or stimulation of signaling pathways with dominant SH2/SH3 adaptor mutants. An SH2/SH3 adaptor (e.g., Grb2) consisting of two SH3 domains and an SH2 domain is depicted diagrammatically. (A) The adaptor normally functions to relocalize SH3-binding proteins to sites of tyrosine phosphorylation that bind the SH2 domain. (BC) Dominant-negative mutants with mutations in the SH2 domain (B) or SH3 domain (C) have very different mechanisms of action when overexpressed. (D) Isolated SH3 domains can be targeted to specific subcellular localizations. If the adaptor normally functions to relocalize proteins to the membrane, then membrane localization of the SH3 domains will mimic tyrosine phosphorylation of SH2-binding sites.

For example, it was shown that the isolated N-terminal SH3 domain of the Crk adaptor protein could block the neurite outgrowth of PC12 cells stimulated by intact Crk protein *(11)*. This experiment firmly implicated the binding of other cellular factors as a requirement for the Crk SH3 to exert its biological activity, as opposed to models in which it played a more passive role (for example, stabilizing the SH2 domain or its binding to tyrosine phosphorylated sites). The observation that the Crk SH3 domain was unable to inhibit neurite outgrowth induced by nerve growth factor (NGF) or by activated Ras demonstrated that binding of endogenous proteins to the Crk SH3 target was required upstream of the activation of Ras in Crk-injected cells, but was not necessary for neurite outgrowth in response to all receptor-mediated signals. This result also provided reassurance that the SH3 domain did not inhibit neurite outgrowth through a nonspecific toxic effect.

A similar approach was used to suggest a role for Grb2 in the internalization of the EGF receptor after ligand stimulation *(12)*. In this case, a pool of different SH2 domains was tested for the ability to block receptor endocytosis, and then the individual domains that comprised the positive pool were assayed until the activity could be uniquely ascribed to the Grb2 SH2 domain. Such an approach, using pools that can then be "sib-selected" to identify the component responsible, might have general applicability in rapidly testing a large number of interaction domains for ability to block a specific effect. This series of experiments also demonstrates that it is possible to circumvent the problem of overlapping binding specificities by injecting a relatively modest amount of protein (several thousand molecules of each SH2 domain per cell in this case).

These experiments implicated a Grb2 SH2-binding site in endocytosis, but did not necessarily imply that Grb2 itself is normally involved. One could imagine the Grb2 SH2 prevented association of some other critical endogenous protein or proteins from associating with the receptor. This question was partially resolved by the demonstration that Grb2 proteins containing a functional C-terminal SH3 domain in addition to the SH2 only weakly inhibited endocytosis, suggesting that these mutant proteins could participate in normal endocytosis. This is far less convincing, however, than if it were possible to demonstrate that injection of the wt protein had no inhibitory effect, or that an excess of the wt could rescue the inhibitory effect of the isolated SH2. However, it must be kept in mind that since the adaptor is presumably functioning as a bifunctional cross-linker, at very high concentrations wt Grb2 would also be predicted to inhibit. This is because the adaptor would be present in excess over both its endogenous SH2-binding and SH3-binding targets, favoring the formation of nonfunctional bimolecular complexes over the biologically active trimolecular complex.

4.2. Transfection

Expression of mutant adaptors by transfection of plasmid DNA permits measurements of a wider range of phenotypic effects and is more convenient than microinjection for large numbers of samples and conditions. If plasmid expressing the dominant negative construct is cotransfected with a reporter plasmid to monitor signal output, it is possible to assay biochemical effects such as kinase activation or changes in transcriptional activity. Such experiments can be very useful to scout for targets to inhibit a specific signaling pathway.

A simple series of such experiments were used to assess the ability of various adaptor protein mutants to inhibit activation of the MAP kinase Erk1 in response to mitogenic signals *(13)*. Mutants of each of the three classes of SH2-SH3 adaptors (Grb2, Crk, and Nck) were constructed such that the binding activity of either their SH2 domain or their SH3 domains was abolished. These mutants were cotransfected into tissue culture cells along with a plasmid expressing a tagged version of the Erk1 kinase. After stimulation, the tagged Erk protein was isolated and its activation state determined. These experiments showed that both the SH2 mutant and SH3 mutants of Grb2 were potent inhibitors of Erk activation in response to EGF *(13)*, whereas Crk and Nck mutants had no inhibitory effect. This demonstrated a requirement both for the tyrosine-phosphorylated sites that bind the Grb2 SH2, and proteins that bind the Grb2 SH3 domain (presumably including the Ras activator Sos), for signal transmission from the growth factor receptor to Ras. By contrast, the results also demonstrated that engagement of proteins that bind the SH2 and SH3 domains of Crk and Nck was not essential for signal transmission.

A more complex pattern of inhibition was noted when Erk activity was stimulated by the nonreceptor tyrosine kinase Abl. In this case, Grb2 mutants still strongly inhibited, but now Crk mutants and in particular a Crk SH3 mutant also inhibited Erk activation. When combinations of Crk and Grb2 mutants were assayed together, a synergistic inhibitory effect was seen with the combination of the Crk SH3 mutant and the Grb2 SH3 mutant. This suggested that signaling from Abl to Ras requires proteins that bind to Crk, and in particular tyrosine-phosphorylated proteins that bind the Crk SH2 must play a critical role in addition to those that bind the Grb2 SH2. These experiments identified a previously unappreciated class of proteins in Abl-transformed cells (those that bind the Crk SH2) that are essential for signal transmission, and provide a means of isolating them biochemically. Another implication is that, if small-molecule competitive inhibitors of specific SH2 domains were available, a combination of inhibitors of the Grb2 SH2 and the Crk SH2 would be more potent and specific for inhibiting signals from Abl than either inhibitor alone.

4.3. Perturbation of Development

Dominant-negative approaches have also been used in much more complicated systems, such as the developing *Xenopus* embryo. It is possible to inject mRNA (or plasmid DNA or even protein) into fertilized *Xenopus* eggs and assess the effects on early development. Early amphibian development is extremely well characterized, and it is possible to assess phenotypic effects on the developmental potential of explants or lineages of cells in the whole embryo. Although the complexity of the signaling events and cell–cell interactions that govern early development can make interpretation of experiments difficult, the fact that such a wide range of signaling mechanisms are required for normal development makes it possible to detect effects of experimental manipulation without preconceived notions of which specific pathways might be affected.

An example of such an approach is the analysis of the SH2-containing protein-tyrosine phosphatase SH-PTP2 *(14)*. In this case it was found that expression of a catalytically inactive form of the phosphatase inhibited mesoderm formation in the early embryo, presumably by binding to tyrosine-phosphorylated sites on proteins such as the FGF receptor and preventing the subsequent activation of MAP kinases. In this case it was possible to demonstrate that the wt protein was able to rescue the inhibitory effects of the catalytically inactive mutant, providing strong evidence that it was SH-PTP2 itself, and not some other endogenous protein that binds to the same tyrosine phosphorylated sites, that was essential for transmitting the signal. The developmental system in this case pointed to a somewhat counterintuitive positive role for a tyrosine phosphatase in a tyrosine-kinase generated signal; a similar positive role for the *Drosophila* homolog of SH-PTP2, Corkscrew, had been suggested by genetic approaches *(15)*.

The *Xenopus* system was also used to explore potential roles for the Nck adaptor and its binding partners. As mentioned above, Nck mutants had no effect on Erk activation in tissue culture cells, suggesting that unlike Grb2 or Crk it might not normally be involved in mitogenic signals *(13)*. Various Nck mutants were expressed in early *Xenopus* embryos and it was found that some mutants induced an anterior truncation phenotype as a consequence of altered dorsoventral patterning in the developing mesoderm *(16)*. In this case, it was possible to deduce the domains involved from the pattern of inhibition using a panel of mutants. All Nck constructs (including the wild type), in which the first and second SH3 domains were intact induced some degree of anterior truncation, whereas all constructs in which either the first or second domain was mutated were inactive. This suggested a role in dorso-ventral patterning for a protein or proteins that bound the first two SH3 domains. Furthermore, the most potent mutant was one in which only the third SH3 domain was mutated, suggesting that proteins binding the third SH3 antagonized the effect of those binding SH3-1 and SH3-2. Finally, a construct containing only the first two SH3 domains fused to a dominant membrane localization signal strongly induced anterior truncation, suggesting that it was membrane localization of proteins binding the first and second SH3s that was responsible for anterior truncation. Once again, by identifying the protein binding domains required for the phenotype, the results immediately suggested the means to isolate the endogenous proteins responsible.

5. TARGETED RELOCALIZATION

A surprising aspect of the latter study was the suggestion that the anterior truncation phenotype was due not to a dominant negative (loss-of-function) effect, but was more likely to be a the result of a gain of function. This was suggested by the ability of overexpressed wild-type Nck to induce the phenotype, and especially by the ability of the membrane-targeted SH3 domains to recapitulate the phenotype. This illustrates the general utility of the experimental re-targeting of protein binding domains as a means of understanding their normal roles in signaling. If, for example, a normal role of Nck is to relocalize (together with its SH3-binding partners) to sites of tyrosine phosphorylation on membranes in response to growth factor stimulation, then it should be possible to mimic that effect by directly targeting the SH3 domains to membranes. The fusion of protein binding domains to ever more specific targeting sequences (for example, targeting focal adhesions, or specific membrane compartments) is a promising approach to dissecting out the specific effects of various components of signaling networks.

Furthermore, if one suspects that a protein-interaction domain is eliciting a specific response via a particular binding partner, that partner can itself be targeted to prove or disprove whether its relocalization is sufficient to induce the response. An illustration is provided by the guanine nucleotide exchange factor Sos. Sos is thought to activate its membrane-bound substrate, Ras, after being recruited to membranes by virtue of its association with the SH3 domains of Grb2. It was possible to demonstrate that direct membrane targeting of Sos (via the addition of myristoylation or farnesylation signals) was sufficient to induce Ras activation *(17)*. Dominant-negative experiments and targeted localization provide complementary lines of evidence that together can firmly establish whether particular interactions are necessary and/or sufficient for a specific signal output.

5.1. Induced Relocalization

One particularly promising approach, which combines dominant-negative and targeted relocalization approaches, involves induced dimerization. Several systems have been developed that allow the inducible crosslinking of two proteins in the cell via a membrane-permeable dimerizing agent. The first such system involved fusion of proteins of interest to a fragment of the immunophilin FKBP, which has high affinity for the immunosuppressive drug FK506. A synthetic, membrane-permeable dimerized derivative of FK506 (termed FK1012) was developed, which induced crosslinking of FKBP-fused proteins within the cell when added to the medium *(18)*. Using such an approach it was possible to demonstrate that induced membrane localization of Sos was sufficient to activate Ras rapidly (and, somewhat surprisingly, induced membrane localization of Grb2 was insufficient for Ras activation) *(19)*. This concept has been refined in systems that drive the heterodimerization of two different fusion proteins (e.g., one targeted to membranes and the other a soluble protein or protein fragment) in the absence of the competing homodimerization reaction *(20,21)*. By permitting the rapid and quantitative relocalization of proteins or domains, this approach can demonstrate the immediate biochemical consequences of relocalization before feedback inhibition or other adaptations modify the response. Depending on the specific fusion constructs, such approaches can generate either conditional dominant negatives or conditional dominant activators, and are likely to prove invaluable in teasing out the initial signal outputs resulting from specific protein–protein complexes (Fig. 2).

6. PEPTIDES AND PEPTIDE MIMETICS

The ability to manipulate the protein–protein complexes involved in signaling would clearly be useful in a variety of clinical settings. This would not only have obvious applications in the treatment of a wide range of human diseases resulting from aberrant or inappropriate signaling, but it would also be useful in some cases to modulate the signaling state of normal cells such as those in the immune system. While the expression of protein binding domains, or dominant negative or targeted mutants of signaling proteins, might provide important information about what interactions are involved in a signaling pathway, these approaches are unlikely to be clinically useful in the near future. Because SH2 and SH3 domains bind small, linear peptides, however, synthetic peptides and peptidomimetic compounds can be used to inhibit their interactions. Such small molecules set the stage for the development of pharmaceuticals targeting protein-interaction domains.

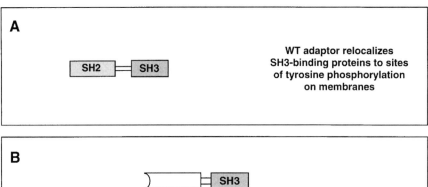

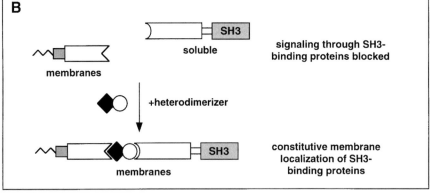

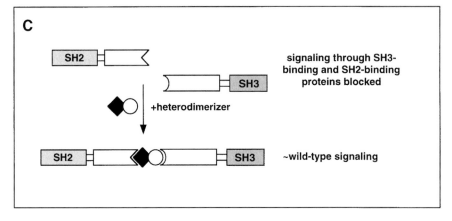

Fig. 2. Inducible manipulation of signaling pathways with an inducible heterodimerization system. (A) Hypothetical SH2/SH3 adaptor consisting of one SH2 and one SH3 domain is depicted. (B) Dominant membrane-targeting fusion protein and an SH3 domain fusion protein are co-expressed at high levels in cells. When membrane-permeable heterodimerizer is added, the two fusion proteins associate and the SH3 domain is inducibly localized to membranes. (C) The SH2 domain and the SH3 domain are overexpressed as separate fusion proteins, which can associate in the presence of heterodimerizer. White boxes, domains that bind with high affinity to the heterodimerizing compound.

Specific peptides that bind with high affinity to protein binding domains have been isolated by a variety of approaches. For SH2 domains the first clues came from sequence inspection of known SH2-binding sites, but the breakthrough came from studies using libraries of random synthetic peptides (with phosphotyrosine in a fixed position) and direct sequencing of the peptides from the library that bound preferentially to specific SH2 domains *(22)*. Using this technique it was possible to generate a consensus sequence for high-affinity binding sites for any SH2 domain. Because this approach averages over many binding sites it is always possible that the highest affinity sites might be obscured, but in practice it has proven quite useful in predicting bona fide binding sites. For SH3 domains, where phosphorylation of the ligand is not required for association, a wider variety of techniques have been applied including the use of expression libraries *(23)*, combinatorial peptide libraries *(24)*, and phage display *(25,26)*. For SH2 and SH3 domains, as well as all other protein-interaction domains that bind relatively short peptide ligands, synthetic peptidomimetic compounds may ultimately provide ligands with even higher affinity or with other useful properties such as membrane permeability.

A number of studies have demonstrated that peptides, when introduced into cells, can block protein–protein interactions critical for signal transmission. This has been most often demonstrated in the case of tyrosine-phosphorylated peptides designed to block SH2–target interactions, presumably because the affinity of SH2-peptide interactions are quite high (dissociation constants of $<10^{-7}$ M). As just one example, in the study mentioned above that demonstrated inhibition of EGF receptor internalization by the SH2 domain of Grb2, the investigators also demonstrated inhibition by microinjection of a tyrosine-phosphorylated peptide based on the known Grb2-binding site on the EGF receptor *(12)*. The unphosphorylated peptide had no effect, as expected if the peptide was exerting its effect by blocking endogenous SH2-phosphotyrosine interactions.

The general usefulness of peptides is compromised by the need to microinject or otherwise mechanically introduce them into cells, making biochemical analysis of signal output difficult, if not impossible. Although one can introduce peptides into permeabilized cells, this raises other difficulties. One alternative approach involves the use of membrane-permeable peptides. It has been found that peptides derived from HIV Tat protein or the *Drosophila* antennapedia gene product can translocate across membranes and deliver covalently linked peptides or proteins to the cytosol *(27,28)*. How these peptides cross the membrane is not completely understood, but the process seems likely to involve a detergent-like micellar structure. The utility of this approach to signal transduction research was demonstrated by the ability of a synthetic tyrosine phosphoryated peptide fused to the antennapedia sequence to inhibit FGF-induced neurite outgrowth in PC12 cells *(29)*. The inhibitory peptide was designed to block association of PLC-γ with the FGF receptor, though of course the possibility that the peptide blocks other associations cannot be ruled out. Whether this approach will be generally applicable to other peptides, and whether the introduced peptides can be further modified (e.g., to restrict their subcellular localization) will determine whether these approaches become widely used.

The inability of most peptides to passively cross the membrane might ultimately be circumvented by using peptidomimetic compound built on a membrane-permeable hydrophobic scaffold. Such inhibitors could be isolated using the powerful techniques of combinatorial chemistry and optimized by high-resolution structural information. The feasibility of constructing nonpeptide inhibitors of protein binding modules has already been demonstrated in the case of SH3 domains, where combinatorial methods were used to construct a library of potential SH3-binding compounds, from which several were isolated with high affinity and specificity for the Src SH3 domain *(30)*. Membrane-permeable peptidomimetic SH2 inhibitors are currently under development by the pharmaceutical industry because of their obvious clinical potential.

Small molecule approaches to inhibiting protein–protein interactions will no doubt evolve further during the next several years. Repeated cycles of library screening and optimization will doubtless increase affinities and specificity for particular domains, making possible ever more precise intervention into signaling networks. Another promising approach to inhibition of proteins containing multiple protein-binding domains is the synthesis of "consolidated" ligands with moieties that simultaneously target different domains on the target molecule. In one study, consolidated ligands designed to bind to both the SH3 and SH2 domains of the non receptor tyrosine kinase Abl were shown to exhibit high affinity and specificity *(31)*. It should be possible to optimize such consolidated ligands by tinkering with the orientation and spacing of the multiple binding elements, thereby generating inhibitors that are extremely specific for the intended target. Getting such relatively large compounds across the membrane, however, might prove more challenging than in the case of smaller inhibitors designed to block a single interaction.

7. CONCLUSION

The realization that protein–protein interactions hold the key to signal transmission presents exciting possibilities for the experimental and clinical manipulation of signaling. The confluence of structural information about binding modules and their ligands, the imminent availability of the sequences of all such binding modules in the genome, novel techniques for generating high-affinity inhibitors of these interactions, and the ability to inducibly re-target binding domains and the other functional domains of proteins that contain them, will ultimately lead to a comprehensive understanding of the logic and connectivity of signaling networks. It is likely that what will emerge will not be merely a series of interconnected, linear pathways, but a more complex set of binding equilibria that will define the signaling state of the cell. A challenge for the next decade is to use this information to be able to predict the behavior of the system and manipulate it in the treatment of disease.

REFERENCES

1. Pawson T. Signaling through scaffold, anchoring, and adaptor proteins. *Science* 1997; 278:2075–2080.
2. Pawson T. Protein modules and signalling networks. *Nature* 1995; 373:573–579.
3. Cohen GB, Baltimore D. Modular binding domains in signal transduction proteins. *Cell* 1995; 80:237–248.
4. Kuriyan J, Cowburn D. Modular peptide recognition domains in eukaryotic signaling. *Annu Rev Biophys Biomol Struct* 1997; 26:259–288.
5. Khwaja A, Hallberg B, Warne PH, Downward, J. Networks of interaction of p120[cbl] and p130[cas] with Crk and Grb2 adaptor proteins. *Oncogene* 1996; 12:2491–2498.

6. Buday L, Khwaja A, Sipeki S, Farago A, Downward J. Interactions of Cbl with two adaptor proteins, Grb2 and Crk, upon T cell activation. *J Biol Chem* 1996; 271:6159–6163

7. Claesson-Welsh L. Signal transduction by the PDGF receptors. *Prog Growth Factor Res* 1994; 5:37–54.

8. Klinghoffer RA, Duckworth B, Valius M, Cantley L, Kaslauskas A. Platelet-derived growth factor-dependent activation of phosphatidylinositol 3-kinase is regulated by receptor binding of SH2-domain-containing proteins which influence Ras activity. *Mol Cell Biol* 1996; 16:5905–5914.

9. Bazenet CE, Gelderloos JA, Kazlauskas A. Phosphorylation of tyrosine 720 in the platelet-derived growth factor alpha receptor is required for binding of Grb2 and SHP-2 but not for activation of Ras or cell proliferation. *Mol Cell Biol* 1996; 16:6926–6936.

10. Segal RA, Bhattacharyya A, Rua LA, Alberta JA, Stephens RM, Kaplan DR, Stiles CD. Differential utilization of Trk autophosphorylation sites. *J Biol Chem* 1996; 271:20,175–20,181.

11. Tanaka S, Hattori S, Kurata T, Nagashima K, Fukui Y, Nakamura S, Matsuda M. Both the SH2 and SH3 domains of human CRK protein are required for neuronal differentiation of PC12 cells. *Mol Cell Biol* 1993; 13:4409–4415.

12. Wang Z, Moran MF. Requirement for the adapter protein GRB2 in EGF receptro endocytosis. *Science* 1996; 272: 1935–1939.

13. Tanaka M, Gupta R, Mayer BJ. Differential inhibition of signaling pathways by dominant-negative SH2/SH3 adapter proteins. *Mol Cell Biol* 1995; 15:6829–6837.

14. Tang TL, Freeman RMJ, O'Reilly AM, Neel BG, Sokol SY. The SH2-containing protein-tyrosine phosphatase SH-PTP2 is required upstream of MAP kinase for early *Xenopus* development. *Cell* 1995; 80:473–483.

15. Perkins LA, Larsen I, Perrimon N. Corkscrew encodes a putative protein tyrosine phosphatase that functions to transduce the terminal signal from the receptor tyrosine kinase torso. *Cell* 1992; 70:225–236.

16. Tanaka M, Lu W, Gupta R, Mayer BJ. Expression of mutated Nck SH2/SH3 adaptor respecifies mesodermal cell fate in *Xenopus laevis* development. *Proc Natl Acad Sci USA* 1997; 94:4493–4498.

17. Aronheim A, Engelberg D, Li N, al-Alawi N, Schlessinger J, Karin M. Membrane targeting of the nucleotide exchange factor Sos is sufficient for activating the Ras signaling pathway. *Cell* 1994; 78:949–961.

18. Spencer DM, Wandless TJ, Schreiber SL, Crabtree GR. Controlling signal transduction with synthetic ligands. *Science* 1993; 262:1019–1024.

19. Holsinger LJ, Spencer DM, Austin DJ, Schreiber SL, Crabtree GR. Signal transduction in T lymphocytes using a conditional allele of Sos. *Proc Natl Acad Sci USA* 1995; 92:9810–9814.

20. Belshaw PJ, Ho SN, Crabtree GR, Schreiber SL. Controlling protein association and subcellular localization with a synthetic ligand that induces heterodimerization of proteins. *Proc Nat Acad Sci USA* 1996; 93:4604–4607.

21. Klemm JD, Beals CR, Crabtree GR. Rapid targeting of nuclear proteins to the cytoplasm. *Curr Biol* 1997; 7:638–644.

22. Songyang Z, Shoelson SE, Chaudhuri M, Gish G, Pawson T, Haser WG, King F, Roberts T, Ratnofsky S, Lechleider RJ, Neel BG, Birge RB, Fajardo JE, Chou MM, Hanafusa H, Shaffhausen B, Cantley LC. SH2 domains recognize specific phosphopeptide sequences. *Cell* 1993; 72:767–778.

23. Ren R, Mayer BJ, Cicchetti P, Baltimore D. Identification of a 10-amino acid proline-rich SH3 binding site. *Science* 1993; 259:1157–1161.

24. Yu H, Chen JK, Feng S, Dalgarno DC, Brauer AW, Schreiber SL. Structural basis for the binding of proline-rich peptides to SH3 domains. *Cell* 1994; 76:933–945.

25. Sparks AB, Rider JE, Hoffman NG, Fowlkes DM, Quilliam LA, Kay BK. Distinct ligand preferences of Src homology 3 domains from Src, Yes, Abl, p53bp, PLC-γ, Crk, and Grb2. *Proc Natl Acad Sci USA* 1996; 93:1540–1544.

26. Rickles RJ, Botfield MC, Zhou X-M, Henry PA, Brugge JS, Zoller MJ. Phage display selection of ligand residues important for Src homology 3 domain binding specificity. *Proc Natl Acad Sci USA* 1995; 92:10,909–10,913.

27. Fawell S, Seery J, Daikh Y, Moore C, Chen LL, Pepinsky B, Barsoum J. Tat-mediated delivery of heterologous proteins into cells. *Proc Natl Acad Sci USA* 1994; 91:664–668.

28. Theodore L, Derossi D, Chassaing G, Llirbat B, Kubes M, Jordan P, Chneiweiss H, Godement P, Prochainz A. Intraneural delivery of protein kinase C pseudosubstrate leads to growth cone collapse. *J Neurosci* 1995; 15:7158–7167.

29. Hall H, Williams EJ, Moore SE, Walsh FS, Prochaintz A, Doherty P. Inhibition of FGF-stimulated neurite outgrowth by a cell-membrane permeable phosphopeptide. *Curr Biol* 1996; 6:580–587.

30. Combs AP, Kapoor TM, Feng S, Chen JK, Daude-Snow LF, Schreiber SL. Protein structure-based combinatorial chemistry: Discovery of non-peptide binding elements to Src SH3 domains. *J Am Chem Soc* 1996; 118:287–288.

31. Cowburn D, Zheng J, Xu Q, Barany G. Enhanced affinities and specificities of consolidated ligands for the Src homology (SH) 3 and SH2 domains of Abelson protein-tyrosine kinase. *J Biol Chem* 1995; 270:26,738–26,741.

25

Protein Tyrosine Kinase Inhibitors as Novel Therapeutic Agents

Alexander Levitzki

1. INTRODUCTION

The malfunctioning of protein tyrosine kinases (PTKs) is the hallmark of numerous diseases. More than 50% of oncogenes and proto-oncogenes involved in human cancers are PTKs. The enhanced activity of PTKs is also implicated in the in nonmalignant diseases, such as psoriasis, papilloma, restenosis, and pulmonary fibrosis. It is therefore not surprising that a surge in publications describing attempts to target PTKs for drug development has occurred over the past decade (see *1* for review). Understanding the molecular pathology of many diseases has progressed at an accelerating pace, and the molecular aberrations that are the hallmarks of an increasing number of pathological states can be identified. Among these molecular hallmarks, the PTKs occupy a prominent position among other signaling elements gone awry. Table 1 summarizes the PTK signaling molecules whose altered activities have been shown to be directly correlated with a human disease. Other PTKs are also implicated but the level of evidence is more correlatory than in the cases summarized in Table 1.

2. UNIVERSAL TARGETS AND SELECTIVE TARGETS

Most proliferative diseases involve more than one signaling pathway; this is especially true in cancers in which many genetic alterations have taken place on the pathway of the cell to its transformed state. Even in benign conditions, such as psoriasis or restenosis, a number of signaling pathways have been implicated. In all these cases, more than one PTK is likely to be involved, although in many instances one PTK can be identified that plays a key role in the disease. Table 1 lists most of these PTKs and the diseases they are associated with. These PTKs identify themselves as targets for drug targeting. PTKs such as IGF-1R and Src family kinases have been implicated in many types of cancer and thus may qualify as *universal targets (1,2)* for the development of PTK inhibitors. Among the PTKs involved in pathophysiological states, a relatively small number of PTKs appear in many cancers and other proliferative states. For example, overexpression of the EGF receptor kinase is the hallmark of most, if not all, epithelial cancers. The overexpression of the EGFR is generally accompanied by the autocrine

From: Signaling Networks and Cell Cycle Control: The Molecular Basis of Cancer and Other Diseases
Edited by: J. S. Gutkind © Humana Press Inc., Totowa, NJ

Table 1
PTKs Whose Enhanced Activities Is Correlated with Specific Diseases

PTK involved	Type of altered activity	Disease implicated
EGFR, unmutated	Overexpression and autocrine stimulation	Epithelial cancers, psoriasis, papilloma
EGFR, truncated	Constitutive activation	Gliomas
PDGFR	Overexpression and autocrine stimulation	Glioblastomas; restenosis, atherosclerosis
	Activation of blood vessel smooth muscle cells in the media	
TEL-PDGFR fusion protein	Constitutive activation of PDGF receptor	Chronic myelomonocytic leukemia
Bcr-Abl	Constitutive activation in the cytoplasm of blood stem cells	Chronic myeloid leukemia (CML)
Jak-2	Persistent activation	Recurrent pre-B acute lymphoid leukemia (pre-B–ALL)
Her-2/neu, Her-3, Her-4 heterodimers	Overexpression	Breast, ovary, lung, gastric cancers
VEGFR/Flk-1/KDR	Activation of tumor vascularization by the anoxic tumor	All cancers
c-Src, C-Yes	Persistently activated	Cancers of the lung, colon, breast, prostate
IGF1-R	Overexpression, autocrine stimulation	Cancers, psoriasis

Abbreviations: PTK, protein tyrosine kinase; EGFR, epidermal growth factor receptor; PDGFR, platelet-derived growth factor receptor.

or paracrine expression of its ligands, producing persistent enhanced stimulation of EGF-dependent pathways. In certain tumors, a truncated persistently active, version of the receptor is overexpressed and induces intense signaling. It is no wonder that attempts to generate EGFR kinase-directed tyrphostins have been pursued since the beginning of the search for PTK inhibitors. One can therefore view the potential success in developing an inhibitor for the EGFR kinase as an important achievement, as it has the chance of becoming a universal inhibitor. The involvement of enhanced EGFR signaling is also the hallmark of papilloma induced by human papillomavirus (HPV) 16/18 *(3)* and of psoriasis *(4)*. Thus, blockers of the EGFR kinase were suggested as potent as antipsoriasis agents *(4,5)* and anti-papilloma agents *(3)*. Indeed, AG 1517 (SU 5271, or PD 153035) has been used in clinical trials since early 1997. Similarly, the involvement of HER-2/neu in breast cancer, ovary cancer, lung cancer, and gastric cancer makes this close relative of the EGFR kinase an attractive target for drug design. In these instances, overexpression of HER-2 occurs in a significant fraction of the cases: 10–35%. In some instances, it is possible to identify a specific PTK whose activity is correlated with the disease. For example, in the chronic phase of chronic myeloid leukemia (CML), the fusion protein Bcr-Abl, the product of the Philadelphia chromosome is implicated as the cause of the leukemia *(6)*. Similarly, TEL-PDGFR *(7)* and Jak-2 *(8)* are associated with other forms of leukemia. In these cases, highly selective inhibitors can be used to inhibit, and even selectively purge, the diseased cells. In most tumors, however, it is expected that one signal transduction inhibitor might not be sufficient by itself to eradicate the disease. Indeed, early in vivo experiments show that tyrphostin RG 13022, an EGFR kinase blocker, is capable of inhibiting the progress of tumor growth and of prolonging the survival of nude mice implanted with a human squamous tumor that overexpresses EGFR. Treatment with RG 13022 by itself, however, does not lead to total eradication of the disease *(9)*. PTK inhibitors may be most efficient in combination with other drugs, such as cytotoxic agents *(10,11)* or antibodies *(9)*.

3. DESIGN AND SYNTHESIS OF PROTEIN TYROSINE PHOSPHORYLATION INHIBITORS

As soon as it became apparent that the enhanced activity of PTKs is a major contributor to oncogenesis, the search for tyrosine kinase inhibitors began. The systematic synthesis of selective PTK inhibitors (tyrosine phosphorylation inhibitors, or tyrphostins) that show selectivity toward the isolated EGFR kinase and that do not inhibit Ter/Thr kinases was reported during the late 1980s *(12)*. It took a few more years to produce highly potent and selective tyrosine kinase inhibitors, mostly by semirational drug design and high-throughput screening *(2,13,14)*. Kinetic analysis of the mode of EGFR kinase action and of pp60^{c-Src} shows that ATP and the substrate bind independently to the kinase domain and that no sequential binding occurs *(15)*. This property simplifies kinetic analysis of the mode of inhibition of PTKs by their inhibitors *(16)*.

One of the most surprising findings on the selectivity of inhibitors discovered so far is the high selectivity displayed by ATP competitive inhibitors. For example, quinoxalines are highly selective inhibitors of PDGFR kinase *(17,18)* and quinozalines for the EGFR kinase *(19* and see below). Further analysis on the mode of tyrosine kinase inhibition shows that the affinity of the inhibitor and its mode of binding to the kinase domain depends on whether the kinase is in its activated form or its basal inactive state. Three examples illustrate this point. Activated Abl kinase, like p210$^{Bcr-Abl}$ and p185$^{Bcr-Abl}$ possesses different affinities to both substrate and inhibitors (tyrphostins) as compared with the their proto-oncogenic form p140^{c-Abl} *(6)*. For example, p210$^{Bcr-Abl}$ and p185$^{Bcr-Abl}$ are inhibited by the tyrphostin AG 957 with K_i values of 0.75 μM and 1.5 μM, as compared with a K_i value of 10.0 μM for the cellular wild-type p140^{c-Abl}. In all these cases, AG 957 is competitive with the substrate and noncompetitive with ATP. The difference between c-Abl and Bcr-Abl is not in the kinase domain, as the Bcr sequence is fused inframe with the intact kinase domain. Thus, tethering the Bcr sequence upstream to the c-Abl appears to alter the conformation of the kinase domain such that it binds more tightly the inhibitor.

The same pattern of behavior is observed with regard to the substrates: the oncogenic forms exhibit lower K_m values toward the substrates, as compared with the proto-oncogenic forms. A similar relationship was found for the mouse proteins, where v-Abl (gagAbl) exhibits higher affinity toward the substrates and inhibitors, as compared with the proto-oncogenic form of the protein. A similar result was recently found for the EGFR kinase; with the receptor truncated at the extracellular domain, EGFRΔ, exhibiting one order of magnitude higher affinity toward quinozalines of the AG 1478 family than the wild-type receptor *(19)*. Kinetic studies show that AG 1478 is a competitive inhibitor with regard to ATP *(20)*. In this case as well, the primary structural alterations do not occur in the kinase domain. However, the structural alterations induced by the truncation alter the conformation within the catalytic domain of the receptor. It is likely, but not proven, that the truncated receptor is a constitutive dimer.

In the case of both Bcr-Abl and the EGFRΔ, these differences can, in principle, be exploited to kill the cancer cell preferentially, which is more sensitive to the agent. Indeed, Ph$^+$ cells can be purged selectively with AG 957 with no significant loss of blood tissue cells in clinical samples from CML patients. In the case of the PDGFR kinase, activation of the receptor also leads to changes in the structure of the kinase domain, but the situation is slightly more complex. Upon activation, the mode of inhibition of the selective inhibitor AG 1296 (or AG 1295) is altered. Whereas the inhibitor is competitive with regard to ATP in the inactive form of the receptor, it binds with higher affinity and becomes mixed competitively with ATP subsequent to receptor activation by PDGF *(22)*. These three examples suggest that this pattern of behavior of PTKs may be a general pattern *(23)*, pointing to the continuing necessity to examine potential PTK inhibitors not only as blockers of PTK autophosphorylation, as is routinely done, but also as blockers of the PTK action on exogenous substrates.

With the advance of X-ray crystallography and the ability to determine the three-dimensional structure of the kinase with the bound inhibitor, drug design has become more precise and rational. The three-dimensional structures of the two tyrosine kinases complexed with kinase inhibitors with inhibitors have already been solved. First, the structure of the EGF receptor with selective and nonselective inhibitors has already been published *(24)*. Second, the Src kinase Hck has been crystallized with the inhibitor complexed with it *(25)*. This structure is currently guiding a number of laboratories in an attempt to design novel, more selective Src kinase inhibitors. An additional challenge is to try to design compounds that block selectively pp60$^{\text{c-Src}}$, Yes, and Fyn, which are activated in many human malignancies (see ref. *26* and references therein), but that do not block significantly other Src family kinases involved in other pathways. Similarly, the availability of the insulin receptor kinase structure in its inactive form *(27)*, as well as its active form complexed with APPNHP and a peptide substrate *(28)*, has led to an informed search for inhibitors for the IGF-1R kinase, which is highly homologous to the insulin receptor kinase. The search has identified AG 538 as a potent inhibitor of the IGF1R kinase (Blum and Levitzky, unpublished). The AG 538 family, identified by this informed search, was designed to find inhibitors that mimic the protein loop encompassing tyrosine state 1158 to tyrosine 1162 and occupying the substrate site in the inactive that become phosphorylated upon activation within the insulin receptor. Indeed, AG 538 is capable to inhibit IGF1R autophosphorylation with an IC$_{50}$ value of 0.4 μM (Blum and Levitzky, unpublished). This series of inhibitors is different from AG 1024 and some of its analogs, which were found by random screening *(29)*. It will be interesting to compare the mode of binding of AG 1024 with AG 538 within the active site of the receptor. Importantly, some of the inhibitors discriminate between the insulin receptor kinase and the IGF1R kinase by a factor of ≤ 8 *(29)*.

It remains a challenge to design inhibitors of IGF1R kinase that differentiate between the two receptor by a wider margin. Figure 1 summarizes the main pharmacophores that have proved effective PTK inhibitors with no significant effects on Ser/The kinases. Figure 2 summarizes the specific compounds that have displayed biological efficacy on the targets quoted.

4. SCREENING FOR TYROSINE KINASE INHIBITORS

The involvement of a number of tyrosine kinases in various cancers requires efficient screening methodologies for the inhibitory compounds. Screening is divided into four steps:

1. *Primary screening:* against the pure isolated PTK in a cell-free system. All cases are prepared for an enzyme-linked immunosorbent assay an (ELISA) format. The compounds are screened against a battery of PTKs and Ser/Ther kinases in order to establish the pattern of selectivity quickly *(2)*.
2. *Secondary screening:* Successful candidates that show high affinity toward the isolated PTK move to this next stage, in which the compound is tested for its potency to inhibit the PTK in the intact cell. Many compounds fail at this stage because they are not permeable, or because they do not reach their target in the intact cell. Compounds that withstand this test are also examined against other kinases within the context of the intact cell. This screening is also conducted in a 96- well format and is therefore amenable to high through-put screening.
3. *Tertiary screening:* Successful compounds are then tested in for the ability to block the growth of the cell, where its growth is driven by the targeted PTK. In many cases, this test is is accompanied by a test that examines the ability of the compound to block the growth of these cells on soft agar. Such potency lends confidence that such compounds may be successful in vivo.
4. *Quaternary screening:* Successful compounds undergo testing in animal models. Animal models range from SCID mice or nude mice harboring the human disease to the inhibition of balloon injury-induced stenosis in the pig as a model for restenosis.

With the availability of chemical libraries, plant and microbial extracts as well as rapid screening methods led to compounds that can be rapidly identified. When the structures of the PTKs are known, optimization by organic synthesis and computer modeling follows. The compounds that prove successful in all the screening tests are ready for evaluation for clinical trials.

5. BIOLOGICAL ACTIVITY OF TYRPHOSTINS

A number of families of PTK inhibitors (tyrphostins) have shown efficacy both in tissue culture and in vivo. *(1)*. A significant number of benzenemalononitriles (BMN) that belong to the first family of PTK inhibitors were found to possess biological activity *(2)*. These include AG 490, AG 126, AG 556, and AG 17 for which promising data in vivo have been reported *(8,30–34)*. Anilidopthalimides, which inhibit EGFR *(35)*, also show efficacy in vivo. Pyrido pyrimidines such as CGP 53716, which inhibit PDGFR *(36)*, have shown efficacy in vivo. A similar compound, CGP 57148B, a pyrazolopyrimidine, blocks Bcr-Abl and shows efficacy in intact cells harboring Bcr-Abl *(37)*. However, this inhibitor also blocks PDGFR and Kit. AG 957, a tyrphostin, derived from Lavendustin A, is highly selective against Bcr-Abl kinase *(6,38)* and has

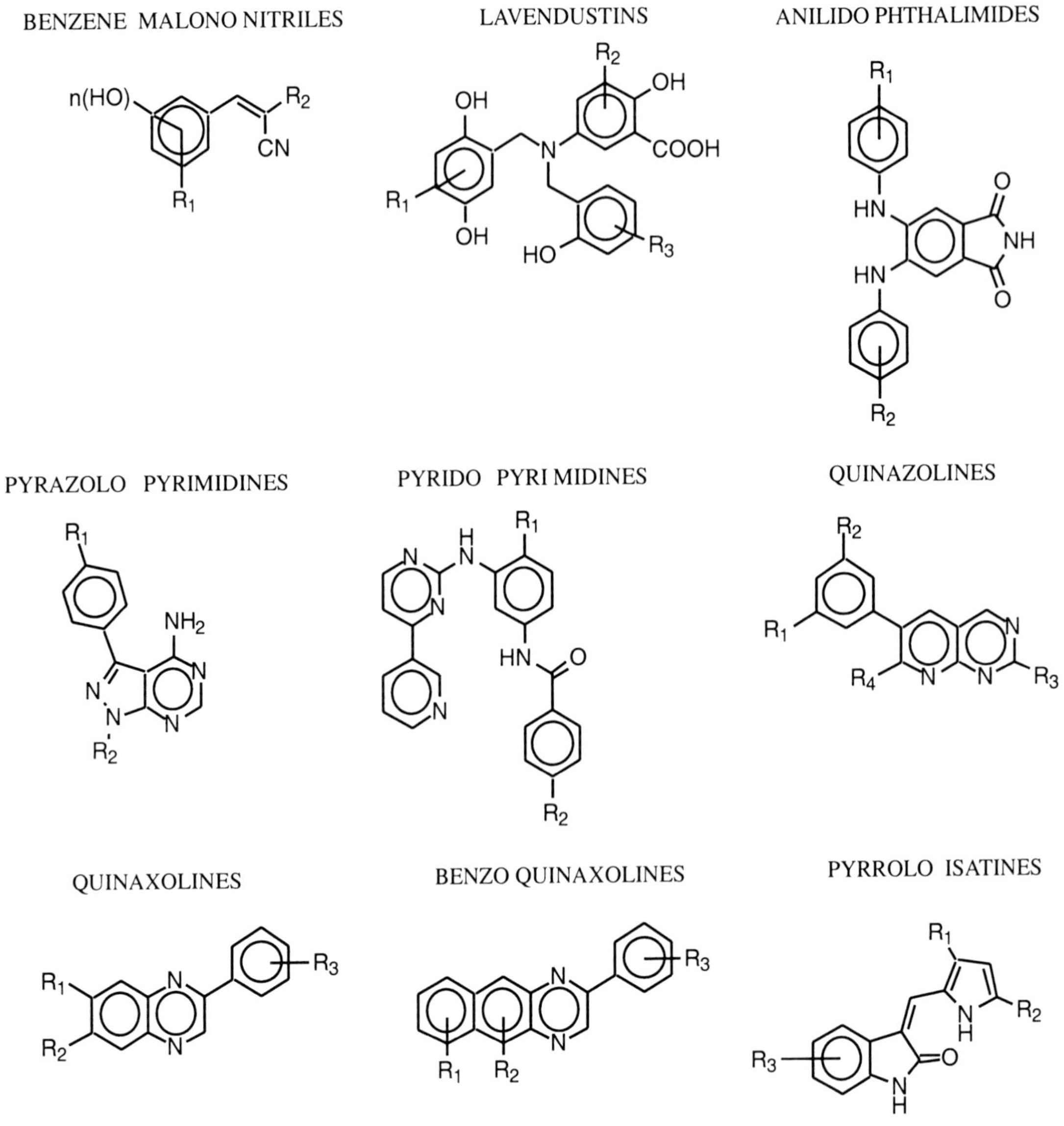

BENZENE MALONO NITRILES   LAVENDUSTINS   ANILIDO PHTHALIMIDES

PYRAZOLO PYRIMIDINES   PYRIDO PYRI MIDINES   QUINAZOLINES

QUINAXOLINES   BENZO QUINAXOLINES   PYRROLO ISATINES

Fig. 1. Lead pharmacophores for PTK inhibitors

been shown to purge selectively Ph$^+$ cells from the blood obtained from CML patients at the chronic phase of the disease *(21)*. Quinoxalines were found to be very selective PDGFR kinase inhibitors with very good efficacy in intact cells *(17,18)*. The quinoxaline AG 1295 has also shown efficacy in vivo by inhibiting balloon injury-induced stenosis in the pig *(39)*. A predictive animal model for restenosis in humans In vivo activity of AG 1295 was also shown in the rat model *(40)*. Quinozalines show good efficacy against the EGFR *(20,41–44)*. AG 1517 *(43)* is identical to PD153035 *(42)*, which is very effective in blocking the growth of psoriatic keratinocytes *(45)*. A related pharmacophore (Fig. 1) that has proved effective against the EGFR kinase is derived

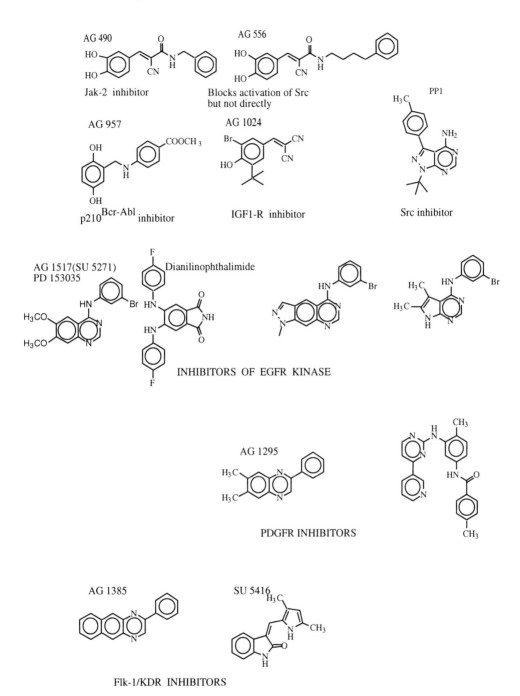

Fig. 2. Tyrphostins with biological activities.

from 4-(phenylamino)pyrrolopyrimidine (*46;* Fig. 2). Another EGF receptor kinase inhibitor is a compound that was designed on the basis of successful inhibitors from the dianilinphthalimide family (*34;* Figs. 1 and 2). Another successful family of EGFR kinase inhibitors were obtained by the fusion of the quinozaline moiety with a third ring (*47;* Figs. 1 and 2).

6. SYNERGISTIC ACTION OF TYRPHOSTINS WITH CYTOTOXIC AGENTS

Enhanced activity of PTKs confers robustness to cancer cells most probably because of the enhancement of antiapoptotic pathways mediated by BclX/Bcl-2 and c-Act/PKB elements. Intensification of antiapoptotic pathways appears to be the predominant factor in the emergence of resistance to cytotoxic drugs and radiation. These inhibitory pathways most probably suppress the stress pathways triggered by cytotoxic agents, preventing cell death. In two instances, this principle has been demonstrated and the molecular mechanism at least partially analyzed. Tyrphostin AG 825 was shown to synergize strongly with cisplatin, etoposide, and doxorubicin, all DNA-damaging agents that trigger the stress pathways (*10*). A series of tumor of non-small lung cancer (NLSC) cell lines with different levels of HER-2/neu overexpression was examined for this effect.

The extent of synergy was found to be dependent on the level of expression of the HER-2/neu receptor. No synergy, but rather additivity, was observed for cells with no overexpression of HER-2/neu, whereas the highest synergy was found in cells with very high expression of HER-2/neu. This was reflected quantitatively in the combination index (Cl) whose value was much lower than 1.0 for the high overexpressors and equal to 1.0 for the cell in which HER-2/neu is not overexpressed (*10*). Apparently, the higher the overexpression of HER-2, the higher the antiapoptotic shield provided by the receptor tyrosine kinase. However, the sensitivity of the cells to stress signaling appears to be enhanced as well with higher expression of HER-2/neu, but its sensitivity to stress signals is masked by the high expression of HER-2/neu. Thus, when the cells are stripped of the robust antiapototic shield, their enhanced vulnerability to stress is exposed.

A similar result was recently obtained with human glioma cells, which overexpress the truncated form of the EGF receptor-EGFRΔ. In this case, EGFR kinase selective agent inhibitors such as AG 1478 or AG 1517 synergize with cisplatin (CDDP). AG 1478 has been demonstrated to reduce the level of expression of Bcl-X$_L$ and to decrease the activity of Caspase 3. The combination of the tyrphostin with cisplatin is lethal to the tumor cells, as it leads to apoptosis (*11*). It seems therefore that EGFRΔ transmits strong antiapoptotic signals that, when inhibited, sensitize the cells to the stress signaling triggered by cisplatin. Because the activated form of EGFR is more sensitive to AG 1478 (*19*) and to some of its analogs (*11*) than is normal wild-type EGFR, it is hoped that EGFR-selective tyrphostins will sensitize the otherwise drug-resistant gliomas to the cytotoxic drugs. Such success will and allow clinical application of these tyrphostins as sensitizers of these tumors to cytotoxic drugs, to which they are normally oblivient.

The combined approach in which a blocker of antiapoptotic signaling is used with a stimulator of stress signaling can prove to be a general approach. Thus, when blockers of Bcl-2/Bcl-X$_L$ proteins and of c-Akt/PKB become available, they are likely to have broad application for cancer therapy. However, because PTKs, especially in tumors are frequently, if not always, the source of antiapoptotic signals, tyrphostins may fulfill this task. In some cases, such as chronic myeloid leukemia (CML) and pre-B-acute lymphoid leukemia (ALL), the selective tyrphostins (AG 490 family and AG 957, respectively) were found sufficient in themselves to induce apoptosis. In these cases, stress signaling appears to be so strong that dismantling of the cells from the antiapoptotic signals is sufficient to induce apoptosis. This possibility is still under investigation.

7. SUCCESS OF TRYPHOSTINS IN VIVO

In a number of cases, the hypothesis that PTK inhibitors should be effective in blocking a proliferative disease or tumor growth in vivo has actually been accomplished in preclinical animal models. These cases are listed below.

7.1. PDGFR Kinase-Directed PTK Inhibitors

Tyrphostin AG 1295 and its close analog, AG 1296, both quinoxalines (Fig. 1), have been shown to block PDGFR kinase selectively with insignificant inhibitory effects on EGFR, Src, Flk-1, HER-2/neu, and IGF1-R. These tyrphostins have also been shown to reverse the transformed phenotype of *cis*-transformed NIH 3T3 cells (*17*) and to slow C6-glioma induced tumors in nude mice (L. Shawver and A. Levitzki, unpublished observations). In recent experiments on pigs, AG 1295 shown to block balloon injury induced stenosis in the femoral artery (*39*). The extent of inhibition is ~50–60%, compared with balloon-injured femoral artery treated with the vehicle alone. Similar results were obtained for rats. AG 17, a nonselective PTK inhibitor was successful in blocking balloon injury-induced stenosis in the rat carotid artery model (*34*) but induced damage in pigs (S. Banai, unpublished observations). The pig model, which is much more faithful and predictive of the human situation, encourages the promotion of AG 1295 and its more potent analogs (Gazit, Banai, and A. Levitzki, in preparation) to undergo testing in the clinical setup. The ability of very selective PDGFR kinase inhibitors to block balloon injury-induced stenosis supports the PDGF hypothesis of the late Russel Ross from 1976 (*48,49*), which implicates this growth factor and its receptor in the process of atherosclerosis and its accelerated form, restenosis. The finding that PDGFR kinase-directed tyrphostins block ~60% stenosis strongly suggests that other signaling pathways should be targeted in an attempt to block the other proliferative signals, such as those elicited by fibroblast growth factor (FGF) and transforming growth factor-α (TGF-α). Because accelerated atherosclerosis in the transplanted heart is the major cause of death of patients undergoing heart transplantation, AG 1295 and its analogs are currently being tested in an animal heart transplant model.

7.2. Jak-2 Inhibitor

Among the many tyrphostins tested, the family of AG 490 have been shown to be potent inhibitors of Jak-2 (*8*) and, to a lesser extent, Jak-3 (*50*). The high potency of AG 490 to block Jak-2 is likely to be the origin of the ability of these agents to block recurrent pre-B-ALL when engrafted in SCID mice (*8*). AG 490 induces apoptotic death in pre-B cells from patients suffering from the disease. In these pre-B cells, Jak-2 is persistently activated, whereas in normal B cells it is not. It is unknown whether the persistent activation of Jak-2 is caused by an activating mutation or to robust autocrine stimulation. The efficacy of AG 490 in vivo is accompanied by the complete absence of toxicity in normal blood tissue. This promising agent is currently undergoing evaluation for clinical trials.

7.3. EGFR Kinase Inhibitors

EGFR kinase blockers from the early tyrphostin family were the first PTK blockers to show efficacy in vivo, in 1991 *(9)*. Because of their unfavorable pharmacokinetic properties, however, they did not make further further progress in preclinical animal models and were later abandoned as possible candidates for the clinical setting. These experiments, however, were a milestone in providing proof of the principle. These experiments showed for the first time that the activity of a tyrphostin identified in a cell-free system culminated in a success in vivo. A few heterocyclic EGFR kinase inhibitors, such as DAPH *(35)* and CGP 59326A, have shown good efficacy in vivo against tumors that overexpress EGFR. Furthermore, the combination of this inhibitor with cytotoxic drugs, such as Adriamycin and vinblastine, induced tumor regression *(51)*. One quinazoline, AG 1517 (SU 5271), is currently being tested as antipsoriatic agent, using topical application. As no animal model is available for psoriasis, the potency of AG 1517 in inhibiting the growth of psoriatic cells and the absence of adverse toxic effects has led to clinical trials using AG 1517. As not only psoriatic cells *(4)*, but HPV (HPV 16)-infected keratinocytes as well, are driven by the EGFR kinase system *(3)*, success may lead to the testing of EGFR-directed PTK inhibitors as anti-papilloma agents *(3)*. As for psoriasis, there is no accepted animal model for papilloma. It is likely that EGFR kinase inhibitors will leap to the clinic, skipping the preclinical animal model. In the case of papilloma, topical application is meant to prevent the transformation of the HPV 16-infected tissue to cervical cancer *(3)*.

7.4. Tyrphostins as Anti-Inflammatory Agents

A number of tyrphostins, such as AG 126 *(33)* and AG 556 *(31,32)*, have shown excellent efficacy as anti-inflammatory agents. The most prominent is AG 556, which was found to be effective as an antisepsis agent in mice *(32)* and dogs *(31)* and very effective in alleviating the symptoms of experimental autoimmune encephalitis, even when administered late in the course of the disease *(52)*. AG 126 was found to be effective in preventing LPS induced mortality in mice *(33)* and to alleviate cirrhosis-like symptoms in rats *(30)*. The search of such compounds within the tyrphostin family was based on scattered reports in the literature that the activation of PTKs is on the pathway of lipopolysaccharidase (LPS)-induced phosphorylation. Similarly, scattered reports suggest that the action of TNF-α involves PTK activation at some point on the overall signaling pathways triggered by the cytokine *(52)*. As no specific molecular target has not been defined, screening for active tyrphostins was based on the potency of compounds tested to block LPS-induced TNF-α production *(33,52)* and TNF-α action *(53)*. It remains to be seen whether the biological activity of this family of tyrphostins is attributable exclusively to the inhibition of PTKs.

REFERENCES

1. Levitzki A. Targeting signal transduction for disease therapy. *Curr Opin Cell Biol* 1996; 8:239–244.
2. Levitzki A, Gazit A. Tyrosine kinases inhibition: An approach to drug development. *Science* 1995; 26:1782–1788.
3. Ben-Bassat H, Rosenbaum-Mitrani S, Hartzstark Z, Shlomai Z, Kleinberger-Doron N, Gazit A, Plowman G, Levitzki R, Tsvieli R, Levitzki A. Blockers of the EGF receptor and of Cdk2 activation induce growth arrest, differentiation, and apoptosis of HPV 16 immortalized human keratinocytes. *Cancer Res* 1997; 57:3741–3750.
4. Ben-Bassat H, Vardi DV, Gazit A, Klaud SN, Chaouat M, Hartzstark Z, Levitzki A. Tyrphostins suppress the growth of psoriatic keratinocytes. *Exp Dermatol* 1995; 113:82–84.
5. Dvir A, Milner Y, Chomsky O, Gilon C, Gazit A, Levitzki A. The inhibition of EGF-dependent proliferation of keratinocytes by tyrosine kinase blockers. *J Cell Biol* 1991; 857–865.
6. Anafi M, Gazit A, Gilon C, Ben-Neriah Y, Levitzki A. Selective Interactions of transforming and normal abl proteins with ATP, tyrosine copolymer substrates and tyrphostins. *J Biol Chem* 1992; 267:4518–4523.
7. Carroll M, Tomasson M, Barker G, Golub T, Gillialand D. The TEL/platelet-derived growth factor beta receptor (PDGF beta R) fusion in chronic myelomonocytic leukemia is a transforming protein that self-associates and activates PDGF beta R kinase-dependent signaling pathways. *Proc Natl Acad Sci USA* 1996; 10:14,845–14,850.
8. Meydan N, Grunberger T, Dadi H, Shahar M, Arpaia E, Lapidot Z, Leader S, Freedman M, Cohen A, Gazit A. Inhibition of recurrent human pre-B acute lymphoblastic leukemia by Jak-2 tyrosine kinase inhibitor. *Nature* 1996; 379:645–648.
9. Yoneda T, Lyall R, M AM, Pearsons PE, Spada AP, Levitzki A, Zilberstein A, Mundy GR. The antiproliferative effects of tyrosine kinase inhibitor tyrphostin on a human squamous cell carcinoma in vitro and in nude mice. *Cancer Res* 1991; 51:4430–4435.
10. Tsai CM, Levitzki A, Wu L-H, Chang K-T, Cheng C-C, Gazit A, Pemg R-P. Enhancement of chemosensitivity by tyrphostin AG 825 in high p185neu expressing non-small cell lung cancer cells. *Cancer Res* 1996; 56:1068–1074.
11. Nagane M, Levitzki A, Cavenee WK, Su Huang H-J. Drug resistance of human glioblastoma cells conferred by a tumor-specific mutant epidermal growth factor receptor through modulation of Bcl-XL and cspase-3-like proteases. *Proc Natl Acad Sci USA* 1998; 95:5724–5729.
12. Yaish P, Gazit A, Gilon C, Levitzki A. Blocking of EGF-dependent cell proliferation by EGF receptor kinase inhibitors. *Science* 1988; 242:933–935.
13. Levitzki A. Tyrphostins: tyrosine kinase blockers as novel antiproliferative agents and dissectors of signal transduction. *FASEB J* 1992; 6:3275–3282.
14. Groundwater PW, Solomons KRH, Drewe JA, Munawar MA. Protein tyrosine kinase inhibitors. *Prog Med Chem* 1996; 33:233–329.
15. Posner I, Engel M, Levitzki A. Kinetic model for the epidermal growth factor (EGF) receptor tyrosine kinase and a possible mechanism of its activation by EGF. *J Biol Chem* 1992; 267:20,638–20,647.
16. Posner I, Engel M, Gazit A, Levitzki A. Kinetics of Inhibition of the tyrosine kinase activity of the epidermal growth factor receptor and Analysis by a new computer program. *Mol Pharmacol* 1994; 45:673–683.
17. Kovalenko M, Gazit A, Bohmer A, Rorsman C, Ronnstrand L, Heldin C, Waltenberger J, FD Bohmer F, Levitzki A. Selective Platelet-derived growth factor receptor kinase blockers reverse sis-transformation. *Cancer Res* 1994; 54:6106–6114.
18. Gazit A, App H, McMahon G, Chen J, Levitzki A, Bohmer FD, Tyrphostin 5.- Potent

Inhibitors of PDGF receptor tyrosine kinase. SAR in quinixalines, quinolines and Indole tyrphostins. *J Med Chem* 1996; 39:2170–2177.

19. Han Y, Caday CG, Nanda A, Cavenee WK, Su Hunag H-J. Tyrphostin AG 1478 preferentially inhibits human glioma cells expressing truncated rather than wild-type epidermal growth factor receptors. *Cancer Res* 1996; 56:3859–3861.

20. Ward WHJ, Cook PN, Slater AM, Davies DH, Holdgate GA, Gree LR. Epidermal Growth factor receptor tyrosine kinase Investigation of catalytic mechanism, structure-based searching an discovery of a potent inhibitor. *Biochem Pharmacol* 1994; 48:639–666.

21. Schindler T, Sicheri F, Pico A, Gazit A, Levitzki A, Kuriyan J. Crystal structure of Hck in complex with a Src family-selective tyrosine kinase inhibitor. *Mol Cell Biol* 1999; 3:639–648.

22. Kovalenko M, Romstrand L, Heldin C-H, Loubochenko M, Gazit A, Levitzki A, Bohmer FD. phosphorylation site-specific inhibition of platelet-derived growth factor b-receptor autophosphorylation by the receptor blocking tyrphostin AG 1296. *Biochemistry* 1997; 36:6260–6269.

23. Levitzki A, Bohmer FD. Altered efficacy and selectivity of tyrosine kinase inhibitors of the activated states of protein tyrosine kinases. *Anticancer Drug Design* 1998; 13:731–734.

24. Mohammadi M, McMahon G, Sun L, Tang C, Hirth P, Yeh BK, Hubbard SR, Schlessinger J. Structure of the tyrosine kinase domain of fibroblast growth factor receptor in complex with inhibitors. *Science* 1997; 276:955–960.

25. Carlos-Stella C, Regazzi E, Sammarelli G, Colla S, Garau D, Gazit A, Savoldo B, Cilloni D, Tabilio A, Levitzki A, Rizzoli V. Effects of the tyrosine kinase inhibitor AG957 and an anti Fas receptor antibody on CD34$^+$ chronic myelogenous leukemia progenitor cells. *Blood* 1999; 93:3973–3982.

26. Levitzki A. SRC as a target for anti-cancer drugs. *Anticancer Drug Design* 1996; 11:175–182.

27. Hubbard SR, Wei L, Ellis L, Hendrickson A. Crystal structure of the tyrosine kianse domain of the human insulin receptor. *Nature* 1994; 372:746–754.

28. Hubbard SR. Crystal structure of the activated insulin receptor tyrosine kinase in complex with peptide substrate and ATP analog. *EMBO J* 1997; 16:5572–5581.

29. Parrizas M, LeRoith D. Insulin-like growth factor-1 inhibition of apoptosis is associated with increased expression of the bcl-xL gene product. *Endocrinology* 1997; 138:1355–1358.

30. Lopez-Talavera JC, Levitzki A, Martinez A, Gazit A, Esteban E, Guardian J. Tyrosine kinase inhibition ameliorates the hyperdynamic state and decreases nitric oxide production in cirrhotic rats with portal hypertension and ascites. *J Clin Invest* 1997; 100:664–670.

31. Sevransky JE, Shaked G, Novogrodsky A, Levitzki A, Gazit A, Hoffman Z, Quezado BD, Tyrphostin AG 556 improves survival and reduces multiorgan failure in canine *E. coli* peritonitis. *J Clin Invest* 1997; 99:1966–1973.

32. Vanichkin A, Palya M, Gazit A, Levitzki A, Novogrodsky A. Late administration of a lipophilic tyrosine kinase inhibitor prevents lipopolysaccharide and *Escherichia coli*-Induced lethal toxicity. *J Infect Dis* 1996; 173:927–933.

33. Novogrodsky A, Vanichkin M, Patya A, Gazit N, Osherov N, Levitzki A. Prevention of LPS-induced lethal toxicity by tyrosine kinase blockers. *Science* 1994; 264:1319–1322.

34. Golomb G, Fishbein I, Banai S, Mishaly D, Msocovitz D, Gertz D, Gazit A, Levitzki A. Controlled delivery of a tyrphostin inhibits intimal hyperplasia in rat carotid artery injury model. *Atherosclerosis* 1996; 125:171–182.

35. Buchdunger E, Mett H, Trinks U, Regenass U, Muller M, Meyer T, Beilstein P, Wirz B, Schneider P, Traxler P. 4,5-Bis(4-fluoroanilino)pthalimide: A selective Inhibitor of the epidermal growth factor receptor signal transduction pathway with potent in vivo antitumor activity. *Clin Cancer Res* 1995; 1:813–821.

36. Buchdunger E, Zimmermann J, Mett H, Meyer T, Muller M, Regenass U, Lydon N. Selective inhibition of the platelet-derived growth factor signal transduction pathway by a protein-

tyrosine kinase inhibitor of the 2-phenylaminopyrimidine class. *Proc Natl Acad Sci USA* 1995; 92:2558–2562.

37. Druker BJ, Tamura S, Buchdunger E, Ohno S, Segal GM, Fanning S, Zimmermann J, Lydon NB. Effects of a selective inhibitor of the Abl tyrosine kinase on the growth of Bcr-Abl positive cells. *Nature Med* 1996; 2:561–566.

38. Kaur G, Gazit A, Levitzki A, Stowe E, Cooney DA, Sausville EA. Tyrphostin induced growth inhibition: correlation with effect on p210[bcr-abl] autokinase activity in K562 chronic myelogenous leukemia. *Anticancer Drugs* 1994; 5:213–222.

39. Banai S, Wolf Y, Golomb G, Pearle A, Waltenberger J, Fishtein I, Schneider A, Gazit A, Perez L, Huber R, Lazarovichi G, Levitzki A, Gertz SD. PDGF-Receptor tyrosine kinase blocker AG 1295 selectively attenuates smooth muscle cell growth in vitro and reduces neointimal formation after balloon angioplasty in swine. *Circulation* 1998; 19:1960–1969.

40. Fishben I, Waltenberger J, Banai S, Rabinovich L, Chorny M, Levitzki A, Gazit A, Huber R, Gertz DS, Golomb G. Local delivery of PDGF receptor-specific tyrphostin inhibits neointimal formation in rats. *Arteriosclerosis Thrombosis Vasc Biol,* in press.

41. Osherov N, Levitzki A. Epidermal growth factor dependent activation of Src family kinases. *Eur J Biochem* 1994; 225:1047–1053.

42. Fry DW, Kraker AJ, McMichael A, Ambroso LA, Nelson JM, Leopold WR, Connors RW, Bridges AJ. A specific inhibitor of the epidermal growth factor receptor tyrosine kinase. *Science* 1994; 265:1093–1095.

43. Gazit A, Chen J, App H, McMahon G, Hirth P, Chen I, Levitzki A. Tyrphostin 4. Highly potent inhibitors of EGF receptor kinase. Structure activity relationship study of 4-anilidoquinazolines. *Biorg Med Chem* 1996; 8:1203–1207.

44. Bridges AJ, Zhou H, Cody DR, Rewcastle GW, McMichael A, Showalter HDH, Fry DW, Kraker AJ, Denny WA. Tyrosine kinase inhibitors. 8. An unusually steep structure–activity relationship for analogues of 4-(3-bromoanilino)-6,7-dimethoxyquinazoline (PD 153035), a potent inhibitor of the epidermal growth factor receptor. *J Med Chem* 1996; 39:267–276.

45. Powell TJ, Chen H, Shenoy N, McCollough J, Narog B, Gazit A, Ben-Bassat H, Harzstark Z, Chauat M, Tang C, McMahon J, Shawver L, Levitzki A. Inhibition of EGF receptor signal transduction and psoriatic keratinocyte growth by 4-(3-bromophenylamino-6,7-dimethoxyquinazoline (SU5271). *Br J Dermatol* 2000, in press.

46. Traxler PM, Furet P, Mett H, Buchdunger E, Meyer T, Lydon N. 4-(Phenylamino)pyrrolopyrimidines: potent and selective, ATP site directed inhibitors of the EGF-receptor protein tyrosine kinase. *J Med Chem* 1996; 39:2285–2292.

47. Rewcastle GW, Palmer BD, Bridges AJ, Showalter HDH, Sun L, Nelson J, McMichael A, Kraker AJ, Fry DW, Denny WA. Tyrosine kinase inhibitors. 9. Synthesis and evaluation of fused tricyclic quinazoline analogues as ATP site inhibitors of the tyrosine kinase activity of the epidermal growth factor receptor. *J Med Chem* 1996; 39:918–928.

48. Ross R, Glomset JA. The pathogenesis of atherosclerosis. *N Engl J Med* 295:369–377.

49. Ross R. The pathogenesis of atherosclerosis—An update. *N Engl J Med* 1986; 314:488–500.

50. Sharfe N, Dadi HK, Roifman CM. JAK 3 protein kinase mediates interleukin-7 induced activation of phosphatidyl inisito-3-kinase. Blood 1995; 86:2077–2085.

51. Lydon NB, Mett H, Muller M, Becker M, Cozens RM, Stover D, Daniels D, Traxler P, Buchdunger E. A potent protein-tyrosine kinase inhibitor which selectively blocks proliferation of EGF receptor expressing tumor cells in vitro and in vivo. *Int J Cancer* 1998; 76:154–163.

52. Brenner T, Poradosu E, Soffer D, Sicsic C, Gazit A, Levitzki A. Suppression of experimental autoimmune encephalomyelitis by tyrphostin AG-556. *Exp Neurol* 1998; 154:489–498.

53. Kelly SA, Goldschmidt-Clermont PJ, Milliken E, Arai T, Smith EH, Bulkley GB. Protien tyrosine phosphorylation mediated TNF-induced endothelial-neutrophil adhesion in vitro. *Am J Physiol* 1998; 43:H513–H519.

26

A Pharmacological Approach
to the MAP Kinase Cascade

David T. Dudley, PhD and Alan R. Saltiel, PhD

1. INTRODUCTION

A wide variety of stimuli activate phosphorylation cascades that regulate subsequent physiological responses. Among the best characterized are the mitogen-activated protein (MAP) kinase cascades. These cascades are characterized by three sequential kinase reactions, often activated downstream of a low-mol-wt G-protein (Fig. 1). These MAP kinase cascades appear to be ubiquitous and are found in such evolutionarily diverse species as nematodes, insects, yeast, and mammals. Although numerous proteins have been identified that participate in these cascades, three clearly recognized MAP kinase pathways have emerged, with distinct physiological consequences and mechanisms of activation. The precise constituents and roles of each of these cascades are discussed in other chapters in this book.

The earliest identified and best studied cascade contains the mammalian kinases Raf1, MEK1 (MAP kinase- or ERK-activating kinase-kinase) and pp44^{MAPK} (ERK1) or pp42^{MAPK} (ERK2). Raf is recruited to the plasma membrane by the small GTPase p21^{ras}, where it can be activated by a mechanism that remains poorly understood. After activation, raf subsequently phosphorylates MEK1 or MEK2 on serine residues 218 and 222. This dual phosphorylation activates MEK, enabling it to phosphorylate ERK1 or ERK2 on both a tyrosine and threonine residue in a signature TEY motif. It remains unknown whether raf can effectively phosphorylate other proteins in vivo. Moreover, although substrate specificity for ERK is reasonably broad, no substrate other than ERK1 and ERK2 (which retain an overall sequence identity of ~90) for MEK1 has been identified. This tight selectivity and the unusual ability to phosphorylate both tyrosine and threonine residues suggest a crucial regulatory role for MEK1 in the pathway.

Clearly, a number of sites in the MAP kinase pathway are amenable to pharmacological intervention. Such agents might be particularly beneficial in targeting tumors that contain activating *ras* mutations. One example of such a compound is PD 098059, identified by screening a library of compounds with an assay consisting of MEK1, ERK1, and myelin basic protein (MBP) *(1)*. The assay was designed so that final

From: Signaling Networks and Cell Cycle Control: The Molecular Basis of Cancer and Other Diseases
Edited by: J. S. Gutkind © Humana Press Inc., Totowa, NJ

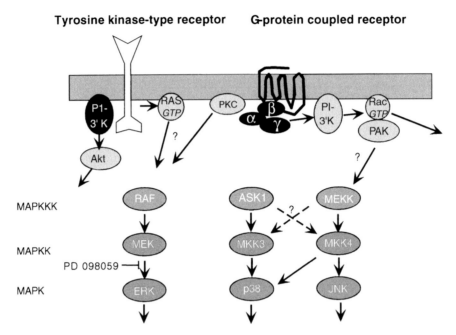

Fig. 1. Schematic representation of the MAP kinase cascades. Each cascade contains three sequential kinases: a MAP kinase kinase kinase (MAPKKK), MAP kinase kinase (MAPKK), and MAP kinase (MAPK). Each set is activated by low-mol-wt G-proteins, such as ras and rac, in an incompletely understood fashion. PD 098059 specifically inhibits activation of the MAPKK, MEK, selectively preventing propagation of a signal through the raf/MEK/erk cascade.

phosphate incorporation into MBP was sensitive to activation of ERK1 by MEK1. Thus, inhibitors of either MEK1 or ERK1 kinase activity would be scored. PD 098059 was subsequently found to be selective for MEK1 and completely inactive against ERK1. The compound has fivefold lower inhibitory activity against the closely related MEK2. Essentially no activity has been noted for inhibition of the related pathways of p38 or jun kinase activation (2). In this regard, PD 098059 does not block the related MEK1 kinases, MKK3, or MKK4. Most important, no other kinase has been found to be substantially inhibited by PD 098059, rendering it unique among kinase inhibitors for its degree of selectivity. Although PD 098059 appears to be exquisitely selective as a kinase inhibitor, it has been identified as an antagonist of the aryl hydrocarbon receptor (3). Whereas this result probably has no impact on most conclusions made by use of PD 098059 to date, it is important to realize that no pharmacological agent has absolute specificity.

   This review focuses on lessons learned from the MEK inhibitor about the biochemistry of MEK and on the cell biology of the MAP kinase pathway. These studies have demonstrated much about molecular interactions of MEK with its upstream regulator and downstream substrate, the importance of cross-talk and feedback loops in the cascade, and the role of the pathway in the actions of a diverse group of extracellular stimuli and biological paradigms.

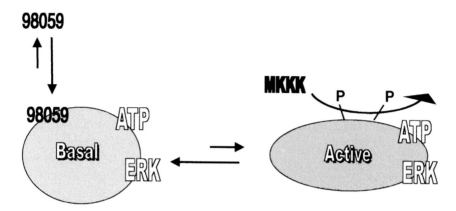

Fig. 2. Proposed mode of PD 098059 inhibition of MEK. PD 098059 preferentially interacts with the basal, nonphosphorylated form of MEK and stabilizes the enzyme in this conformation. Dissociation of the inhibitor permits of MEK phosphorylation by the MKKK, RAF-1, resulting in activation. PD 098059 does not inhibit phosphorylated MEK.

2. MECHANISM OF MEK ACTIVATION

MEK is activated by phosphorylation on serine residues 218 and 222 within a regulatory loop between kinase subdomains VII and VIII *(4,5)*. Partial activation is achieved by substitution of acidic residues in this region *(6,7)*. Further, activation is sensitive to the presence of residues 32–51, as deletion of this region coupled with aspartate substitution at 218 and 222 results in a fully activated enzyme. Thus, MEK exhibits an unusual mechanism for activation that involves conformational changes within a regulatory region mediated by electrostatic interactions and secondary structural changes at the N-terminus *(6,7)*.

The degree of specificity for MEK exhibited by PD 098059 suggested that the compound might inhibit at a unique site. Kinetic analysis showed that PD 098059 does not compete for either the ATP or ERK binding site on MEK1. In addition, prior activation of MEK1 through phosphorylation by raf renders the enzyme insensitive to inhibition by PD 098059 *(2)*. This aspect of PD 098059 activity is also observed when tested against various mutants of MEK1. PD 098059 inhibits the partially activated MEK-2E mutant (serines 218 and 222 converted to glutamate), is weaker against the more activated MEK-2D mutant (serines 218 and 222 converted to aspartate), and is inactive against the fully activated ΔN/2D construct (aspartate at 218 and 222 coupled with deletion of residues 32–51). Together, these data suggest that the binding site on MEK1 for PD 098059 is sensitive to the conformational change MEK1 undergoes upon activation. Further, PD 098059 may inhibit by stabilizing the inactive form of MEK1, perhaps by interacting with an allosteric regulatory site on the enzyme (Fig. 2).

The exact site of interaction is unknown, but it is tempting to speculate that PD 098059 may bind to MEK at or near the N-terminus of the protein. Recent studies have indicated that this domain may play an important regulatory role. Ahn and colleagues. *(6,7)* have identified an α-helical region from residues 44–51 that stabilizes

MEK in an inactive conformation. Deletion of this region results in activation. However, the presence of N-terminal residues 1–32 are obligatory for activation, as deletion of this region yields an enzyme with much lower basal activity, and much lower activation after phosphorylation of serines 218 and 222. A recent report indicates that residues 1–7 are necessary for activity *(8)*. Within this span of 7 amino acids lie three consecutive lysines in MEK1 and an RRK stretch in MEK2. Interestingly, replacement of ser218 and 222 with acidic amino acids enhances activation, and substitution of 4 aspartate residues from 218–222 results in the strongest activation. One possibility is that the N-terminal basic residues interact with the acidic residues in the regulatory loop (or negatively charged phosphates in naturally activated MEK). This interaction, which could be disrupted by PD 098059, may control activation.

3. FUNCTIONAL EFFECTS OF MAP KINASE CASCADE

PD 098059 has become a useful tool to block the MAP kinase cascade selectively in cultured cells in a simple, convenient manner. Although a comprehensive review of all experimental settings in which the inhibitor has been used is beyond the scope of this chapter, some of the salient features of the MAP kinase pathway demonstrated by use of this compound are highlighted.

3.1. The MAP Kinase Pathway in Insulin Action

MAP kinase was first discovered as an insulin-sensitive enzyme *(9)*, leading many investigators to suspect an important role in insulin action. PD 098059 has been used to evaluate the role of the MAP kinase pathway in a variety of cellular effects of insulin. In particular, the inhibitor can block the activation of pathways that correspond to the growth-promoting effects of the hormone, including stimulation of protein synthesis *(10)*, initiation factor eIF4e *(11)*, pp90rsk *(12)*, farnesyl transferase phosphorylation *(13)*, cyclic adenosine monophosphate (cAMP)-response element binding protein (CREB) phosphorylation and transcriptional activation *(14)*, c-fos and egr-1 *(12,15)* transcription, and DNA synthesis *(16)*. However, cellular actions of insulin that are related to its physiological effects on metabolism remain completely unaffected by the MEK inhibitor, including glucose uptake *(12,17,18)*, glycogen synthesis *(12,18–20)*, lipogenesis *(12)*, protein phosphatase 1 activation *(12)*, amino acid transport *(21)*, and phosphodiesterase 3B phosphorylation and activation *(22)*, as well as expression of hexokinase II *(23)* and phosphoenolpyruvate carboxykinase *(24)*. Thus, PD 098059 has been used to demonstrate that the MAP kinase pathway does not play an important role in insulin action.

3.2. The MAP Kinase Pathway in Cellular Growth and Differentiation

As essentially all growth factors have been shown to activate the MAP kinase pathway, it is reasonable to assume this pathway plays an important role in the control of cell growth, survival or cell cycle progression. PD 098059 blocks growth of a wide variety of tumor cell lines in culture or soft agar, including small cell lung cancer controlled by small peptides or TPA *(25)*, pancreatic cancer *(26,27)*, renal cells *(28)*, glioma *(29)*, and astrocytoma *(30)*. In general, the drug appears to exert a cytostatic,

80. Downey GP, Butler JR, Tapper H, Fialkow L, Saltiel AR, Rubin BB, Grinstein S. Importance of MEK in neutrophil microbicidal responsiveness. *J Immunol* 1998; 160:434–443.
81. Mayer AM, Brenic S, Glaser KB. Pharmacologicaltargeting of signaling pathways in protein kinase C-stimulated superoxide generation in neutrophil-like HL-60 cells: effect of phorbol ester, arachidonic acid and inhibitors of kinase(s), phosphatase(s) and phospholipase A2. *J Pharmacol Exp Ther* 1996; 279:633–644.
82. Kuroki M, O'Flaherty JT. Differential effects of a mitogen-activated protein kinase kinase inhibitor on human neutrophil responses to chemotactic factors. *Biochem Biophys Res Commun* 1997; 232:474–477.
83. Mocsai A, Banfi B, Kapus A, Farkas G, Geiszt M, Buday L, Farago A, Ligeti E. Differential effects of tyrosine kinase inhibitors and an inhibitor of the mitogen-activated protein kinase cascade on degranulation and superoxide production of human neutrophil granulocytes. *Biochem Pharmacol* 1997; 54:781–789.
84. Coffer PJ, Geijsen N, M'Rabet L, Schweizer RC, Maikoe T, Raaijmakers JA, Lammers JW, Koenderman L. Comparison of the roles of mitogen-activated protein kinase kinase and phosphatidylinositol 3-kinase signal transduction in neutrophil effector function. *Biochem J* 1998; 329:121–130.
85. Zu YL, Qi J, Gilchrist A, Fernandez GA, Vazquez Abad D, Kreutzer DL, Huang CK, Sha'afi RI. p38 mitogen-activated protein kinase activation is required for human neutrophil function triggered by TNF-alpha or FMLP stimulation. *J Immunol* 1998; 160:1982–1989.
86. Knall C, Worthen GS, Johnson GL. Interleukin 8-stimulated phosphatidylinositol-3-kinase activity regulates the migration of human neutrophils independent of extracellular signal-regulated kinase and p38 mitogen-activated protein kinases. *Proc Natl Acad Sci USA* 1997; 94:3052–3057.
87. Haneda M, Araki S, Togawa M, Sugimoto T, Isono M, Kikkawa R. Mitogen-activated protein kinase cascade is activated in glomeruli of diabetic rats and glomerular mesangial cells cultured under high glucose conditions. *Diabetes* 1997; 46:847–853.
88. Huwiler A, Staudt G, Kramer RM, Pfeilschifter J. Cross-talk between secretory phospholipase A2 and cytosolic phospholipase A2 in rat renal mesangial cells. *Biochim Biophys Acta* 1997; 1348:257–272.
89. Xing M, Insel PA. Protein kinase C-dependent activation of cytosolic phospholipase A2 and mitogen-activated protein kinase by alpha 1-adrenergic receptors in Madin-Darby canine kidney cells. *J Clin Invest* 1996; 97:1302–1310.
90. Xing M, Firestein BL, Shen GH, Insel PA. Dual role of protein kinase C in the regulation of cPLA2-mediated arachidonic acid release by P2U receptors in MDCK-D1 cells: Involvement of MAP kinase-dependent and -independent pathways. *J Clin Invest* 1997; 99:805–814.
91. Wheeler Jones C, Abu Ghazaleh R, Cospedal R, Houliston RA, Martin J, Zachary I. Vascular endothelial growth factor stimulates prostacyclin production and activation of cytosolic phospholipase A2 in endothelial cells via p42/p44 mitogen-activated protein kinase. *FEBS Lett* 1997; 420:28–32.
92. Patel V, Brown C, Goodwin A, Wilkie N, Boarder MR. Phosphorylation and activation of p42 and p44 mitogen-activated protein kinase are required for the P2 purinoceptor stimulation of endothelial prostacyclin production. *Biochem J* 1996; 320:221–226.
93. Muthalif MM, Benter IF, Uddin MR, Malik KU. Calcium/calmodulin-dependent protein kinase IIalpha mediates activation of mitogen-activated protein kinase and cytosolic phospholipase A2 in norepinephrine-induced arachidonic acid release in rabbit aortic smooth muscle cells. *J Biol Chem* 1996; 271:30,149–30,157.
94. Muthalif MM, Benter IF, Uddin MR, Harper JL, Malik KU. Signal transduction mechanisms involved in angiotensin-(1–7)-stimulated arachidonic acid release and prostanoid synthesis in rabbit aortic smooth muscle cells. *J Pharmacol Exp Ther* 1998; 284:388–398.
95. Pyne NJ, Tolan D, Pyne S. Bradykinin stimulates cAMP synthesis via mitogen-activated

protein kinase-dependent regulation of cytosolic phospholipase A2 and prostaglandin E2 release in airway smooth muscle. *Biochem J* 1997; 328:689–694.

96. Chen WC, Chen CC. ATP-induced arachidonic acid release in cultured astrocytes is mediated by Gi protein coupled P2Y(1) and P2Y(2) receptors. *Glia* 1998; 22:360–370.

97. Hernandez M, Burillo SL, Crespo MS, Nieto ML. Secretory phospholipase A2 activates the cascade of mitogen-activated protein kinases and cytosolic phospholipase A2 in the human astrocytoma cell line 1321N1. *J Biol Chem* 1998; 273:606–612.

98. Borsch Haubold AG, Kramer RM, Watson SP. Inhibition of mitogen-activated protein kinase kinase does not impair primary activation of human platelets. *Biochem J* 1996; 318:207–212.

99. Bianchini L, L'Allemain G, Pouyssegur J. The p42/p44 mitogen-activated protein kinase cascade is determinant in mediating activation of the Na$^+$/H$^+$ exchanger (NHE1 isoform) in response to growth factors. *J Biol Chem* 1997; 272:271–279.

100. Aharonovitz O, Granot Y. Stimulation of mitogen-activated protein kinase and Na$^+$/H$^+$ exchanger in human platelets. Differential effect of phorbol ester and vasopressin. *J Biol Chem* 1996; 271:16,494–16,499.

101. Garnovskaya MN, Mukhin Y, Raymond JR. Rapid activation of sodium-proton exchange and extracellularsignal-regulated protein kinase in fibroblasts by G protein-coupled 5-HT1A receptor involves distinct signalling cascades. *Biochem J* 1998; 1:489–495.

102. Cohen DM. Urea-inducible Egr-1 transcription in renal inner medullary collecting duct (mIMCD3) cells is mediated by extracellular signal-regulated kinase activation. *Proc Natl Acad Sci USA* 1996; 93:11,242–11,247.

103. Johnson CM, Hill CS, Chawla S, Treisman R, Bading H. Calcium controls gene expression via three distinct pathways that can function independently of the Ras/mitogen-activated protein kinases (ERKs) signaling cascade. *J Neurosci* 1997; 17:6189–6202.

104. Muller JM, Krauss B, Kaltschmidt C, Baeuerle PA, Rupec RA. Hypoxia induces c-fos transcription via a mitogen-activated protein kinase-dependent pathway. *J Biol Chem* 1997; 272:23,435–23,439.

105. Pende M, Fisher TL, Simpson PB, Russell JT, Blenis J, Gallo V. Neurotransmitter- and growth factor-induced cAMP response element binding protein phosphorylation in glial cell progenitors: Role of calcium ions, protein kinase C, and mitogen-activated protein kinase/ribosomal S6 kinase pathway. *J Neurosci* 1997; 17:1291–1301.

106. Sato N, Kamino K, Tateishi K, Satoh T, Nishiwaki Y, Yoshiiwa A, Miki T, Ogihara T. Elevated amyloid beta protein(1-40) level induces CREB phosphorylation at serine-133 via p44/42 MAP kinase (Erkl/2)-dependent pathway in rat pheochromocytoma PC12 cells. *Biochem Biophys Res Commun* 1997; 232:637–642.

107. Hu E, Kim JB, Sarraf PS, Spiegelman BM. Inhibition of adipogenesis through MAP kinase-mediated phosphorylation of PPARγ. *Science* 1996; 274:2100–203.

108. Camp HS, Tafuri SR. Regulation of peroxisome proliferator-activated receptor—activity by mitogen-activated protein kinase. *J Biol Chem* 1997; 272:10,811–10,816.

109. Wartmann M, Cella N, Hofer P, Groner B, Liu X, Hennighausen L, Hynes NE. Lactogenic hormone activation of Stat5 and transcription of the beta-casein gene in mammary epithelial cells is independent of p42 ERK2 mitogen-activated protein kinase activity. *J Biol Chem* 1996; 271:31,863–31,868.

110. Kirken RA, Malabarba MG, Xu J, DaSilva L, Erwin RA, Liu X, Hennighausen L, Rui H, Farrar WL. Two discrete regions of interleukin-2 (IL2) receptor beta independently mediate IL2 activation of a PD98059/rapamycin/wortmannin-insensitive Stat5a/b serine kinase. *J Biol Chem* 1997; 272:15,459–15,4565.

111. Nishiya T, Uehara T, Edamatsu H, Kaziro Y, Itoh H, Nomura Y. Activation of Stat1 and subsequent transcription of inducible nitric oxide synthase gene in C6 glioma cells is independent of interferon-gamma-induced MAPK activation that is mediated by p21ras. *FEBS Lett* 1997; 408:33–38.

112. Pircher TJ, Flores Morales A, Mui AL, Saltiel AR, Norstedt G, Gustafsson JA, Haldosen LA. Mitogen-activated protein kinase kinase inhibition decreases growth hormone stimulated transcription mediated by STAT5. *Mol Cell Endocrinol* 1997; 133:169–176.

113. Bhat GJ, Baker KM. Angiotensin II stimulates rapid serine phosphorylation of transcription factor Stat3. *Mol Cell Biochem* 1997; 170:171–176.

114. Ceresa BP, Horvath CM, Pessin JE. Signal transducer and activator of transcription-3 serine phosphorylation by insulin is mediated by a Ras/Raf/MEK-dependent pathway. *Endocrinology* 1997; 138:4131–4137.

115. Langlois WJ, Sasaoka T, Saltiel AR, Olefsky JM. Negative feedback regulation and desensitization of insulin- and epidermal growth factor-stimulated p21(ras) activation. *J Biol Chem* 1995; 270:25,320–25,323.

116. Chen D, Waters SB, Holt KH, Pessin JE. SOS phosphorylation and disassociation of the Grb2-SOS complex by the ERK and JNK signaling pathways. *J Biol Chem* 1996; 271:6328–6332.

117. Vanderkuur JA, Butch ER, Waters SB, Pessin JE, Guan KL, Carter Su C. Signaling molecules involved in coupling growth hormone receptor to mitogen-activated protein kinase activation. *Endocrinology* 1997; 138:4301–4307.

118. Kao AW, Waters SB, Okada S, Pessin JE. Insulin stimulates the phosphorylation of the 66- and 52-kilodalton Shc isoforms by distinct pathways. *Endocrinology* 1997; 138:2447–2480.

119. Okada S, Kao AW, Ceresa BP, Blaikie P, Margolis B, Pessin JE. The 66-kDa Shc isoform is a negative regulator of the epidermal growth factor-stimulated mitogen-activated protein kinase pathway. *J Biol Chem* 1997; 272:28,042–28,049.

120. Wartmann M, Hofer P, Turowski P, Saltiel AR, Hynes NE. Negative modulation of membrane localization of the Raf-1 protein kinase by hyperphosphorylation. *J Biol Chem* 1997; 272:3915–3923.

121. Bokemeyer D, Sorokin A, Dunn MJ. Differential regulation of the dual-specificity protein-tyrosine phosphatases CL100, B23, and PAC1 in mesangial cells. *J Am Soc Nephrol* 1997; 8:40–50.

122. Brondello JM, Brunet A, Pouyssegur J, McKenzie FR. The dual specificity mitogen-activated protein kinase phosphatase-1 and -2 are induced by the p42/p44MAPK cascade. *J Biol Chem* 1997; 272:1368–1376.

123. Cook SJ, Beltman J, Cadwallader KA, McMahon M, McCormick F. Regulation of mitogen-activated protein kinase phosphatase-1 expression by extracellular signal-related kinase-dependent and Ca^{2+}-dependent signal pathways in Rat-1 cells. *J Biol Chem* 1997; 272: 13,309–13,319.

124. Franklin CC, Kraft AS. Conditional expression of the mitogen-activated protein kinase (MAPK) phosphatase MKP-1 preferentially inhibits p38 MAPK and stress-activated protein kinase in U937 cells. *J Biol Chem* 1997; 272:16,917–16,423.

27

Specific Inhibitors of p38 MAP Kinase

Peter R. Young

1. INTRODUCTION

Over the past few years there has been a considerable increase in our understanding of how various stimuli result in alterations of cellular phenotype through intracellular signaling pathways, as a result of the identification of the molecular components of each pathway and their regulation in response to stimulus. Among the components of each pathway, several have the potential for being targets for pharmacological intervention in various disease pathologies, and this is particularly true of protein kinases. However, it is becoming increasingly clear that in any pathway there are often several components that have multiple isoforms or homologues which can act in parallel, and this complicates the task of selecting the "right" target.

To date, most of the characterization of signaling pathways relies on comparison of in vitro and in vivo substrate phosphorylation patterns, kinetics of phosphorylation, biochemical fractionation, and overexpression of active and inactive or dominant negative forms of individual components. Whereas these methods can often suggest the contribution of the molecule under study to particular known downstream pathways and exclude others, they can also be misleading. For example, a dominant negative form of a kinase may prevent not only binding of the endogenous, active form of the kinase, but the binding of other kinases that bind to the same site as well, only one of which may ultimately be the one responsible for the effect seen.

Another approach to evaluating different signaling pathways is to develop specific, membrane permeable low-mol-wt inhibitors of particular molecular components that appear to play a pivotal role. Most commonly, a molecular target is picked and an assay developed that can detect inhibitors of its activity. In the case of protein kinases, inhibitors have typically been discovered either through the use of a high throughput kinase assay that can be used to screen a large compound collection or through structure-based design. An alternative approach has been to look for inhibitors of a particular cellular readout, such as the expression of a particular gene product or reporter gene, and then to attempt to discover the target through biochemical or genetic means. While this can be more technically challenging, it has the advantage of finding the most relevant molecular target for achieving the desired physiological effect. This latter

From: Signaling Networks and Cell Cycle Control: The Molecular Basis of Cancer and Other Diseases
Edited by: *J. S. Gutkind © Humana Press Inc., Totowa, NJ*

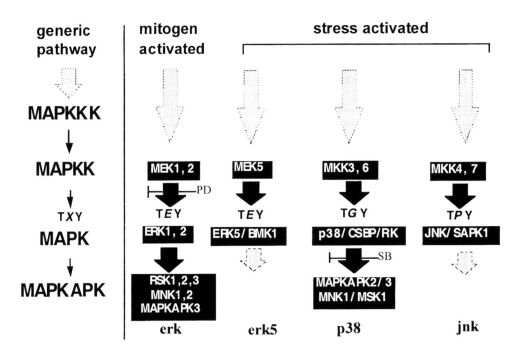

Fig. 1. MAP kinase cascades. The candidate MAPKKKs for each pathway have been excluded for clarity. The steps blocked by PD98059 and SB203580/SB202190 are marked by PD and SB, respectively.

approach was used to discover compounds that inhibited the production of interleukin-1 (IL-1) and tumor necrosis factor (TNF) from lipopolysaccharide (LPS)-stimulated human monocytes. Purification of the target led to the discovery that these compounds were inhibitors of p38 mitogen-activated protein (MAP) kinase *(1)*. As described further below, these inhibitors have allowed further understanding of the physiological role of p38 and represent a potentially exciting new avenue for the treatment of several diseases with an inflammatory component.

2. MAP KINASE PATHWAYS

The MAP kinases are a family of proline directed serine-threonine protein kinases. The term MAP kinase is derived from the observation that the earliest discovered members responded to mitogenic stimuli. Since then, the family has come to include several other homologues that respond to both mitogenic and nonmitogenic stimuli (Fig. 1). In response to a suitable stimulus, all MAP kinases are phosphorylated on a threonine and tyrosine in an activation loop (Thr Xaa Tyr, where Xaa is one of three amino acids) close to the active site. This results in a conformational change and activation of the kinase activity of the MAP kinase, which then can phosphorylate a number of specific substrates, including other kinases, enzymes, cytoskeletal proteins, and transcription factors *(2)*.

MAP kinases can be broadly divided into three families: ERK, JNK/SAPK (also known as SAPK1), and p38 (also known as CSBP, RK, SAPK2a). These differ in primary sequence by the nature of the Xaa amino acid in the Thr Xaa Tyr motif in the activation loop: ERK is Glu, JNK/SAPK is Pro, and p38 is Gly. They also differ in the length of the activation loop itself. However, these differences do not seem to determine directly the most distinctive feature of the three families, which is their phosphorylation and activation by different MAP kinase kinases in response to the appropriate cell stimulus *(3,4)*. Rather, this seems to be determined by other regions of each MAP kinase *(3)*. As a result, the ERKs are activated by MEK1 and 2 (MAP or ERK kinase), the JNK/SAPKs by MKK4/SEK and MKK7, and the p38s by MKK3, MKK4 and MKK6 *(5–19)*. The MAP kinase kinases are in turn activated by phosphorylation on two serines by the MAP kinase kinase kinases (MAPKKK), which include the MEKKs, MLKs, ASK1, Tp12, and a number of other candidates *(20–25)*, although the specific physiological involvement of each of these kinases is still under investigation *(26)*.

The existence of these largely parallel pathways containing homologous kinases has led to them being referred to as the ERK, JNK/SAPK, and p38 MAP kinase pathways respectively. The JNK/SAPK and p38 pathways are often distinguished from the ERK pathway because the former are found to respond to various stress stimuli and are therefore referred to as stress-activated protein kinases (SAPKs), whereas the ERK pathway is largely associated with mitogenic stimuli. However, this distinction breaks down with the newest ERK member, ERK5 (or BMK), which by primary sequence is an ERK, yet it responds to oxidative stress *(27,28)*. The distinctions further break down as individual stimuli are examined in detail, leaving a picture that is somewhat more complicated.

3. p38 MAP KINASE

3.1. Splice Variants and Homologs of p38 MAP Kinase

There are three different splice forms of p38. Two forms, CSBP1 and 2 *(1)*, are a result of alternate splicing of two internal 25 amino acid regions encoded by adjacent exons (P. McDonnell, unpublished data) conserved in mice and humans (D. Woolf, unpublished data). A third form, Mxi2 *(29)*, was discovered through a yeast two-hybrid screen with the transcription factor Max as the bait, and results in a protein lacking the C-terminal 65 amino acids. No known functional differences in mammalian cells have been ascribed to CSBP1 and 2, and there has been limited characterization of Mxi2.

A search of EST databases revealed three additional members of the p38 MAP kinase family, all of which contain the TGY motif *(30–39)*. These are known by a number of different names. Table 1 lists alternative names. One of the homologs appears to have two alternative forms, p38β and p38β2, which differ by the presence of an 8 amino acid insertion, but only p38β2 which lacks this insertion has significant kinase activity *(30,34–36,38)*. p38 is activated by MKK3, 4 and 6, but the homologus show some selectivity. For example, p38β2 is preferentially activated by MKK6 *(38)*.

3.2. Stimulation of p38 MAP Kinase

p38 MAP kinase is activated in response to a number of different stimuli. Consistent with its designation as a stress activated protein kinase, p38 is activated by chemical, heat, osmotic, pH, oxidative and ischemic stress, growth factor withdrawal, high or low glucose, ultraviolet (UV) irradiation, and photodynamic therapy *(1,40–50)*. Among

Table 1
Members of the p38 MAP Kinase Family

Name	p38	p38β/β2	p38γ	p38δ
Alternative names	SAPK2a CSBP, RK	SAPK2b p38-2	SAPK3 ERK6	SAPK4
% amino acid identity to p38	100	73	63	61
Size	360	372/364	367	365
Chromosomal location	6p21 (123)	—	22q13.3 (124)	—
mRNA expression	Ubiquitous	Ubiquitous	Skeletal muscle	Testes, pancreas, prostate, small intestine
Stimulation by PMA[a]	No	No	Yes	Yes
Substrates	MAPKAPK2/3 ATF2, MBP, Elk1, SAP-1a, MNK1, MSK1	MAPKAPK2/3 ATF2, MBP, Elk1	ATF2, MBP ?	ATF2, MBP ?
Inhibition by SB203580 or SB202190	Yes	Yes	No	No

[a]In HeLa cells transfected with epitope-tagged versions of each kinase *(34)*. There are some exceptions.

the chemical stimulants are arsenite *(41,51)* and cytotoxic compounds such as MMS *(43)*, tunicamycin *(43)*, cycloheximide, and anisomycin *(52,53)*. Interestingly, the effects of anisomycin do not appear to be attributable to its ability to inhibit protein translation since p38 is activated at much lower concentrations than those required to inhibit translation. However, p38 is also stimulated by agents that mediate the initial physiological response to local and systemic "stress," which in its more general form covers injury, infection and inflammation. These include LPS and the proinflammatory cytokines IL-1, TNF, FasL, CD40L, and TGFβ1 *(1,42,54–58)* and cross-linking of the T- and B-cell antigen receptors *(57)*. Similarly, a number of G-protein-coupled seven-transmembrane receptors such as thrombin, thromboxane, f-Met-Leu-Phe, muscarinic, and β-adrenergic, which can influence these responses, can activate p38 *(59–63)*. However, this neat association of p38 with stress, even in its most general definition, is probably an oversimplification, as a number of growth factors are known to activate p38 in some cells, including granulocyte-colony-stimulating factor (G-CSF), IL-3, SCF, FGF, VEGF, and NGF *(64–67)*. Furthermore, whereas (PMA) phorbol myristate acetate is generally not considered a major stimulator of p38, it was recently shown to be a stimulator in the squamous cell carcinoma UM-SCC-1 *(43)* and a co-stimulator with calcium ionophore in Jurkat cells *(68)*. These multiple stimuli emphasize the need to evaluate the role of p38 activation on a case-by-case basis.

Fewer studies have been conducted with the p38 homologs, but the limited evidence to date suggests that they are activated by similar cellular stresses and proinflammatory cytokines. One difference that does seem to have emerged is the ability of p38γ and p38δ to be activated by PMA, whereas this activation is weak for p38 and p38β2 *(34)*, with the exceptions noted above. Also, bradykinin was found to preferentially activate p38β2 over p38 in neuroblastoma × glioma hybrid cells *(69)*.

3.3. Substrates of p38

A number of potential substrates of p38 have been determined from in vitro and in vivo studies. p38 can phosphorylate and activate the serine-threonine protein kinases MAPKAP kinase-2, MAPKAP kinase-3, MAPKAP kinase-5, MNK1, and MSK1 *(70–76)*. MAPKAP kinases-2 and -3 phosphorylate Hsp27 and LSP-1, which regulate cytoskeletal changes *(41,51,54,71,77–79)*. MAPKAP kinase-2 also phosphorylates tyrosine hydroxylase, the rate-limiting enzyme in catecholamine synthesis *(80)*. MNK1 phosphorylates eIF2, and may therefore regulate protein translation *(72)*. MSK1 phosphorylates the transcription factor CREB, and stimulates its activity *(76)*. p38 can also directly phosphorylate several transcription factors, including ATF2, MEF-2C, CHOP, Elk1, and SAP-1a, and regulate their activity *(43,81–85)*. However, p38 does not directly regulate the activation of NF-κB *(42,86)*. p38 also phosphorylates the intracellular enzyme $cPLA_2$ *(60)*.

Where it has been tested, p38β2 phosphorylates the same in vitro substrates as p38, including ATF2, myelin basic protein (MBP), Elk1, SAP-1a, and the MAPKAP kinases-2/3 *(34,36,38)*. Whereas p38γ and p38δ phosphorylate ATF2, Elk1, PHAS-1 and MBP, they differ from p38 and p38β2 in being unable to phosphorylate MAPKAP kinases-2/3 *(34,35,37,39,87)*. It is likely that they will differ in their activity toward further substrates.

The selectivity of p38 for its targets is probably not just determined by its recognition of the target substrate Ser/Thr-Pro sequence, since unactivated p38 also associates with MAPKAP kinase-2 and MAPKAP kinase-3 in cells *(63,71)*. Furthermore, interaction with substrate appears to be required before ATP can bind *(88)*. In vitro the interaction of p38 with MAPKAP kinase-3 is of low nM affinity (M. Doyle, personal communication) and appears to be dependent on p38 residues not important for kinase activity *(88a)*. A similar "docking" interaction site has been identified in JNK2 *(89)*.

4. INHIBITORS OF p38 MAP KINASE

4.1. Discovery and Mechanism of Action

The discovery of inhibitors of p38 MAP kinase emanated from an effort to find the molecular target of a series of pyridinyl imidazoles (SB CSAIDs), which inhibited the production of IL-1 and TNF-α from LPS-treated human monocytes and monocytic cell lines. Through the use of labeled and radiophotoaffinity versions of these compounds, the target was identified as CSAID binding protein (CSBP), which turned out to be identical to the independently isolated murine p38 MAP kinase *(1)*. Subsequent work has elucidated the mechanism by which these compounds work.

The pyridinyl imidazoles, as exemplified by SB203580 and SB202190 (Fig. 2), work by binding to the ATP site and inhibiting the kinase activity of p38 MAP kinase *(90)*. A direct pharmacological association was established by the close correlation of the IC_{50} of the compounds in binding and inhibiting p38 with their potency in inhibiting cytokine production from LPS treated human monocytes. The inhibitors bind to both

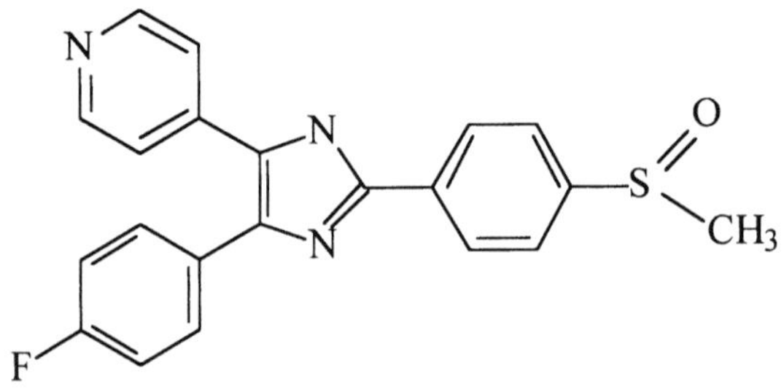

SB203580

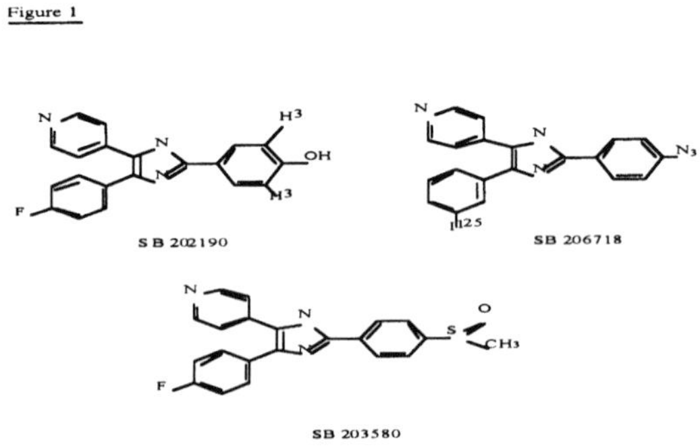

Figure 1

SB202190

Fig. 2. Chemical structure of the p38 inhibitors SB203580 and SB202190.

the inactive and active forms with comparable affinity, and this is seen for compounds spanning a wide range of potency, suggesting that the final bound form of the compound in both cases is very similar. Although the compounds bind to the inactive form of p38, they do not appear to inhibit its enzymatic activation by MKKs as judged by their lack of effect on its phosphorylation and the activity of kinase isolated from treated cells in vitro *(90)*. Some investigators have seen inhibition of p38 activation isolated from treated cells, but this often occurs at significantly higher concentrations of inhibitor which may therefore be retained in immunoprecipitates. It may also reflect a contribution of autophosphorylation *(4)*.

4.2. Selectivity of p38 MAP Kinase Inhibitors

When tested on different serine-threonine and tyrosine protein kinases, many of the pyridinyl imidazoles appear to have significant selectivity *(51)*. In particular, the inhibitor SB203580 does not inhibit several other protein kinases in the MAP kinase signaling pathway and does not inhibit most other MAP kinase members, such as the ERKs and

JNK1 variants at doses $100 \times$ the dose required to inhibit p38 kinase. More detailed in vitro analysis with immunoprecipitated recombinant JNK isoforms transiently expressed in mammalian cells suggested that SB203580 could partially inhibit two of the JNK2 splice variants at 10 μM and completely inhibit them at 100 μM, whereas inhibition of p38 was complete at 1 μM (IC_{50} = 0.1 μM) *(85)*, and similar data have been obtained from endogenous JNK isoforms *(91)*. By contrast, SB 203580 was unable to inhibit the two p38 homologues p38γ and p38δ at 100 μM, whereas p38β2 was inhibited with a similar IC_{50} value to p38 *(34,35,37,87)*. More recent data suggest that TGFβR type I and some tyrosine kinases such as Lck may also be partially inhibited in vitro at higher concentrations (IC_{50} = 20–50 μM) *(92)*. However, the sensitivity of kinases other than p38 to SB203580 has not been determined in viable cells.

These data have suggested that SB203580 is highly selective and have encouraged its use in assessing the role of p38 in various in vitro biological assays. However, it is clear that at higher concentrations one may not assume that all the effects that are seen are necessarily through inhibition of p38 kinase. Indeed, the related SB202190 was found to induce apoptosis at 50 μM some 100-fold higher than the concentrations needed to inhibit p38 in vivo *(93);* this could be through the inhibition of a number of protein kinases, including tyrosine kinases required for growth. SB203580 is also able to inhibit leukotriene synthesis at higher concentrations *(94)*. Furthermore, related pyridinyl imidazoles may not maintain the selectivity of SB203580. We have found that small changes in structure can reduce the level of selectivity toward other protein kinases, as illustrated by the ability of one of these compounds to bind and inhibit ERK *(95)*. These complications may be avoided by only using the inhibitor at doses required to inhibit p38 in viable cells.

4.3. Basis for Selectivity of Pyridinyl Imidazole Inhibitors of p38

The basis for the selectivity of the pyridinyl imidazoles has been revealed through mutagenesis and X-ray crystallographic structures of p38 MAP kinase: inhibitor complexes *(92,95–98)*. All these structures involve binding of the inhibitor to the unactivated form of p38. Active protein kinases typically consist of an β-sheet-rich N-terminal domain and an α-helical rich C-terminal domain whose interface forms the ATP binding site. The unactivated form of p38 exhibits a structure similar to ERK2 in which the amino and C-terminal domains are misaligned so that ATP binds only weakly *(99–101)*. Furthermore, the nonphosphorylated activation loop occupies the substrate peptide binding channel. Both alterations presumably contribute to the low activity of the nophosphorylated p38. In the p38:inhibitor structures, the pyridinyl imidazoles bind in the back of the ATP pocket close to the crossover connection between the two domains and overlapping the region where the adenosine ring of ATP would sit, but forming several other side chain interactions, some of which result from localized conformational changes *(95–97)*. By analogy to the homolog ERK2, whose active structure has been solved crystallographically *(102)*, dual phosphorylation of p38 is expected to alter the conformation of the activation loop, and allow the two domains to come together to form a catalytically active ATP site. Because these conformational changes are mostly at the opposite end of the ATP binding site to the inhibitor binding region, it is easy to see how a similar inhibitor binding site could be accommodated in both the inactive and active forms. In addition to supporting the similar binding characteristics for the two forms, the similarity of the inhibitor–complex structure to the inactive form of p38 suggests that inhibitor binding might drive the active form to the inactive state. This may account for some of the selectivity of the pyridinyl imidazoles.

While some of the residues which bind to the inhibitors are conserved in many kinases, others are unique *(98)*. In particular, there is a pocket at the back of the ATP site which binds the fluorophenyl ring of the inhibitors but does not bind any part of ATP. This pocket is dependent on the small Thr at position 106. When this residue is changed to a larger amino acid, it occludes this pocket and reduces binding of the pyridinyl imidazoles, whereas smaller residues increase binding *(92,96,98)*. Adjacent amino acids, especially His107 and Leu108, may also contribute to drug binding, particularly in mammalian cells *(98)*.

Interestingly, these are the very amino acids that are different in p38γ and p38δ, and when they are substituted with the amino acids from p38, these two kinases become as sensitive as p38 to inhibition by SB203580. Furthermore, when these same residues are substituted into the equivalent position in the more evolutionarily distant JNK1, it too becomes sensitive to SB203580 *(92,98)*. This suggests that some of the kinases that may be sensitive to SB203580 and other pyridinyl imidazoles with a 4-fluorophenyl group will be recognizable by the presence of Thr or smaller residue at position 106. This has been shown to be the case for the TGFβRI and RII kinases and for the tyrosine kinase Lck *(92)*. However, these kinases are still 100-fold less sensitive to SB203580 than is p38.

These mutated MAP kinases may have further utility in evaluating MAP kinase pathways, since the introduction of SB203580-insensitive forms of p38 into cells may allow further validation of the role of p38 in particular cell-mediated events. Likewise, the introduction of SB203580-sensitive forms of the MAP kinases into knockout trans-genic mice or cells may enable the evaluation of other pathways with the p38 inhibitors.

5. USE OF p38 INHIBITORS

5.1. In Vivo Substrates

Historically, the biggest concern with interpreting the results of in vivo kinase inhibitor studies has been the potential for the effects observed to be mediated through a different kinase from the one thought to be targeted, and there are several examples of this. Hence, despite the selectivity of the p38 inhibitor SB203580, this may not hold at concentrations of >10 μ*M* as noted above. Further confidence may be obtained by comparing the dose response of the kinase inhibitor in inhibiting the phosphorylation or activation of a known in vivo substrate to the physiological response being measured in the cell of interest.

It has now been clearly established that MAPKAP kinase-2 is an in vivo substrate of p38 in response to physiological stimuli *(51)*. Of the four p38 homologs, only p38 and p38β2 can phosphorylate and activate MAPKAP kinase in vitro, and these are also the only two inhibited by SB203580 *(34)*. When used in vivo, SB203580 inhibits the activation of MAPKAP kinase-2 by all the stimuli that have been monitored suggesting that p38/p38β are the sole enzymes responsible for this process. Furthermore, SB203580 also inhibits phosphorylation of the small heat shock protein hsp27 in vivo, which is a known in vitro substrate of MAPKAP kinase-2. Therefore, these two events constitute an internal control for the use of SB203580 in vivo and should help define the dose range within which the compound is active.

Several other proteins have now been established as in vivo substrates of p38. These include the MAPKAP kinase-2-related MAPKAP kinase-3 and MNK1, and the p90rsk-related MSK1 and 2 *(70–76)*. These kinases seem to form complexes with unactivated p38 and dissociate upon activation, whereupon they phosphorylate different substrates (Section 3.3.). Inhibition of the activation of these kinases leads to effects on transcription and cytoskeleton and may affect protein translation.

5.2. Role of p38 in Transcription Regulation

As mentioned above, several transcription factors are also substrates of p38α/β/β2 in vivo. These include Elk1, Sap-1a, CHOP, and MEF2C *(43,81–85)*. Direct phosphorylation of MEF2C and Elk1/Sap-1a, as well as indirect phosphorylation of CREB/ATF1 *(65,76,103)* in response to stress leads to the production of c-fos and c-jun and their homologs, which are the components of AP-1 and whose formation is inhibited by SB203580 *(52,81,104)*. Although ATF2 is an in vitro substrate of p38 and can be activated in vivo upon overexpression of a constitutively active form of MKK6, its phosphorylation is not inhibited by SB203580 in vivo in response to more physiological stimuli *(52)*, suggesting that its phosphorylation may be mediated by p38γ/p38δ at least in the cells studied to date. Although SB203580 does not inhibit NF-κB activation, consistent with the finding that IκB is not an in vitro substrate *(86)*, it can inhibit some NF-κB-mediated transcription *(86,105,106)*, although the mechanism is unclear. It is possible that p38 may regulate the functional interaction of NF-κB with other transcription factors. From several studies with SB203580, it is clear that although it is completely able to inhibit transcription mediated by these transcription factors under some circumstances, in other cases other MAP kinase members may be involved. For example, some combination studies of SB203580 with the MEK inhibitor PD98059 have indicated that both ERK and p38 are required for UV activation of c-fos transcription *(82)*. Other transcription factors regulated by the p38 kinase pathway include IUF1 *(49)* and NFAT *(68)*.

5.3. Time Course Studies

One additional area in which inhibitors have been useful is in examining the time course of the critical p38 signaling event that affects a particular cellular response. Because the compound is taken up by cells in a matter of minutes, by varying the time of addition it is possible to determine the exact time after which p38 is important. In LPS stimulated monocytes, the time course of inhibition of IL-1 and TNF by SB203580 overlapped the time course of inhibition by cycloheximide and occurred later than inhibition by actinomycin D, supporting other data suggesting that the effects were at the translational level *(107–109)*. In UV-induced HIV LTR-dependent transcription, SB203580 could be added a few hours after UV treatment, indicating that the critical role of p38 occurred well after the initial activation of its kinase activity and suggesting some intermediate signaling events *(105)*.

5.4. Regulation of Cytokine and Proinflammatory Enzymes

SB203580 has proved useful in determining the role of p38 in gene expression. As noted above, the pyridinyl imidazoles were originally discovered for their effect on LPS-stimulated IL-1 and TNF *(1)*, and we now know that the production of several other inflammatory cytokines can be inhibited by SB203580, including IL-6, IL-8, granulocyte-macrophage colony-stimulating factor (GM-CSF), interferon-γ (IFN-γ), and CD23 *(86,110–112)*. These cytokines are involved in stimulating the infiltration of circulating leukocytes to localized disease areas and in Th1-mediated cellular immune responses *(110)*. These effects can occur at both the transcription and translation levels, with the former likely resulting from effects on both AP-1 and NF-κB. Interestingly, the inhibitors suppress not only the production of proinflammatory cytokines, but also some of their actions on immune and nonimmune cells. SB203580 also inhibits the production of IL-2 and IL-7 in T cells *(68,113)*, although no inhibition was seen in various in vitro T-cell proliferation assays at doses known to inhibit p38 *(114)*.

p38 also plays a role in regulating the activity of various inflammatory enzymes. Thus SB203580 inhibits the production of cyclo-oxygenase-2 and inducible nitric oxide synthase *(115–117)*, and inhibits the activation of PLA2 *(60)*. It also inhibits the aggregation of platelets in response to thromboxane and collagen *(61)*.

5.5. Regulation of Cell Death and Survival by p38

Several studies have suggested that p38 may play a role in both cell survival and apoptosis depending on the stimulus and the cell type. Thus in Fas induced apoptosis of Jurkat cells, p38 inhibition does not block apoptosis *(55,118)*, whereas in neural and fibroblast cell lines in which growth factor is withdrawn, p38 may contribute to survival *(44,48)*. A criticism of many of these studies is that they are conducted in cell lines adapted to long term growth. However, the same dichotomy seems evident in cells isolated from natural sources, since LPS-induced eosinophil apoptosis, B-cell apoptosis induced by crosslinking of the B-cell antigen receptor, and anisomycin-induced apoptosis in cardiac myocytes are not inhibited by SB203580 *(57,106)*, whereas p38 inhibition does prevent stress induced apoptosis in neutrophils *(119)*. There is some evidence that this dichotomy may be caused by an underlying pro-apoptotic p38 activity and anti-apoptotic p38β/β2 activity and that the effects of inhibition by pyridinyl imidazole inhibitors may depend on which activity predominates *(93,120)*.

These data suggest a significant role for p38 during injury and infection, and this may also be true for certain viral infections. SB203580 was shown to directly inhibit the transcription of human immunodeficiency virus (HIV) LTR transcription and p24 production in response to stress or cytokine stimulation *(105,121)*, suggesting that the p38 MAP kinase pathway may play a role in the etiology of HIV.

5.6. Therapeutic Potential of p38 Inhibitors

Even before p38 was discovered as their target, the pyridinyl imidazoles such as SB203580 had already shown promise in animal models of inflammation. SB203580 and related pyridinyl imidazoles demonstrate the ability to inhibit LPS induced TNF production in vivo in both rats and mice, consistent with their pharmacokinetic profile *(94,114)*. The compounds have also shown efficacy in models of such as adjuvant arthritis, collagen-induced arthritis, endotoxin shock, skin inflammation, phenylbenzo-quinine hyperalgesia, bone resorption, and angiogenesis, suggesting that suitable clinical candidates could show promise in treating several of these and other diseases with a significant inflammatory cytokine component *(94,114,122)*.

6. SUMMARY AND PROSPECTIVE

The unexpected selectivity of the pyridinyl imidazoles toward a single protein kinase, p38, has contributed to the renewed enthusiasm for protein kinases as targets for drug discovery. It is now clear that the ATP binding site of at least some protein kinases may offer important differences in local conformation that can lead to selectivity. As more protein kinases are screened against large compound banks, we might expect to learn how often selective inhibitors can be obtained and whether p38 is atypical.

The exciting profile of the p38 inhibitors in disease models has led to considerable further interest in this target from many pharmaceutical companies. While it is tempting to believe that all the effects seen in vivo are attributable to p38 inhibition, it is actually hard to prove that this is the case. All the inhibitors that we have tested show ability to inhibit TNF production in animals and are active in inflammatory disease models but, until multiple structural classes of inhibitors have been tested, it is possible that individual compounds may demonstrate slightly different profiles as a result of differences in pharmacokinetics, distribution, and interaction with other molecular targets.

Now that several of the components of the stress-activated protein kinase pathways have been discovered, we can begin to evaluate their relative importance through mouse transgenic knockout or dominant negative studies. As part of this exercise, it is likely that inhibitors for some of these molecules will emerge, which should permit further understanding of their role in stress-induced responses and pathology. Some of these may also lead to novel therapeutic entities.

REFERENCES

1. Lee JC, Laydon JT, McDonnell PC, Gallagher TF, Kumar S, Green D, McNulty D, Blumenthal MJ, Heys JR, Landvatter SW, Strickler JE, McLaughlin MM, Siemens IR, Fisher SM, Livi GP, White JR, Adams JL, Young PR. A protein kinase involved in the regulation of inflammatory cytokine biosynthesis. *Nature* (1994); 372:739–746.
2. Cobb MH, Goldsmith EJ. How MAP kinases are regulated. *J Biol Chem* 1995; 270:14,843–14,846.
3. Brunet A, Pouyssegur J. Identification of MAP kinase domains by redirecting stress signals into growth factor responses. *Science* 1996; 272:1652–1655.
4. Jiang Y, Li Z, Schwarz EM, Lin A, Guan K, Ulevitch RJ, Han J. Structure-function studies of p38 mitogen-activated protein kinase. Loop 12 influences substrate specificity and autophosphorylation, but not upstream kinase selection. *J Biol Chem* 1997; 272:11,096–11,102.
5. Sanchez I, Hughes RT, Mayer BJ, Yee K, Woodgett JR, Avruch J, Kyriakis JM, Zon LI. Role of SAPK/ERK kinase-1 in the stress-activated pathway regulating transcription factor c-jun. *Nature* 1994; 372:794–798.
6. Derijard B, Raingeaud J, Barrett T, Wu I-H, Han J, Ulevitch RJ, Davis RJ. Independent human MAP kinase signal transduction pathways defined by MEK and MKK Isoforms. *Science* 1995; 267:682–685.

7. Lin A, Minden A, Martinetto H, Claret F-X, Lange-Carter C, Mercurio F, Johnson GL and Karin M. Identification of a dual specificity kinase that activates the Jun kinases and p38-Mpk2. *Science* 1995; 268:286–290.

8. Han J, Lee JD, Jiang Y, Li Z, Feng L, Ulevitch RJ. Characterization of the structure and function of a novel MAP kinase kinase (MKK6). *J Biol Chem* 1996; 271:2886–2891.

9. Moriguchi T, Kuroyanagi N, Yamaguchi K, Gotoh Y, Irie K, Kano T, Shirakabe K, Muro Y, Shibuya H, Matsumoto K, Nishida E, Hagiwara M. A novel kinase cascade mediated by mitogen-activated protein kinase kinase 6 and MKK3. *J Biol Chem* 1996; 271:13,675–13,679.

10. Stein B, Brady H, Yang MX, Young DB, Barbosa MS. Cloning and characterization of MEK6, a novel member of the mitogen-activated protein kinase kinase cascade. *J Biol Chem* 1996; 271:11,427–11,433.

11. Cuenda A, Alonso G, Morrice N, Jones M, Meier R, Cohen P, Nebreda AR. Purification and cDNA cloning of SAPKK3, the major activator of RK/p38 in stress- and cytokine-stimulated monocytes and epithelial cells. *EMBO J* 1996; 15:4156–4164.

12. Tournier C, Whitmarsh AJ, Cavanagh J, Barrett T, Davis RJ. Mitogen-activated protein kinase kinase 7 is an activator of the c-Jun NH2-terminal kinase. *Proc Natl Acad Sci USA* 1997; 94:7337–7342.

13. Holland PM, Suzanne M, Campbell JS, Noselli S, Cooper JA. MKK7. *J Biol Chem* 1997; 272:24,994–24,998.

14. Moriguchi T, Toyoshima F, Masuyama N, Hanafusa H, Gotoh Y, Nishida E. A novel SAPK/JNK kinase, MKK7, stimulated by TNFalpha and cellular stresses. *EMBO J* 1997; 16:7045–7053.

15. Lu X, Nemoto S, Lin A. Identification of c-Jun NH$_2$-terminal protein kinase (JNK)-activating kinase 2 as an activator of JNK but not p38. *J Biol Chem* 1997; 272:24,751–24,754.

16. Wu Z, Wu J, Jacinto E, Karin M. Molecular cloning and characterization of human JNKK2, a novel Jun NH$_2$-terminal kinase-specific kinase. *Mol Cell Biol* 1997; 17:7407–7416.

17. Lawler S, Cuenda A, Goedert M, Cohen P. SKK4, a novel activator of stress-activated protein kinase-1 (SAPK1/JNK). *FEBS Lett* 1997; 414:153–158.

18. Yao Z, Diener K, Wang XS, Zukowski M, Matsumoto G, Zhou G, Mo R, Sasaki T, Nishina H, Hui CC, Tan TH, Woodgett JP, Penninger JM. Activation of stress-activated protein kinases/c-Jun N-terminal protein kinases (SAPKs/JNKs) by a novel mitogen-activated protein kinase kinase. *J Biol Chem* 1997; 272:32,378–32,383.

19. Foltz IN, Gerl RE, Wieler JS, Luckach M, Salmon RA, Schrader JW. Human mitogen-activated protein kinase kinase 7 (MKK7) is a highly conserved c-Jun N-terminal kinase/stress-activated protein kinase (JNK/SAPK) activated by environmental stresses and physiological stimuli. *J Biol Chem* 1998; 273:9344–9351.

20. Ichijo H, Nishida E, Irie K, ten Dijke P, Saitoh M, Moriguchi T, Takagi M, Matsumoto K, Miyazono K, Gotoh Y. Induction of apoptosis by ASK1, a mammalian MAPKKK that activates SAPK/JNK and p38 signaling pathways. *Science* 1997; 275:90–94.

21. Tibbles LA, Ing YL, Kiefer F, Chan J, Iscove N, Woodgett JR, Lassam NJ. MLK-3 activates the SAPK/JNK and p38/RK pathways via SEK1 and MKK3/6. *EMBO J* 1996; 15:7026–7035.

22. Hirai S, Katoh M, Terada M, Kyriakis JM, Zon LI, Rana A, Avruch J, Ohno S. MST/MLK2, a member of the mixed lineage kinase family, directly phosphorylates and activates SEK1, an activator of c-Jun N-terminal kinase/stress-activated protein kinase. *J Biol Chem* 1997; 272:15,167–15,173.

23. Rana A, Gallo K, Godowski P, Hirai S, Ohno S, Zon L, Kyriakis JM, Avruch J. The mixed lineage kinase SPRK phosphorylates and activates the stress-activated protein kinase activator, SEK-1. *J Biol Chem* 1996; 271:19,025–19,028.

24. Blank JL, Gerwins P, Elliott EM, Sather S, Johnson GL. Molecular cloning of mitogen-activated protein/ERK kinase kinases (MEKK) 2 and 3. Regulation of sequential phosphorylation pathways involving mitogen-activated protein kinase and c-Jun kinase. *J Biol Chem* 1996; 271:5361–5368.

25. Salmeron A, Ahmad TB, Carlile GW, Pappin D, Narsimhan RP, Ley SC. Activation of MEK-1 and SEK-1 by Tpl-2 proto-oncoprotein, a novel MAP kinase kinase kinase. *EMBO J* 1996; 15:817–826.

26. Kyriakis JM, Avruch J. Sounding the alarm: protein kinase cascades activated by stress and inflammation. *J Biol Chem* 1996; 271:24,313–24,316.

27. Zhou G, Bao ZQ, Dixon JE. Components of a new human protein kinase signal transduction pathway. *J Biol Chem* 1995; 270:12,665–12,669.

28. Abe J, Kusuhara M, Ulevitch RJ, Berk BC, Lee JD. Big mitogen-activated protein kinase 1 (BMK1) is a redox-sensitive kinase. *J Biol Chem* 1996; 271:16,586–16,590.

29. Zervos AS, Faccio L, Gatto JP, Kyriakis JM, Brent R. Mxi2, a mitogen-activated protein kinase that recognizes and phosphorylates Max protein. *Proc Natl Acad Sci USA* 1995; 92:10,531–10,534.

30. Jiang Y, Chen C, Li Z, Guo W, Gegner JA, Lin S, Han J. Characterization of the structure and function of a new mitogen-activated protein kinase (p38β). *J Biol Chem* 1996; 271:17,920–17,926.

31. Lechner C, Zahalka MA, Giot J-F, Moller NPH, Ullrich A. ERK6, a mitogen-activated protein kinase involved in C2C12 myoblast differentiation. *Proc Natl Acad Sci USA* 1996; 93:4355–4359.

32. Li Z, Jiang Y, Ulevitch RJ, Han J. The primary structure of p38 gamma: a new member of p38 group of MAP kinases. *Biochem Biophys Res Commun* 1996; 228:334–340.

33. Mertens S, Craxton M, Goedert M. SAP kinase-3, a new member of the family of mammalian stress-activated protein kinases. *FEBS Lett* 1996; 383:273–276.

34. Kumar S, McDonnell PC, Gum RJ, Hand AT, Lee JC, Young PR. Novel homologues of CSBP/p38 MAP kinase: activation, substrate specificity and sensitivity to inhibition by pyridinyl imidazoles. *Biochem Biophys Res Commun* 1997; 235:533–538.

35. Goedert M, Cuenda A, Craxton M, Jakes R, Cohen P. Activation of the novel stress-activated protein kinase SAPK4 by cytokines and cellular stresses is mediated by SKK3 (MKK6); comparison of its substrate specificity with that of other SAP kinases. *EMBO J* 1997; 16:3563–35671.

36. Stein B, Yang MX, Young DB, Janknecht R, Hunter T, Murray BW, Barbosa MS. p38-2, a novel mitogen-activated protein kinase with distinct properties. *J Biol Chem* 1997; 272:19,509–19,517.

37. Jiang Y, Gram H, Zhao M, New L, Gu J, Feng L, Di Padova F, Ulevitch RJ, Han J. Characterization of the structure and function of the fourth member of p38 group mitogen-activated protein kinases, p38delta. *J Biol Chem* 1997; 272:30,122–30,128.

38. Enslen H, Raingeaud J, Davis RJ. Selective activation of p38 mitogen-activated protein (MAP) kinase isoforms by the MAP kinase kinases MKK3 and MKK6. *J Biol Chem* 1998; 273:1741–1748.

39. Wang XS, Diener K, Manthey CL, Wang S, Rosenzweig B, Bray J, Delaney J, Cole CN, Chan Hui PY, Mantlo N, Lichenstein HS, Zukowski M, Yao Z. Molecular cloning and characterization of a novel p38 mitogen-activated protein kinase. *J Biol Chem* 1997; 272:23,668–23,674.

40. Han J, Lee JD, Bibbs L, Ulevitch RJ. A MAP kinase targeted by endotoxin and hyperosmolarity in mammalian cells. *Science* 1994; 265:808–811.

41. Rouse J, Cohen P, Trigon S, Morange M, Alonso-Llamazares A, Zamanillo D, Hunt T, Nebreda AR. Identification of a novel protein kinase cascade stimulated by chemical stress and heat shock which activates MAP kinase-activated protein MAPKAP kinase-2 and induces phosphorylation of the small heat shock proteins. *Cell* 1994; 78:1027–1037.

42. Raingeaud J, Gupta S, Rogers JS, Dickens M, Han J, Ulevitch RJ, Davis RJ. Pro-inflammatory cytokines and environmental stress cause p38 mitogen-activated protein kinase activation by dual phosphorylation on tyrosine and threonine. *J Biol Chem* 1995; 270:7420–7426.

43. Wang XZ, Ron D. Stress-induced phosphorylation and activation of the transcription factor CHOP (GADD153) by p38 MAP kinase. *Science* 1996; 272:1347–1349.

44. Xia Z, Dickens M, Raingeaud J, Davis RJ, Greenberg ME. Opposing effects of ERK and JNK-p38 MAP kinases on apoptosis. *Science* 1996; 270:1326–1331.

45. Bogoyevitch MA, Gillespie Brown J, Ketterman AJ, Fuller SJ, Ben Levy R, Ashworth A, Marshall CJ, Sugden PH. Stimulation of the stress-activated mitogen-activated protein kinase subfamilies in perfused heart. p38/RK mitogen-activated protein kinases and c-Jun N-terminal kinases are activated by ischemia/reperfusion. *Circ Res* 1996; 79:162–173.

46. Yin T, Sandhu G, Wolfgang CD, Burrier A, Webb RL, Rigel DF, Hai T, Whelan J. Tissue-specific pattern of stress kinase activation in ischemic/reperfused heart and kidney. *J Biol Chem* 1997; 272:19943–19950.

47. Clerk A, Fuller SJ, Michael A, Sugden PH. Stimulation of "stress-regulated" mitogen-activated protein kinases (stress-activated protein kinases/c-Jun N-terminal kinases and p38-mitogen-activated protein kinases) in perfused rat hearts by oxidative and other stresses. *J Biol Chem* 1998; 273:7228–7234.

48. Kummer JL, Rao PK, Heidenreich KA. Apoptosis induced by withdrawal of trophic factors is mediated by p38 mitogen-activated protein kinase. *J Biol Chem* 1997; 272:20,490–20,494.

49. Macfarlane WM, Smith SB, James RF, Clifton AD, Doza YN, Cohen P, Docherty K. The p38/reactivating kinase mitogen-activated protein kinase cascade mediates the activation of the transcription factor insulin upstream factor 1 and insulin gene transcription by high glucose in pancreatic beta-cells. *J Biol Chem* 1997; 272:20,936–20,944.

50. Tao J, Sanghera JS, Pelech SL, Wong G, Levy JG. Stimulation of stress-activated protein kinase and p38 HOG1 kinase in murine keratinocytes following photodynamic therapy with benzoporphyrin derivative. *J Biol Chem* 1996; 271:27,107–27,115.

51. Cuenda A, Rouse J, Doza YN, Meier R, Cohen P, Gallagher TF, Young PR, Lee JC. SB 203580 is a specific inhibitor of a MAP kinase homologue which is stimulated by cellular stresses and interleukin-1. *FEBS Lett* 1995; 364:229–233.

52. Hazzalin CA, Cano E, Cuenda A, Barratt MJ, Cohen P, Mahadevan LC. p38/Rk is essential for stress-induced nuclear responses: Jnk/Sapks and c-Jun/Atf-2 phosphorylation are insufficient. *Curr Biol* 1996; 6:1028–1031.

53. Hazzalin CA, Le Panse R, Cano E, Mahadevan LC. Anisomycin selectively desensitizes signalling components involved in stress kinase activation and fos and jun induction. *Mol Cell Biol* 1998; 18:1844–1854.

54. Freshney NW, Rawlinson L, Guesdon F, Jones E, Cowley S, Hsuan J, Saklatvala J. Interleukin-1 activates a novel protein kinase cascade that results in the phosphorylation of Hsp27. *Cell* 1994; 78:1039–1049.

55. Juo P, Kuo CJ, Reynolds SE, Konz RF, Raingeaud J, Davis RJ, Biemann HP, Blenis J. Fas activation of the p38 mitogen-activated protein kinase signalling pathway requires ICE/CED-3 family proteases [published erratum appears in *Mol Cell Biol* 1997; Mar;17:1757]. *Mol Cell Biol* 1997; 17:24–35.

56. Sutherland CL, Heath AW, Pelech SL, Young PR, Gold MR. Differential activation of the ERK, JNK, and p38 mitogen-activated protein kinases by CD40 and the B cell antigen receptor. *J Immunol* 1996; 157:3381–3390.

57. Salmon RA, Foltz IN, Young PR, Schrader JW. The p38 mitogen-activated protein kinase is activated by ligation of the T or B lymphocyte antigen receptors, Fas or CD40, but suppression of kinase activity does not inhibit apoptosis induced by antigen receptors. *J Immunol* 1997; 159:5309–5317.

58. Hannigan M, Zhan L, Ai Y, Huang CK. The role of p38 MAP kinase in TGFβ1-induced signal transduction in human neutrophils. *Biochem Biophys Res Commun* 1998; 246:55–58.
59. Kramer RM, Roberts EF, Strifler BA, Johnstone EM. Thrombin induces activation of p38 MAP kinase in human platelets. *J Biol Chem* 1995; 270:27,395–27,398.
60. Kramer RM, Roberts EF, Um SL, Borsch Haubold AG, Watson SP, Fisher MJ, Jakubowski JA. p38 mitogen-activated protein kinase phosphorylates cytosolic phospholipase A2 (cPla2) in thrombin-stimulated platelets. Evidence that proline-directed phosphorylation is not required for mobilization of arachidonic acid by cPla2. *J Biol Chem* 1996; 271:27,723–27,729.
61. Saklatvala J, Rawlinson L, Waller RJ, Sarsfield S, Lee JC, Morton LF, Barnes MJ, Farndale RW. Role for p38 mitogen-activated protein kinase in platelet aggregation caused by collagen or a thromboxane analogue. *J Biol Chem* 1996; 271:6586–6589.
62. Yamauchi J, Nagao M, Kaziro Y, Itoh H. Activation of p38 mitogen-activated protein kinase by signaling through G protein-coupled receptors. Involvement of $G_{\beta\gamma}$ and $G_{\alpha q}11$ subunits. *J Biol Chem* 1997; 272:27,771–27,777.
63. Krump E, Sanghera JS, Pelech SL, Furuya W, Grinstein S. Chemotactic peptide N-formyl-met-leu-phe activation of p38 mitogen-activated protein kinase (MAPK) and MAPK-activated protein kinase-2 in human neutrophils. *J Biol Chem* 1997; 272:937–944.
64. Foltz IN, Lee JC, Young PR, Schrader JW. Hemopoietic growth factors with the exception of interleukin-4 activate the p38 mitogen-activated protein kinase pathway. *J Biol Chem* 1997; 272:3296–3301.
65. Tan Y, Rouse J, Zhang A, Cariati S, Cohen P, Comb MJ. FGF and stress regulate CREB and ATF-1 via a pathway involving p38 MAP kinase and MAPKAP kinase-2. *EMBO J* 1996; 15:4629–4642.
66. Rousseau S, Houle F, Landry J, Huot J. p38 Map kinase activation by vascular endothelial growth factor mediates actin reorganization and cell migration in human endothelial cells. *Oncogene* 1997; 15:2169–2177.
67. Xing J, Kornhauser JM, Xia Z, Thiele EA, Greenberg ME. Nerve growth factor activates extracellular signal-regulated kinase and p38 mitogen-activated protein kinase pathways to stimulate CREB serine 133 phosphorylation. *Mol Cell Biol* 1998; 18:1946–1955.
68. Matsuda S, Moriguchi T, Koyasu S, Nishida E. T lmphocyte activation signals for interleukin-2 production involve activation of MKK6-p38 and MKK7-SAPK/JNK signaling pathways sensitive to cyclosporin A. *J Biol Chem* 1998; 273:12,378–12,382.
69. Wilk Blaszczak MA, Stein B, Xu S, Barbosa MS, Cobb MH, Belardetti F. The mitogen-activated protein kinase p38-2 is necessary for the inhibition of N-type calcium current by bradykinin. *J Neurosci* 1998; 18:112–118.
70. Stokoe D, Engel K, Campbell DG, Cohen P, Gaestel M. MAPKAP kinase-2; a novel protein kinase activated by mitogen-activated protein kinase. *FEBS Lett* 1992; 313:307–313.
71. McLaughlin MM, Kumar S, McDonnell PC, Van Horn S, Lee JC, Livi GP, Young PR. Identification of mitogen-activated protein (MAP) kinase-activated protein kinase-3, a novel substrate of CSBP p38 MAP kinase. *J Biol Chem* 1996; 271:8488–8492.
72. Waskiewicz AJ, Flynn A, Proud CG, Cooper JA. Mitogen-activated protein kinases activate the serine/threonine kinases Mnk1 and Mnk2. *EMBO J* 1997; 16:1909–1920.
73. Fukunaga R, Hunter T. MNK1, a new MAP kinase-activated protein kinase, isolated by a novel expression screening method for identifying protein kinase substrates. *EMBO J* 1997; 16:1921–1933.
74. Ni H, Wang XS, Diener K, Yao Z. MAPKAPK5, a novel mitogen-activated protein kinase (MAPK)-activated protein kinase, is a substrate of the extracellular-regulated kinase (ERK) and p38 kinase. *Biochem Biophys Res Commun* 1998; 243:492–496.
75. New L, Jiang Y, Zhao M, Liu K, Zhu W, Flood LJ, Kato Y, Parry GCN, Han J. PRAK, a novel protein kinase regulated by the p38 MAP kinase. *EMBO J* 1998; 17:3372–3384.
76. Deak M, Clifton AD, Lucocq JM, Alessi DR. Mitogen and stress activated protein kinase

(MSK1) is directly activated by MAPK and SAPK2/p38, and may mediate activation of CREB. *EMBO J* 1998; 17:4426–4441.

77. Landry J, Huot J. Modulation of actin dynamics during stress and physiological stimulation by a signaling pathway involving p38 MAP kinase and heat-shock protein 27. *Biochem Cell Biol* 1995; 73:703–707.

78. Huang C-K, Zhan L, Ai Y, Jongstra J. LSP1 is the major substrate for mitogen-activated protein kinase-activated protein kinase 2 in human neutrophils. *J Biol Chem* 1997; 272:17–19.

79. Ludwig S, Engel K, Hoffmeyer A, Sithanandam G, Neufeld B, Palm D, Gaestel M, Rapp U.R. 3pK, a novel mitogen-activated protein (MAP) kinase-activated protein kinase, is targeted by three MAP kinase pathways. *Mol Cell Biol* 1996; 16:6687–6697.

80. Thomas G, Haavik J, Cohen P. Participation of a stress-activated protein kinase cascade in the activation of tyrosine hydroxylase in chromaffin cells. *Eur J Biochem* 1997; 247:1180–1189.

81. Han J, Jiang Y, Li Z, Kravchenko VV, Ulevitch RJ. Activation of the transcription factor MEF2C by the MAP kinase p38 in inflammation. *Nature* 1997; 386:296–299.

82. Price MA, Cruzalegui FH, Treisman R. The p38 and ERK MAP kinase pathways cooperate to activate ternary complex factors and c-fos transcription in response to UV light. *EMBO J* 1996; 15:6552–6563.

83. Janknecht R, Hunter T. Convergence of MAP kinase pathways on the ternary complex factor Sap-1a. *EMBO J* 1997; 16:1620–1627.

84. Raingeaud J, Whitmarsh AJ, Barrett T, Derijard B, Davis RJ. MKK3- and MKK6-regulated gene expression is mediated by the p38 mitogen-activated protein kinase signal transduction pathway. *Mol Cell Biol* 1996; 16:1247–1255.

85. Whitmarsh AJ, Yang S-H, Su MSS, Sharrocks AD, Davis RJ. Role of p38 and JNK mitogen-activated protein kinases in the activation of ternary complex factors. *Mol Cell Biol* 1997; 17:2360–2371.

86. Beyaert R, Cuenda A, Vanden Berghe W, Plaisance S, Lee JC, Haegeman G, Cohen P, Fiers W. The p38/RK mitogen-activated protein kinase pathway regulates interleukin-6 synthesis in response to tumor necrosis factor. *EMBO J* 1996; 15:1914–1923.

87. Cuenda A, Cohen P, Buee Scherrer V, Goedert M. Activation of stress-activated protein kinase-3 (SAPK3) by cytokines and cellular stresses is mediated via SAPKK3 (MKK6); comparison of the specificities of SAPK3 and SAPK2 (RK/p38). *EMBO J* 1997; 16:295–305.

88. LoGrasso PV, Frantz B, Rolando AM, O'Keefe SJ, Hermes JD, O'Neill EA. (1997) Kinetic mechanism for p38 MAP kinase. *Biochemistry* 1997; 36:10,422–10,427.

88a. Gum RJ, Young PR. Identification of two distinct regions of p38 MAPK required for substrate binding and phosphorylation. *Biochem Biophys Res,* in press.

89. Kallunki T, Su B, Tsigelny I, Sluss HK, Derijard B, Moore G, Davis R, Karin M. JNK2 contains a specificity-determining region responsible for efficient c-jun binding and phosphorylation. *Genes Dev.* 1994; 8:2996–3007.

90. Young PR, McLaughlin MM, Kumar S, Kassis S, Doyle ML, McNulty D, Gallagher TF, Fisher S, McDonnell PC, Carr SA, Huddleston MJ, Seibel G, Porter TG, Livi GP, Adams JL, Lee JC. Pyridinyl imidazole inhibitors of p38 mitogen-activated protein kinase bind in the ATP site. *J Biol Chem* 1997; 272:12,116–12,121.

91. Clerk A, Sugden PH. The p38-MAPK inhibitor, SB203580, inhibits cardiac stress-activated protein kinases/c-Jun N-terminal kinases (SAPKs/JNKs). *FEBS Lett* 1998; 426:93–96.

92. Eyers PA, Craxton M, Morrice N, Cohen P, Goedert M. Conversion of SB 203580-insensitive MAP kinase family members to drug-sensitive forms by a single amino acid substitution. *Chem Biol* 1998; 5:321–328.

93. Nemeto S, Xiang J, Huang S, Lin A. Induction of Apoptosis by SB202190 through inhibition of p38β mitogen activated protein kinase. *J Biol Chem* 1998; 273:16,415–16,420.

94. Griswold DE, Young PR. Pharmacology of cytokine suppressive anti-inflammatory drug binding protein (CSBP), a novel stress induced kinase. *Pharmacol Commun.* 1996; 7:323–329.

95. Wang Z, Canagarajah BJ, Boehm JC, Kassis S, Cobb MH, Young PR, Adams JL, Goldsmith EJ. (1998) How protein kinases can be specific. *Structure* 1998; 6:1117–1128.

96. Wilson KP, McCaffrey PG, Hsiao K, Pazhanisamy S, Galullo V, Bemis GW, Fitzgibbon MJ, Caron PR, Murcko MA, Su MSS. The structural basis for the specificity of pyridinylimidazole inhibitors of p38 MAP kinase. *Chem Biol* 1997; 4:423–431.

97. Tong L, Pav S, White DM, Rogers W, Crane KM, Cywin CL, Brown ML, Pargellis CA. A highly specific inhibitor of human p38 MAP kinase binds in the ATP pocket. *Nature Struct Biol* 1997; 4:311–316.

98. Gum RJ, McLaughlin MM, Kumar S, Wang Z, Bower MJ, Lee JC, Adams JL, Livi GP, Goldsmith EJ, Young PR. Acquistion of sensitivity of stress-activated protein kinases to the p38 inhibitor, SB 203580, by alteration of one or more amino acids within the ATP binding pocket. *J Biol Chem* 1998; 273:15,605–15,610.

99. Wilson KP, Fitzgibbon MJ, Caron PR, Griffith JP, Chen W, McCaffrey PG, Chambers SP, Su MS. Crystal structure of p38 mitogen-activated protein kinase. *J Biol Chem* 1996; 271:27,696–27,700.

100. Wang Z, Harkins PC, Ulevitch RJ, Han J, Cobb MH, Goldsmith EJ. The structure of mitogen-activated protein kinase p38 at 2.1-Å resolution. *Proc Natl Acad Sci USA* 1997; 94:2327–2332.

101. Zhang F, Strand A, Robbins D, Cobb MH, Goldsmith E. Atomic structure of the MAP kinase ERK2 at 2.3A resolution. *Nature* 1994;367:704–710.

102. Canagarajah BJ, Khokhlatchev A, Cobb MH, and Goldsmith EJ. (1997) Activation mechanism of the MAP kinase ERK2 by dual phosphorylation. *Cell,* 90:859–869.

103. Iordanov M, Bender K, Ade T, Schmid W, Sachsenmaier C, Engel K, Gaestel M, Rahmsdorf HJ, Herrlich P. CREB is activated by UVC through a p38/HOG-1-dependent protein kinase. *EMBO J* 1997; 16:1009–1022.

104. Hazzalin CA, Cuenda A, Cano E, Cohen P, Mahadevan LC. Effects of the inhibition of p38/RK MAP kinase on induction of five fos and jun genes by diverse stimuli. *Oncogene* 1997; 15:2321–2331.

105. Kumar S, Orsini MJ, Lee JC, McDonnell PC, Debouck C, Young PR. Activation of the HIV-1 long terminal repeat by cytokines and environmental stress requires an active CSBP/p38 MAP kinase. *J Biol Chem* 1996; 271:30,864–30,869.

106. Zechner D, Craig R, Hanford DS, McDonough PM, Sabbadini RA, Glembotski CC. MKK6 activates myocardial cell NF-kappaB and inhibits apoptosis in a p38 mitogen-activated protein kinase-dependent manner. *J Biol Chem* 1998; 273:8232–8239.

107. Young P, McDonnell P, Dunnington D, Hand A, Laydon J, Lee J. Pyridinyl imidazoles inhibit IL-1 and TNF production at the protein level. *Agents Actions* 1993; 39:C67–C69.

108. Prichett W, Hand A, Sheilds J, Dunnington D. Mechanism of action of bicyclic imidazoles defines a translational regulatory pathway on tumor necrosis factor α. *J Inflamm* 1995; 45:97–105.

109. Perregaux DG, Dean D, Cronan M, Connelly P, Gabel CA. Inhibition of Interleukin-1β production by SKF86002: evidence of two sites of in vitro activity and of a time and system dependence. *Mol Pharmacol* 1995; 48:433–442.

110. Rincon M, Enslen H, Raingeaud J, Recht M, Zapton T, Su MS-S, Penix LA, Davis RJ, Flavell RA. Interferon g expression by Th1 effector T cells mediated by the p38 MAP kinase signaling pathway. *EMBO J.* 1998; 17:2817–2829.

111. Marshall LA, Hansbury MJ, Bolognese BJ, Gum RJ, Young PR, Mayer RJ. Inhibitors of the p38 mitogen-activated kinase modulate interleukin-4 induction of low affinity IgE receptor (CD23) in human monocytes. *J Immunol* 1998; 161:6005–6013.

112. Shapiro L, Dinarello CA. Osmotic regulation of cytokine synthesis in vitro. *Proc Natl Acad Sci USA* 1995; 92:12, 230–12,234.

113. Crawley JB, Rawlinson L, Lali FV, Page TH, Saklatvala J, Foxwell BM. T cell proliferation in response to interleukins 2 and 7 requires p38MAP kinase activation. *J Biol Chem* 1997; 272:15,023–15,027.

114. Badger AM, Bradbeer JN, Votta B, Lee JC, Adams JL, Griswold DE. Parmacological profile of SB 203580, a selective inhibitor of cytokine suppressive binding protein/p38 kinase, in animal models of arthritis, bone resorption, endotoxin shock and immune function. *J Pharmacol Exp Ther* 1996; 279:1453–1461.

115. Ridley SH, Sarsfield SJ, Lee JC, Bigg HF, Cawston TE, Taylor DJ, DeWitt DL, Saklatvala J. Actions of IL-1 are selectively controlled by p38 mitogen-activated protein kinase: regulation of prostaglandin H synthase-2, metalloproteinases, and IL-6 at different levels. *J Immunol* 1997; 158:3165–3173.

116. Guan Z, Baier LD, Morrison AR. p38 mitogen-activated protein kinase down-regulates nitric oxide and up-regulates prostaglandin E2 biosynthesis stimulated by interleukin-1beta. *J Biol Chem* 1997; 272:8083–8089.

117. Badger AM, Cook MN, Lark MW, Newmann-Tarr TM, Swift BA, Nelson AH, Barone FC, Kumar S. SB 203580 inhibits p38 mitogen-activated protein kinase, nitric oxide production, and inducible nitric oxide synthase in bovine cartilage-derived chondrocytes. *J Immunol* 1998; 161:467–473.

118. Huang S, Jiang Y, Li Z, Nishida E, Mathias P, Lin S, Ulevitch RJ, Nemerow GR, Han J. Apoptosis signaling pathway in T cells is composed of ICE/Ced-3 family proteases and MAP kinase kinase 6b. *Immunity* 1997; 6:739–749.

119. Frasch SC, Nick JA, Fadok VA, Bratton DL, Worthen GS, Henson PM. p38 mitogen-activated protein kinase-dependent and -independent intracellular signal transduction pathways leading to apoptosis in human neutrophils. *J Biol Chem* 1998; 273:8389–8397.

120. Wang Y, Huang S, Sah VP, Ross J Jr, Brown JH, Han J, Chien KR. Cardiac muscle cell hypertrophy and apoptosis induced by distinct members of the p38 mitogen-activated protein kinase family. *J Biol Chem* 1998; 273:2161–2168.

121. Shapiro L, Heidenreich KA, Meintzer MK, Dinarello CA. Role of p38 mitogen-activated protein kinase in HIV type 1 production in vitro. *Proc Natl Acad Sci USA* 1998; 95:7422–7426.

122. Jackson JR, Bolognese B, Hillegass L, Kassis S, Adams J, Griswold DE, Winkler JD. Pharmacological effects of SB 220025, a selective inhibitor of P38 mitogen-activated protein kinase, in angiogenesis and chronic inflammatory disease models. *J Pharmacol Exp Ther* 1998; 284:687–692.

123. McDonnell PC, DiLella AG, Lee JC, Young PR. Localization of the human stress responsive MAP kinase-like CSAIDs binding protein (CSBP) gene to chromosome 6q21.3/21.2. *Genomics* 1995; 29:301–302.

124. Goedert M, Hasegawa J, Craxton M, Leversha MA, Clegg S. Assignment of the human stress-activated protein kinase-3 gene (SAPK3) to chromosome 22q13.3 by fluorescence in situ hybridization. *Genomics* 1997; 41:501–502.

28

Farnesyltransferase Inhibitors

Anti-Ras or Anticancer Drugs?

Adrienne D. Cox and Channing J. Der

1. INTRODUCTION

Oncogenic *ras* mutations and aberrant Ras function are important in many human tumors, so blocking the activity of oncogenic Ras has been a significant priority in recent drug discovery efforts toward novel cancer chemotherapeutic agents. These efforts have included attempts designed specifically to inhibit the active, guanosine triphosphate (GTP)-bound form of Ras, to reduce the total amount of GTP-bound Ras, to interfere with Ras binding to its downstream targets or to interfere with those targets themselves, or to prevent Ras from associating with the plasma membrane. Of these approaches, the last has been the most successful to date. Ras and other farnesylated proteins require modification by a farnesyl isoprenoid lipid for correct subcellular localization and biological activity. Farnesyltransferase (FTase), the enzyme that attaches the isoprenoid to the C-terminus of Ras, has been a target for rational drug design since its cloning in 1991, and FTase inhibitors (FTIs) are now in early phases of clinical trials as anticancer agents.

FTIs have been developed from natural products, by screening of existing or novel combinatorial chemical libraries, and by rational drug design based on molecular mimicry of Ras CAAX target sequences. Such inhibitors have been shown to inhibit the processing and biological activity of Ras proteins in tissue culture and animal model systems. Proof of principle has been established for the function of these compounds as inhibitors of FTase, and their mechanism of action was thought to be well understood. Currently, advanced preclinical studies and phase I clinical trials are underway for several of these compounds. Surprising results have emerged from several of these studies, prompting considerable debate and speculation regarding the biological consequences of inhibiting FTase activity, and a large number of questions regarding the optimal refinement and clinical success of FTIs in cancer treatment remain to be answered. This review will give a brief overview of the history of FTI development, describe new findings regarding FTase and FTIs, and discuss some of the most intriguing aspects of current investigation: alternative prenylation of some Ras proteins, non-Ras

From: Signaling Networks and Cell Cycle Control: The Molecular Basis of Cancer and Other Diseases
Edited by: J. S. Gutkind © Humana Press Inc., Totowa, NJ

targets of FTIs, inhibitors of the related prenyltransferase GGTase I, and prospects for the clinical value of FTase inhibitors.

2. Ras AND HUMAN CANCERS

The three human *ras* genes encode proteins that regulate diverse signaling pathways important for normal cellular proliferation, differentiation, and apoptosis *(1,2)*. Owing to alternative splicing of the Kirsten *ras* gene, there are four Ras proteins altogether: the H-, K4A-, K4B-, and N-Ras proteins share >90% amino acid identity, differing mainly in the final 20 residues. These proteins exhibit the same potent transforming action in experimental cell culture and animal studies, and it has been assumed that their biochemical and biological properties are also essentially identical. However, recent evidence from a number of fields, including farnesyltransferase inhibitor studies, has begun to show evidence that potentially important differences do exist. The characterization of such differences will be critical to understanding the exact role of Ras in normal and diseased cells.

Mutated versions of *ras* genes can be found in approximately 30% of all human cancers, suggesting an important role for aberrant Ras function in carcinogenesis *(3,4)*. However, the frequency of mutations is not uniform with respect to type of *ras* gene or tumor. K-*ras* is most frequently mutated, and those mutations occur most frequently in carcinomas (i.e., tumors of epithelial cell origin). In particular, carcinomas of the pancreas, colon and lung have high incidences of K-*ras* mutations, and have been considered particularly good targets for anti-Ras drugs. N-*ras* mutations are most frequently found in hematopoietic malignancies, whereas H-*ras* mutations, although relatively rare compared to those of K- and N-*ras,* are found in head and neck tumors. By contrast, carcinomas of the breast, ovary and cervix, for example, rarely exhibit *ras* mutations. However, overexpression of the HER2/Neu/ErbB2 or EGF receptor tyrosine kinases is common in breast cancers, and their transforming actions are dependent on signaling through Ras proteins *(5)*. Thus, the findings of aberrant Ras function in the absence of mutations in *ras* itself suggests that the importance of Ras in a given tumor cannot be predicted solely on the basis of *ras* mutation status. This has important implications for the use of anti-Ras drugs.

3. FTIs AS INHIBITORS OF Ras PROCESSING AND FUNCTION

Although Ras proteins require lipid modification for their correct plasma membrane localization and biological activity, they are initially synthesized as biologically inactive, cytosolic precursors *(6–8)* (Fig. 1). Within minutes after synthesis, they become post-translationally modified on their C-terminal consensus tetrapeptide sequences, generally referred to as the CAAX box or CAAX motif, consisting of cysteine followed by two aliphatic amino acids and a terminal X amino acid that is methionine or serine. The cytoplasmic enzyme FTase catalyzes a thioether linkage of a C15 farnesyl isoprenoid moiety from a farnesyl diphosphate (FPP) donor to the cysteine residue of the CAAX motif. This modification is followed rapidly by proteolytic removal of the AAX residues and carboxylmethylation of the now farnesylated cysteine residue. Compounds that interfere with the protease and methyltransferase enzymes are currently under investigation as possible anti-Ras drugs *(9)*. In H-, N-, and K-Ras4A (but not K4B) proteins, the

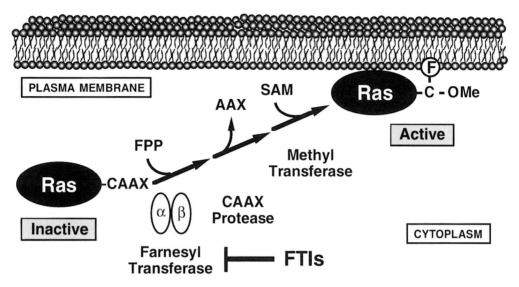

Fig. 1. Ras processing and membrane association is critical for Ras transforming activity. Ras proteins are initially synthesized as cytosolic, inactive proteins. Within minutes, Ras proteins undergo a series of CAAX-signaled posttranslational modifications that promote translocation and stable association with the inner surface of the plasma membrane. The first modification is catalyzed by farnesyltransferase to cause covalent addition of the farnesol group from farne-sylpyrophosphate (FPP) onto the cysteine residue of the CAAX sequence. Proteolytic degradation to remove the AAX residues, followed by carboxylmethylation of the farnesyl-cysteine residue (donor: S-adenosyl methionine, SAM), complete the CAAX-signaled modifications. FTI inhibition of Ras farnesylation renders Ras completely cytosolic and nontransforming.

palmitoylation of upstream cysteines also contributes to hydrophobicity and membrane interaction in a dynamic and regulatable manner *(10),* and this process, too, may be a target for rational drug design. Because farnesylation is required for the additional, later processing steps *(11),* and alone is sufficient to confer significant membrane association and transforming potential *(12),* blocking this step is a potent means of blocking Ras processing and function.

Several classes of FTIs have been developed, including those derived from natural compounds, random screening of existing or novel combinatorial chemical libraries, and rational drug design based on lipid and protein substrates of FTase *(13,14).* Because the CAAX tetrapeptide is both necessary and sufficient for farnesylation *(15,16),* the K-Ras CAAX sequence CVIM formed the basis for the original FTI inhibitors. It was quickly discovered that the potent nonsubstrate CVFM could provide a good starting point *(17).* However, peptides are poor drug candidates due to their poor cellular uptake and rapid proteolytic degradation. To avoid these problems, most current FTIs are based on CAAX peptidomimetics that are improved in these properties. Discussions of FTI development from a medicinal chemistry point of view can be found in several recent reviews *(13,14,18,19).*

During the initial development stages, the ability of different classes of FTIs to block Ras processing and transformation was tested widely in rodent fibroblasts transformed by Ras proteins *(20–26).* Characterization of H-Ras processing in such cells clearly indicated the ability of FTIs to inhibit H-Ras farnesylation potently and specifically, without affecting the modification of geranylgeranylated proteins, such as Rap1a or genetically engineered H-Ras-GG mutants *(23,26,27)*. Further, Ras activation of the Raf/MAP kinase pathway and signaling to a variety of transcription factors was shown to be inhibited specifically by these FTIs *(23,26,27)*. Therefore, it seemed clear that FTIs could block Ras lipid modification and biology in predictable ways.

4. FTIs AS ANTICANCER AGENTS

The ability of Ras-transformed murine cells to grow in soft agar or as tumors in nude mice was in many cases inhibited dramatically by FTI treatment, suggesting that FTIs might indeed be developed into potent anticancer drugs. Further investigation showed that a wide variety of human tumor cell lines were also inhibited by FTIs in anchorage-independent growth in tissue culture *(21,23–25,28–31)* and in nude mouse xenografts *(28,32–34)*. In an effort to use systems more relevant to human cancers, some investigators turned to transgenic animals. In two types of H-*ras* transgenic mice, structurally different FTIs were shown to cause regression of established mammary and/or salivary tumors, by mechanisms thought to include induction of apoptosis *(35)*. Even tumors from transgenic animals with multiple genetic defects, such as crosses between H-*ras* and p53 or myc mutant animals, regressed in response to FTI treatment *(36)*. Thus, it has been straightforward to demonstrate a good correlation between FTI inhibition of H-Ras processing, signaling and transformation. All these findings continued to suggest the eventual clinical value of FTIs, and drug development efforts over the past 4 or 5 years have been intense.

However, several results greatly slowed the translation of drug discovery efforts to successful drug development, as the pharmaceutical and academic research communities have attempted to understand, account for, and use a variety of unpredicted findings. First, although FTIs were developed originally as cancer chemotherapeutics for the large number of tumors in which Ras is believed to be important, *ras* mutation status was determined not to be predictive of FTI sensitivity or resistance in human tumor cells *(30)*. Possible bases for, and consequences of, this lack of correlation are discussed in greater detail below. In addition, K-Ras4B protein in particular was very resistant to FTI inhibition of processing, and K-*ras*-transformed cells were frequently resistant to FTI inhibition of growth and transformation *(37)*. Because most human cancers that contain oncogenic *ras* mutations have mutated K-Ras or N-Ras proteins *(3,4)*, not the H-*ras* proteins that were the subject of such simply interpreted results as described above, these new findings appeared to be cause for consternation. Nevertheless, in many cases it was indeed possible to inhibit tumor cell growth using FTIs, despite a failure to inhibit Ras prenylation *(37)*. These findings led to the conclusion that additional research to understand the mechanism of FTI action might be important to improving drug development efforts.

Because it is clear that FTIs inhibit the action of FTase to farnesylate both Ras and other normally farnesylated proteins, the main biological questions to be answered presently concern the role of targets other than Ras in the cellular response to FTIs and how FTI responsiveness can be predicted. In terms of drug development, what features should be incorporated into the next generation of FTIs to improve their eventual clinical value, and how can clinical trials be designed most effectively to take advantage of FTI activity while minimizing any FTI problems?

5. NEW DEVELOPMENTS IN FTIs

Over the last year or so, several recent developments have made it possible to understand more clearly the biochemistry and pharmacology, if not the biological consequences, of FTI activity. First, structure–function studies of the FTase enzyme itself have shown progress *(18,19)*. FTase is a metalloenzyme composed of a 45-kDa α and a 48-kDa β subunit; enzymatic activity requires both Zn^{2+} and Mg^{2+}. The α subunit is shared with the highly related enzyme geranylgeranyltransferase I (GGTase I), whereas the β subunit is specific to FTase. The crystal structure of the heterodimeric FTase has been resolved to 2.25 Å and shown to be composed of an unusual crescent-shaped seven-helical hairpin domain and an α-α barrel domain structure that also shows exactly how the isoprenoid and protein substrates bind *(38)*. The cocrystal structure of FTase complexed with a farnesyl diphosphate substrate has also been determined *(39)*. Along with mutational analyses of FTase from several laboratories *(40,41)*, this crystallographic information has shown the importance of particular residues for specific binding and utilization of FPP and for coordination of the zinc ion. Interaction of CAAX-competitive FTIs with FTase indicate which residues are likely to be important for binding the protein substrate. For a further discussion of these parameters, readers are referred to recent reviews *(18,19)*.

Second, a better understanding of the kinetics of the reaction has shown an ordered mechanism by which an enzyme–FPP–protein substrate complex is formed, with substrate binding required for release of product *(42)*. Further, differences in FPP and GGPP binding to their respective prenyl transferases have been described that have implications for improving the specificity of inhibitors for FTase versus GGTase *(43)*.

Third, new FTIs are continually being synthesized or isolated from natural products including plants and fungi, and natural compounds are often subjected to additional modifications by medicinal chemistry *(13)*. For example, the prototype for one such series of compounds (SCH-44342-SCH 66336) was originally developed not as an FTI, but for its antihistaminic properties. Unlike most CAAX- or FPP-based compounds, members of these series were early nonpeptide, nonthiol, noncarboxylic acid-containing tricyclic inhibitors of FTase *(44)*. One of these series is now in clinical trials in the United States and Europe, as are rationally designed FTIs. An understanding of the biochemistry of FTase enzyme activity should continue to lead to new improvements in FTIs.

6. RESISTANCE OF K-Ras

One of the biggest surprises to come from FTI studies has been the high level of resistance of K-Ras to inhibition of processing even by the most potent FTIs available *(45)*. This development was greeted with dismay because K-Ras is the form of Ras most commonly mutated in human tumors. Although it has long been appreciated that the affinity of K-Ras4B for the FTase enzyme is considerably higher than that of H-Ras *(15)*, with N-Ras intermediate, the 20-fold difference in FTase affinity between H-Ras and K-Ras is not sufficient to explain the much greater than 20-fold difference

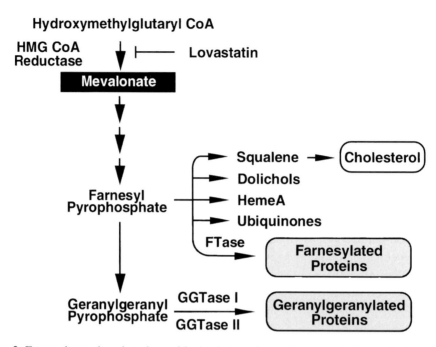

Fig. 2. Farnesylpyrophosphate is a critical substrate for protein prenylation and other cellular metabolites. Mevalonate is the essential precursor for all isoprenoid biosynthesis, including farnesyl pyrophosphate (FPP). FPP is required for production of GGPP, and both FPP and GGPP are used by three protein prenyltransferases for protein prenylation. FPP is also used for the biosynthesis of cholesterol and other byproducts of the mevalonate biosynthetic pathways. Whereas compactin and lovastatin block all isoprenoid biosynthesis, FTIs selectively block the farnesylation of Ras and other CAAX (where X = S, M, and C) terminating proteins. GGTase I (CAAX, where X = L and F) and GGTase II (CC, CXC, and CCXX terminating members of the Rab family of Ras-related proteins) catalyze the geranylgeranylation of proteins.

in FTI sensitivity. Earlier studies showed that K-Ras processing could only be blocked by levels of FTI that also resulted in cross-inhibition of the closely related prenyl transferase GGTase I (Fig. 2). GGTase I is responsible for the prenylation of CAAX-terminating (where X=L) geranylgeranylated proteins, which are much greater in number than farnesylated proteins and which include many members of the Ras superfamily. It turns out that, whereas FTI alone can completely block H-Ras processing, it takes a combination of FTI and GGTI to efficiently block processing of K-Ras4B *(37,46)*. This is explained by in vitro *(47,48)* and in vivo *(49,50)* data showing that, in the absence of FTase activity, K-Ras (4B), as well as N-Ras and K-Ras (4A), are substrates for alternative prenylation by GGTase I. Thus, under conditions of FTase inhibition, all the Ras proteins except H-Ras can escape loss of prenylation by becoming geranylgeranylated. However, either FTIs or GGTIs can inhibit tumor cell growth when used as single agents *(46),* presumably as a result of inhibiting a different set of prenylated proteins important for proliferation. These findings have a potentially huge impact on strategies for FTI development and use.

In the past, FTIs have been designed to be as specific for FTase versus GGTase I as possible, with the main goals thereafter being improvements in potency and pharmacokinetics (PK). Should this strategy be revised? The consensus seems to be that it should not. Rather, increased efforts have been devoted to understanding the biology and consequences of alternative prenylation and to the possibility that Ras proteins are not the most important targets of FTase inhibition in terms of cancer chemotherapy.

7. ALTERNATIVE PRENYLATION

Alternative prenylation of normal, endogenous K-Ras4B by GGTase I in the presence of FTIs has been invoked as an explanation for the unexpected lack of FTI toxicity to normal cells, where growth factor-stimulated proliferative pathways continue to function despite FTI treatment. The resistance of K-Ras-transformed cells to FTI inhibition of transformation suggests that sufficient function is retained by the geranylgeranylated oncogenic form to allow continued transformation. It is known that geranylgeranylated forms of oncogenic K-Ras4B, when overexpressed, are indeed transforming in rodent fibroblasts *(12,51)*. It is unknown whether this is also true at single-copy levels in human tumor cells. Certainly not all the geranylgeranylated Ras is functionally identical to farnesylated Ras, as a significant portion is mislocalized to internal membranes *(51)* (A.D. Cox, unpublished observations), and plasma membrane localization is an absolute requirement for proper function.

However, clearly some cells that contain activated K-Ras are sensitive to FTIs *(30,46)*. Is alternative prenylation less efficient in sensitive cells? Are the levels or regulation of K-Ras proteins different in sensitive cells? Does alternative prenylation of normal K-Ras4B explain the lack of toxicity to normal cells? Is the inhibition of processing of another target besides K-Ras more critical for FTI sensitivity of transformed cells? The answers to these questions are unknown. Because different FTIs comprising a wide variety of structures all tend to affect cells in the same manner, it appears likely that the response to FTIs is largely mechanism based, that is, caused by inhibition of FTase, and generally that the explanation for sensitivity versus resistance will also be mechanism based. Therefore, understanding the cellular consequences of FTase inhibition will be key to improving FTI sensitivity.

8. NON-Ras TARGETS

The originally heretical concept that, in terms of cellular transformation, Ras might not be the most important farnesylated protein whose processing is inhibited by FTIs is now increasingly accepted. Evidence in support of non-Ras targets includes the failure of *ras* mutation status to predict FTI sensitivity or resistance and the lack of correlation between inhibition of Ras processing and inhibition of transformed growth properties. Thus, the collective experience with a large number of tumor cell lines has shown that some tumors containing *ras* mutations are FTI sensitive, whereas others are resistant; conversely, tumors without mutated *ras* can be either sensitive or resistant *(30,46)*.

Clearly, the relative importance of mutated Ras to the transformed phenotype may vary from tumor to tumor or from cell line to cell line. However, differing cellular reliance on oncogenic Ras for transformation has failed to provide a satisfactory prediction of FTI sensitivity. In only two tumor cell lines are matched pairs with and without mutated *ras* available: the HT1080 fibrosarcoma with or without activated N-*ras* (52), and the DLD-1 colon carcinoma with or without activated K-*ras (53)*. Direct comparison of FTI sensitivity between these pairs showed that the HT1080 cells containing activated N-Ras are approx 10-fold more FTI sensitive than those without (A.D. Cox, unpublished observations). However, DLD-1 cells are resistant to FTIs, regardless of *ras* mutation status. Thus, some other predictor of FTI sensitivity must be sought.

8.1. Target X?

What might such a non-Ras target of FTase be? Is there a single target X, or does each cell line or tumor have a different target X, depending on its milieu? No consensus is readily available, other than that the function of such a protein must be required for transformation and that it must be a physiological substrate of FTase. It is likely that a true target X is not alternatively prenylated, or at least that the alternatively prenylated form is functionally distinct from the farnesylated form.

Farnesylated proteins include not only Ras family members, but the nuclear lamins, several retinal signal transducing heterotrimeric G proteins, protein and lipid phosphatases, kinases, nuclear hormone receptors or their partners, cytokine-inducible proteins, heat-shock proteins and a host of proteins that remain uncharacterized functionally (Table 1). The search for farnesylated proteins has been undertaken by expression cloning *(54)*, two-dimensional gel electrophoresis of extracts from prenoid precursor-labeled cells *(55)*, and computer data base searching for CAAX-containing proteins *(56)*. Which of these proteins are logical candidates for physiologically important FTI targets? Although the potential functional control by farnesylation of many of these proteins is likely to be important for different disease states, clearly not all farnesylated proteins are likely to have functions relevant to the responses of tumor cells to FTIs.

Although no truly convincing target X protein has emerged to date, the most interesting candidates so far include RhoB, RhoE, and related proteins, the growth-related phosphatases and lipid kinases. Evidence for the importance of RhoB in the response to FTI includes the finding that a myristylated form can abrogate the sensitivity of Ras-transformed cells to FTIs *(57)*. RhoB is normally both farnesylated (F) and geranyl-geranylated (GG) *(58)*, but FTI treatment shifts all the lipid to the geranylgeranyl form. RhoB-F and RhoB-GG apparently are not functionally equivalent *(59)*, supporting a role for RhoB as target X. However, the expression pattern of RhoB does not correlate with FTI sensitivity in human tumor cell lines, and inhibition of RhoB alone does not appear to be able to account for all the functional consequences of inhibiting FTase. Therefore, it is likely that target X remains to be identified.

Other possible targets X include members of the RhoE family, including Rho6, Rho7 and Rho8/RhoE. These proteins are farnesylated and are constitutively GTP-bound *(60–62)*, suggesting the likelihood of regulation at a level other than GTP cycling. Two recent studies showed that RhoE family proteins function in disrupting cytoskeletal organization. If, like other members of the Rho family, they also participate in cell cycle regulation and transformation, their importance as potential target X proteins would increase. The consequences to cellular transformation of inhibiting RhoE function are currently unknown.

The Ras-related protein Rheb has been shown to antagonize Ras transformation, and FTI treatment inhibits its farnesylation and membrane localization *(63)*. It is unknown

Table 1
Farnesylated Proteins: Potential Target X?

Protein	*(C/K/R)* CAAX[b]	Function	*Entrez Prot. No.[c]/* Nucleotide Acc. No.	PubMed UI[d]
H-Ras	C C CVLS	Signaling for growth/ diff/death	131869 Swiss P01112	83141783 (seq)
N-Ras	C CVVM	Signaling for growth/ diff/death	131883 Swiss P01111	84002264 (seq)
K-Ras4A (2A)	C K CIIM	Signaling for growth/ diff/death	131875 Swiss P01116	83271513 (seq)
K-Ras4B (2B)	K CVIM	Signaling for growth/ diff/death	131879 Swiss P01118	83271513 (seq)
Lamin A	-CSIM	Nuclear membrane arch.	124962 Swiss P02545	86313596 (seq)
Lamin B1	-CAIM	Nuclear membrane arch.	125953 Swiss P20700	90062174 (F)
Lamin B2	-CYVM	Nuclear membrane arch.	547822 Swiss P03252	92334349 (seq)
RhoB	C CCKVL	Cytoskeletal org.; immed/early	132542 Swiss P01121	88203210 (seq)
RhoE/Rho8	K CTVM	Cytoskeletal org.; cell cycle control?	1839517 Genbank S82240	96220452 (S, F)
Rho6	K CSIM	Cytoskeletal org.; cell cycle control?	2500182 Swiss Q92730	98198477
Rho7	K CNLM	Cytoskeletal org.; cell cycle control?	2168149	98198477
Rheb	-CSVM	Unknown; antagonist of Ras	2136086 PIR S68419	96128233 (seq) 97256779 (F)
Rap2A	C CNIQ	Golgi loc.; unknown fcn.	131852 Swiss P10114	88319657 (seq) 93143700 (F)
PRL-1/ hPTPCAAX1	R CCIQ	Tyrosine phosphatase	2961199 GenB AF051160	94254833 (mouse seq)
IP3 5-PTPase	-CCVVQ	Inositol lipid metabolism/Ca^{2+} signaling	631267 PIR S45721	94283632 (seq) 96215347 (F)
Rhodopsin kinase	-CLVS	Photoreceptor S/T kinase	2833269 Swiss Q15835	97172975 (seq)
Transducin γ	-CVIS	Photoreceptor GTPase	585181 Swiss Q08447	93272877 (seq)
cGMP PDEα	-CCIQ	Retinal PDE	2851392 Swiss P16499	90169986 (seq)
DnaJ homolog	-CQTS	Heat shock/ chaperone	1706474 Swiss P31689	93326630 (seq)
PxF/HK33	-CLIM	Peroxisomal metabolism	72923 Swiss P40855	97480732 (seq) 94245743 (F)
Phosphorylase B kinase α L (liver form) (PHKA)	-CQMQ	Glycogen metab.	1170685 Swiss P46019	94043107 (seq)
Phosphorylase B kinase α M (skeletal muscle form)	-CAMQ	Glycogen metab.	1170683 Swiss P46020	94043107 (seq)

(continued)

Table 1 *(continued)*

Protein	(C/K/R) CAAX[b]	Function	Entrez Prot. No.[c]/ Nucleotide Acc. No.	PubMed UI[d]
Phosphorylase B kinase β (PHKB)	-CLIS	Glycogen metab.	2499582 Swiss Q93100	9628381 (seq)
IFN-GBP1-I	R CTIS	Cytokine mediator	183002 GenB M55542	91342675
Dexras1 (mouse)	K CVIS	Dexamethasone-inducible prot.	2253713 GenB AF009246	98123070 (S)
Batten disease protein CLN3	-CQLS	Lysosomal storage	2498243 Swiss Q13286	96016090
TTF	R CKIF	Hemat. only	2500200 Swiss Q13286	95303479 (seq)
RhoD	-CVVT	Endosome transport	3024539 Swiss O00212	97236425 (seq)
RhoM (mouse)	R CCLAT	Unknown	1752825 DDBJD89821	T. Endo (unpublished observations)
TC10	C CCLIT	Unknown	134080 Swiss P17081	90205863 (seq)
TC21 (placental form)	K C CVIF	Growth/diff.	2507282 Swiss P17082	90205863 (seq)

[a]Human form is given unless otherwise specified. Human CAAX sequences are not always identical to those of other species. References cited in support of farnesylation (F) may or may not refer directly to the human form of the protein. Proteins may have more than one entry, depending on the database used; in such cases, the entry chosen for this table was based on priority or correctness of human sequence. Not all farnesylated proteins have been identified or characterized.

[b]C/K/R CAAX shows the CAAX motif as well as upstream second signals of additional (potentially palmitoylatable) cysteine(s) or at least three lysine (K) or arginine (R) residues. In conjunction with X = M, upstream K/R residues may help signal alternative prenylation, as may C immediately adjacent to the CAAX motif.

[c]Entrez prot. #, the unique accession number for the Entrez browser's protein search engine; Nucleotide acc. #, the unique accession number for the original sequence database source; PubMed UI, the unique identifier for the Entrez browser's literature search engine PubMed.

[d]Accession numbers and unique identifiers are all from the National Center for Biotechnology Information at the National Library of Medicine's Entrez browser for protein, nucleotide, and literature databases. These can be accessed at: http://www.ncbi.nlm.nih.gov.

whether FTI action can cause Rheb to become a super-repressor of Ras or of some other protein important for transformation.

In addition to Ras superfamily members, known farnesylated proteins include tyrosine phosphatases such as PRL-1/hPTP(CAAX1), which appear to be involved in growth control *(54,64,65)*. As expected given its X = Q motif, FTI treatment has been shown to inhibit hPTP/CAAX1-mediated transformation of rodent fibroblasts. Further studies to determine whether this is a physiologically relevant target X protein are underway.

Type I inositol phosphate 3 5-phosphatase (IP3 5-PTPase) is a farnesylated lipid phosphatase *(66)* that alters intracellular calcium mobilization and inositol lipid binding to the IP4 receptor protein GAP1[IP4BP], which exhibits GAP activity for some Ras family members. Whether this PTPase is important for the response of normal or transformed cells to FTIs also remains to be determined.

Newly discovered farnesylated proteins now include those inducible by steroid hormones and cytokines, such as the IFN-inducible GBP1 *(67)*. Dexras1 was found by differential display analysis to be induced by dexamethasone in a mouse adrenocorticotrophic cell line *(68)*. Although Ras family members play an important role in insulin signaling, and Dexras1 may be important in glucocorticoid action, it is unclear whether such a protein is likely to have a role in transformation. Nevertheless, as more farnesylated proteins are identified, understanding their function may provide insight as to which are likely target X proteins. Perhaps target X will be found in Table 1, or perhaps it or they have yet to be identified.

9. INHIBITORS OF GGTaseI

Alternative prenylation of K-Ras and N-Ras proteins by GGTase I in the presence of FTIs has focused interest on inhibitors of GGTase I (GGTIs) as agents capable of synergizing with FTIs to provide complete inhibition of Ras processing. K-Ras processing can indeed be completely blocked by a combination of FTI and GGTI *(46)*, although either inhibitor alone is capable of inhibiting tumor cell growth in vivo, presumably via different mechanisms. The consequences of inhibiting GGTase I include blocking the prenylation and thus the signaling and function of many Ras-related proteins, particularly Rho family members important in cytoskeletal organization and cell cycle progression *(69)*. The potential cellular toxicity of GGTase I inhibitors is thought to be much greater than that of FTIs, in part because of the higher number of geranylgeranylated proteins compared with farnesylated proteins, and in part because of the emerging notion that geranylgeranylated proteins (e.g., Rac1, RhoA, and Cdc42) play a particularly critical role in cell cycle regulation *(69)*.

Evidence for the role of geranylgeranylated proteins in cell cycle control has come from both rescue and inhibitor experiments. First, mevalonate and geranylgeraniol (or GGPP), but not farnesol (or FPP), can restore cell cycle progression to cells treated with inhibitors of HMG CoA reductase such as lovastatin, mevastatin, and simvastatin *(70,71)*. Second, although Ras proteins have been shown by multiple means to be required for the G1/S transition, GGTI but not FTI confers a G1 arrest *(72,73)*. Several lines of evidence are emerging to suggest that Ras control of the cell cycle, as in so many other functions, is a consequence of the confluence of multiple signaling pathways. Thus, Ras can activate both ERK and Rho pathways to induce cyclin D1 and degrade the CDK inhibitor p27[KIP], respectively *(74)*. The possibility that RhoA itself may cycle off membranes during G1 and reassociate during the G1/S transition is another bit of evidence that RhoA may be a direct target relevant for antiproliferative effects of the statins and of GGTIs *(75)*. In fact, several studies have indicated the possibility that these agents may have useful antiatherosclerotic properties because of their antiproliferative effects on endothelial cells important for intimal hyperplasia *(76,77)*. Thus, both GGTIs and FTIs may be useful for inhibiting aberrant proliferative pathways, but GGTIs may be most useful in cardiovascular disease whereas FTIs may be most useful in cancer.

10. LABORATORY USE AS ANTI-Ras REAGENTS

FTIs were originally developed with the intent to inhibit Ras processing and function, but they are clearly specific inhibitors of FTase, not of Ras. FTIs should not be used as specific inhibitors of Ras signaling and function. The use of FTIs to prevent Raf-1 activation, to block Ras-mediated activation of the Raf/MEK/MAPK cascade, and to inhibit transcriptional activation of Ras-responsive promoters has been very useful for inhibiting H-Ras signaling in model systems where H-Ras drives the readout of interest. However, in all other cases, caution must be used in interpreting the results of FTI treatment for these reasons: (1) FTIs inhibit FTase, and therefore it is likely that FTIs block the processing of other physiologically important farnesylated targets at doses that influence Ras processing, signaling, and transformation; (2) N-Ras and K-Ras can escape inhibition of prenylation by FTIs; and (3) inhibition of K-Ras biology, particularly transformation, does not require inhibition of K-Ras processing. Therefore, FTIs can be highly useful to determine the relevance of farnesylated proteins to the biological function of interest, but caution should be exercised in ascribing functions inhibited by FTIs to Ras-driven pathways.

In addition to the likelihood of physiologically important non-Ras targets, it is possible that there is an as yet unknown form of modification that occurs in the presence of FTase inhibition. Such a possibility could explain the ability, for example, of nuclear lamins to fail to be prenylated and yet still be functionally capable of forming appropriate nuclear architecture *(78)*. This could also help explain why many cell types fail to show a complete Ras-processing gel-shift or aqueous/detergent fractionation under conditions of apparently complete inhibition of FTase. However, the possibility of a novel type of modification is highly controversial, and further study will be required to determine whether it exists.

11. PROSPECTS FOR CLINICAL USE AS ANTICANCER DRUGS

The encouraging results in animal models suggest the possibility that FTIs may indeed find value in the clinic. However, it is not unusual for compounds performing well in animal studies ultimately to fail to yield positive results in actual patients. It is not yet known whether FTIs will fall in the first or second group, but results from the first clinical trials are imminent. Several issues remain outstanding in terms of FTI development and use.

First, given the facts described above, what tumor types should be targeted for FTI treatment? It was originally expected that tumors containing a high percentage of mutated *ras,* such as pancreatic cancers (90% mutated K-*ras*), might be ideal targets for FTIs. However, we have seen that *ras* mutation status is not predictive of FTI sensitivity, and that Ras is not likely to be the most important target of FTI inhibition of farnesylation. The transformation of at least some FTI-sensitive tumors may be driven by upregulation of Ras signaling in the absence of mutations in *ras* itself, for example by upregulation of growth factor receptor tyrosine kinases, but this is unlikely to explain the majority of responses to FTIs. Absent the ability to predict which parameters indicate FTI sensitivity, this remains one of the most important problems to be solved before FTIs can be targeted to the appropriate patient population.

Second, these compounds have long been expected to be cytostatic, rather than cytotoxic, requiring continuous dosing. An apparent exception to the cytostatic rule is the case in the H-*ras* transgenic animals, in which impressive regression of established tumors was shown to occur, depending on other genetic alterations, by mechanisms including the induction of apoptosis *(35,36)*. A recent comparable study on N-*ras* transgenic animals showed excellent FTI inhibition of tumor growth but little regression *(79)*. If continuous dosing is required *(35,80)*, the development of resistance will likely be of more concern than if intermittent dosing is useful. These questions will be explored in ongoing and upcoming clinical trials.

Third, what treatment regimens will be most useful for FTI inhibition of tumor growth? Although tumor regression resulting from FTI treatment alone has been shown in the H-*ras* transgenic animal models, FTIs may find the most clinical value when used in combination with other treatment modalities. For example, FTIs alone have been shown to be modest radiosensitizers in H-Ras-transformed rodent cell systems *(81)* and in human tumor cell lines containing oncogenic H-Ras, where they were able to inhibit Ras processing. In human tumor cell lines containing oncogenic K-Ras, FTI together with an inhibitor of GGTase I could inhibit K-Ras processing and increase radiosensitization *(82)*. Tumor cells lacking oncogenic Ras proteins were not radiosensitized by FTIs *(82)*. In each case, the radiosensitization effect has been ascribed to blocking oncogenic Ras function, which causes radioresistance in many tumor cells.

Other possible combinations include taxol, which has been shown recently to synergize with FTIs to inhibit tumor cell growth in vitro *(83)*. Synergy of FTIs with agents that cause microtubule depolymerization may be due to blockade of Ras or of some other farnesylated protein that controls the mitotic check point. Taxol has also been shown to inhibit prenylation, possibly by altering isoprenoid metabolism, and to increase apoptosis *(84)*, possibly as an indirect result of interference with geranylgeranylated proteins. These characteristics may also contribute to the ability to synergize with FTIs. A recent study showing that the subcellular localization to plasma membranes of K-Ras, but not H-Ras, is altered by taxol treatment *(85)* suggests the possibility of an additional functional effect on Ras signaling that is not directly related to inhibition of processing.

Finally, FTIs may be combined with other novel inhibitors of signal transduction pathways leading to increased proliferation, including those of tyrosine kinase growth factor receptors such as EGFR or of the Raf/MEK/MAPK pathway, of other MAPK family pathways, such as JNK or p38, or to pathways controlling angiogenesis, invasion, and metastasis.

12. SUMMARY

Inhibitors of FTase, the enzyme that attaches the farnesyl isoprenoid lipid to Ras and other farnesylated proteins, can block H-Ras processing, signaling, and transformation. Because the other Ras family members can escape inhibition of prenylation by becoming substrates for the highly related enzyme GGTase I, it seems likely that there are other physiologically important farnesylated proteins that help to determine the sensitivity of non-H-Ras-driven tumor cells to FTIs. Understanding the biological consequences of FTase inhibition and characterizing the functions of other farnesylated cellular proteins will permit generation of specific inhibitors of appropriate signaling pathways, and will improve the potential clinical value of FTIs as a novel class of anticancer therapy.

REFERENCES

1. Barbacid M. *ras* genes. *Annu Rev Biochem* 1987; 56:779–827.
2. Khosravi-Far R, Der CJ. The Ras signal transduction pathway. *Cancer Metastas Rev* 1994; 13:67–89.
3. Bos JL. *ras* oncogenes in human cancer: A review. *Cancer Res* 1989; 49:4682–4689.
4. Clark GJ, Der CJ, Dickey BF, Birnbaumer L, eds. GTPases, in *Biology*. vol I. *Oncogenic Activation of Ras Proteins*. Springer-Verlag, 1993, Berlin, 108, pp 259–288.
5. Pazin MJ, Williams LT. Triggering signaling cascades by receptor tyrosine kinases. *Trends Biochem Sci* 1992; 17:374–378.
6. Maltese WA. Posttranslational modification of proteins by isoprenoids in mammalian cells. *FASEB J* 1990; 4:3319–3328.
7. Cox AD, Der CJ. Protein prenylation: More than just glue? *Curr Opin Cell Biol* 1992; 4:1008–1016.
8. Magee AI, Newman CMH, Giannakouros T, Hancock JF, Fawell E, Armstrong J. Lipid modifications and function of the *ras* superfamily of proteins. *Biochem Soc Trans* 1992; 20:497–499.
9. Boyartchuk VL, Ashby MN, Rine J. Modulation of Ras and α-factor function by carboxyl-terminal proteolysis. *Science* 1997; 275:1796–1800.
10. Magee AI, Gutierrez L, McKay IA, Marshall CJ, Hall A. Dynamic fatty acylation of p21^{N-ras}. *EMBO J* 1987; 6:3353–3357.
11. Willumsen BM, Christensen A, Hubbert NL, Papageorge AG, Lowy DR. The p21 *ras* C-terminus is required for transformation and membrane association. *Nature* 1984; 310:583–586.
12. Kato K, Cox AD, Hisaka MM, Graham SM, Buss JE, Der CJ. Isoprenoid addition to Ras protein is the critical modification for its membrane association and transforming activity. *Proc Natl Acad Sci USA* 1992; 89:6403–6407.
13. Sattler I, Tamanoi F. Prenylation of Ras and inhibitors of prenyltransferases, in *Regulation of the RAS Signaling Network*. Maruta H, Burgess AW, eds. RG Landes, Austin, TX, pp. 95–137.
14. Cox AD, Der CJ. Farnesyltransferase inhibitors and cancer treatment: Targeting simply Ras? *Biochim Biophys Acta* 1997; 1333:F51–F71.
15. Reiss Y, Goldstein JL, Seabra MC, Casey PJ, Brown MS. Inhibition of purified p21^{ras} farnesyl:protein transferase by Cys-AAX tetrapeptides. *Cell* 1990; 62:81–88.
16. Moores SL, Schaber MD, Mosser SD, Rands E, O'Hara MB, Garsky VM, Marshall MS, Pompliano DL, Gibbs JB. Sequence dependence of protein isoprenylation. *J Biol Chem* 1991; 266:14,603–14,610.
17. Goldstein JL, Brown MS, Stradley SJ, Reiss Y, Gierasch LM. Nonfarnesylated tetrapeptide inhibitors of protein farnesyltransferase. *J Biol Chem* 1991; 266:15,575–15,578.
18. Omer CA, Kohl NE. CA1A2X-competitive inhibitors of farnesyltransferase as anti-cancer agents. *Trends Pharmacol Sci* 1997; 18:437–444.
19. Sebti S, Hamilton AD. Inhibitors of prenyl transferases. *Curr Opin Oncol* 1997; 9:557–561.
20. James GL, Goldstein JL, Brown MS, Rawson TE, Somers TC, McDowell RS, Crowley CW, Lucas BK, Levinson AD, Marsters JC, Jr. Benzodiazepine peptidomimetics: potent inhibitors of Ras farnesylation in animal cells. *Science* 1993; 260:1937–1942.
21. Kohl NE, Mosser SD, deSolms SJ, Giuliani EA, Pompliano DL, Graham SL, Smith RL, Scolnick EM, Oliff A, Gibbs JB. Selective inhibition of *ras*-dependent transformation by a farnesyltransferase inhibitor. *Science* 1993; 260:1934–1937.
22. Garcia AM, Rowell C, Ackermann K, Kowalczyk JJ, Lewis MD. Peptidomimetic inhibitors of *ras* farnesylation and function in whole cells. *J Biol Chem* 1993; 268:18,415–18,418.
23. Cox AD, Garcia AM, Westwick JK, Kowalczyk JJ, Lewis MD, Brenner DA, Der CJ. The

CAAX peptidomimetic compound B581 specifically blocks farnesylated, but not geranylgeranylated or myristylated, oncogenic Ras signaling and transformation. *J Biol Chem* 1994; 269:19,203–19,206.

24. Manne V, Yan N, Carboni JM, Tuomari AV, Ricca CS, Brown JG, Andahazy ML, Schmidt RJ, Patel D, Zahler R, Weinmann R, Der CJ, Cox AD, Hunt JT, Barbacid M, Seizinger BR. Bisubstrate inhibitors of farnesyltransferase: a novel class of specific inhibitors of Ras transformed cells. *Oncogene* 1995; 10:1763–1779.

25. Carboni JM, Yan N, Cox AD, Bustelo X, Graham SM, Lynch MJ, Weinmann R, Seizinger BR, Der CJ, Barbacid M, Manne V. Farnesyltransferase inhibitors are inhibitors of Ras, but not R-Ras/TC21, transformation. *Oncogene* 1995; 10:1905–1913.

26. Lerner EC, Qian L, Blaskovich MA, Fossum RD, Vogt A, Sun J, Cox AD, Der CJ, Hamilton AD, Sebti SM. Ras CAAX peptidomimetic FTI-277 blocks oncogenic Ras signaling by inducing cytoplasmic accumulation of inactive Ras/Raf complexes. *J Biol Chem* 1995; 270:26,802–26,806.

27. James GL, Brown MS, Cobb MH, Goldstein JL. Benzodiazepine peptidomimetic BZA-5B interrupts the MAP kinase activation pathway in H-Ras-transformed Rat-1 cells, but not in untransformed cells. *J Biol Chem* 1996; 269:27,705–27,714.

28. Kohl NE, Wilson FR, Mosser SD, Giuliani E, deSolms SJ, Conner MW, Anthony NJ, Holtz WJ, Gomez RP, Lee T, Smith RL, Graham SL, Hartman GD, Gibbs JB, Oliff A. Protein farnesyltransferase inhibitors block the growth of *ras*-dependent tumors in nude mice. *Proc. Natl. Acad. Sci. USA* 1994; 91:9141–9145.

29. Yan N, Ricca C, Fletcher J, Glover T, Seizinger BR, Manne V. Farnesyltransferase inhibitors block the neurofibromatosis type 1 (NF1) malignant phenotype. *Cancer Res* 1995; 55:3569–3575.

30. Sepp-Lorenzino L, Ma Z, Rands E, Kohl NE, Gibbs JB, Oliff A, Rosen N. A peptidomimetic inhibitor of farnesyl:protein transferase blocks the anchorage-dependent and -independent growth of human tumor cell lines. *Cancer Res* 1995; 55:5302–5309.

31. Hunt JT, Lee VG, Leftheris K, Seizinger B, Carboni J, Mabus J, Ricca C, Yan N, Manne V. Potent, cell active, non-thiol tetrapeptide inhibitors of farnesyltransferase. *J Med Chem* 1996; 39:353–358.

32. Leftheris K, Kiline T, Vite GD, Cho YH, Bhide RS, Patel DV, Patel MM, Schmidt RJ, Weller HN, Andahazy ML, Carboni JM, Gullo-Brown JL, Lee FYF, Ricca C, Rose WC, Yan N, Barbacid M, Hunt JT, Meyers CA, Seizinger BR, Zahler R, Manne V. Development of highly potent inhibitors of Ras farnesyl transferase possessing cellular and in vivo activity. *J Med Chem* 1996; 39:224–236.

33. Nagasu T, Yoshimatsu K, Rowell C, Lewis MD, Garcia AM. Inhibition of human tumor xenograft growth by treatment with the farnesyl transferase inhibitor B956. *Cancer Res* 1995; 55:5310–5314.

34. Sun J, Qian Y, Hamilton AD, Sebti SM. Ras CAAX peptidomimetic FTI-276 selectively blocks tumor growth in nude mice of a human lung carcinoma with K-Ras mutation and p53 deletion. *Cancer Res* 1995; 55:4243–4247.

35. Kohl NE, Omer CA, Conner MW, Anthony NJ, Davide JP, deSolms SJ, Giuliani EA, Gomez RP, Graham SL, Hamilton K, Handt LK, Hartman GD, Koblan KS, Kral AM, Miller PJ, Mosser SD, O'Neill TJ, Rands E, Schaber MD, Gibbs JB, Oliff A. Inhibition of farnesyltransferase induces regression of mammary and salivary carcinomas in *ras* transgenic mice. *Nature Med* 1995; 1:792–797.

36. Barrington RE, Subler MA, Rands E, Omer CA, Miller PJ, Hundley JE, Koester SK, Troyer DA, Bearss DJ, Conner MW, Gibbs JB, Hamilton K, Koblan KS, Mosser SD, O'Neill TJ, Schaber MD, Senderak ET, Windle JJ, Oliff A, Kohl NE. A farnesyltransferase inhibitor induces tumor regression in transgenic mice harboring multiple oncogenic mutations by mediating alterations in both cell cycle control and apoptosis. *Mol Cell Biol* 1998; 18:85–92.

37. Lerner EC, Zhang TT, Knowles DB, Qian Y, Hamilton AD, Sebti SM. Inhibition of the prenylation of K-Ras, but not H- or N-Ras, is highly resistant to CAAX peptidomimetics and requires both a farnesyltransferase and a geranylgeranyltransferase I inhibitor in human tumor cell lines. *Oncogene* 1997; 15:1283–1288.

38. Park HW, Boduluri SR, Moomaw JF, Casey PJ, Beese LS. Crystal structure of protein farnesyltransferase at 2.25 Å resolution. *Science* 1997; 275:1800–1804.

39. Long SB, Casey PJ, Beese LS. Cocrystal structure of protein farnesyltransferase complexed with a farnesyl diphosphate substrate. *Biochemistry* 1998; 37: 9612–9618.

40. Del Villar K, Mitsuzawa H, Yang W, Sattler I, Tamanoi F. Amino acid substitiutions that convert the protein substrate specificity of farnesyltransferase to that of geranylgeranyltransferase type I. *J Biol Chem* 1997; 272:680–687.

41. Kral AM, Diehl RE, deSolms SJ, Williams TM, Kohl NE, Omer CA. Mutational analysis of conserved residues of the beta-subunit of human farnesyl:protein transferase. *J Biol Chem* 1997; 272:27,319–27,323.

42. Tschantz WR, Furfine ES, Casey PJ. Substrate binding is required for release of product from mammalian protein farnesyltransferase. *J Biol Chem* 1997; 272:9989–9993.

43. Yokoyama K, Zimmerman K, Scholten J, Gelb MH. Differential prenyl pyrophosphate binding to mammalian protein geranylgeranyltransferase-I and protein farnesyltransferase and its consequence on the specificity of protein prenylation. *J Biol Chem* 1997; 272:3944–3952.

44. Njoroge FG, Vibulbhan B, Pinto P, Bishop WR, Bryant MS, Nomeir AA, Lin C, Liu M, Doll RJ, Girijavallabhan V, Ganguly AK. Potent, selective, and orally bioavailable tricyclic pyridyl acetamide N-oxide inhibitors of farnesyl protein transferase with enhanced in vivo antitumor activity. *J Med Chem* 1998; 41:1561–1567.

45. James GL, Goldstein JL, Brown MS. Resistance of K-rasB[V12] proteins to farnesyltransferase inhibitors in Rat-1 cells. *Proc Natl Acad Sci USA* 1996; 93:4454–4458.

46. Sun J, Qian Y, Hamilton AD, Sebti SM. Both farnesyltransferase and geranylgeranyltransferase I inhibitors are required for inhibition of oncogenic K-Ras prenylation but each alone is sufficient to suppress human tumor growth in nude mouse xenografts. *Oncogene* 1998; 16:1467–1473.

47. James GL, Goldstein JL, Brown MS. Polylysine and CVIM sequences of K-RasB dictate specificity of prenylation and confer resistance to benzodiazepine peptidomimetic in vitro. *J Biol Chem* 1995; 270:6221–6226.

48. Zhang FL, Kirschmeier P, Carr D, James L, Bond RW, Wang L, Patton R, Windsor WT, Syto R, Zhang R, Bishop WR. Characterization of Ha-Ras, N-Ras, Ki-Ras4A, and Ki-Ras4B as in vitro substrates for farnesyl protein transferase and geranylgeranyl protein transferase type I. *J Biol Chem* 1997; 272:10,232–10,239.

49. Rowell CA, Kowalczyk JJ, Lewis MD, Garcia AM. Direct demonstration of geranylgeranylation and farnesylation of Ki-Ras in vivo. *J Biol Chem* 1997; 272:14,093–14,097.

50. Whyte DB, Kirschmeier P, Hockenberry TN, Nunez-Oliva I, James L, Catino JJ, Bishop WR, Pai JK. K- and N-Ras are geranylgeranylated in cells treated with farnesyl protein transferase inhibitors. *J Biol Chem* 1997; 272:14,459–14,464.

51. Hancock JF, Cadwallader K, Paterson H, Marshall CJ. A CAAX or a CAAL motif and a second signal are sufficient for plasma membrane targeting of *ras* proteins. *EMBO J* 1991; 10:4033–4039.

52. Plattner R, Anderson MJ, Sato KY, Fasching CL, Der CJ, Stanbridge EJ. Loss of oncogenic *ras* expression does not correlate with loss of tumorigenicity in human cells. *Proc Natl Acad Sci USA* 1996; 93:6665–6670.

53. Shirasawa S, Furuse M, Yokoyama N, Sasazuki T. Altered growth of human colon cancer cell lines disrupted at activated Ki-*ras*. *Science* 1993; 260:85–88.

54. Cates CA, Michael RL, Stayrook KR, Harvey KA, Burke YD, Randall SK, Crowell PL, Crowell DN. Prenylation of oncogenic human PTP(CAAX) protein tyrosine phosphatases. *Cancer Lett* 1996; 110:49–55.

55. James GL, Goldstein JL, Pathak RK, Anderson RG, Brown MS. PxF, a prenylated protein of peroxisomes. *J Biol Chem* 1994; 269:14,182–14,190.

56. Kaminski JJ, Rane DF, Snow ME, Weber L, Rothofsky ML, Anderson SD, Lin SL. Identification of novel farnesyl protein transferase inhibitors using three-dimensional database searching methods. *J Med Chem* 1997; 40:4103–4112.

57. Lebowitz PF, Davide JP, Prendergast GC. Evidence that farnesyltransferase inhibitors suppress Ras transformation by interfering with Rho activity. *Mol Cell Biol* 1995; 15:6613–6622.

58. Adamson P, Marshall CJ, Hall A, Tilbrook PA. Post-translational modifications of p21[rho] proteins. *J Biol Chem* 1992; 267:20,033–20,038.

59. Lebowitz PF, Casey PJ, Prendergast GC, Thissen JA. Farnesyltransferase inhibitors alter the prenylation and growth-stimulating function of RhoB. *J Biol Chem* 1997; 272:15,591–15,594.

60. Foster R, Hu K-Q, Lu Y, Nolan KM, Thissen J, Settleman J. Identification of a novel human Rho protein with unusual properties: GTPase deficiency and in vivo farnesylation. *Mol Cell Biol* 1996; 16:2689–2699.

61. Nobes CD, Lauritzen I, Mattei MG, Paris S, Hall A, Chardin P. A new member of the Rho family, Rnd1, promotes disassembly of actin filament structures and loss of cell adhesion. *J Cell Biol* 1998; 141:187–197.

62. Guasch RM, Scambler P, Jones GE, Ridley AJ. RhoE regulates actin cytoskeleton organization and cell migration. *Mol Cell Biol* 1998; 18:4761–4771.

63. Clark GJ, Kinch MS, Rogers-Graham K, Sebti SM, Hamilton AD, Der CJ. The Ras-related protein Rheb is farnesylated and antagonizes Ras signaling and transformation. *J Biol Chem* 1997; 272:10,608–10,615.

64. Diamond RH, Cressman DE, Laz TM, Abrams CS, Taub R. PRL-1, a unique nuclear protein tyrosine phosphatase, affects cell growth. *Mol Cell Biol* 1994; 14: 3752–3762.

65. Diamond RH, Peters C, Jung SP, Greenbaum LE, Haber BA, Silberg DG, Traber PG, Taub R. Expression of PRL-1 nuclear PTPase is associated with proliferation in liver but with differentiation in intestine. *Am J Physiol* 1996; 271:G121–129.

66. De Smedt F, Boom A, Pesesse X, Schiffmann SN, Erneux C. Post-translational modification of human brain type I inositol-1,4,5-triphosphate 5-phosphatase by farnesylation. *J Biol Chem* 1996; 271:10,419–10,424.

67. Nantais DE, Schwemmle M, Stickney JT, Vestal DJ, Buss JE. Prenylation of an interferon-gamma-induced GTP-binding protein: The human guanylate binding protein, huGBP1. *J Leukoc Biol* 1996; 60:423–431.

68. Kemppainen RJ, Behrend EN. Dexamethasone rapidly induces a novel *ras* superfamily member-related gene in AtT-20 cells. *J Biol Chem* 1998; 273:3129–3131.

69. Olson MF, Ashworth A, Hall A. An essential role for Rho, Rac and Cdc42 GTPases in cell cycle progression through G_1. *Science* 1995; 269:1270–1272.

70. Crick DC, Andres DA, Waechter CJ. Geranylgeraniol promotes entry of UT-2 cells into the cell cycle in the absence of mevalonate. *Exp Cell Res* 1997; 231:302–307.

71. Raiteri M, Arnaboldi L, McGeady P, Gelb MH, Verri D, Tagliabue C, Quarato P, Ferraboschi P, Santaniello E, Paoletti R, Fumagalli R, Corsini A. Pharmacological control of the mevalonate pathway: Effect on arterial smooth muscle cell proliferation. *J Pharmacol Exp Ther* 1997; 281:1144–1153.

72. Vogt A, Qian Y, McGuire TF, Hamilton AD, Sebti SM. Protein geranylgeranylation, not farnesylation, is required for the G1 to S phase transition in mouse fibroblasts. *Oncogene* 1996; 13:1991–1999.

73. Miquel K, Pradines A, Sun J, Qian Y, Hamilton AD, Sebti SM, Favre G. GGTI-298 induces G0-G1 block and apoptosis whereas FTI-277 causes G2-M enrichment in A549 cells. *Cancer Res* 1997; 57:1846–1850.

74. Weber JD, Hu W, Jefcoat SC Jr, Raben DM, Baldassare JJ. Ras-stimulated extracellular

signal-related kinase 1 and RhoA activities coordinate platelet-derived growth factor-induced G1 progression through the independent regulation of cyclin D1 and p27. *J Biol Chem* 1997; 272:32,966–32,971.

75. Noguchi Y, Nakamura S, Yasuda T, Kitagawa M, Kohn LD, Saito Y, Hirai, A. Newly synthesized Rho A, not Ras, is isoprenylated and translocated to membranes coincident with progression of the G1 to S phase of growth-stimulated rat FRTL-5 cells. *J Biol Chem* 1998; 273:3649–3653.

76. Flint OP, Masters BA, Gregg RE, Durham SK. HMG CoA reductase inhibitor-induced myotoxicity: Pravastatin and lovastatin inhibit the geranylgeranylation of low-molecular-weight proteins in neonatal rat muscle cell culture. *Toxicol Appl Pharmacol* 1997; 145:99–110.

77. Stark WW Jr, Blaskovich MA, Johnson BA, Qian Y, Vasudevan A, Pitt B, Hamilton AD, Sebti SM, Davies P. Inhibiting geranylgeranylation blocks growth and promotes apoptosis in pulmonary vascular smooth muscle cells. *Am J Physiol* 1998; 275:L55–63.

78. Dalton MB, Fantle KS, Bechtold HA, DeMaio L, Evans RM, Krystosek A, Sinensky M. The farnesyl protein transferase inhibitor BZA-5B blocks farnesylation of nuclear lamins and p21^{ras} but does not affect their function and localization. *Cancer Res* 1995; 55:3295–3304.

79. Mangues R, Corral T, Kohl NE, Symmans WF, Lu S, Malumbres M, Gibbs JB, Oliff A, Pellicer A. Antitumor effect of a farnesyl-protein transferase inhibitor in mammary and lymphoid tumors overexpressing N-*ras* in transgenic mice. *Cancer Res* 1998; 58:1253–1259.

80. Prendergast GC, Davide JP, Lebowitz PF, Wechsler-Reya R, Kohl NE. Resistance of a variant *ras*-transformed cell line to phenotypic reversion by farnesyl transferase inhibitors. *Cancer Res* 1996; 56:2626–2632.

81. Bernhard EJ, Kao G, Cox AD, Sebti SM, Hamilton AD, Muschel RJ, McKenna WG. The farnesyltransferase inhibitor FTI-277 radiosensitizes H-*ras*-transformed rat embryo fibroblasts. *Cancer Res* 1996; 56:1727–1730.

82. Bernhard EJ, McKenna WG, Hamilton AD, Sebti SM, Qian Y, Wu JM, Muschel RJ. Inhibiting Ras prenylation increases the radiosensitivity of human tumor cell lines with activating mutations of *ras* oncogenes. *Cancer Res* 1998; 58:1754–1761.

83. Moasser MM, Sepp-Lorenzino L, Kohl NE, Oliff A, Balog A, Su DS, Danishefsky SJ, Rosen N. Farnesyl transferase inhibitors cause enhanced mitotic sensitivity to taxol and epothilones. *Proc Natl Acad Sci USA* 1998; 95:1369–1374.

84. Danesi R, Figg WD, Reed E, Myers CE. Paclitaxel (taxol) inhibits protein isoprenylation and induces apoptosis in PC-3 human prostate cancer cells. *Mol Pharmacol* 1995; 47:1106–1111.

85. Thissen JA, Gross JM, Subramanian K, Meyer T, Casey PJ. Prenylation-dependent association of K-Ras with microtubules: Evidence for a role in subcellular trafficking. *J Biol Chem* 1997; 272:30,362–30,370.

29

Targeted p53 Gene Therapy-Mediated Radiosensitization and Chemosensitization

Esther H. Chang, PhD, Liang Xu, MD, PhD, and Kathleen F. Pirollo, PhD

1. INTRODUCTION

Gene therapy is based on restoring a missing or defective cellular function by delivering and expressing a gene encoding the protein responsible for that function. Initially, gene therapy was envisioned as a potential means to correct inherited monogenic defects. This remains an active area of research, and a number of human clinical trials of this approach are ongoing *(1–3)*. In addition to inherited monogenic defects, gene therapy is being applied to other types of diseases. This chapter describes gene therapy, as it is being used in the armamentarium of the war against cancer. More than 100 oncology-related clinical trials involving gene therapy have been approved worldwide *(4)*. These therapeutic protocols include the expression of cytokines to enhance cellular immunogenicity, the expression of genes encoding prodrug activating enzymes, the expression of genes resulting in increased drug sensitivity (e.g., HSV-TK/gancyclovir), or drug resistance (e.g., MDR-1 to protect normal bone marrow cells) *(5)* and the restoration of the function(s) of tumor suppressor genes. In addition to trials wherein an exogenous gene is being expressed with therapeutic intent, a number of other trials involving the suppression of gene expression (e.g., with antisense molecules targeting oncogenes) are also ongoing. The focus of the current chapter is the nonviral delivery of a functional tumor suppressor gene (encoding p53) to cancer cells.

2. DELIVERY SYSTEMS FOR GENE THERAPY

2.1. Viral Vectors for Gene Delivery

The development of various strategies to introduce genes into cells has made cancer treatment involving gene therapy a reality. The ideal therapeutic for cancer would be one that selectively targets a cellular pathway responsible for the tumor phenotype and would be nontoxic to normal cells. To date, this ideal therapeutic remains largely just that—an ideal. Although cancer treatments involving gene therapy hold substantial promise, many issues need to be addressed before this promise can be realized. Perhaps foremost among the issues associated with macromolecular treatments is the efficient

From: Signaling Networks and Cell Cycle Control: The Molecular Basis of Cancer and Other Diseases
Edited by: J. S. Gutkind © Humana Press Inc., Totowa, NJ

delivery of the therapeutic molecules to the site(s) in the body where they are needed. In the case of cancer therapy, the ideal would be to deliver the exogenous gene to all cancer cells (primary tumor and metastases) and only to cancer cells. A variety of delivery systems have been tried. These approaches can be divided into two broad categories: viral and nonviral vectors.

Retroviruses, adenoviruses, and herpes virus are currently the most frequently used viral vectors in gene therapy. By far the largest number of approved clinical protocols involve retroviruses. Adeno-associated, pox, vaccinia, and baculovirus have also been studies for their potential use in gene delivery. However, viral delivery systems have significant drawbacks. Retroviruses have low transduction efficiencies and their insert size is limited. They also require active cell division, which may be advantageous in some cases. Moreover, with retroviral vectors, there is always the potential for unwanted insertional mutagenesis and of random deletion of the transgene. Adenovirus have a sufficiently high capacity to accommodate most cDNAs and can infect both replicating and quiescent cells. In genereal, adenoviral vectors can deliver DNA with higher efficiency *(6)*. The major disadvantage for adenoviral delivery systems is their tendency to be immunogenic and to induce a nonspecific inflammatory response and antiviral cellular immunity *(7–10)*. In the case of herpes virus vectors, their neurotropism, which accounts for its successful application in treating brain cancer, is also its greatest limitation, with potential for severe host toxicity.

The major shortcoming to all these viral systems is their lack of specificity for cancer cells. Currently, none has tumor targeting capability, although investigations are ongoing to develop new ways to alter viral coat proteins to achieve tumor specificity. For example, a retroviral vector has been targeted to cells expressing a specific cellular antigen by replacing the N-terminal SU peptide of the Moloney murine leukemia virus (Mo-MuLV) envelope protein with a single-chain antibody derivative (designated scFv) *(11–13)*. Retroviruses have also been engineered to target lung cancer cells through replacement of the viral envelope protein with heregulin, a ligand for EGF-R and the related HER-2 receptor, which is overexpressed in certain tumors, including most lung cancer cells *(14)*. Efforts are also underway to redirect adenoviral vectors to fibroblast growth factor (FGF) receptors using a bifunctional antibody directed against the adenoviral knob protein and FGF *(15,16)*.

2.2. Nonviral Vectors for Gene Delivery

The infectivity that makes viruses attractive as delivery vectors also poses their greatest drawback—safety or, more precisely, the potential lack thereof. The theoretically possible generation of novel viruses with new targets for infection has been a concern in the relatively short history of gene therapy. The concern has been that, once introduced into patients, these viruses could be transformed via genetic alteration into new human pathogens. Even without invoking this worst-case scenario, the introduction of viral vectors are subject to attack by the immune system of the patient. Other practical issues need to be addressed for any viral delivery system as well, such as the capacity of the virus to carry foreign DNA. Consequently, a significant amount of attention has been directed at developing delivery systems for cancer gene therapy, which could circumvent some of the problems associated with viral vectors. These systems consist primarily of naked plasmid DNA or liposomes.

The delivery of simple plasmid DNA, without benefit of any additional vector, is one method of nonviral gene transfer. The lack of immunogenicity caused by the absence of foreign (i.e., viral) components is an attractive feature of this approach. Here the DNA is delivered via mechanical methods, such as direct injection into the tissue, or particle bombardment of tissues or tumors with DNA-coated gold particles using a "gene gun" *(17)*. The direct transfection of cytokine genes into tumors in vivo by the gene gun has been reported to inhibit tumor growth in mice *(18,19)*. The gene transfer efficiency of plasmid DNA has also been improved by taking advantage of receptor mediated endocytosis. Cell surface receptors provide a means by which some measure of selectivity can be achieved since certain receptors are elevated on specific tumor cell types. By linking the plasmid encoding a putative therapeutic gene to a ligand for a receptor elevated on tumor cells, tumor targeting might be achieved. Antibodies to tumor cell surface antigens also provide a means to achieve targeting. An interesting variation on this theme involves the use of adenoviruses to assist in the escape of nonviral DNA from endosomes after receptor-mediated endocytosis of the DNA *(20,21)*.

Liposomes are essentially phospholipid bilayer vessicles with an internal space that makes them potential vehicles for delivery of drugs *(22)*. The basis for their attractiveness as delivery vehicles are the low intrinsic level of toxicity of the lipid components as well as their versatility. Features of liposomes that make them versatile and attractive for DNA delivery include simplicity of preparation; the ability to complex large amounts of DNA; use with any type and size of DNA or RNA; the ability to transfect many different types of cells, including nondividing cells; and a relative lack of immunogenicity or biohazardous activity *(23)*. Liposomes can also be formulated in a large range of sizes and chemical components *(24)*. However, conventional neutral liposomes have proved inefficient for delivery of anticancer drug to the cells. Therefore, specialized liposomes are currently being developed to advance efficiency and cell-specific targeting. These specialized liposmomes include cationic liposmes as well as sterically stabilized, fusogenic, and pH- or thermosensitive liposomes. Immunoliposomes, liposomes incorporating antibodies for targeting, are also being tested. Combinations and permutations of these specialized types of liposomes are being tested to achieve higher efficiency of gene delivery and better tumor targeting and have recently been reviewed by Dass et al. *(24)*.

More than 20 clinical protocols using liposomes for cancer gene therapy have been approved, and more than a dozen trials are now under way *(4,25)*. Such trials have been stimulated in part by the fact that liposomes for delivery of small molecule therapeutics (e.g., antifungal agents and conventional cancer chemotherapeutic agents) are already on the market suggesting that liposomes can be safe and effective agents for delivery *(22)*. In the case of the liposomal drugs that are on the market, however, the function of the liposome is to reduce the toxicity of the agent that they contain. None of these liposmal drugs involves targeted delivery to a specific cell type. Thus, a major shortcomings of most lipid delivery systems for gene therapy remains a lack tumor specificity, as well as a relatively low transfection efficiency when compared to viral vectors *(26)*. However, as discussed below, these shortcomings can be dramatically alleviated when liposomes are complexed to a ligand recognized by cell surface receptors.

The remainder of this chapter focuses on the use of a cationic liposomal delivery system and its potential for tumor-targeted gene delivery by receptor-mediated endocytosis. We concentrate on the gene augmentation approach in which liposomes are used to deliver a gene encoding wild-type (wt) p53 to tumor cells, with the net result the restoration of the normal p53 function that many tumors lack. This restoration has a profound effect on the ability to treat the tumors. This approach has exciting potential as a novel means of treating a variety of human cancers.

3. THE p53 GENE AND CANCER

A role for the tumor suppressor gene p53 in many critical cellular pathways, particularly in the cell's response to DNA damage has been well established. These pathways include not only gene transcription, DNA repair, genomic stability, chromosomal segregation, and senescence, but also regulation of cell cycle events and the modulation of programmed cell death (apoptosis). For its role in monitoring DNA damage, p53 has been christened "guardian of the genome" (27). Cancer cells are characterized by genetic instability, and mutations in p53 have been found to occur with extremely high frequency in almost all types of human cancers. Indeed, quantitative or qualitative alterations in the p53 gene are suggested to play a role in over half of all human malignancies (28). Moreover, mechanisms other than mutation of the p53 gene itself may also result in loss of wtp53 function and thereby also contribute to tumorigenesis. Functional inactivation can occur, for example, through amplification of the MDM-2 protein as is the case in approximately one-third of sarcomas (29,30) and a subset (<10%) of breast, lung, brain, and bladder cancers (31), or through binding to the E6 protein of HPV (32,33). This latter mechanism may play a role in cervical carcinomas, the majority of which are HPV positive. The presence of p53 mutations in the most common types of human tumors has been found to be associated with poor clinical prognosis (34–36). Moreover, mutant (mt) p53 is rarely found in some of the more curable forms of cancer, such as Wilms tumor, retinoblastoma, testicular cancer, neuroblastoma, and acute lymphoid leukemia (37–42).

Abnormalities in p53 function may also contribute to angiogenesis, the process of new blood vessel formation by which solid tumors derive nutrients essential for tumor growth. A growing number of genes have been shown to be transcriptionally regulated (both activated and repressed) by p53. (For reviews covering these genes, see *43* and *44.*) Among these are secreted proteins, which inhibit angiogenesis, such as thrombospondin (45) and IGF-BP3 (46), which inhibits the IGF pathway, as well as angiogenic factors FGF (47) and VEGF (48,49). It has also been suggested that the development of the angiogenic phenotype in human fibroblasts occurs in a stepwise fashion and is dependent on the loss of both alleles of the p53 gene (50). Further evidence for the role of wtp53 in controlling angiogenesis is found in a recent report that wtp53 expression by an adenoviral vector was able to downregulate VEGF expression in human colon cancer cells in vitro, and to inhibit tumor cell-induced angiogenesis in vivo (51).

Numerous studies have reported that the expression of wtp53 has suppressed both in vitro and in mouse xenograft models, the growth of various malignancies, such as prostate (52,53), head and neck (54–56), colon (57–59), cervical (60), and lung (61–63) tumor cells. This subject has recently been fully reviewed (64). It has also been reported that a p53–liposome complex partially inhibited the growth of human glioblastoma *(65)* and human breast cancer *(66)* xenografts in mice. In addition, Seung et al. *(67)* used liposome-mediated intratumoral introduction of a radiation-inducible construct expressing tumor necrosis factor-α (TNF-α) to inhibit growth of a murine fibrosarcoma xenograft after exposure to ionizing radiation *(67)*. However, p53 expression alone, although able to inhibit tumor growth partially, has not been shown to eliminate established tumors in the long term. This observation has led our laboratory and others to explore p53 gene therapy in combination with more conventional cancer therapeutic modalities.

The normal development of mice lacking wtp53 *(68)* and the observations of a post irradiation G1 block in p53-expressing cells, suggests that wtp53 functions in the regulation of the cell after DNA damage or stress rather than during proliferation and development. As it appears that many conventional anticancer therapies (chemotherapeutics and radiation) induce DNA damage and appear to work by inducing apoptosis *(69)*, alterations in the p53 pathway could conceivably lead to failure of therapeutic regimens. Indeed, a direct link has been suggested between mutations in the p53 gene and resistance to cytotoxic cancer treatments, (both chemo-and radiotherapy) *(70)*. It had been suggested earlier that the loss of wtp53, which is essential for the effective activation of apoptosis after irradiation or treatment with chemotherapeutic agents, may contribute to the crossresistance to anticancer agents observed in some tumor cells *(71)*. Various laboratories have established the correlation between the presence of mtp53 and chemoresistance in mouse fibrosarcomas *(72,73)* and in primary tumor cultures from human gastric, esophageal, and breast carcinomas, as well as B-cell chronic lymphoid leukemia *(42,74,75)*. The status of p53 has also been associated with the effectiveness of chemotherapeutic agents in ovarian teratocarcinomas *(76)*, testicular carcinomas *(77)*, and breast cancer *(78)*.

Lack of wtp53 function has also been associated with an increase in radiation resistance. Thymocytes from knockout mice that lack wtp53 were found to be deficient in apoptosis in response to γ-radiation or etoposide, a topoisomerase II inhibitor *(79–82)*. The presence of mtp53 and the consequent absence of a G1 block have also been found to correlate with increased radiation resistance in some human tumors and cell lines *(83, 84)*. These include human tumor cell lines representative of head and neck, lymphoma, bladder, breast, thyroid, ovary, and brain cancer *(85–90)*. Moreover, McIlwrath et al. *(87)* measured the G1 arrest in 12 human tumor cell lines displaying a wide range of radioresponsiveness. These investigators found a significant inverse correlation between the level of ionizing radiation-induced G1 arrest and the radiation-resistant phenotype, that is, cell lines lacking the G1 arrest were radioresistant. However, the relationship between p53 status and the radiation resistance phenotype is not entirely clear and may not completely or directly correlate with fibroblast cells or all tumor cell lines *(137,138)*. These results collectively suggest that cells with functional p53 respond to DNA damage by undergoing apoptosis, whereas cells lacking functional p53 may continue to divide and accumulate genetic damage (Fig. 1A).

On the basis of these considerations, gene therapy to restore wtp53 function in tumor cells should reestablish the p53-dependent cell cycle checkpoints and the apoptotic pathway thus leading to the reversal of the chemo- and radioresistant phenotypes (Fig. 1B). Consistent with this model, chemosensitivity, along with apoptosis, was restored

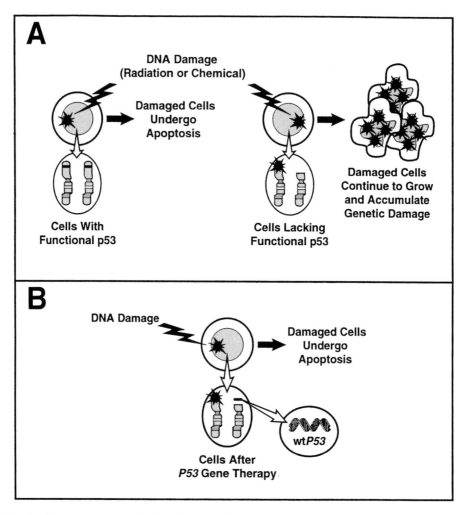

Fig. 1. p53 and response to DNA damage. Cells with functional p53 respond to DNA damage caused by radiation or chemicals (e.g., chemotherapeutic agents) by undergoing apoptosis. In contrast cells lacking functional p53 fail to respond appropriately to DNA damage, continue to grow and accumulate additional genetic damage. Such cells give rise to tumors that are often relatively resistant to conventional cancer therapy regimens. **(A)** Depicted on the left is a normal cell with two copies of the p53 gene on chromosome 17. Depicted on the right is a cell that has one copy of the p53 gene altered by mutation and the other copy deleted. **(B)** Restoration of p53 function restores appropriate response to DNA damage. When the p53 gene is introduced via gene therapy and expressed, the restoration of p53 function results in cells that undergo apoptosis in response to DNA-damaging radiation or chemicals.

by expression of wtp53 in non-small cell lung carcinoma mouse xenografts carrying mtp53 (62,139). Chemosensitivity of xenografts involving the p53-null lung tumor cell line H1299 *(91)* and T98G glioblastoma cells *(139)* and sensitivity of WiDr colon cancer xenografts *(92)* to cisplatin has been demonstrated. Increased cell killing by doxorubicin or mitomycin C was also shown in SK-Br-3 breast tumor cells by adenoviral transduction of wtp53 *(93)*. However, the presence of some conflicting reports *(94,95)* indicates that the relationship between p53 expression and chemoresistance may have a tissue or cell type-specific component. The transfection of wtp53 by an adenoviral vector has also been shown to sensitize ovarian *(96)* and colorectal *(97)* tumor cells to radiation. It has also been reported that adenoviral-mediated wtp53 delivery did restore functional apoptosis in a radiation-resistant squamous cell carcinoma of the head and neck (SCCHN) tumor line, resulting in radiosensitization of these cells in vitro *(98)*. More significantly, the combination of intratumorally injected adeno-wtp53 and radiation led to complete and long-term tumor regression of established SCCHN xenograft tumors *(99)*.

4. TUMOR-TARGETED CATIONIC LIPOSOMES

The vast majority of the p53 gene therapy studies have employed adenoviral vectors for delivery. However, as previously discussed, there are currently no efficient means of targeting adenovirus specifically to tumor cells in vivo. For the most part, adenoviral gene delivery involves intratumoral injection. For many primary tumors, this is a serious shortcoming, but it has an even greater impact on the treatment of metastatic cancer. For primary cancers and especially for metastatic disease, a systemic delivery system capable of tumor targeting is imperative.

Receptor mediated endocytosis *(100–102)* is one mechanism that is currently being exploited for cell-specific targeting. This physiological process represents a highly efficient internalization mechanism present in eukaryotic cells exhibiting high transport capacity, in addition to ligand-dependent cell specificity. Conjugation to a therapeutic gene or gene carrier of a ligand with affinity to a specific cell surface membrane receptor can serve to provide cell selective uptake of molecules which would otherwise be excluded from the cell *(102–108)*. The addition of a ligand, commonly through a cationic linker such as polylysine or protamines, has already demonstrated some potential in targeting DNA to cells in vivo *(101)*. Despite the attractiveness of liposomes as a delivery system for gene therapy, their major weakness is their relatively low transfection efficiency and lack of tumor specificity. However, recent reports have demonstrated that by taking advantage of receptor mediated endocytosis both of these obstacles can be overcome.

Cationic liposomes were developed for the transfer of DNA into cells. The lipid–DNA complex is formed by a combination of electrostatic attraction and hydrophobic interaction *(109)*. The excess positive charge of the complex permits DNA transfection of the cells *(110)*. Cationic liposomes are composed of positively charged lipid bilayers and can be complexed to negatively charged naked DNA by simple mixing of lipids and DNA, such that the resulting complex has a net positive charge. The complex is easily bound and taken up by cells with high transfection efficiency *(111)*. More importantly, from the perspective of human cancer therapy, cationic liposomes have been proven to be safe and efficient for in vivo gene delivery *(111,112)*.

Two ligands, folate and transferrin, have demonstrated their liposome-targeting ability both in vitro and in vivo. Folic acid enters the cell through two mechanisms: facilitated transport *(113,114)* or through the folate binding protein, a membrane-associated folate receptor that functions through receptor-mediated endocytosis *(100,115)*. Conjugation of folate to macromolecules or liposomes by its γ-carboxyl group results in loss of recognition by the folate transport system. The conjugated ligand can still be recognized by the folate binding protein and these folate conjugates are selectively taken up by cells that express this membrane folate receptor *(103,116)*. This is advantageous for cancer gene therapy, as the level of this receptor has been found to be elevated in a variety of human cancers, including ovarian, colon, breast, cervical, renal, and oral *(117–123)*. Moreover, the folate receptor recycles during the internalization of folate in rapidly dividing cells such as cancer cells *(124)*, which may also increase uptake of receptor-bound molecules, even in cancer cells not expressing elevated receptor levels. Folate-conjugated macromolecules and liposomes have been shown to be specifically taken up in vitro by receptor-bearing tumor cells *(125–127)*.

The plasma glycoprotein transferrin is the major mechanism by which cells acquire iron, using receptor-mediated endocytosis to internalize the transferrin–iron complex. The receptor for transferrin is displayed on the surface of proliferating cells. There is evidence that the receptor is also more highly expressed on tumor cells, including oral *(128)*, prostate *(129)*, and breast cancer *(130)* cells, as compared with normal cells *(131)*. Levels of transferrin receptor have also been found to correlate with the aggressive and proliferative ability of tumor cells *(132)*. Therefore, the level of transferrin receptor, like the folate receptor, can be considered a prognostic tumor marker. In addition, the transferrin receptor may also be exploited for tumor-specific delivery. Various laboratories have made use of the transferrin ligand–receptor interaction to use monoclonal antibodies against transferrin as anticancer agents *(133)* or to facilitate uptake of antibody–toxin conjugates *(134)*.

Recently, our group has been developing a novel approach for cancer gene therapy that draws on the knowledge gained in the field over the past decade to devise a systemic delivery system that specifically targets tumor cells and results in a more effective cancer treatment modality. This approach uses a ligand-directed cationic liposome system to deliver wtp53 to the tumor cells (Fig. 2). The inclusion of either the folate or transferrin ligand to the liposome–DNA complex takes advantage of the tumor-targeting facet and receptor-mediated endocytosis associated with these two ligands to introduce wtp53 efficiently and specifically to the tumor cells. The consequence of this restoration of wtp53 function is an increase in sensitization to conventional radiation and chemotherapies thereby increasing their efficacy.

The liposome composition used was based on the cationic lipid DOTAP and fusogenic neutral lipid DOPE, either conjugated to folic acid *(105)* or simply mixed with iron-saturated transferrin *(135)*. The ratio of lipids themselves, as well as the lipid-to-DNA ratio, was optimized for different tumor cell types, such as adenocarcinoma versus squamous cell carcinoma. In vitro studies demonstrated that the addition of the ligand significantly increased the transfection efficiency of tumor cells as compared with the liposome alone in even in the presence of high levels of serum *(135,136)*. Transfection of wtp53 by this method resulted in significant radiosensitization of a previously radiation resistant SCCHN cell line in vitro *(135,136)*. The in vivo tumor targeting capability of this system was assessed using the β-galactosidase reporter gene in three different types of cancer: SCCHN, breast cancer, and prostate cancer. These studies demonstrated that, after intravenous administration, only the tumors were transfected, with an efficiency of 50–70%, while normal organs and tissues, including the highly proliferative bone marrow and intestinal crypt cells, showed no signs of reporter gene

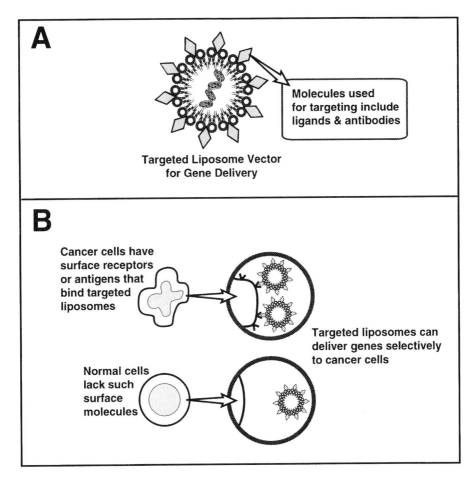

Fig. 2. (A) Targeted liposomes for gene therapy. Liposomes represent non-viral vectors for gene therapy. Liposomes can be constructed such that they have on their surface molecules that can result in targeted delivery of the liposomes and their contents to specific cell types. These targeting molecules may be ligands recognized by cell surface receptors or antibodies that recognize cell surface antigens. **(B)** Selective gene delivery to cancer cells. Cancer cells have on their surface elevated levels of certain receptors and antigens compared to their normal counterparts. These surface molecules can be exploited for selective delivery of therapeutic genes, such as p53.

expression *(136)*. Some ligand–liposome–DNA complex was evident in macrophages. Most significantly, even micrometastases in the lung, spleen and lymph nodes showed evidence of very highly efficient and specific transfection.

When the systemically delivered ligand–liposome wtp53 complex was administered, in combination with radiation, to mice bearing radiation-resistant human SCCHN xenografts, these tumors regressed completely (Fig. 3). Histological examination of the area of the former tumor showed only normal and scar tissue remaining, with no evidence of live tumor cells. This was in contrast to the tumors from animals treated only with the ligand–liposome–p53 complex or only with radiation. In these animals, some cell death was evident. However, nests of live tumor cells remained, resulting in the regrowth

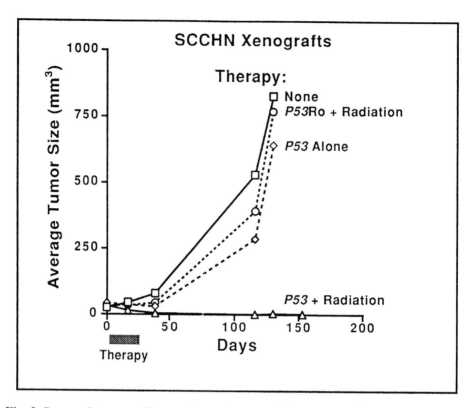

Fig. 3. Synergy between p53 gene therapy by targeted liposomes and conventional radiation therapy. Mice bearing xenografts of human head and neck cancer cells were treated with the indicated regimens (none; *P53* alone; *P53*Ro + radiation, or *P53* + radiation) and the size of their tumors measured over time. Mice were euthanized when their tumor burden became excessive. The wild-type p53 gene was delivered by intravenous injection in liposomes targeting the transferrin receptor. *P53*Ro denotes a plasmid wherein the p53 gene is in a reverse orientation to serve as a control for no expression of p53 (thus, *P53*Ro + Radiation represents the effect of radiotherapy in the absence of p53 expression).

of the tumors in these animals. Strikingly, no recurrence of the tumors was evident in the animals receiving the combination therapy, even 1 year after the end of treatment *(136)*. Similar results were observed in mice bearing radiation resistant human prostate tumor xenografts *(136)*. Consequently, this system, which augments conventional treatments, yields a more effective form of cancer therapy.

5. SUMMARY AND PERSPECTIVE

It appears that the ligand-directed liposome delivery system we have employed may be represent significant advance towards achieving one of the goals of human cancer gene therapy, that of tumor specific targeting. The selectivity of gene expression has been demonstrated using a reporter gene and the gene of interest (p53). The approach described represents a coupling of an efficient gene delivery system with a growing understanding of the function of the p53 gene. The role of p53 in the cellular response to DNA damage underlies the use of p53 gene therapy in combination with DNA-damaging agents (chemotherapeutics and radiation). Tumor cells that are relatively resistant to these agents are rendered sensitive by p53 gene therapy. In the general field of cancer therapeutics, there is a growing use of combination therapies, including the use of more than one chemotherapeutic agent and of chemotherapy in conjunction with radiotherapy. Our results suggest that, in the future, gene therapy will take its place in the armentarium against cancer. While gene therapy may have uses in isolation, our results suggest that its more profound impact on cancer treatment may be as an addition to more conventional treatments.

6. ACKNOWLEDGMENTS

Portions of the authors' research described here was supported by a sponsored research agreement with SynerGene Therapeutics, Inc. We also thank Dr. Joe Harford of the National Cancer Institute for critical reading of the manuscript.

REFERENCES

1. Blaese RM, Culver KW, Miller AD, Carter CS, Fleisher T, Clerici M, Shearer G, Chang L, Chiang Y, Tolstoshev P, et al. T lymphocyte-directed gene therapy for ADA-SCID: Initial trial results after 4 years. *Science* 1995; 270:475–480.
2. Kiem HP, von Kalle C, Schuening F, Storb R. Gene therapy and bone marrow transplantation. *Curr Opin Oncol* 1995; 7:107–114.
3. Medin JA, Karlsson S. Viral vectors for gene therapy of hematopoietic cells. *Immunotechnology* 1997; 3:3–19.
4. Roth JA, Cristiano RJ. Gene therapy for cancer: What have we done and where are we going? *J Natl Cancer Inst* 1997; 89:21–39.
5. Licht T, Herrmann F, Gottesman MM, Pastan I. (1997). In vivo drug-selectable genes: a new concept in gene therapy. *Stem Cells* 1997; 15:104–111.
6. Bramson JL, Graham FL, Gauldie J. The use of adenoviral vectors for gene therapy and gene transfer in vivo. *Curr Opin Biotechnol* 1995; 6:590–595.
7. Smith TA, Mehaffey MG, Kayda DB, Saunders JM, Yei S, Trapnell BC, McClelland A, Kaleko M. Adenovirus mediated expression of therapeutic plasma levels of Human Factor IX in mice. *Nature Genet* 1993; 5:397–402.
8. Setoguchi Y, Jaffe HA, Chu, CS, Crystal RG. Intraperitoneal in vivo gene therapy to deliver Alpha 1-Antitrypsin to the systemic circulation. *Am J Respir Cell Mol Biol* 1994; 10:369–377.
9. Yang Y, Nunes FA, Berencsi K, Furth EE, Gonczol E, Wilson JM. Cellular immunity to viral antigens limits E1-deleted adenoviruses for gene therapy. *Proc Natl Acad Sci USA* 1994; 91:4407–4411.
10. Yang Y, Li Q, Ertl HC, Wilson JM. Cellular and humoral immune responses to viral antigens create barriers to lung-directed gene therapy with recombinant adenoviruses. *J Virol* 1995; 69:2004–2015.
11. Russell SJ, Hawkins RE, Winter G. Retroviral vectors displaying functional antibody fragments. *Nucleic Acids Res* 1993; 21:1081–1085.
12. Chu TH, Martinez I, Sheay WC, Dornburg R. Cell targeting with retroviral vector particles containing antibody-envelope fusion proteins. *Gene Ther* 1994; 1:292–299.
13. Kasahara N, Dozy AM, Kan YW. Tissue-specific targeting of retroviral vectors through ligand–receptor interactions. *Science* 1994; 266:1373–1376.
14. Han X, Kasahara N, Kan YW. Ligand-directed retroviral targeting of human breast cancer cells. *Proc Natl Acad Sci USA* 1995; 92:9747–9751.

15. Sosnowski BA, Gonzalez AM, Chandler LA, Buechler YJ, Pierce GF, Baird A. Targeting DNA to cells with basic fibroblast growth factor (FGF2). *J Biol Chem* 1996; 271:33647–33653.

16. Goldman CK, Rogers BE, Douglas JT, Sosnowski BA, Ying W, Siegal GP, Baird A, Campain JA, Curiel DT. Targeted gene delivery to Kaposi's sarcoma cells via the fibroblast growth factor receptor. *Cancer Res* 1997; 57:1447–1451.

17. Cotten M, Wagner E. Non-viral approaches to gene therapy. *Curr Opin Biotechnol* 1993; 4:705–710.

18. Sun WH, Burkholder JK, Sun J, Culp J, Turner J, Lu XG, Pugh TD, Ershler WB, Yang NS. In vivo cytokine gene transfer by gene gun reduces tumor growth in mice. *Proc Natl Acad Sci USA* 1995; 92:2889–2893.

19. Rakhmilevich AL, Turner J, Ford MJ, McCabe D, Sun WH, Sondel PM, Grota K, Yang NS. Gene gun-mediated skin transfection with Interleukin 12 gene results in regression of established primary and metastatic murine tumors. *Proc Natl Acad Sci USA* 1996; 93:6291–6296.

20. Curiel DT, Wagner E, Cotten M, Birnstiel ML, Agarwal S, Li CM, Loechel S, Hu PC. High-efficiency gene transfer mediated by adenovirus coupled to DNA–polylysine complexes. *Hum Gene Ther* 1992; 3:147–154.

21. Cristiano RJ, Smith LC, Kay MA, Brinkley BR, Woo SL. Hepatic gene therapy: Efficient gene delivery and expression in primary hepatocytes utilizing a conjugated adenovirus–DNA complex. *Proc Natl Acad Sci USA* 1993; 90:11,548–11,552.

22. Allen TM. Liposomes. Opportunities in drug delivery. *Drugs* 1997; 54(suppl 4):8–14.

23. Farhood H, Gao X, Son K, Yang YY, Lazo JS, Huang L, Barsoum J, Bottega R, Epand RM. Cationic liposomes for direct gene transfer in therapy of cancer and other diseases. *Ann NY Acad Sci* 1994;716:23–34; discussion 34,35.

24. Dass CR, Walker TL, Burton MA, Decruz EE. Enhanced anticancer therapy mediated by specialized liposomes. *J Pharm Pharmacol* 1997; 49:972–975.

25. Zhang WW, Fujiwara T, Grimm EA, Roth JA. Advances in cancer gene therapy. *Adv Pharmacol* 1995; 32:289–341.

26. Wolff JA, Budker V. Cationic lipid-mediated gene transfer. In: Sobol RE, Scanlon KJ, eds. Internet book of gene therapy. Stanford, CT: Appleton & Lange, 1995 65–73.

27. Lane DP. Cancer. p53, guardian of the genome. *Nature* 1992; 358:15,16.

28. Hollstein M, Rice K, Greenblatt MS, Soussi T, Fuchs R, Sorlie T, Hovig E, Smith-Sorensen B, Montesano R, Harris CC. Database of p53 gene somatic mutations in human tumors and cell lines. *Nucleic Acids Res* 1994; 22:3551–3555.

29. Oliner JD, Kinzler KW, Meltzer PS, George DL, Vogelstein B. Amplification of a gene encoding a p53-associated protein in human sarcomas. *Nature* 1992; 358:80–83.

30. Leach FS, Tokino T, Meltzer P, Burrell M, Oliner JD, Smith S, Hill DE, Sidransky D, Kinzler KW, Vogelstein B. *P53* mutation and MDM2 amplification in human soft tissue sarcomas. *Cancer Res* 1993; 53:2231–2234.

31. Sidransky D, Hollstein M. Clinical implications of the p53 gene. *Annu Rev Med* 1996; 47:285–301.

32. Scheffner M, Werness BA, Huibregtse JM, Levine AJ, Howley PM. The E6 oncoprotein encoded by human papillomavirus types 16 and 18 promotes the degradation of p53. *Cell* 1990; 63:1129–1136.

33. Scheffner M, Huibregtse JM, Vierstra RD, Howley PM. The HPV-16 E6 and E6–AP complex functions as a ubiquitin-protein ligase in the ubiquitination of p53. *Cell* 1993; 75:495–505.

34. Harris CC, Hollstein M. Clinical implications of the p53 tumor-suppressor gene. *N Engl J Med* 1993; 329:1318–1327.

35. Harris CC. Structure and function of the p53 tumor suppressor gene: Clues for rational cancer therapeutic strategies. *J Natl Cancer Inst* 1996a; 88:1442–1455.

36. Harris CC. *P53* tumor suppressor gene: From the basic research laboratory to the clinic— An abridged historical perspective. *Carcinogenesis* 1996b; 17:1187–1198.

37. Heimdal K, Lothe RA, Lystad S, Holm R, Fossa SD, Borresen AL. No germline tp53 mutations detected in familial and bilateral testicular cancer. *Genes Chromosom Cancer* 1993; 6:92–97.

38. Wada M, Bartram CR, Nakamura H, Hachiya M, Chen DL, Borenstein J, Miller CW, Ludwig L, Hansen-Hagge TE, Ludwig WD. Analysis of p53 mutations in a large series of lymphoid hematologic malignancies of childhood. *Blood* 1993; 82:3163–3169.

39. Bardeesy N, Falkoff D, Petruzzi MJ, Nowak N, Zabel B, Adam M, Aguiar MC, Grundy P, Shows T, Pelletier J. Anaplastic Wilms' tumour, a subtype displaying poor prognosis, harbours p53 gene mutations. *Nature Genet* 1994; 7:91–97.

40. Faraldi F, Calzolari A, Alfieri E, Mincione GP, Mincione F. Lack of detection of p53 expression in retinoblastoma tumor cells. *Pathologica* 1994; 86:401–402.

41. Malkin D, Sexsmith E, Yeger H, Williams BR, Coppes MS. Mutations of the p53 tumor suppressor gene occur infrequently in Wilms' tumor. *Cancer Res* 1994; 54:2077–2079.

42. Nabeya Y, Loganzo F Jr, Maslak P, Lai L, de Oliveira AR, Schwartz GK, Blundell ML, Altorki NK, Kelsen DP, Albino AP. The mutational status of p53 protein in gastric and esophageal adenocarcinoma cell lines predicts sensitivity to chemotherapeutic agents. *Int J Cancer* 1995; 64:37–46.

43. Ko LJ, Prives C. P53: Puzzle and paradigm. *Genes Dev* 1996; 10:1054–1072.

44. Velculescu VE, El-Deiry WS. Biological and clinical importance of the p53 tumor suppressor gene. *Clin Chem* 1996; 42:858–868.

45. Dameron KM, Volpert OV, Tainsky MA, Bouck N. Control of angiogenesis in fibroblasts by p53 regulation of thrombospondin-1. *Science* 1994; 265:1582–1584.

46. Buckbinder L, Talbott R, Velasco-Miguel S, Takenaka I, Faha B, Seizinger BR, Kley N. Induction of the growth inhibitor IGF-binding protein 3 by p53. *Nature* 1995; 377:646–649.

47. Ueba T, Nosaka T, Takahashi JA, Shibata F, Florkiewicz RZ, Vogelstein B, Oda Y, Kikuchi H, Hatanaka M. Transcriptional regulation of basic fibroblast growth factor gene by p53 in human glioblastoma and hepatocellular carcinoma cells. *Proc Natl Acad Sci USA* 1994; 91:9009–9013.

48. Mukhopadhyay D, Tsiokas L, Sukhatme VP. Wild-Type p53 and v-*src* exert opposing influences on human vascular endothelial growth factor gene expression. *Cancer Res* 1995; 55:6161–6165.

49. Enholm B, Paavonen K, Ristimaki A, Kumar V, Gunji Y, Klefstrom J, Kivinen L, Laiho M, Olofsson B, Joukov V, Eriksson U, Alitalo K. Comparison of VEGF, VEGF-B, VEGF-C and ANG-1 mRNA regulation by serum, growth factors, oncoproteins and hypoxia. *Oncogene* 1997; 14:2475–2483.

50. Volpert OV, Dameron KM, Bouck N. Sequential development of an angiogenic phenotype by human fibroblasts progressing to tumorigenicity. *Oncogene* 1997; 14:1495–1502.

51. Bouvet M, Ellis LM, Nishizaki M, Fujiwara T, Liu W, Bucana CD, Fang B, Lee JJ, Roth JA. Adenovirus-mediated wild-type p53 gene transfer down-regulates vascular endothelial growth factor expression and inhibits angiogenesis in human colon cancer. *Cancer Res* 1998; 58:2288–2292.

52. Yang C, Cirielli C, Capogrossi MC, Passaniti A. Adenovirus-mediated wild-type p53 expression induces apoptosis and suppresses tumorigenesis of prostatic tumor cells. *Cancer Res* 1995; 55:4210–4213.

53. Srivastava S, Katayose D, Tong YA, Craig CR, McLeod DG, Moul JW, Cowan KH, Seth P. Recombinant adenovirus vector expressing wild-type p53 is a potent inhibitor of prostate cancer cell proliferation. *Urology* 1995; 46:843–848.

54. Liu TJ, Zhang WW, Taylor DL, Roth JA, Goepfert H, Clayman GL. Growth suppression of human head and neck cancer cells by the introduction of a wild-type p53 gene via a recombinant adenovirus. *Cancer Res* 1994; 54:3662–3667.

55. Liu TJ, el-Naggar AK, McDonnell TJ, Steck KD, Wang M, Taylor DL, Clayman GL. Apoptosis induction mediated by wild-type p53 adenoviral gene transfer in squamous cell carcinoma of the head and neck. *Cancer Res* 1995; 55:3117–3122.

56. Clayman GL, el-Naggar AK, Roth JA, Zhang WW, Goepfert H, Taylor DL, Liu TJ. In vivo molecular therapy with p53 adenovirus for microscopic residual head and neck squamous carcinoma. *Cancer Res* 1995; 55:1–6.

57. Shaw P, Bovey R, Tardy S, Sahli R, Sordat B, Costa J. Induction of apoptosis by wild-type p53 in a human colon tumor-derived cell line. *Proc Natl Acad Sci USA* 1992; 89:4495–4499.

58. Spitz FR, Nguyen D, Skibber JM, Cusack J, Roth JA, Cristiano RJ. In vivo adenovirus-mediated p53 tumor suppressor gene therapy for colorectal cancer. *Anticancer Res* 1996; 16:3415–3422.

59. Harris MP, Sutjipto S, Wills KN, Hancock W, Cornell D, Johnson DE, Gregory RJ, Shepard HM, Maneval DC. Adenovirus-mediated p53 gene transfer inhibits growth of human tumor cells expressing mutant p53 protein. *Cancer Gene Ther* 1996; 3: 121–130.

60. Hamada K, Alemany R, Zhang WW, Hittelman WN, Lotan R, Roth JA, Mitchell MF. Adenovirus-mediated transfer of a wild-type p53 gene and induction of apoptosis in cervical cancer. *Cancer Res* 1996; 56:3047–3054.

61. Fujiwara T, Grimm EA, Mukhopadhyay T, Cai DW, Owen-Schaub LB, Roth JA. A retroviral wild-type p53 expression vector penetrates human lung cancer spheroids and inhibits growth by inducing apoptosis. *Cancer Res* 1993; 53:4129–4133.

62. Fujiwara T, Grimm EA, Mukhopadhyay T, Zhang WW, Owen-Schaub LB, Roth JA. Induction of chemosensitivity in human lung cancer cells in vivo by adenovirus-mediated transfer of the wild-type p53 gene. *Cancer Res* 1994; 54:2287–2291.

63. Zhang WW, Fang X, Mazur W, French BA, Georges RN, Roth JA. High-efficiency gene transfer and high-level expression of wild-type p53 in human lung cancer cells mediated by recombinant adenovirus. *Cancer Gene Ther* 1994; 1:5–13.

64. Nielsen LL, Maneval DC. P53 tumor suppressor gene therapy for cancer. *Cancer Gene Ther* 1998; 5:52–63.

65. Hsiao M, Tse V, Carmel J, Tsai Y, Felgner PL, Haas M, Silverberg GD. Intracavitary liposome-mediated p53 gene transfer into glioblastoma with endogenous wild-type p53 in vivo results in tumor suppression and long-term survival. *Biochem Biophys. Res Commun* 1997; 233:359–364.

66. Xu M, Kumar D, Srinivas S, Detolla LJ, Yu SF, Stass SA, Mixson AJ. Parenteral gene therapy with p53 inhibits human breast tumors in vivo through a bystander mechanism without evidence of toxicity. *Hum Gene Ther* 1997; 8:177–185.

67. Seung LP, Mauceri HJ, Beckett MA, Hallahan DE, Hellman S, Weichselbaum RR. Genetic radiotherapy overcomes tumor resistance to cytotoxic agents. *Cancer Res* 1995; 55:5561–5565.

68. Donehower LA, Harvey M, Slagle BL, McArthur MJ, Montgomery CA Jr, Butel JS, Bradley A. Mice deficient for p53 are developmentally normal but susceptible to spontaneous tumours. *Nature* 1992; 356:215–221.

69. Kerr JF, Winterford CM, Harmon BV. Apoptosis. its significance in cancer and cancer therapy. *Cancer* 1994; 73:2013–2026.

70. Lowe SW. Cancer therapy and p53. *Curr Opin Oncol* 1995; 7:547–553.

71. Johnson P, Gray D, Mowat M, Benchimol S. Expression of wild-type p53 is not compatible with continued growth of p53-negative tumor cells. *Mol Cell Biol* 1991; 11:1–11.

72. Lowe SW, Bodis S, Bardeesy N, McClatchey A, Remington L, Ruley HE, Fisher DE, Jacks T, Pelletier J, Housman DE. Apoptosis and the prognostic significance of p53 mutation. *Cold Spring Harb Symp Quant Biol* 1994; 59:419–426.

73. Lowe SW, Bodis S, McClatchey A, Remington L, Ruley HE, Fisher DE, Housman DE, Jacks T. P53 status and the efficacy of cancer therapy in vivo. *Science* 1994; 266:807–810.

30

Treatment of p53-Deficient Cancers by Adenovirus E1B-Region Mutants
From Basic Research to the Clinic

David H. Kirn, MD

1. INTRODUCTION

The vast majority of human cancers are incurable once they have become metastatic. Chemotherapy and radiotherapy can induce tumor growth inhibition or regression in some cases, but solid tumor progression and resistance to these standard therapeutic modalities inevitably develop. Further dose escalation to overcome resistance is generally limited by the resultant toxicity to normal tissues. Clearly, new agents with larger therapeutic indices between cancer cells and normal cells are needed. Such agents would have improved efficacy and reduced toxicity as compared with currently available modalities.

Viruses have been used as gene delivery vectors to cause cancer cell inhibition or killing. These viruses have been constructed to deliver tumor suppressor genes, antisense constructs for specific oncogenes, immunostimulatory genes, or drug activating enzymes. A major difficulty with this approach is the daunting goal of delivering genes to every cancer cell in the body. Although local effects on noninfected tumor cells (i.e., bystander effects) might be possible with drug-activating enzyme systems *(1)* or immunostimulatory gene therapy, most approaches to gene therapy will have effects that are limited almost exclusively to cells that are initially infected.

By contrast, a replicating viral therapeutic can overcome this limitation. Viral replication in a small fraction of the tumor cells leads to amplification and spread of the antitumoral effect *(2)*. Cell killing can be attributable to viral replication and cell lysis exclusively, or this could be augmented by including additional immunostimulatory or toxin-producing genes *(3)*. Over the last several decades, there has been an explosion of knowledge in molecular biology. Many viruses have been characterized genetically and the specific gene products responsible for necessary viral functions identified. For example, the genes necessary for control of the cell cycle, pathogenesis, and avoidance of cellular immunity have been identified for a number of viruses. Genetic engineering of viruses is now possible, allowing deletion or augmentation of specific viral functions. The development of virus purification and concentration techniques has facilitated large

From: Signaling Networks and Cell Cycle Control: The Molecular Basis of Cancer and Other Diseases
Edited by: J. S. Gutkind © Humana Press Inc., Totowa, NJ

scale production of high titer purified virus in many cases. The increase in our knowledge of immunology will permit identification of the mechanisms limiting virus efficacy *(4)*. The virus and host mechanisms that modulate the immune response may be modified in order to decrease antiviral immunity, and consequently to enhance efficacy.

2. ADENOVIRUS

Adenoviruses are nonintegrating double-stranded DNA viruses that infect a broad range of human cell types. Infections with human adenoviruses are mild and widespread, with 70–80% of adults having evidence of antibodies directed against adenovirus serotypes 2 or 5, or both, which usually arose during childhood infections. Exposure to wild-type adenovirus can lead to self-limited symptoms, such as upper respiratory tract infection, bronchitis, gastroenteritis, conjunctivitis, and cystitis *(5)*. Other favorable attributes of adenovirus as an oncolytic agent include its well-described genome, its ability to infect both dividing and nondividing cells, and its amenability to high-titer manufacturing and purification *(3)*.

3. PRECLINICAL DEVELOPMENT OF ONYX-015

3.1. Background

p53 is mutated in roughly 50% of all human cancers, including non-small cell lung (60%), colon (50%), breast (40%), head and neck (60%), and ovarian (60%) cancers in the advanced stages *(6–10)*. Loss of p53 function is associated with resistance to chemotherapy or decreased survival, or both, in numerous tumor types, including breast, colon, bladder, ovarian, and non-small cell lung cancers *(7,11)*. Effective therapies for tumors that lack functional p53 are clearly needed.

p53 mediates cell cycle arrest or apoptosis, or both, in response to DNA damage (e.g., due to chemotherapy or radiation) or foreign DNA synthesis (e.g., during viral replication) *(12)*. Consequently, DNA tumor viruses such as adenovirus, SV40, and human papillomavirus (HPV) encode for proteins that inactivate p53, permitting efficient viral replication *(13–15)*. For example, the adenovirus E1B-region 55-kDa protein binds and inactivates p53, in complex with the E4orf6 protein *(14,15)* (Figs. 1 and 2). Theoretically, because p53 is inactivated during efficient viral replication, McCormick et al. hypothesized that an adenovirus lacking E1B 55-kDa gene expression might be severely limited in its ability to replicate in normal cells. Cancer cells that lack p53 function should support viral replication and resultant cell destruction.

3.2. In Vitro Studies With ONYX-015 (dl1520)

ONYX-015 (ONYX Pharmaceuticals, Richmond, CA) is an attenuated adenovirus type 2/5 chimera (dl1520) with two mutations in the early-region E1B 55 kDa gene; this virus was created in the laboratory of Dr. Arnie Berk *(15)*. The cytopathic effects of wild-type adenovirus and ONYX-015 were studied on a pair of cell lines that were identical, except for p53 function: the RKO human colon cancer cell line with normal p53 function (the parental line), and an RKO subclone transfected with dominant-negative p53 (courtesy of Dr. Michael Kastan) *(2,16)* (Fig. 2). As predicted, ONYX-015 induced cytopathic effects similar to wild-type adenovirus in the subclone lacking

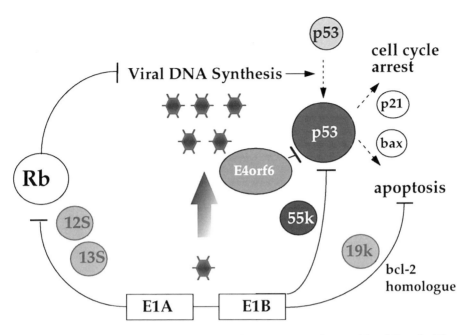

Fig. 1. Interaction of adenovirus early region-1 gene products with pAB and p53.

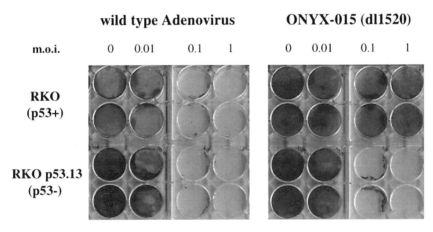

Fig. 2. Enhanced sensitivity of p53(−) tumor cells to ONYX-015 compared to p53(+) tumor cells (m.o.i., multiplicity of infection, is the ratio of infectious virus to cells).

functional p53, whereas cytopathic effects with ONYX-015 were reduced by approximately two orders of magnitude in the parental tumor line harboring normal p53 (Fig. 2). Subsequently, a tumor cell line that was resistant to ONYX-015 because of normal p53 function (U2OS) became sensitive to ONYX-015 after transfection and expression of the E1B 55-kDa gene. Subsequently, separate groups have confirmed these findings in other matched pairs of cell lines, both with and without p53 function (R. Brown and I. Ganley, unpublished data). Therefore, ONYX-015 is able to replicate selectively in p53-deficient cancer cells because of a deletion in the E1B 55-kDa gene.

Subsequent experiments demonstrated that primary (nonimmortalized) human endothelial cells, fibroblasts, small airway cells, and mammary epithelial cells are relatively resistant to ONYX-015 replication and cytolysis, in contrast to effects seen with wild-type adenovirus *(17)*. Replication-dependent cytopathic effects were demonstrated in human tumor cell lines of many different histologies after infection with ONYX-015. Tumor cells that lack p53 function through different mechanisms (p53 gene mutation or deletion, or both, or p53 degradation by HPV E6 protein) were shown to be destroyed by ONYX-015. In addition, several carcinoma lines with normal p53 gene sequence, including two chemotherapy-resistant ovarian cancer subclones, were efficiently lysed *(17)*. Subsequent reports from other groups have confirmed that p53 gene sequence does not predict sensitivity to ONYX-015.

3.3. In Vivo Studies with ONYX-015

ONYX-015 exhibited significant in vivo antitumoral activity against subcutaneous human tumor xenografts in nude mice after intratumoral or intravenous injection; the in vivo efficacy against each tumor type correlated with the in vitro sensitivity of the cell line to ONYX-015. Efficacy against intraperitoneal carcinoma was documented after administration of intraperitoneal virus (C. Heise and D. Kirn, submitted for publication). Owing to the lack of efficient replication in rodent cells, however, immuno-competent (syngeneic) tumor models have not been useful for studying replication-dependent effects. Therefore, the role of the antiviral and antitumoral immune responses may only be determined in cancer patients until a novel model is developed.

4. PRINCIPLES OF ANTITUMORAL EFFICACY WITH REPLICATING VIRUSES

The antitumoral efficacy of replicating viruses can be augmented by several mechanisms. First, we have shown that the intratumoral distribution of ONYX-015 has a significant impact on efficacy. Techniques that lead to enhanced intratumoral distribution will result in improved efficacy. For example, divided dosing is superior to single doses with the same total dose of virus. Increasing the suspension volume in which the virus is administered also improves distribution and consequently efficacy (C. Heise and D. Kirn, submitted for publication).

We have also shown that the efficacy of ONYX-015 can be augmented by combining it with systemic chemotherapeutic agents. Because chemotherapeutic and viral agents have different mechanisms of action and nonoverlapping toxicities, the combination of these agents is attractive. We have documented additive or synergistic effects when combining ONYX-015 with a variety of agents in vitro or in vivo, or both, including 5-fluorouracil (5-FU), cisplatin, taxol, gemcitabine, and irinotecan *(17)* (D. Kirn, unpublished data). Preliminary experiments in nude mouse–human tumor xenografts studied the optimal sequencing of viral and chemotherapeutic treatments. Regimens using simultaneous treatment or virus, followed by chemotherapy, were equivalent; both regimens were superior to chemotherapy, followed by virus. Future studies will attempt to elucidate the mechanism(s) leading to improved efficacy, as well as studying the influence of genetic factors within the tumor on the efficacy seen with combination therapy.

5. CLINICAL DEVELOPMENT OF ONYX-015

5.1. Development Approach

ONYX-015 is a novel agent with a novel mechanism of action. We hypothesized that both toxicity and efficacy would be dependent on the following variables: (1) the intrinsic ability of a given tumor to replicate the virus, (2) the ability of the virus to spread within the tumor microenvironment (e.g., fibrosis secondary to radiation therapy might decrease the efficiency of viral spread), (3) the location of the tumor to be treated (e.g., intracranial vs peripheral), and (4) the route of administration of the virus (e.g., intratumoral, intraperitoneal, or intravascular). In addition, data on viral replication, antiviral immune responses, and their relationship to antitumoral efficacy were critical during the early stages of development.

We therefore elected to treat patients with recurrent head and neck carcinomas initially. The rationale for targeting this population is as follows. These tumors are frequently amenable to direct injection and biopsy in the outpatient clinic setting. p53 abnormalities are very common; gene mutations or deletions are present in up to 70% of recurrent tumors *(10,18)*. Other p53-inactivating mechanisms, such as mdm-2 overexpression and HPV E6 expression, appear to be present in another 15–20% of these tumors *(11)*. Finally, most patients suffer severe morbidity, and even mortality, from the local/regional progression of these tumors. Up to two-thirds of these patients die as a result of local complications *(10)*. Therefore, local therapy might lead to significant palliation, and even to prolonged survival.

5.2. Phase I Trial: Head and Neck Cancer

5.2.1. Trial Design

Patients enrolled onto the phase I trial had recurrent squamous cell carcinoma of the head and neck that was not surgically curable and had failed either prior radiation or chemotherapy *(19,20)*. p53 gene sequence and immunohistochemical staining were determined on all tumors but were not used as entry criteria. Other baseline tests included lymphocyte subsets (CD3, 4, 8), delayed-type hypersensitivity (DTH) skin testing (including mumps and *Candida*), and neutralizing antibodies to ONYX-015. Six patient cohorts received single intratumoral injections of ONYX-015 every 4 wk (until progression) at doses of 10^7–10^{11} plaque-forming units (pfu) per dose. Two additional cohorts received five consecutive daily doses of 10^9 or 10^{10} (total dose 5×10^9 or 5×10^{10}) every 4 wk (multidose cohorts). After treatment, patients were observed for toxicity and for target (injected) tumor response. Additional biological endpoints included changes in neutralizing antibodies, the presence of virus in the blood (PCR d 3 and 8), viral replication within the injected tumor (in tumor biopsies on d 8 and 22), and associated immune cell infiltration.

5.2.2. Trial Results

No significant toxicity was seen in any of the 32 patients treated. Flu-like symptoms were noted in approximately one-half of patients on the single-dose regimen and in two-thirds of patients on the multidose regimen. No toxicity occurred in the adjacent normal tissues. Neutralizing antibodies were positive in approx 70% of cases before treatment. After treatment, all patients had positive antibody titers, and all patients had an increase in antibody titer. Replication was identified infrequently on d 8 tumor biopsies in patients on the single-injection protocol, whereas d 8 biopsies were uniformally positive in evaluable tumor biopsies from patients on the multidose regimen.

Three of the 23 patients on the single dose regimen had partial repressions (PR) of the injected tumor and nine had tumor stabilization (8+ to 16+ wk). In addition, three patients with stable disease had ≥50% necrosis of the injected tumor. By contrast, two of nine patients on the multidose regimen had PR's and an additional five had tumor stabilization (four of whom had significant necrosis); two patients had progressive disease. One patient received seven treatments over 7 mo while maintaining a partial remission. Responding patients included some with positive baseline neutralizing antibodies.

5.3. Phase II Trials: Head and Neck Cancer

5.3.1. Trial Design and Preliminary Results

On the basis of these results, two phase II trials in head and neck cancer patients were initiated. In the first study, ONYX-015 was injected intratumorally for 5 consecutive days (10^{10} pfu/d) in patients with recurrent refractory squamous cell carcinoma of the head and neck. Patients had unresectable tumors that had progressed despite chemotherapy or radiation, or both, after tumor recurrence. p53 sequencing was performed on all tumors. Treatment cycles were repeated every 3 wk. Primary endpoints include the target (injected) tumor regression rate, time to target tumor progression and safety.

Thirty patients were treated. Significant tumor regressions, including complete regressions, have been documented. Final data on the response rate and response duration are unavailable pending final data analysis. Correlations of regression with baseline tumor size, p53 gene sequence, and neutralizing antibody levels will be performed. Mild flu-like symptoms have been seen in most patients. No other toxicity related to ONYX-015 has been seen to date. ONYX-015 has been well tolerated and displays antitumoral activity in refractory recurrent head and neck cancer patients.

5.3.2. Intratumoral Injection Technique

The tumor injection protocol used in phase I was changed slightly for the phase II protocol. Changes in injection technique were made in order to compensate for asymmetric tumor necrosis after ONYX-015 injection in the phase I trial. Some tumors displayed central necrosis, for example, after centralized injections. In order to target ONYX-015 to the advancing, invasive rim of the tumor primarily, injections were initiated near the tumor's edge. Needle tracts were directed out to, and just beyond, the edge into normal tissue, in addition to several centrally directed tracts. These changes in technique resulted in more symmetric tumor shrinkage without central necrosis or toxicity to adjacent normal tissues.

5.3.3. ONYX-015 in Combination With Chemotherapy

In a second phase II trial, patients are being treated simultaneously for 5 d with ONYX-015 intratumorally (as above) and standard chemotherapy intravenously: cisplatin (d 1 bolus) and continuous infusion 5-fu (d 1–5). This is based on preclinical results showing additive efficacy in vivo when ONYX-015, cisplatin, and 5-FU are coadministered *(17)*. These patients are all chemotherapy-naive in the setting of recurrent disease. Thirty evaluable patients have been enrolled, and final data analysis is pending.

5.4. Other Tumor Targets for Clinical Development

Additional local or regional tumor targets include ovarian cancer (phase I intraperitoneal injection trial), pancreatic cancer (phase I intratumoral injection completed), colorectal liver metastases (hepatic arterial infusion trial to be initiated in 1998), superficial recurrent bladder cancer (intravesical administration), and malignant astrocytomas (including glioblastoma multiforme).

6. SUMMARY

Selectively replicating viruses may become a new platform for cancer treatment. If successful in clinical trials, these agents will constitute a new category in the antitumoral armamentarium. Many viruses are currently being studied. An adenovirus (ONYX-015) entered clinical trials in 1996, and herpesvirus agents entered clinical trials in 1998. Critical issues need to be addressed if the clinical value of these agents is to be optimized. For each virus, the effect of antiviral immunity on antitumoral efficacy must be better understood. For all viruses, physical barriers to spread within tumors (e.g., fibrosis, pressure gradients) must be overcome. Although proof of concept experiments with chemotherapy and ONYX-015 has been encouraging, further studies may be required to determine optimal sequencing of the treatment regimen. Combination studies with radiation therapy are also under way with ONYX-015. Finally, modification of these agents may enhance their efficacy against systemic metastases after intravenous administration.

Second-generation virus constructs will be developed on the basis of clinical and preclinical data. Enhanced replication and virulence against tumor cells will be a major goal. The necessary degree of selectivity for tumor cells versus normal cells will depend on the route of administration. Normal tissue will be exposed to much higher doses of virus after intravenous injection than intratumoral injection, for example. Finally, replicating viruses that carry genes encoding prodrug activating enzymes (e.g., cytosine deaminase or thymidine kinase) or immunomodulatory cytokines, for example, have been constructed. This approach will allow the beneficial attributes of gene therapy agents to be combined with the advantages of selectively replicating vectors.

REFERENCES

1. Trinh QT, Austin EA, Murray DM, Knick VC, Huber BE. Enzyme/prodrug gene therapy: Comparison of cytosine deaminase/5-fluorocytosine versus thymidine kinase/ganciclovir enzyme/prodrug systems in a human colorectal carcinoma cell line. *Cancer Res* 1995; 55:4808–4812.
2. Bischoff JR, Kirn DH, Williams A, Heise C, Horn S, Muna M, Ng L, Nye JA, Sampson-Johannes A, Fattaey A, McCormick F. An adenovirus mutant that replicates selectively in p53-deficient human tumor cells *Science* 1996; 274:373–376.
3. Kirn DH. Selectively replicating viral agents for cancer. *Expert Opin Investigational Drugs* 1996; 5:753–762.
4. Zinkernagel RM. Immunology taught by viruses. *Science* 1996; 271:173–178.

5. Ginsberg HS, Prince GA. The molecular basis of adenovirus pathogenesis. *Infect Agents Dis* 1994; 3:1–8.

6. Eliopoulos AG, Kerr DJ, Herod J, Hodgkins L, Krajewski S, Reed JC, Young LS. The control of apoptosis and drug resistance in ovarian cancer: influence of p53 and Bcl-2. *Oncogene* 1995; 11:1217–1228.

7. Bergh J, Norberg T, Sjogren S, Lindgren A. Holmberg L. Complete sequencing of the p53 gene provides prognostic information in breast cancer patients, particularly in relation to adjuvant systemic therapy and radiotherapy. *Nature Med* 1995; 1:1029–1034.

8. Rodrigues NR, Rowan A, Smith ME, Kerr IB, Bodmer WF, Gannon JV, Lane DP. p53 mutations in colorectal cancer. *Proc Natl Acad Sci USA* 1990; 87:7555–7559.

9. Chung KY, Mukhopadhyay T, Kim J, Casson A, Ro JY, Goepfert H, Hong WK, Roth JA. Discordant p53 gene mutations in primary head and neck cancers and corresponding second primary cancers of the upper aerodigestive tract. *Cancer Res* 1993; 53:1676–1683.

10. Boyle JO, Hakim J, Koch W, van der Riet P, Hruban RH, Roa RA, Correo R, Eby YJ, Ruppert JM, Sidransky D. The incidence of p53 mutations increases with progression of head and neck cancer. *Cancer Res* 1993; 53:4477–4480.

11. Chang F, Syrjanen S, Syrjanen K. Demonstration of human papillomavirus (HPV) type 30 in esophageal squamous-cell carcinomas by in situ hybridization [letter]. *J Clin Oncol* 1995; 13:1009–1022.

12. Kastan MB, Onyekwere O, Sidransky D, Vogelstein B, Craig RW. Participation of p53 protein in the cellular response to DNA damage. *Cancer Res* 1991; 51:6304–6311.

13. Scheffner M, Werness BA, Huibregtse JM, Levine AJ, Howley PM. The E6 oncoprotein encoded by human papillomavirus types 16 and 18 promotes the degradation of p53. *Cell* 1990; 63:1129–1136.

14. Dobner T, Horikoshi N, Rubenwolf S, Shenk T. Blockage by adenovirus E4orf6 of transcriptional activation by the p53 tumor suppressor. *Science* 1996; 272:1470–1473.

15. Barker DD, Berk AJ. Adenovirus proteins from both E1B reading frames are required for transformation of rodent cells by viral infection and DNA transfection. *Virology* 1987; 156:107–121.

16. Slichenmyer WJ, Nelson WG, Slebos RJ, Kastan MB. Loss of a p53-associated G1 checkpoint does not decrease cell survival following DNA damage. *Cancer Res* 1993; 53:4164–4169.

17. Heise C, Sampson JA, Williams A, McCormick F, Von HD, Kirn DH. ONYX-015, an E1B gene-attenuated adenovirus, causes tumor-specific cytolysis and antitumoral efficacy that can be augmented by standard chemotherapeutic agents. *Nature Med* 1997; 3:639–645.

18. Brennan JA, Boyle JO, Koch WM, Goodman SN, Hruban RH, Eby YJ, Couch MJ, Forastiere AA, Sidransky D. Molecular assessment of histopathological staging in squamous-cell carcinoma of the head and neck. *N Engl J Med* 1995; 332:712–717.

31

The Cell Cycle Inhibitor p27 as a Prognostic Marker in Human Tumors and a Novel Target for Therapeutic Intervention

Michele Pagano, MD and Katya Ravid, PhD

1. REGULATION OF THE CELL CYCLE BY CYCLIN-DEPENDENT KINASES

The cell cycle in eukaryotic cells has traditionally been divided into two major phases: interphase and mitosis (M phase). Interphase is composed of three subphases: G1, S, and G2. During M phase, the duplicated chromosomes segregate and the cell undergoes cytokinesis, giving rise to two daughter cells. Intracellular components during G1 phase are active in preparing the cells to replicate their genome (during S phase), whereas those of cells in G2 phase prepare the cells for entry into M.

The regulation of the cell division cycle involves a complex network of molecular interactions. Each phase of the cell cycle is controlled by the sequential activation of various cyclin-dependent kinases (Cdks). The rise and fall of Cdk activity are attributable to the synthesis and degradation of positive (cyclins) and negative Cdk inhibitors regulators and to activating and inhibitory phosphorylations. Although more than a dozen distinct cyclin–Cdk complexes exist in mammalian cells, a role in the regulation of the cell cycle has been well documented for only a few: Cdk4 association with D-type cyclins is essential for G1 phase progression; Cdk2 association with cyclin A and cyclin E is essential for the G1 to S transition and for S phase progression (*1,2;* Fig. 1); activity of the mitosis-promoting kinase, Cdkl (also called Cdc2), requires binding to a B-type cyclin *(3).* Because of their stimulatory action on the cell cycle, some cyclins can act as oncogenes *(4).*

The Ckis mediate cell cycle arrest by binding to and inhibiting the activity of Cdks. So far, based on their sequence homology, two families of Ckis have been identified in mammalian cells: the Cip/Kip family, which includes p21, p27, and p57, and the Ink family, which includes p15, p16, p18, and p20 *(5).* Ckis are upregulated in response to various antiproliferative signals such as growth factor deprivation, cytokines, DNA damage, contact inhibition, and lack of adhesion. Because of their negative action on the cell cycle, Ckis have potential roles as tumor suppressors *(4).*

From: Signaling Networks and Cell Cycle Control: The Molecular Basis of Cancer and Other Diseases
Edited by: J. S. Gutkind © Humana Press Inc., Totowa, NJ

2. REGULATION OF THE CELL CYCLE BY p27

The Cki p27 is a potent inhibitor of the Cdk2-cyclin E and Cdk2-cyclin A complexes, which are essential for DNA replication. p27 was identified in extracts derived from G1 cells as an activity able to inhibit Cdk activities in vitro *(6–8)*. The *p27* gene was then cloned by the ability of its protein product to interact with Cdks. It was found to share homology with p21 and, when overexpressed in mammalian cells, to block the cell cycle in G1 *(9,10)*. The p27 protein level and/or its binding to Cdks increase in cells treated with cyclic adenosine monophosphate (cAMP) *(11)*, lovastatin *(7)*, rapamycin *(12)*, or transforming growth factor-β (TGF-β) *(8,13)*, and this increase appears to be involved in the G1 block induced by these agents. Furthermore, p27 has been found to be expressed at high levels in quiescent cells, probably playing an important role in maintaining cells in G0 *(12,14–16)*. Similarly, cell contact and lack of cell adhesion upregulate p27 levels *(8,14,17,18)*. Finally, p27 levels increase in cells undergoing differentiation *(19–21)*. In contrast to the protein, p27 mRNA levels do not change under the conditions listed above. Indeed, cellular abundance of p27 is controlled not by transcription, but at the level of translation *(22)* and degradation *(23)*. The ubiquitin pathway controls the downregulation of p27 that occurs during late G1 (Fig. 1), whereas an increase in mRNA association to the polyribosomes is observed during the induction of differentiation *(24)*, indicating that p27 translation and degradation are regulated by different pathways. Recently, it has been shown that the F-box protein Skp2 functions as the substrate-specific subunits of an ubiquitin ligase enzyme for p27 both in vivo *(25,25a)* and in vitro *(25,25b)*. Recognition of p27 by Skp2 requires phosphorylation of p27 at threonine-187 *(25c)*.

p27-deficient mice develop tumors of the pituitary pars intermedia with 100% penetrance. Because p27$^{-/-}$ cells have shorter and more numerous cell cycles than those of wild-type cells, mutant mice show generalized hyperplasia *(26–28)*. In addition, irradiation or carcinogen treatment induces significantly more tumors in p27$^{-/-}$ and p27$^{+/-}$ than in control mice *(28a)*. This phenotype confirms the importance of p27 in controlling cellular proliferation. Finally, p27 is a target of oncogenes as illustrated by the fact that the adenovirus E1A protein *(29)*, the human papilloma viral (HPV) E7 protein *(30)*, as well as the proto-oncogene c-Myc *(31,32)*, target and inactivate p27 by dissociating it from cyclin–Cdk complexes.

Taken together, these results suggest a role for p27 as a tumor suppressor. However, no structural alterations of the p27 gene and only very rare genetic mutations which do not affect its function have been identified in human tumors *(33–37)*. The following sections review recent studies that show p27 to be a target of oncogenic events that ultimately result in eliminating p27 protein from tumor cells.

3. p27 AS A PROGNOSTIC MARKER
IN HUMAN BREAST CARCINOMAS

Breast cancer is the most common cancer among women in the United States, and its incidence is increasing. It is an important public health problem, considering that the actuarial lifelong risk of breast cancer is approx 1 in 9 women. It is estimated that half a million women will die from breast cancer during the 1990s. According to the

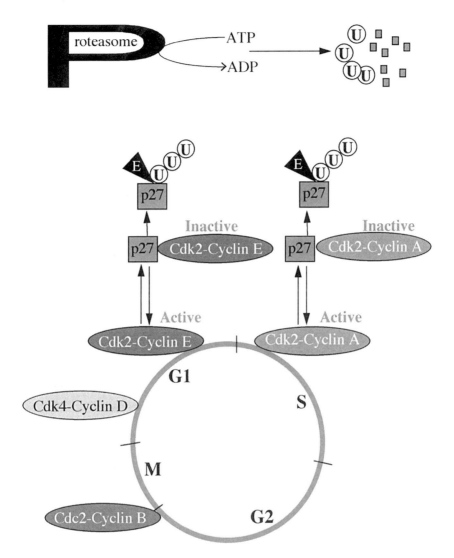

Fig. 1. The cell cycle kinase Cdk2, when bound to specific cyclins (E and A), promotes the G1/S transition and progression through the S phase. p27 is a specific inhibitor of Cdk2-cyclin E and Cdk2-cyclin A complexes. Degradation of p27 by specific ubiquitinating enzymes (E), followed by ubiquitination (U) and targeting to the proteasome (P), frees Cdk2 complexes to promote cell cycle progression. Mitogenic stimuli induce and antimitogenic stimuli inhibit p27 degradation. Enhanced p27 degradation pathway could lead to uncontrolled cellular proliferation.

American Cancer Society (ACS) approx 180,000 cases of breast cancer will be diagnosed in 1998 and 44,000 lives will be lost.

The prognosis of breast cancer after surgical resection depends on pathologic grading and clinical staging. However, with the current staging system, the survival within the different categories ranges substantially. Lymph node involvement remains the only prognostic factor routinely used. However, 30% of lymph node-negative patients will suffer recurrence. No reliable prognostic test has so far been identified that is capable of identifying those lymph node-negative patients who will relapse. In 1988, the National Cancer Institute (NCI) recommended that all lymph node-negative patients undergo adjuvant treatment (e.g., chemotherapy). This means that 70% of lymph node-negative patients are needlessly suffering the debilitating and costly effects of additional therapy, costing the U.S. health care system more than $0.5 billion each year. The need to define which of the node-negative patients could be managed without chemotherapy is therefore urgent.

For historical and pragmatic reasons (i.e., the need of large specimens for surgical pathological diagnosis) much of the available information on breast lesions is derived from tumors >2 cm in diameter, which represent advanced stages of disease. Patients with small primary tumors (≤1 cm in size, T1a,b) have only a 10–20% relapse rate; however, disease relapse almost always leads to death. Traditional prognostic factors (size, presence of metastasis) are, for obvious reasons, less informative in this subset of tumors. In addition, commonly accepted prognostic markers (e.g., p53 and erbB2) do not appear to be of great value in small breast tumors *(38–40)*. Clearly, there is an urgent need to find new molecular markers to identify patients with small primary tumors who are most at risk and therefore need more aggressive treatment. Analysis of gene products by immunohistochemistry provides a potentially rapid and cost-effective prognostic test and may ensure that adjuvant therapy is given to those patients who are most likely to benefit from it.

An impressive body of evidence points to a role for cell cycle regulatory proteins in breast tumorigenesis. This is particularly true for cyclin D1 and cyclin E for two reasons. First, overexpression of an MMTV-cyclin D1 *(41)* or an MMTV-cyclin E *(42)* transgene in female mice induce ductal hyperplasia of the breast and a predisposition to developing breast adenocarcinoma later in life; (2) cyclin D1-deficient mice show severe abnormalities of the mammary gland during pregnancy and lactation *(43,44)*. In addition, *cyclin D1* gene amplification *(45,46)* and cyclin D1 mRNA overexpression in often observed in human breast carcinomas *(45,47,48)* and human breast tumor cell lines *(45,49)*. In addition, cyclin D1 and cyclin E protein overexpression is often detected in human breast cancer *(50–55)*. Notably, the overexpression of cyclin D1 mRNA can distinguish invasive and *in situ* breast carcinomas from nonmalignant lesions *(56)*.

Because it counteracts cyclin action, the Cki p27 plays an important role in the regulation of mammary cell proliferation. Indeed, levels of p27 decrease when breast cancer cells are stimulated to reenter the cell cycle with estradiol treatment *(57)*, whereas they increase when inhibition of cell cycle progression is achieved with anti-estrogens *(58)*. p27 may be an excellent candidate as a molecular prognostic marker for human breast cancer.

Three retrospective immunohistochemical studies have evaluated p27 levels in a total of 648 patients with breast carcinomas (of which 202 were T1a/b, 163 from node-negative patients, and 278 were from premenopausal women) *(55,59,60)*. These studies show that loss or diminished levels of p27 are associated with poor prognosis. By multivariate analysis, p27 was found to be an independent prognostic marker for these tumors. Cancer patients with tumors expressing low levels or lacking p27 had an approximately threefold higher risk of death, as compared with patients with tumors expressing high levels of this protein. More recent studies have shown that as compared with the primary tumors, a further reduction in p27 abundance is often observed in metastatic lymph nodes of breast carcinomas (J. Slingerland, personal communication).

The fact that similar results were obtained from studies performed on three distinct breast cancer patient populations derived from geographically distinct centers, indicates that immunohistochemical assessment of p27 levels is a reproducible assay with considerable potential for routine practical use as a prognostic indicator in breast cancer patients. Interestingly, in all three studies, p27 expression did not correlate with proliferative activity, as measured by expression of cyclin A, PCNA, or KI-67, indicating that lack of p27 is not simply an indicator of increased proliferation.

4. p27 AS A PROGNOSTIC MARKER IN HUMAN COLON CARCINOMA

Despite considerable progress in the elucidation of the molecular mechanisms responsible for colonic malignancies, colorectal cancer remains one of the three most common causes of cancer death in the United States *(61,62)*. The prognosis of colorectal cancer after resection depends on pathologic and clinical staging. Currently, the outlook for resected colorectal carcinoma depends primarily on the analysis of standard clinical and pathological variables *(61)*. However, although predicting outcome in patients with stage I and IV cancer is straightforward, the present staging method creates broad groups of patients within stage II and III whose survival may vary at more than 40% at 5 years *(62)*. Improved predictive value may be derived from evaluating the expression of molecular markers in tumor samples *(63)*.

In a retrospective series of 149 patients with colorectal carcinomas (of which 32 and 65 were in stage I and II, respectively), we have recently shown that p27 is an independent prognostic marker and that lack of p27 (10% of patients) is associated with poor prognosis *(64)*. In fact, as compared with p27 expressors, this group had a 2.88-fold higher risk of dying from stage II colorectal carcinoma. In addition, as compared with high p27 expressors, lack of p27 expression and poor p27 expression are associated with a 32.3- and 12.4-fold increased risk of dying from stage II colorectal carcinomas, respectively. Thus, assessment of p27 expression can be used as an independent prognostic marker for stage II colorectal carcinomas. Furthermore, our study suggests that adjuvant therapy, which benefits patients with stage III cancer, may also be appropriate for patients with stage II disease whose colorectal tumors express little or no p27.

In contrast to what has been observed in several other human tumors, the proliferative state of colorectal carcinomas, assessed by Ki-67 expression *(65)*, flow cytometry *(65)*, and bromodeoxyuridine incorporation *(66)* does not correlate with prognosis. Thus, the prognostic value of p27 expression is not likely to reflect its role as an inhibitor of proliferation.

Several genetic alterations also have prognostic value in patients with colorectal cancers. These include deletion of DCC (deleted in colorectal cancer) gene and the linked allelic loss of chromosome 18q *(67–71)*; mutation/deletion of p53 tumor suppressor gene and the linked allelic loss of chromosome 17p *(72–76)*; mutation of MCC (mutated in colorectal cancer) gene and the linked allelic loss of chromosome 5q *(77,78);* activating mutations of *ras* proto-oncogene *(79,80);* deletion of nm23 gene *(81);* aneuploidy *(82);* microsatellite instability *(83–85);* and fractional allelic loss *(86,87).* However, compared with the evaluation of these other parameters, p27 assessment has the added advantage of being not only rapid and inexpensive, but also easy to perform in the clinical setting, as it is based on a simple immunohistochemical stain in formalin-fixed, paraffin-embedded archival material. In addition, the current availability of automated processors permits fast, direct, and standardized comparison of protein levels from case to case. Finally, p27 yields better prognostic value as compared with disaccharidase sucrase-isomaltase, another colorectal immunohistochemical marker *(88)* (M. Pagano and M. Loda, unpublished results).

5. p27 AS A PROGNOSTIC MARKER IN OTHER HUMAN CANCERS

p27 has been implicated as a powerful prognostic marker in several human cancers. It has been shown that loss of p27 is an independent prognostic marker in gastric nonsmall-cell lung *(89),* and prostate *(90,91)* carcinomas and in Barrett's associated adenocarcinomas of the esophagus *(92).* Another study has shown low p27 expression in benign and malignant endocrine neoplasms as compared with normal endocrine tissues *(93).* Interestingly, whereas adenomas and hyperplastic tissues expressed similar Ki-67 levels, the latter tissues had threefold more p27-positive cells than adenomas, suggesting that p27 evaluation may be useful in distinguishing between these two conditions.

6. THE UBIQUITIN PATHWAY AND CANCER

The activity of a Cdk–cyclin complex is regulated both by phosphorylation events *(94)* and by a controlled degradation of cyclins and Ckis via the ubiquitin-proteasome pathway *(95).* This latter process represents the major nonlysosomal proteolytic pathway which controls the timed destruction of cellular regulatory proteins, including the Cki p27, the tumor suppressor p53, the cyclins, the proto-oncogenes c-Myc, c-Jun, c-Fos, and the transcription factors NF-κB and E2F.

Ubiquitin is a 76-amino acid polypeptide that is abundantly present in all eukaryotic cells. Substrates recognized by the proteasome pathway are marked by the covalent binding of a chain of ubiquitin molecules. Conjugation of ubiquitin to substrate proteins requires adenosine triphosphate (ATP) and the involvement of a ubiquitin-activating enzyme (E1), a ubiquitin-conjugating enzyme (E2 or Ubc), and a ubiquitin-ligase (E3). Both E2 and E3 proteins exist as large families, different combinations of E2s with E3 proteins are thought to define the substrate specificity *(96).*

Is the ubiquitin–proteasome pathway altered in cancer? Untimely disruption of cell cycle regulatory proteins may result in deregulated proliferation typical of cancer cells. Carcinoma cells with low or absent p27 protein displayed enhanced proteolytic activity specific for p27 *(64),* suggesting that low p27 expression in these tumors results from enhanced proteasome-mediated degradation rather than diminished gene/protein expression. A deregulation of the ubiquitin–proteasome-mediated degradation of other negative (e.g., p53) and positive (e.g., cyclins, β-catenin) regulators of proliferation has also been correlated with tumorigenesis (reviewed in refs. *95,97,98*). Thus, aggressive tumors may result through selection of cells that (1) lack tumor suppressor proteins because of an increase in their ubiquitin-mediated degradation; and/or (2) overexpress oncogenic proteins because of a decrease in their ubiquitin-mediated degradation.

7. CONCLUDING REMARKS

Acting through its function as a Cdk inhibitor, p27 may have an important role as a tumor suppressor. However, unlike many well-known tumor suppressors, such as p53 and p16, the *p27* gene does not appear to be a frequent target for inactivating mutations. Still, levels of p27 protein have been found reduced or absent in a variety of tumor types. Indeed, studies reviewed here have shown that examination of p27 protein levels by simple immunohistochemistry is able to provide independent prognostic information for neoplasias of the breast, colon, stomach, lung, prostate, and esophagus. Furthermore, recent evidence suggests that low levels of p27 in these tumors may result from specific alterations in the degradation of the protein by the ubiquitin-proteasome pathway.

These recent findings should stimulate new strategies for therapeutic intervention. For example, a drug capable of inhibiting p27 degradation should result in a block to proliferation, especially in tumors in which a loss of p27 is a result of enhanced activity of the ubiquitin-proteasome pathway. Such a drug may be designed (1) to inhibit the specific ubiquitin ligase, yet to be identified, which selectively targets p27 for degradation; and (2) to block the specific binding site within p27, which may be essential for its recognition by the ubiquitin proteasome pathway. It is hoped that modulation of the p27 degradation process may lead to improved therapeutic control over several human cancers.

ACKNOWLEDGMENTS

We thank Massimo Loda and Elizabeth Newcomb for critically reading the manuscript. We apologize to colleagues whose work has not been cited, or cited indirectly through other articles, owing to space limitations. M.P. is in part supported by the grants CA66229-02 and CA57587-01 from the National Institutes of Health. K.R., an Established Investigator with the American Heart Association, is in part supported by an grants HL58547 and HL53080 from the National Institutes of Health.

REFERENCES

1. Dutta A. The cell cycle, in *Results and Problems in Cell Differentiation,* (Pagano M, ed), Springer-Verlag, Berlin, 1998; pp. 33–56.
2. Sheaff RJ, Roberts J. The cell cycle, in *Results and Problems in Cell Differentiation* (Pagano M, ed), Springer-Verlag, 1998; pp. 1–34.
3. Pines J. The cell cycle, in *Results and Problems in Cell Differentiation* (Pagano M, eds), Springer-Verlag, Berlin, 1998; pp. 57–78.
4. Sherr C. Cancer cell cycles. *Science* 1996; 274:1672–1677.
5. Sherr C, Roberts J. Inhibitors of mammalian G1 cyclin-dependent kinases. *Genes Dev* 1995; 9:1149–1163.
6. Hengst L, Dulic V, Slingerland J, Lees E, Reed S. A cell cycle regulated inhibitor of cyclin-dependent kinases. *Proc Natl Acad Sci USA* 1994; 91:5291–5295.
7. Slingerland J, Hengst L, Pan C, Alexander D, Stampfer M, Reed S. A novel inhibitor

of cyclin-Cdk activity detected in TGFβ-arrested epitehelial cells. *Mol Cell Biol* 1994; 14:3683–3694.

8. Polyak K, Kato M, Solomon MJ, Sherr CJ, Massague J, Roberts JM, Koff A. p27[Kip1], a cyclin-Cdk inhibitor, links TGF-β and contact inhibition to cell cycle arrest. *Genes Dev* 1994; 8:9–22.

9. Polyak K, Lee M, Erdjement-Bromage H, Koff A, Roberts J, Tempst P, Massague J. Cloning of p27[kip1], a cyclin-dependent kinase inhibitor and a potential mediator of extracellular antimitogenic signals. *Cell* 1994; 79:59–66.

10. Toyoshima H, Hunter T. p27, a novel inhibitor of G1-cyclin-cdk protein kinase activity, is related to p21. *Cell* 1994; 78:67–74.

11. Kato J, Matsuoka M, Polyak K, Massague J, Sherr CJ. Cyclic AMP-induced G1 phase arrest mediated by an inhibitor (p27[kip1]) of cyclin-dependent kinase-4 activation. *Cell* 1994; 79:487–496.

12. Nourse J, Firpo E, Flanagan M, Coats S, Polyak C, Lee M, Massague J, Crabtree G, Roberts J. Interleukin-2-mediated elimination of p27Kip1 cyclin-dependent kinase inhibitor prevented by rapamycin. *Nature* 1994; 372:570–573.

13. Reynisdottir I, Polyak K, Iavarone A, Massague J. Kip/cip and Ink4 Cdk inhibitors cooperate to induce cell cycle arrest in response to TGF-beta. *Genes Dev* 199; 9;1831–1845.

14. Fang F, Orend G, Watanabe N, Hunter T, Ruoslahti E. Dependence of cyclin E-CDK2 kinase activity on cell anchorage. *Science* 1996; 271:499–502.

15. Firpo EJ, Koff A, Solomon M, Roberts J. Inactivation of a Cdk2 inhibitor during interleukin 2-induced proliferation of human T lymphocytes. *Mol Cell Biol* 1994; 14: 4889–4901.

16. Pagano M, Beer-Romero P, Glass S, Tam S, Theodoras A, Rolfe M, Draetta G. Targeting ubiquitin-mediated degradation for proliferation inhibitors, in *Cancer Genes: Functional Aspects,* Vol 7 (Mihich E, Housman D, eds), Plenum, New York, 1996; pp. 241–254.

17. Croix B, Florenes V, Rak J, Flanagan M, Bhattacharya N, Slingerland J, Kerbel R. Impact of the cylin-dependent kinasee inhibitor p27 on adhesion-dependent resistance of tumor cells to anticancer agents. *Nature Med* 1996; 2:1204–1210.

18. Schulze A, Zerfass-Thome K, Berges J, Middendorp S, Jansen-Durr P, Henglein B. Anchorage-dependent transcription of the cyclin A gene. *Mol Cell Biol* 1996; 16:4632–4638.

19. Halevy O, Novitch B, Spicer D, Skapek S, Rhee J, Hannon G, Beach D, Lassar A. Correlation of terminal cell cycle arrest of skeletal muscle with induction of p21 by MyoD. *Science* 1995; 267:1018–1021.

20. Kranenburg O, Scharnhorst V, Van der Eb A, Zantema A. Inhibition of Cyclin-dependent kinase activity triggers neuronal differntiation of mouse neuroblastoma cells. *J Cell Biol* 1995; 131:227–234.

21. Liu M, Lee M, Cohen M, Bommakanti M, LF. Transcriptional activation of the Cdk inhibitor p21 by vitamin D3 leads to the induced differentiation of the myelomonocytic cell line U937. *Genes Dev* 1996; 10:142–153.

22. Hengst L, Reed S. Translation control of p27[Kip1] accumulation during the cell cycle. *Science* 1996; 271:1861–1864.

23. Pagano M, Tam SW, Theodoras AM, Romero-Beer P, Del Sal G, Chau V, Yew R, Draetta G, Rolfe M. Role of the ubiquitin-proteasome pathway in regulating abundance of the cyclin-dependent kinase inhibitor p27. *Science* 1995; 269:682–685.

24. Millard S, Yan J, Nguyen H, Pagano M, Kiyokawa H, Koff A. Enhanced ribosomal association of p27 mRNA is a mechanism contributing to accumulation during growth arrest. *J Biol Chem* 1997; 272:7093–7098.

25. Carrano AC, Eytan E, Hershko A, Pagano M. Skp2 is required for the ubiquitin-mediated degradation of the Cdk-inhibitor p27. *Nature Cell Biol* 1999; 1:193–199.

25a. Sutterlüty H, Chatelain E, Marti A, Wirbelauer C, Senften M, Müller U, Krek W. p45 SKP2 promotes p27 Kip1 degradation and induces S phase in quiescent cells. *Nature Cell Biol* 1999; 1:207–214.

25b. Tsvetkov LM, Yeh KH, Lee S, Sun H, Zhang H. p27Kip1 ubiquitination and degradation is regulated by the SCFSkp2 complex through phosphorylated Thr187 in p27. *Current Biology* 1999; 661–664.

25c. Montagnoli A, Fiore F, Eytan E, Carrano C, Draetta G, Hershko A, Pagano M. Ubiquitination of p27 is regulated by Cdk-dependent phosphorylation and trimeric complex formation. *Genes & Development* 1999; 13:1181–1189.

26. Fero M, Rivkin M, Tasch M, Porter P, Carow C, Firpo E, Tsai L, Broudy V, Perlmutter R, Kaushansky K, Roberts J. A syndrome of muti-organ hyperplasia with features of gigantism, tumorigenesis and female sterility in p27[Kip1]-deficient mice. *Cell* 1996;85:733–744.

27. Kiyokawa H, Kineman R, Manova-Todorova K, Soares V, Hoffman E, Onoi M, Hayday A, Frohman D, Koff A. Enhancehd growth of mice lacking the cyclin-dependent kinase inhibitor function of p27Kip1. *Cell* 1996; 85:721–732.

28. Nakayama K, Ishida N, Shirane M, Inomata A, Inoue T, Shishido NIH, Loh D. Nakayama K. Mice lacking p27 disply inceased body size, multiple organ hyperplasia, retinal dysplasia, and pituitary tumors. *Cell* 1996; 85:707–720.

28a. Fero ML, Randel E, Gurley KE, Roberts JM, Kemp CJ. The murine gene p27Kip1 is haplo-insufficient for tumour suppression. *Nature* 1998; 396:177–180.

29. Mal A, Poon R, Howe P, Toyoshima H, Hunter T, Harter, M. Inactivation of p27kip1 by the viral E1A oncoprotein in TGFβ-treated cells. *Nature* 1996; 380:262–265.

30. Zerfass K, Zwerschke W, Mannhardt B, Tindle R, Botz J, Jansen-Dürr P. Inactivation of the cdk inhibitor p27[Kip1] by the human papillomavirus 16 E7 oncoprotein. *Oncogene* 1996; 13:2323–2330.

31. Steiner P, Philipp A, Lukas J, D, G-K, Pagano M, Mittnacht S, Bartek J, Eilers M. Identification of a Myc-dependent step during the assembly of active cyclin/cdk complexes. *EMBO J* 1995; 14:4814–4826.

32. Vlach J, Hennecke S, Amati B. Phosphorylation-dependent of the cyclin-dependent kinase inhibitor p27Kip1. *EMBO J* 1997; 16:5334–5344.

33. Kawamat AN, Morosetti R, Miller C, Park D, Spirin K, Nakamaki T, Takeuchi S, Hatta Y, Simpson J, Wilczynski S, Lee Y, Bartram C, Koeffler H. Molecular analysis of the cyclin-dependent kinase inhibitor gene p27/kip1 in human malignancies. *Cancer Res* 1995; 55:2266–2269.

34. Pietenpol J, Bohlander S, Sato Y, Papadopoulos N, Liu B, Friedman C, Trask B, Roberts J, Kinzler K, Rowley J, Vogelstein B. Assignment of the human *p27[Kip1]* gene to 12p13 and its analysis in leukemias. *Cancer Res* 1995; 55:1206–1210.

35. Ponce-Castañeda V, Lee M, Latres E, Polyak K, Lacombe L, Montgomery K, Mathew S, Krauter K, Sheinfeld J, Massague J, Cordon-Cardo C. *p27[Kip1]*: Chromosomal mapping to 12p12–12p13.1 and absence of mutations in human tumors. *Cancer Res* 1995; 55:1211–1214.

36. Spirin K, Simpson J, Tacheuchi S, Kawamata N, Miller C, Koeffler H. p27/Kip1 mutation found in breast cancer. *Cancer Res* 1996; 56:2400–2404.

37. Stegmaier K, Takeuchi S, Golub T, Bhohlander S, Bartram C, Koeffler P, Gilliland G. Mutational analysis of the candidate tumor suppressor genes Tel and Kip1 in childhood acute lymphoblastic leukemia. *Cancer Res* 1996; 56:1413–1417.

38. Porter-Jordan K, Lippman M. Overview of the biologic markers of breast cancer. *Hematol Oncol Clin North Am* 1994; 8:73–100.

39. Shackney S, Pollice A, Smith C, Alston L, Singh S, Janocko L, Brown K, Petruolo S, Groft D, Yakulis R, Hartsock R. The accumulation of multiple genetic abnormalities in individual tumor cells in human breast cancers: Clinical prognostic implications. *Cancer J Sci Am* 1996; 2:106–119.

40. Shackney S, Shankey T. Common patterns of genetic evolution in human solid tumors. *Cytometry* 1997; 29:1–27.

41. Wang TC, Cardiff RD, Zukerberg L, Lees E, Arnold A, Schmidt EV. Mammary hyperplasia and carcinoma in MMTV-cyclin D1 transgenic mice. *Nature* 1994; 369:669–671.

42. Bortner DM, Rosenberg MP. Induction of mammary gland hyperplasia and carcinomas in transgenic mice expressing human cyclin E. *Mol Cell Biol* 1997; 17:453–459.

43. Fantl V, Stamp G, Andrews A, Rosewell I, Dickson C. Mice lacking cyclin D1 are small and show defects in eye and mammary gland development. *Genes Dev* 1995; 9:2364–2372.

44. Sicinski P, Donaher J, Parker S, Li T, Fazeli A, Gardner H, Haslam S, Bronson R, Elledge S, Weinberg R. Cyclin D1 provides a link between development and oncogenesis in the retina and breast. *Cell* 1995; 82:621–630.

45. Lammie G, Fantl V, Smith R, Schuuring E, Brookes S, Michalides R, Dickson C, Arnold A, Peters G. D11S287, a putative oncogene on chromosome 11q13, is amplified and expressed in squamous cell and mammary carcinimas and linked to BCL-1. *Oncogene* 1991; 6:439–444.

46. Schuuring E, Verhoeven E, van Tinteren H, Peterse J, Nunnink B, Thunnissen F, Devilee P, Cornelisse C, van de Vijver M, Mooi W, Michalides R. Amplification of genes within the chromosome 11q13 region is indicative of poor prognosis in patients with operable breast cancer. *Cancer Res* 1992; 52:5229–5234.

47. Jiang W, Kahan S, Tomita N, Zhang Y, Lu S, Weinstein B. Amplification and expression of the human cyclin D gene in esophageal cancer. *Cancer Res* 1992; 52:2980–2983.

48. Rosenberg CL, Motokura T, Kronenberg HM, Arnold A. Coding sequence of the overexpressed transcript of the putative oncogene PRAD1/cyclin D1 in two primary human tumors. *Oncogene* 1993; 8:519–521.

49. Seto M, Yamamoto K, Iida S, Akao Y, Utsumi KR, Kubonishi I, Miyoshi I, Ohtsuki T, Yawata Y, Namba M, Motokura T, Arnold A, Takahashi T, Ueda, R. Gene rearrangement and overexpression of PRAD1 in lymphoid malignancy with t(11;14)(q13;q32)translocation. *Oncogene* 1992; 7:1401–1406.

50. Bartkova J, Lukas J, Muller H, Lutzhoft D, Strauss M, Bartek J. Cyclin D1 protein expression and function in human breast cancers. *Int J Cancer* 1994; 57:353–361.

51. Buckley MF, Sweeney KJE, Hamilton JA, Sini RL, Manning DL, Nicholson RI, deFazio A, Watts CKW, AME, Sutherland RL. Expression and amplification of cyclin genes in human breast cancer. *Oncogene* 1993; 8:2127–2133.

52. Dutta A, Chandra R, Leiter L, Lester S. Cyclins as markers of tumor proliferation: Immunocytochemical studies in breast cancer. *Proc Natl Acad Sci USA* 1995; 92:5386–5390.

53. Keyomarsi K, Pardee A. Redundant cyclin overexpression and gene amplification in breast cancer cells. *Proc Natl Acad Sci USA* 1993; 90:1112–1116.

54. Keyomarsi K, Pardee A. Cyclin E—A better prognostic marker for breast cancer than Cyclin D? *Nature Med* 1996; 2:254.

55. Porter P, Malone K, Heagerty P, Alexander G, Gatti L, Firpo EJ, Daling J, Roberts J. Expression of cell-cycle regulators p27Kip1 and Cyclin E, alone and in combination, correlate with survival in young breast cancer patients. *Nature Med* 1997; 3:222–225.

56. Weinstat-Saslow D, Merino M, Manrow R, Lawrence J, Bluth R, Wittenbel K, Simpson J, Page D, Steeg P. Overexpression of cyclin D1 mRNA distinguishes inavasive and *in situ* breast carcinomas from non-malignant lesions. *Nature Med* 1995; 1:1257–1260.

57. Foster J, Wimalasena J. Estrogen regulates activity of cyclin-dependent kinases and retinoblastoma protein phosphorylation in breast cancer cells. *Mol Endocrinol* 10: 488–496.

58. Watts CKW, Brady A, Sarcevic B, deFazio A, Sutherland, RL. Antiestrogens inhibition of cell cycle progression in breast cancer cells is associated with inhibition of cyclin-dependent kinase activity and decreased retinoblastoma protein phosphorylation. *Mol Endocrinol* 1996; 9:1804–1813.

59. Catzavelos C, Bhattacharya N, Ung Y, Wilson J, Roncari L, Sandhu C, Shaw P, Yeger H, Morava-Protzner I, Kapusta L, Franssen E, Pritchard K, Slingerland J. Decreased levels

of the cell-cycle inhibitor p27Kip1 protein: Prognostic implications in primary breast cancer. *Nature Med* 1997; 3:227–230.

60. Tan P, Cady B, Wanner M, Worland P, Cukor B, Fiorentino M, Magi-Galluzzi C, Lavin P, Pagano M, Loda M. The cell cycle inhibitor p27 is an independent prognostic marker in small (T1a,b) invasive breast carcinomas. *Cancer Res* 1997; 57:1259–1263.

61. Deans G, Parks T, Rowlands B, Spence R. Prognostic factors in coloreactal cancer. *Br J Surg* 1992; 79:608–613.

62. Statement CDC Adjuvant therapy for patients with colon and rectal cancers. *JAMA* 1990; 264:1444–1450.

62. Cancer AJCO. *Manual for Staging of Cancer,* 4th ed, JB Lippincott, Philadelphia, 1993.

63. Vogelstein B, Fearon E, Hamilton S. Genetic alteration during colorectal tumor development. *N Engl J Med* 1988; 319:525–532.

64. Loda M, Cukor B, Tam S, Lavin P, Fiorentino M, Draetta G, Jessup J, Pagano M. Increased proteasome-dependent degradation of teh cyclin-dependent kinase inhibitor p27 in aggressive colorectal carcinomas. *Nature Med* 1997; 3:231–234.

65. Sahin A, Brown R, Ordonez N, Cleary K, el-Naggar A, Wilson P, Ayala A. Assesment of Ki-67-derived tumor proliferative activity in colorectal adenocarcinomas. *Mod Pathol* 1994; 7:17–22.

66. Risio M, Coverlizza S, Ferrari A, Candelaresi G, Rossini S. Immunohistochemical study of epithelial cell proliferation in hyperplastic polyps, adenomas, and adenocarcinomas of the large bowel. *Gastroenterology* 1988; 94:899–906.

67. Fearon E, Cho K, Nigro J. Identification of a chromosome 18q gene that is altered in colorectal cancers. *Science* 1990; 247:49–56.

68. Hedrick L, Cho K, Vogelstein B. Cell adhesion molecules as tumour suppressors. *Trends Cell Biol* 1993; 3:36–39.

69. Jen J, Kim H, Piantadosi S, Liu Z, Levitt R, Sistonen P, Kinzler K, Vogelstein B, Hamilton S. Allelic loss of chromosome 18q and progression in colorectal cancer. *N Engl J Med* 1994; 331:213–221.

70. Nigam A, Savage F, Boulos P, Stamp G, Liu D, Pignatelli M. Loss of cell–cell and cell–matrix adhesion molecules in colorectal cancer. *Br J Cancer* 1993; 68:507–514.

71. Wielenga V, Heider K, Offerhaus G. Expression of CD44 variant proteins in human colorectal cancer is related to tumor progression. *Cancer Res* 1993; 53:4754–4756.

72. Baas I, Mulder J, Offerhaus G, Vogelstein B, Hamilton S. An evaluation of six antibodies for immunohistochemistry of mutant p53 gene product in archival colorectal neoplasms. *J Pathol* 1994; 172:5–12.

73. Baker SJ, Fearon ER, Nigro JM, Hamilton SR, Preisinger AC, Jessup JM, VanTuinen P, Ledbetter DH, Barker DF, Nakamura Y, White R, Vogelstein B. Chromosome 17 deletions and p53 gene mutations in colorectal carcinomas. *Science* 1989; 244:217–221.

74. Hamelin R, Laurent-Puig P, Olschwang S. Association of *p53* mutations with short survival in colorectal cancer. *Gastroenterology* 1994; 106:42–48.

75. Harris C, Hollstein M. Clinical implications of the *p53* tumor-suppressor gene. *N Engl J Med* 1993; 329:1318–1327.

76. Nigro J, Baker S, Preisinger A. Mutations in the p53 gene occur in diverse human tumour types. *Nature* 1989; 342:705–708.

77. Groden J, Thliveris A, Samowitz W, Carlson M, Gelbert L, Albertsen H, Joslyn G, Stevens J, Spirio L, Robertson M, et al. Identification and characterization of the familial adenomatous polyposis coli gene. *Cell* 1991; 66:589–600.

78. Kinzler K, Nilbert M, Su L, Vogelstein B, Bryan T, Levy D, Smith KAP, Hedge P, McKechnie D, et al. Identification of FAP locus genes from chromosome 5q21. *Science* 1991; 253:661–665.

79. Bell S, Scott N, Cross D. Prognostic value of p53 overexpression and c-Ki-*ras* gene mutations in colorectal cancer. *Gastroenterology* 1993; 104:57–64.

80. Finkelstein S, Sayegh R, Bakker A, Swalsky, P. Determination of tumor aggressiveness in colorectal cancer by K-*ras*-2 analysis. *Arch Surg* 1993; 128:526–532.

81. Cohn K, Wang F, DeSoto-LaPaix F. Association of *nm23*-H1 allelic deletions with distant metastases in colorectal carcinoma. *Lancet* 1991; 338:722–724.

82. Jass J, Mukawa K, Goh H, Love S, Capellaro D. Clinical importance of DNA content in rectal cancer measured by flow cytometry. *J Clin Pathol* 1989; 42:254–259.

83. Kim H, Jen J, Vogelstein B, Hamilton SR. Clinical and pathologiccal characteristics of sporadic colorectal carcinomas with DNA replication errors in microsatellite sequences. *Am J Pathol* 1994; 145:146–156.

84. Liu B, Parson R, Papadopulos N, Nicolaides N, Lynch H, Watson P, Jass, J, Dunlop M, Wyllie A, De La Chapelle A, Hamilton S, Volgestein B, Kinzler K. Analysis of mismatch repair genes in hereditary non-polyposis colorectal cancer patients. Nature Med 1996; 2:169–174.

85. Thibodeau S, Bren G, Schaid D. Microsatellite instability in cancer of the proximal cancer. *Science* 1993; 260:816–819.

86. Offerhaus G, De Feyter E, Cornelisse C. The relationship of DNA aneuploidy to molecular genetic alterations in colorectal carcinoma. *Gastroenterology* 102:1612–1619.

87. Vogelstein B, Fearon E, Kern S. Allelotype of colorectal carcinomas. *Science* 1989; 244:207–211.

88. Jessup J, Lavin PT, Andrews CJ, Loda M, Mercurio A, Minsky B, Mies C, Cukor B, Bleday R, Steele GJ. Sucrase-Isomaltase is an independent prognostic market for colorectal cancer. *Dis Colon Rectum* 1995; 38:1257–1264.

89. Mori M, Mimori K, Shiraishi T, Tanaka S, Ueo H, Sugimachi K, Akiyosji T. p27 expression and gastric carcinoma. *Nature Med* 1997; 3:593.

89. Esposito V, Baldi A, DeLuca A, Sgaramella G, Giordano GG, Caputi M, Baldi F, Pagano M, Giordano A. Prognostic role of the cell cycle inhibitor p27 in non small cell lung cancer. *Cancer Res* 1997; 57:3381–3385.

90. Tsihlias J, Kapusta L, Morava-Protzner I, Bhattacharya N, Catzavelos C, Klotz L, Slinger-land J. Loss of Cdk inhibitor p27 is a novel prognostic factor in localized human prostate adenocarcinoma. *Cancer Res* 1998; 58:542–548.

91. Yang R, Naitoh J, Philpson J, Wang H, Loda M, Reiter R. Low levels of p27 protein expression predict poor desease-free survival in patients with pathological T2a-T3b adeno-carcinomas of the prostate. *J Urol* 1998; 159:941–945.

92. Singh S, Lipman J, Goldman H, Ellis FH Jr, Aizenman L, Cangi MG, Signoretti S, Chaur DS, Pagano M, M. Loda, M. Loss or altered subcellular localization of p27 in Barret's associated adenocarcinoma. *Cancer Res* 1998; 58:1730–1735.

93. Lloyd CW, Pearce KJ, Rawlins DJ, Ridge RW, Shaw PJ. Endoplasmic microtubules connect the advancing nucleus to the tip of legume root hairs, but f-actin is involved in basipetal migration. *Cell Motil* 1987; 8:27–36.

94. Solomon MJ, Kaldis P. Cell cycle control, in *Results and Problems in Cell Differentiation* (Pagano M, ed), Vol 22, Springer-Verlag, Berlin, 79–110.

95. Pagano M. Regulation of cell cycle regulatory proteins by the ubiquitin pathway. *FASEB J* 1997; 11:1067–1075.

96. Rolfe M, Chiu I, Pagano M. The ubiquitiin-mediated proteolytic pathway as a therapeutic aerea. *J Mol Med* 1997; 75:5–17.

97. Brown J, Pagano M. The mechanism of p53 degradation. *Biochim Biophys Acta* 1997; 1332:1–6.

98. Peifer M. β-Catenin as oncogene: The smoking gun. *Science* 1997; 275:1752, 1753.

32

Chemical Cyclin-Dependent Kinase Inhibitors

Therapeutic Implications

Edward A. Sausville, MD, PhD
and Adrian M. Senderowicz, MD

1. INTRODUCTION

As reviewed in other chapters of this book, the regulation of the eukaryotic cell cycle machinery is closely controlled by proteins whose levels of expression vary (cyclins) and that serve as activators of a unique family of protein kinases, by catalytic subunits (cyclin-dependent kinases [CDKs]), by endogenous CDK inhibitors (CKI), and by posttranslational modifications of these complexes *(1–3)*. An abnormality in any component of this machinery could lead to deregulation in proper cell cycle progression, abnormal cell proliferation, and ultimately disease *(3)*.

Several disease entities are known to be associated with aberrations in cell cycle regulation. Theoretically, the use of cyclin-dependent kinase modulators in these diseases could potentially have a therapeutic role. Examples of non-neoplastic diseases entities that fit this description include angiogenic processses, such as diabetic retinopathy and coronary atherosclerosis/restenosis after coronary angioplasty *(4,5)*, and neurodegenerative diseases such as Alzheimer's disease, where brain tissues recovered from afflicted patients demonstrate abnormality in expression of cell cycle-related proteins *(6,7)*. Moreover, in in vitro models, the use of inhibitors of CDKs was able to prevent neuronal cell apoptosis secondary to growth factor deprivation *(8)*. Abnormal cellular proliferation and expression of cyclins or CDKs have also been observed in experimental models of glomerulopathies and renal tubule regeneration *(9,10)*. Again, inhibitors of CDK1 and CDK2 prevented the development of experimental proliferative glomerulonephritis *(11)*, substantiating a potentially therapeutic role for CDKs in these diseases. Other disease entities in which aberrant cell proliferation and abnormal expression of cell cycle-related proteins are observed are inflammatory disorders, psoriasis, degenerative muscle disorders, and pulmonary fibrosis, among others *(12–15)*.

Neoplastic diseases represent the most readily recognized and numerically significant category of disorders with alteration on cell-cycle control *(3,16–18)*. It has been known for decades that neoplastic cells have intrinsic derangements in the progression of the normal cell cycle *(16,19)*. In contrast to normal cells, tumor cells are unable to stop

From: Signaling Networks and Cell Cycle Control: The Molecular Basis of Cancer and Other Diseases
Edited by: J. S. Gutkind © Humana Press Inc., Totowa, NJ

at predetermined points of the cell cycle, so-called checkpoints. These delays or pauses in the cell cycle are necessary to verify the integrity of the genome before cells advance to the next phase *(20,21)*. With the discovery of the function of oncogenes and tumor suppressor genes, it was evident that tumor cells frequently acquire either mutations or deletions in those genes important to tumorigenesis. Some of these regulatory genes are necessary to regulate these checkpoints. Specifically, most, if not all, tumor types have an abnormality in some component of the retinoblastoma gene product (Rb) pathway, including CDK4 or CDK6, cyclin D1, D2, D3, and Rb *(3,22)*. As a consequence of these cell cycle alterations, tumor cells are able to transverse the S phase of the cell cycle, in a way that ignores growth factor signals, because of a lack of G1 checkpoints *(3)*. Certainly, specific inhibitors of the Rb pathway, including CDK4 or CDK6, could prevent cells from entering S phase, inducing cell cycle arrest with consequent beneficial antiproliferative effect *(23,24)*. In cells that have bypassed the necessity for these G1 kinases *(25)*, the development of CDK2 inhibitors could alternatively act efficiently to prevent S phase progression *(26,27)*. Another strategy to develop antiproliferative drugs with altered potential CDK regulation as targets would be to abrogate the remaining intact cell cycle checkpoints with small molecules *(28)*. Thus, the abrogation of intact checkpoints could induce the inappropriate acceleration of certain phases of the cell cycle, including premature mitosis, in the case of G2 checkpoint abrogation, with consequent apoptosis. The last strategy is of particular interest in sensitizing cells to agents that would normally cause pause or arrest in G2. In either case, modulators of the cyclin-dependent kinases are unique novel targets for cancer chemotherapy.

We can classify the available chemical CDK inhibitors into two groups. The first are the classic direct chemical inhibitors that directly interact with the CDK holoenzyme. Examples include flavopiridol congeners, polysulfates, butyrolactone I, 9-hydroxyellipticine, toyocamycin derivatives, and purine derivatives. This chapter focuses on this group. The second group is composed of agents that indirectly downregulate the activity of the CDKs by interacting with upstream pathways necessary for CDK activation or interaction with proteins/cofactors necessary for the catalytic activity of these enzymes. There is a long list of agents with these properties, including vitamin D3 and its analogs, rapamycin and lovastatin, among others *(29–31)*. Moreover, we could include in this latter group the endogenous CDK inhibitors (CKIs) such as p21, p16, and p27 that interact with components of the CDK complex resulting in CDK inhibition *(17)*. Intense efforts are being undertaken to introduce these CKIs into tumor tissues to induce local cell cycle arrest and apoptosis *(32)*. The results of these efforts are still too premature to draw any conclusions.

2. BIOCHEMICAL PROPERTIES OF CDK INHIBITORS

Chemical (small molecule) CDK inhibitors (CDKI) can be subdivided into seven families (Fig. 1): (1) purine derivatives (isopentenyladenine, 6-dimethyl aminopurine, olomucine, roscovitine, and CVT-313), (2) butyrolactone I, (3) flavopiridols (flavopiridol and deschloroflavopiridol), (4) staurosporines (staurosporine and UCN-01), (5) toyocamycin, (6) 9-hydroxyellipticine, and (7) polysulfates (suramin). Not all CDKI are specific to CDKs; staurosporine, UCN-01, suramin, 6-dimethylaminopurine, and

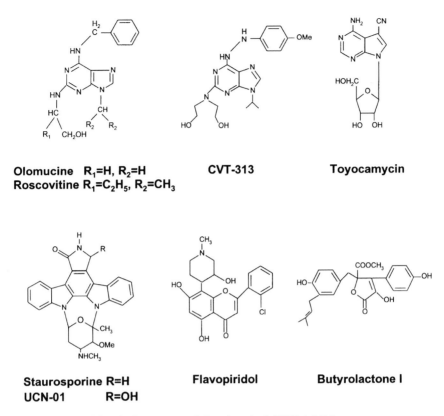

Olomucine   R₁=H, R₂=H
Roscovitine R₁=C₂H₅, R₂=CH₃   CVT-313   Toyocamycin

Staurosporine R=H   Flavopiridol   Butyrolactone I
UCN-01   R=OH

Fig. 1. Structures of the chemical CDK inhibitors.

isopentenyladenine are relatively nonspecific protein kinase inhibitors. By contrast, flavopiridol, butyrolactone I, olomucine, roscovitine, and CVT-313 are more selective for CDKs. Actually, butyrolactone I, olomucine, roscovitine, and CVT-313 are very specific for CDK1 and 2, with relative inactivity against CDK4 and CDK6. By contrast, flavopiridol showed similar activity against all CDKs tested so far (A. Senderowicz, unpublished results) *(26,33)*. The degree of selectivity of toyocamycin and 9-hydroxyellipticine has not yet been defined *(34)*.

2.1. Olomucine, Roscovitine, and Derivatives

The first CDK inhibitor discovered was dimethylaminopurine *(35)*. This compound was initially shown to inhibit cell cycle progression in embryos. Later, it was identified as an inhibitor of CDK1 (p34^{cdc2}) (IC$_{50}$ = 120 μM) *(34)*. Subsequent studies showed it to be relatively nonspecific. Isopentenyladenine, a derivative of this compound, was somewhat more potent and specific for the CDKs (IC$_{50}$: 55 μM) *(36)*. Other purine structures were obtained after intense screening to obtain more specific and potent CDK inhibitors. Olomucine displayed a potent ability to inhibit CDK1 and CDK2 (IC$_{50}$ = 7 nM) *(36,34)*. Roscovitine, an even more potent CDK inhibitor (IC$_{50}$ values for CDK1/CDK2 = 0.7 μM), was derived from the olomucine structure *(34)*. When the crystal structure of CDK2 in complex with isopentenyladenine, olomucine, or roscovitine were resolved, it was clear that all three inhibitors can bind to the ATP site *(37,38)*. Finally, CVT-313, a novel purine analog, was obtained using a combinatorial library strategy and knowledge of the crystal structure of CDK2. Similar to the previous analogs, CVT-313 was specific for CDK1 and CDK2 with IC_{50} values of 4.2 and 1.5 μM respectively *(39)*.

As expected for compounds that inhibit CDK1 and CDK2, exposure of cells to purine inhibitors induced G1 and/or G2/M arrest *(27,39,40)*. Interestingly, the antiproliferative effect was accompanied, in the case of olomucine and roscovitine, by the induction of apoptosis *(8,27)*. No immediate clinical trials are planned with these compounds, but they serve as important tools in dissecting cellular effects caused by CDK action.

2.2. Butyrolactone I

Butyrolactone I compound was originally identified from *Aspergillus terreus* var. *africans*. It inhibits CDKs with IC_{50} of 0.6–1.5 μM for CDK1 and CDK2, respectively *(41)*. Not only is this compound specific for CDKs, but it is completely inactive against CDK4 *(34,42)*. Butyrolactone I inhibits CDK2 in a manner competitive with ATP *(41)*. It has modestly potent antiproliferative activity against a panel of human lung carcinoma cell lines, with an IC_{50} of 20–80 μM *(43)*. Butyrolactone I induced a prominent G2/M block, concordant with the compounds' potent CDK1 inhibition *(43)*. In the HL-60 cell line, butyrolactone induced apoptosis at concentrations within the ~60-μM range, similar to concentrations required for CDK inhibition *(44)*. There is no recorded intent of clinical trials with this agent.

2.3. Flavopiridol

Flavopiridol, also known as L86-8275, is a semisynthetic flavonoid derived from rohitukine, an alkaloid isolated from a plant indigenous to India *(24)*. In initial studies, flavopiridol was found to be a potent in vitro EGF receptor tyrosine kinase (EGFR) and protein kinase A (PKA) inhibitor (IC_{50}-21 and 122 μM, respectively) *(24)*. However, when the compound was tested in the NCl 60 cell line anticancer drug screen panel, the IC_{50} for growth inhibition was 66 nM, approx 1000 times lower than the concentration required to inhibit PKA and EGFR *(24,45)*.

Moreover, the antiproliferative effect did not correlate with the presence of EGFR *(45)*. Further studies in our laboratory demonstrated that flavopiridol could induce cell cycle arrest during either G1 or G2/M. When MDA-MB 468 cells were synchronized at G2/M with nocodazole and released into media containing either vehicle or flavopiridol, there was evidence of flavopiridol-induced G1 arrest. If the same MDA-MB 468 cells were synchronized at the G1/S boundary with aphidocolin, flavopiridol-treated cells were arrested in G2/M, concordant with the ability of flavopiridol to inhibit both CDK2 and CDK1, respectively *(26,33,45)*.

MDA-MB 468 cells treated with flavopiridol showed a decrease in immunoprecipitated CDK1 H1 kinase activity, reflecting CDK1 activity. In addition, a decline in tyrosine and threonine phosphorylation in CDK1 immunoprecipitates was observed at same time points, suggesting functional CDK1 inactivation *(46)*. Further studies using purified CDKs showed that flavopiridol inhibits CDK 1, 2, and 4 in a competitive manner with respect to ATP, with a K_i value of 41 nM *(26,33)*. When the crystal structure of deschloroflavopiridol and CDK2 was resolved, it was evident that flavopiridol binds to the ATP binding pocket, with the benzopyran occupying the same region as the purina ring of ATP *(47)*. This observation was concordant with our prior biochemical studies with the compound *(26,33)*. Flavopiridol inhibits the CDKs examined thus far (IC$_{50}$ ~100 n*M*) *(26,33)*. For CDK7 (CDK-activating kinase), potency is somewhat diminished (IC$_{50}$ ~300 n*M*) *(23)*.

Another aspect of the cell cycle regulatory properties of flavopiridol is the downregulation of cyclin D1 protein levels in several tumor cell lines *(48)*. This decline occurred within 3 h of exposure and was not accompanied by shortening cyclin D1 protein half-life. No other G1 cyclin (D2, D3, or E) appeared to be decreased at the same time points. Cyclin D1 mRNA steady-state levels declined within 2 h of treatment with flavopiridol. In summary, flavopiridol could induce cell cycle arrest by at least three different mechanisms: first, by the direct inhibition of CDKs, competitive with respect with ATP; second, by preventing necessary threonine phosphorylation of CDKs; and finally, in the case of the G1, by downregulation of cyclin D1, an important cofactor for CDK4 and CDK6 activation. The relationship of this last activity to CDK effects is unknown and is the subject of ongoing experiments.

Another feature of the action of flavopiridol is the induction of apoptosis in several tumor cell lines *(49,50)*. In one example, susceptibility to apoptosis by flavopiridol varied depending on the growth state of the cells. Thus, postmitotic nondividing PC-12 cells were protected from apoptosis-induced by nerve growth factor (NGF) deprivation by the presence of flavopiridol or olomucine. By contrast, cycling PC-12 cells were not protected from NGF withdrawal but actually were induced to undergo apoptosis after exposure to flavopiridol *(8)*. The specific mechanism(s) for flavopiridol-induced apoptosis is still unknown. There is evidence that in some systems neither BCL-2/ BAX nor p53 pathways are involved *(49)*, whereas in other systems bcl-2 is downregulated *(51)*. When flavopiridol was tested in head and neck cell lines, it showed notable cell cycle arrest/apoptosis in all cell lines tested, including a cell line (HN30) that was refractory to XRT and bleomycin. Moreover, this effect was independent of p53 status and was also associated with depletion of cyclin D1 *(52)*.

Based on the notable activity observed in lymphoid xenografts when flavopiridol was administered intraperitoneally route every day for 5 d for only one cycle *(53)*, we used a similar schedule using a refractory head and neck xenograft with mutated p53 (HN12 cell line). Significant antitumor activity sustained for at least 10 wk was observed after only one cycle of flavopiridol. Tumor tissues obtained from these animals showed not only frank apoptosis but specific cyclin D1 depletion as well *(52)*. Moreover, when flavopiridol is combined with standard chemotherapeutic agents, there is evidence of synergistic cytotoxic effects *(54,55)*.

Initial phase I clinical trials in humans were recently completed and are be discussed below.

2.4. Staurosporine/ UCN-01

Staurosporine is a nonspecific protein kinase inhibitor that shows cell cycle arrest in transformed and nontransformed cells at 1–100 n*M* *(56)*. At similar concentrations, staurosporine has the capacity to inhibit CDK1 *(36,57)*. In order to increase the specificity of staurosporine, several analogs have been synthesized or isolated from natural product sources. One of them, UCN-01 (7-hydroxystaurosporine), has potent activity against several PKC isoenzymes *(58)*, similarly to staurosporine. In addition to the effects on PKC, UCN-01 shows prominent effects on cell cycle and antiproliferative activity in several human tumor cell lines *(59)*. By contrast, another highly selective potent PKC inhibitor, GF 109203X shows no potent antiproliferative effect despite similar capacity to inhibit PKC. Taken together, these results suggest that the antiproliferative effect of UCN-01 is not explained solely by inhibition of PKC. In seeking to define the mechanism(s) for cell cycle arrest, UCN-01 displayed moderately potent inhibition of immunoprecipitated CDK1 and CDK2 (IC_{50}-300–600 n*M*), and caused inappropriate activation of the same kinases in tissue culture cells *(59)*. These observations were concordant with the parallel observation that UCN-01 abrogated the G2 checkpoint after DNA damage (γ irradiation) again caused by CDK1 inappropriate activation *(28)*. Preliminary data showed that this effect was accompanied by CDK1 tyrosine dephosphorylation, which was evident at lower concentrations than the concentrations required to inhibit the CDKs in vitro *(59,60)*. Thus, UCN-01 directly inhibits CDKs, but in cells more potently affects their upstream regulation by action on targets that remain to be defined.

2.5. Other CDK Inhibitors

Suramin inhibits the p34^{cdc2} kinase (CDK1) *(61)*. Many nuclear enzymes and protein kinases are also inhibited by suramin at similar concentration *(62)*. Clinical trials with this agent have demonstrated marginal activity in patients with refractory prostate cancer *(63,64)*. During screening of soil microrganisms for in vitro CDK1 and CDK2 kinase inhibition, *Streptomyces* sp. LPL931 was found to have potent CDK1 and CDK2 inhibitory activity *(65)*. When purified, the compound was identical to toyocamycin, a nucleoside analog with antiviral and antiproliferative activity in mammalian cells. Moreover, toyocamycin is able to inhibit multiple protein kinases at high micromolar concentration *(65)*. Toyocamycin effects on other CDKs are still unknown. Likewise, the specificity of 9-hydroxyellipticine *(66)*, another CDK inhibitor, is unknown *(34)*.

3. CLINICAL EXPERIENCE WITH CDK INHIBITORS

3.1. Flavopiridol Phase I Clinical Trial

Flavopiridol has good antitumor activity in several tumor xenografts (e.g., colon and prostate cancer) *(24)*, especially with protracted schedules of drug exposure. Based on these encouraging preclinical data, two clinical trials of flavopiridol have recently been completed *(67,68)*. Flavopiridol was administered by a 72-h continuous infusion. Seventy-six patients were treated in the National Cancer Institute (NCI) phase I trial of infusional flavopiridol. Dose-limiting toxicity (DLT) was secretory diarrhea, maximal tolerated dose (MTD), 50 mg/m^2/d × 3. Patients receiving more than 50 mg/m^2/d × 3 received antidiarrhea prophylaxis. This allowed a second MTD of 78 mg/m^2/d × 3 to be defined. The dose-limiting toxicity at the higher dose level consisted of reversible hypotension and a significant pro-inflammatory syndrome. No myelotoxicity was observed. Some patients, particularly those with with non-Hodgkin's lymphoma, colon, prostate and kidney cancer may have experienced clinical benefit. Moreover, 14 patients received flavopiridol for more than 6 mo without evidence of tumor progression, including one patient with refractory renal cancer who achieved a partial response (shrinkage of >50% masses); five patients who received flavopiridol for more than 1 yr and one patient who received flavopiridol for more than 2 yr. This potential for disease stabilization noted in this trial is concordant with the preclinical models, in which tumor stasis was observed.

Appropriate metrics of cytostatic effect is necessary to confirm that CDK inhibition might be relatable to this clinical outcome. Plasma flavopiridol concentrations of 300–500 nM, effective to inhibit CDK in vitro were safely achieved during our trial *(67)*. Efforts to determine whether these concentrations induced CDK inhibition in tissues from patients in this trial are being undertaken.

In a complementary phase I trial also exploring the use of a 72-h continuous infusion, Thomas et al. *(68)* found that the DLT is diarrhea, as demonstrated in the NCl experience. Moreover, plasma flavopiridol concentrations of 300–500 nM were also observed.

Phase II trials in patients with non-Hodgkin's lymphoma, colon, prostate, and kidney cancer, among others, and phase I trials with novel schedules are warranted *(49,53)*.

3.2. UCN-01 Phase I Clinical Trial

Based on the antitumor activity observed in preclinical models and unique mechanism of action, we began a phase I trial of infusional UCN-01 in patients with refractory neoplasms. At this writing, 26 patients have been treated with UCN-01. Unique clinical features observed in this initial human experience included an unexpectedly prolonged half-life (~30 d), 100 times longer than the half-life observed in preclinical models, probably because of very avid plasma protein binding *(69,70)*. This has resulted in a relative lack of myelotoxicity or gastrointestinal toxicity, prominent side effects observed in animal models, despite very high plasma concentrations achieved (~50 μM) *(71)*. Poorly defined muscle toxicity, characterized by muscle cramps in the lower extremities, has also been observed. MTD of UCN-01 is yet to be achieved.

In summary, several chemical CDK inhibitors have been discovered or developed during the last decade. Two inhibitors, flavopiridol and UCN-01, are being tested in early phase clinical trials. In the near future, great efforts will be expanded to define novel specific CDK inhibitors (e.g., specific CDK4 or CDK6 inhibitors). These compounds will be potentially useful in a variety of different clinical settings where abnormal proliferation is seen, besides cancer. These compounds will allow us to test the hypothesis that restoration of a "more normal" cell cycle regulation in human disease is possible. It is hoped that they will convey benefit to all patients with diseases of cell cycle regulation.

REFERENCES

1. Morgan DO. Principles of CDK regulation. *Nature* 1995; 374:131–134.
2. Pines J. Cyclins and cyclin-dependent kinases: A biochemical view. *Biochem J* 1995; 308:697–711.
3. Sherr CJ. Cancer cell cycles. *Science* 1996; 274:1672–1677.
4. Wei GL, Krasinski K, Kearney M, Isner JM, Walsh K, Andres V. Temporally and spatially coordinated expression of cell cycle regulatory factors after angioplasty. *Circ Res* 1997; 80:418–426.
5. Yang ZY, Simari RD, Perkins ND, San H, Gordon D, Nabel GJ, Nabel EG. Role of the p21 cyclin-dependent kinase inhibitor in limiting intimal cell proliferation in response to arterial injury. *Proc Natl Acad Sci USA* 1996; 93:7905–7910.
6. McShea A, Harris PL, Webster KR, Wahl AF, Smith MA. Abnormal expression of the cell

cycle regulators P16 and CDK4 in Alzheimer's disease. *Am J Pathol* 1997; 150:1933–1939.

7. Liu WK, Williams RT, Hall FL, Dickson DW, Yen SH. Detection of a Cdc2-related kinase associated with Alzheimer paired helical filaments. *Am J Pathol* 1995; 146:228–238.

8. Park DS, Farinelli SE, Greene LA. Inhibitors of cyclin-dependent kinases promote survival of post-mitotic neuronally differentiated PC12 cells and sympathetic neurons. *J Biol Chem* 1996; 271:8161–8169.

9. Park SK, Kang SK, Lee DY, Kang MJ, Kim SH, Koh GY. Temporal expressions of cyclins and cyclin dependent kinases during renal development and compensatory growth. *Kidney Int* 1997; 51:762–769.

10. Shankland SJ, Hugo C, Coats SR, Nangaku M, Pichler RH, Gordon KL, Pippin J, Roberts JM, Couser WG, Johnson RJ. Changes in cell-cycle protein expression during experimental mesangial proliferative glomerulonephritis. *Kidney Int* 1996; 50:1230–1239.

11. Pippin JW, Qu Q, Meijer L, Shankland SJ. Direct in vivo inhibition of the nuclear cell cycle cascade in experimental mesangial proliferative glomerulonephritis with Roscovitine, a novel cyclin-dependent kinase antagonist. *J Clin Invest* 1997; 100:2512–2520.

12. Sugiyama M, Tsukazaki T, Yonekura A, Matsuzaki S, Yamashita S, Iwasaki K. Localisation of apoptosis and expression of apoptosis related proteins in the synovium of patients with rheumatoid arthritis. *Ann Rheum Dis* 1996; 55:442–449.

13. Chilosi M, Doglioni C, Menestrina F, Lestani M, Piazzola E, Benedetti A, Pedron S, Montagna L, Pizzolo G, Mariuzzi GM, Janossy G. Expression of extracellular matrix molecules, proliferation markers and cyclin-dependent kinase inhibitors in inflamed tissues. *Biochem Soc Trans* 1997; 25:524–8.

14. Inohara S, Kitano Y. Immunohistochemical detection of cyclin D and cyclin A in human hyperproliferative epidermis. *Arch Dermatol Res* 1994; 288:504–506.

15. Gadbois DM, Lehnert BE. Cell cycle response to DNA damage differs in bronchial epithelial cells and lung fibroblasts. *Cancer Res* 1997; 57:3174–3179.

16. Hartwell LH, Kastan MB. Cell cycle control and cancer. *Science* 1994; 266:1821–1828.

17. Harper J, Elledge S. Cdk inhibitors in development and cancer. *Curr Opin Genet Dev* 1996; 6:56–64.

18. Cordon-Cardo C. Mutations of cell cycle regulators. Biological and clinical implications for human neoplasia. *Am J Pathol* 1995; 147:545–560.

19. Pardee S. A restriction point for control of normal animal cell proliferation. *Proc Natl Acad Sci USA* 1974; 71:1286–1290.

20. Elledge SJ. Cell cycle checkpoints: Preventing an identity crisis. *Science* 1996; 274:1664–1672.

21. Paulovich A, Toczyski D, Hartwell L. When checkpoints fail. *Cell* 1997; 88:315–321.

22. Hirama T, Koeffler H. Role of the cyclin-dependent kinase inhibitors in the development of cancer. *Blood* 1995; 86:841–854.

23. Carlson B, Pearlstein R, Naik R, Sedlacek H, Sausville E, Worland P. Inhibition of CDK2, CDK4 and CDK7 by flavopiridol and structural analogs. *Proc Am Assoc Cancer Res* 1996;

24. Sedlacek HH, Czech J, Naik R, Kaur G, Worland P, Losiewicz M, Parker B, Carlson B, Smith A, Senderowicz A, Sausville E. Flavopiridol (L86-8275, NSC-649890), a new kinase inhibitor for tumor therapy. *Int J Oncol* 1996; 9:1143–1168.

25. Lukas J, Bartkova J, Rohde M, Strauss M, Bartek J. Cyclin D1 is dispensable for G1 control in retinoblastoma gene-deficient cells independently of cdk4 activity. *Mol Cell Biol* 1995; 15:2600–2611.

26. Carlson BA, Dubay MM, Sausville EA, Brizuela L, Worland PJ. Flavopiridol induces G1 arrest with inhibition of cyclin-dependent kinase (CDK) 2 and CDK4 in human breast carcinoma cells. *Cancer Res* 1996; 56:2973–2978.

27. Meijer L, Borgne A, Mulner O, Chong JP, Blow JJ, Inagaki N, Inagaki M, Delcros JG,

Moulinoux JP. Biochemical and cellular effects of roscovitine, a potent and selective inhibitor of the cyclin-dependent kinases cdc2, cdk2 and cdk5. *Eur J Biochem* 1997; 243:527–536.

28. Wang Q, Fan S, Eastman A, Worland PJ, Sausville EA, O'Connor P. UCN-01: a potent abrogator of G2 checkpoint function in cancer cells with disrupted p53. *J Natl Cancer Inst* 1996; 88:956–965.

29. Morice WG, Wiederrecht G, Brunn GJ, Siekierka JJ, Abraham RT. Rapamycin inhibition of interleukin-2-dependent p33cdk2 and p34cdc2 kinase activation in T lymphocytes. *J Biol Chem* 1993; 268:22,737–22,745.

30. Wang QM, Jones JB, Studzinski GP. Cyclin-dependent kinase inhibitor p27 as a mediator of the G1-S phase block induced by 1,25-dihydroxyvitamin D3 in HL60 cells. *Cancer Res* 1996; 56:264–267.

31. Keyomarsi K, Sandoval L, Band V, Pardee AB. Synchronization of tumor and normal cells from G1 to multiple cell cycles by lovastatin. *Cancer Res* 1991; 51:3602–3609.

32. Roth JA, Cristiano RJ. Gene therapy for cancer: What have we done and where are we going? *J Natl Cancer Inst* 1997; 89:21–39.

33. Losiewicz MD, Carlson BA, Kaur G, Sausville EA, Worland PJ. Potent inhibition of CDC2 kinase activity by the flavonoid L86-8275. *Biochem Biophys Res Commun* 1994; 201:589–595.

34. Meijer L, Kim SH. Chemical inhibitors of cyclin-dependent kinases. *Methods Enzymol* 1997; 283:113–128.

35. Meijer L, Pondaven P. Cyclic activation of histone H1 kinase during sea urchin egg mitotic divisions. *Exp Cell Res* 1988; 174:116–129.

36. Rialet V, Meijer L. A new screening test for antimitotic compounds using the universal M phase-specific protein kinase, p34^{CDC2}/cyclin Bcdc13, affinity-immobilized on p13suc1-coated microtitration plates. *Anticancer Res* 1991; 11:1581–1590.

37. Schulze-Gahmen U, Brandsen J, Jones HD, Morgan DO, Meijer L, Vesely J, Kim SH. Multiple modes of ligand recognition: Crystal structures of cyclin-dependent protein kinase 2 in complex with ATP and two inhibitors, olomoucine and isopentenyladenine. *Proteins* 1995; 22:378–391.

38. De Azevedo WF, Leclerc S, Meijer L, Havlicek L, Strnad M, Kim SH. Inhibition of cyclin-dependent kinases by purine analogues: Crystal structure of human cdk2 complexed with roscovitine. *Eur J Biochem* 1997; 243:518–526.

39. Brooks EE, Gray NS, Joly A, Kerwar SS, Lum R, Mackman RL, Norman TC, Rosete J, Rowe M, Schow SR, Schultz PG, Wang X, Wick MM, Shiffman D. CVT-313, a specific and potent inhibitor of CDK2 that prevents neointimal proliferation. *J Biol Chem* 1997; 272:29,207–29,211.

40. Buquet-Fagot C, Lallemand F, Montagne M, Mester J. Effects of olomucine, a selective inhibitor of cyclin-dependent kinases, on cell cycle progression in human cancer cell lines. *Anticancer Drugs* 1997; 8:623–631.

41. Kitagawa M, Okabe T, Ogino H, Matsumoto H, Suzuki-Takahashi I, Kokubo T, Higashi H, Saitoh S, Taya Y, Yasuda H, et al. Butyrolactone I, a selective inhibitor of cdk2 and cdc2 kiness. *Oncogene* 1993; 8:2425–2432.

42. Kitagawa M, Higashi H, Takahashi IS, Okabe T, Ogino H, Taya Y, Hishimura S, Okuyama A. A cyclin-dependent kinase inhibitor, butyrolactone I, inhibits phosphorylation of RB protein and cell cycle progression. *Oncogene* 1994; 9:2549–2557.

43. Nishio K, Ishida T, Arioka H, Kurokawa H, Fukuoka K, Nomoto T, Fukumoto H, Yokote H, Saijo N. Antitumor effects of butyrolactone I, a selective cdc2 kinuse inhibitor, on human lung cancer cell lines. *Anticancer Res* 1996; 16:3387–3395.

44. Shibata Y, Nishimura S, Okuyama A, Nakamura T. p53-independent induction of apoptosis by cyclin-dependent kinase inhibition. *Cell Growth Diff* 1996; 7:887–891.

45. Kaur G, Stetler-Stevenson M, Sabers S, Worland P, Sedlacek H, Myers C, Czech J, Naik

R, Sausville E. Growth inhibition with reversible cell cycle arrest of carcinoma cells by flavone L86-8275. *J Natl Cancer Inst* 1992; 84:1736–1740.

46. Worland PJ, Kaur G, Stetler-Stevenson M, Sebers S, Sartor O, Sausville EA. Alteration of the phosphorylation state of p34cdc2 kinase by the flavone L86-8275 in breast carcinoma cells. Correlation with decreased H1 kinase activity. *Biochem Pharmacol* 1993; 46:1831–1840.

47. De Azevedo, WF Jr, Mueller-Dieckmann HJ, Schulze-Gahmen U, Worland PJ, Sausville E, Kim SH. Structural basis for specificity and potency of a flavonoid inhibitor of human CDK2, a cell cycle kinase. *Proc Natl Acad Sci USA* 1996; 93:2735–2740.

48. Carlson B, Lahusen T, Singh S, Loaiza-Perez A, Worland PJ, Restell R, Albanese C, Sausville EA, Senderowicz AM. Down regulation of cyclin D1 by transcriptional repression in MCF-7 human breast carcinoma cells induced by flavopiridol. *Cancer Res* 1999; 59:4634–4641.

49. Parker B, Kaur GA, Nieves-Neira W, Taimi M, Kolhagen G, Shimizu T, Pommier Y, Sausville E, Senderowicz AM. Early induction of apoptosis in hematopoietic cell lines after exposure to flavopiridol. *Blood* 1998; 91:458–465.

50. Bible KC, Kaufmann SH. Flavopiridol: A cytotoxic flavone that induces cell death in noncycling A549 human lung carcinoma cells. *Cancer Res* 1996; 56:4856–4861.

51. Konig A, Schwartz GK, Mohammad RM, Al-Katib A, Gabrilove JL. The novel cyclin-dependent kinase inhibitor flavopiridol downregulates Bcl-2, and induces growth arrest and apoptosis in chronic B-cell leukemia lines. *Blood* 1997; 90:4307–4312.

52. Patel V, Senderowicz AM, Pinto DJ, Igishi T, Ensley JF, Sausville EA, Gutkind JS. Flavopiridol, a novel cyclin-dependent kinase inhibitor prevents the growth of head and neck squamous cell carcinomas by inducing apoptosis. *J Clin Inves* 1998; 58:3248–3353.

53. Arguello F, Alexander M, Sterry J, Tudor G, Smith E, Kalavar N, Greene J, Koss W, Morgan D, Stinson S, Siford T, Alvord W, Labansky R, Sausville E. Flavopiridol induces apoptosis of normal lymphoid cells, causes immunosuppression, and has potent antitumor activity in vivo against human and leukemia xenografts. *Blood* 1998; 91:2482–2490.

54. Bible KC, Kaufmann SH. Cytotoxic synergy between flavopiridol (NSC 649890, L86-8275) and various antineoplastic agents: The importance of sequence of administration. *Cancer Res* 1997; 57:3375–3380.

55. Schwartz G, Farsi K, Maslak P, Kelsen D, Spriggs D. Potentiation of apoptosis by flavopiridol in mitomycin-C-treated gastric and breast cancer cells. *Clin Cancer Res* 1997; 3:1467–1472.

56. Crissman HA, Gadbois DM, Tobey RA, Bradbury EM. Transformed mammalian cells are deficient in kinase-mediated control of progression through the G1 phase of the cell cycle. *Proc Natl Acad Sci USA* 1991; 88:7580–7584.

57. Gadbois DM, Hamaguchi JR, Swank RA, Bradbury EM. Staurosporine is a potent inhibitor of p34cdc2 and p34cdc2-like kinases. *Biochem Biophys Res Commun* 1992; 184:80–85.

58. Seynaeve CM, Kazanietz MG, Blumberg PM, Sausville EA, Worland PJ. Differential inhibition of protein kinase C isozymes by UCN-01, a staurosporine analogue. *Mol Pharmacol* 1994; 45:1207–1214.

59. Wang Q, Worland PJ, Clark JL, Carlson BA, Sausville EA. Apoptosis in 7-hydroxystaurosporine-treated T lymphoblasts correlates with activation of cyclin-dependent kinases 1 and 2. *Cell Growth Diff* 1995; 6:927–936.

60. Yu L, Orlandi L, Wang P, Orr M, Senderowicz AM, Sausville EA, Silvestrini RA, O'Connor P. UCN-01 abrogates G2 arrest through a cdc2-dependent pathway that involves inactivation of the Wee1Hu kinase. *J Biol Chem* 1998; 273:33,455–33,464.

61. Nomoto T, Nishio K, Saijo N. Cell cycle regulation by anticancer agent. (In Japanese.) *Gan To Kagaku Ryoho* 1995; 22:1719–1723.

62. Meijer L. *Chemical Inhibitors of Cyclin-Dependent Kinases.* Plenum Press, New York.

63. Dawson NA, Figg WD, Cooper MR, Sartor O, Bergan RC, Senderowicz AM, Steinberg

SM, Tompkins A, Weinberger B, Sausville EA, Reed E, Myers CE. Phase II trial of suramin, leuprolide, and flutamide in previously untreated metestatic prostate cancer. *J Clin Oncol* 1997; 15:1470–1477.

64. Dawson N, Figg W, Brawley O, Bergan R, Cooper M, Senderowicz AM, Headlee D, Steinber S, Sutherland M, Patronas N, Sausville E, Linehan W, Reed E, Sartor O. Phase II study of suramin plus aminoglutethimide in two cohorts of patients with androgen-independent prostate cancer: Simultaneous antiandrogen withdrawal and prior antiandrogen withdrawal. *Clin Cancer Res* 1998; 4:37–44.

65. Park S, Cheon J, Lee Y, Park Y, Lee K, Lee C, Lee S. A specific inhibitor of Cyclin-dependent protein kinases, CDC2 and CDK2. *Mol Cells* 1996; 6:679–683.

66. Ohashi M, Sugikawa E, Nakanishi N. Inhibition of p53 protein phosphorylation by 9-hydroxyellipticine: A possible anticancer mechanism. *Jpn J Cancer Res* 1995; 86:819–827.

67. Senderowicz AM, Headlee D, Stinson S, Lush R, Kalil N, Villalba L, Hill K, Steinberg S, Figg W, Tompkins A, Arbuck S, Sausville EA. A phase I trial of continuous infusion flavopiridol, a novel cyclin-dependent kinase inhibitor, in patients with refractory neoplasms. *J Clin Oncol* 1998; 16:2986–2999.

68. Thomas J, Cleary J, Tutsch K, Arzoomanian R, Alberti D, Simon K, Feierabend D, Morgan K, Wilding G. (1997) Phase I clinical and pharmacokinetic trial of flavopiridol, in *Proceedings of the 88th Annual Meeting of the American Association of Cancer Research,* San Diego, CA.

69. Sausville EA, Lush R, Headlee D, Smith A, Figg W, Arbuck S, Senderowicz AM, Fuse E, Tanii H, Kuwabara T, Kobayashi S. Clinical pharmacology of UCN-01: Initial observations and comparison to preclinical models. *Cancer Chemother Pharmacol* 1998; 425:554–559.

70. Fuse E, Tanii H, Kurata N, Kobayashi H, Shimada Y, Tamura T, Sasaki Y, Tanigawara Y, Lush RD, Headlee D, Figg W, Arbuck SG, Senderowicz AM, Sausville EA, Akinaga S, Kuwabara T, Kobayashi S. Unpredicted clinical pharmacology of UCN-01 caused by specific binding to human alpha1-acid glycoprotein. *Cancer Res* 1998; 58:3248–3253.

71. Senderowicz AM, Headlee D, Lush R, Bauer K, Figg W, Murgo AS, Arbuck S, Inoue K, Kobashi S, Kuwabara T, Sausville E. Phase I trial of infusional UCN-01, a novel protein kinase inhibitor, in patients with refractory neoplasms: in *10th National Cancer Institute—European Organization for Research on Treatment of Cancer Symposium Proceedings,* Amsterdam, Holland.

Index